Evidence-Based Urology

EDITED BY

Philipp Dahm MD, MHSc, FACS
Associate Professor of Urology
Director of Clinical Research
Department of Urology
University of Florida
Gainesville, FL, USA

Roger R. Dmochowski MD
Professor of Urology
Director of Female Pelvic Medicine and Reconstruction
Department of Urologic Surgery
Vanderbilt University Medical Center
Nashville, TN, USA

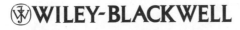WILEY-BLACKWELL   BMJ|Books

A John Wiley & Sons, Ltd., Publication

Library of Congress Cataloging-in-Publication Data
Evidence-based urology / edited by Philipp Dahm, Roger R. Dmochowski.—2nd ed.
      p. ; cm.
   Includes bibliographical references and index.
   ISBN 978-1-4051-8594-3
   1. Urology.   2. Evidence-based medicine.   I. Dahm, Philipp.
II. Dmochowski, Roger R.
   [DNLM: 1. Urologic Diseases.   2. Evidence-Based Medicine.
WJ 140 E93 2010]
   RC870.E95   2010
   616.6—dc22

                                                                        2010006118

ISBN: 9781405185943

A catalogue record for this book is available from the British Library.

Set in 9.25/12pt Palatino by MPS Limited, A Macmillan Company
Printed in Singapore by Fabulous Printers Pte Ltd
1   2010

Evidence-Based Urology

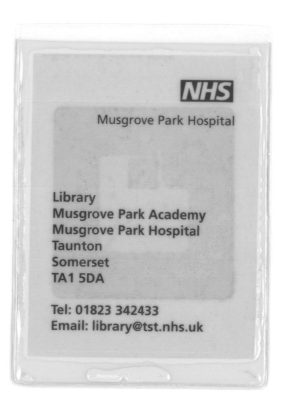

Contents

Contents

Evidence-Based Medicine Series

Updates and additional resources for the books in this series are available from:
www.evidencebasedseries.com

List of contributors

Anthony Addesa
Department of Radiation Oncology, Virginia Commonwealth University, Richmond, VA, USA

Ashok Agarwal
Center for Reproductive Medicine, Glickman Urological and Kidney Institute, The Cleveland Clinic, Cleveland, OH, USA

Mitchell Anscher
Department of Radiation Oncology, Virginia Commonwealth University, Richmond, VA, USA

Daniel A. Barocas
Department of Urologic Surgery, Vanderbilt University Medical Center, Nashville, TN, USA

Jeanette Buckingham
John W. Scott Health Sciences Library, University of Alberta, Alberta, Canada

Benjamin K. Canales
Department of Urology, University of Florida, Gainesville, FL, USA

Sam S. Chang
Department of Urologic Surgery, Vanderbilt University Medical Center, Nashville, TN, USA

Christopher R. Chapple
Sheffield Teaching Hospital NHS Trust, Royal Hallamshire Hospital, Urology Research, Sheffield, UK

Peter Chung
Department of Radiation Oncology, University of Toronto, and the Radiation Medicine Program, Princess Margaret Hospital, Toronto, Canada

J. Quentin Clemens
Department of Urology, University of Michigan, Ann Arbor, MI, USA

Michael S. Cookson
Department of Urologic Surgery, Vanderbilt University Medical Center, Nashville, TN, USA

Jonathan C. Craig
School of Public Health, University of Sydney, New South Wales, Australia

Philipp Dahm
Department of Urology, University of Florida, Gainesville, FL, USA

Fnu Deepinder
Center for Reproductive Medicine, Glickman Urological and Kidney Institute, The Cleveland Clinic, Cleveland, OH, USA

Roger R. Dmochowski
Department of Urologic Surgery, Vanderbilt University, Nashville, TN, USA

Sean P. Elliott
Department of Urologic Surgery, University of Minnesota, Minneapolis, MN, USA

Martha M. Faraday
Four Oaks, LLC; Keedysville, MD, USA

Fernando Ferrer
Department of Urology, Connecticut Children's Medical Center, Hartford, CT, USA

Susan F. Fesperman
Department of Urology, University of Florida, Gainesville, FL, USA

Robert A. Figlin
City of Hope National Medical Center, Department of Medical Oncology and Therapeutics Research, City of Hope Comprehensive Cancer Center, Duarte, CA, USA

John M. Fitzpatrick
Department of Urology and Surgical Professional Unit, Mater Misericordiae University Hospital, Dublin, Ireland

Alexander Gomelsky
Department of Urology, Louisiana State University Health Sciences Center, Shreveport, LA, USA

Michael Hagan
Department of Radiation Oncology, Virginia Commonwealth University, Richmond, VA, USA

John M. Hollingsworth
University of Michigan, Department of Urology, Division of Health Services Research, Ann Arbor, MI, USA

Ryan Hutchinson
Department of Urologic Surgery, Vanderbilt Medical Center, Nashville, TN, USA

Alexander Karl
Department of Urology, School of Medicine, University of California-San Francisco, San Francisco, CA, USA

Melissa R. Kaufman
Department of Urologic Surgery, Vanderbilt University, Nashville, TN, USA

Bodo E. Knudsen
Department of Urology, Ohio State University Medical Center, Columbus, OH, USA

Badrinath R. Konety
Department of Urology, University of Munich LMU, Munich, Germany

Zoe S. Kopp
Pfizer Inc, New York, NY, USA

Jeffrey C. LaRochelle
Institute of Urologic Oncology and Department of Urology, David Geffen School of Medicine, University of California, Los Angeles, CA, USA

Ngoc-Bich Le
Department of Urology, University of Florida, Gainesville, FL, USA

Yair Lotan
Department of Urology, University of Texas Southwestern Medical Center at Dallas, TX, USA

Rustom P. Manecksha
Department of Urology and Surgical Professional Unit, Mater Misericordiae University Hospital, Dublin, Ireland

Malcolm D. Mason
Cochrane Urological Cancers Unit, Velindre NHS Trust, Cardiff, UK

Philip Masson
Department of Renal Medicine, Royal Infirmary of Edinburgh, Edinburgh, Scotland

Bahaa S. Malaeb
Department of Urologic Surgery, University of Minnesota, Minneapolis, MN, USA

S.L. Matheson
Centre for Kidney Research, The Children's Hospital at Westmead, Westmead, New South Wales, Australia

Jack W. McAninch
Department of Urology, San Francisco General Hospital, San Francisco, CA, USA

James M. McKiernan
Department of Urology, Columbia University Medical Center, New York, NY, USA

Chris G. McMahon
University of Sydney, Australian Centre for Sexual Health, Sydney, Australia

Priya Mitra
Department of Radiation Oncology, Virginia Commonwealth University, Richmond, VA, USA

Adam C. Mues
Department of Urology, Ohio State University Medical Center, Columbus, OH, USA

Alana M. Murphy
Department of Urology, Columbia University Medical Center, New York, NY, USA

Dominic Muston
Health Economic Modelling Unit, Heron Evidence Development Ltd, Luton, UK

Michael Myers
Department of Radiation Oncology, Virginia Commonwealth University, Richmond, VA, USA

J. Curtis Nickel
Department of Urology, Queen's University, Kingston, Ontario, Canada

Regina D. Norris
University of Pittsburgh Medical Center, Children's Hosptial of Pittsburgh, Pittsburgh, PA, USA

Susan L. Norris
Department of Medical Informatics and Clinical Epidemiology, Oregon Health and Science University, Portland, OR, USA

Ann Oldendorf
Department of Urology, University of Michigan, Ann Arbor, MI, USA

Allan J. Pantuck
Institute of Urologic Oncology and Department of Urology, David Geffen School of Medicine, University of California, Los Angeles, CA, USA

Dipen J. Parekh
Department of Urology, University of Texas Health Sciences Center at San Antonio, San Antonio, TX, USA

Margaret S. Pearle
Department of Urology, University of Texas Southwestern Medical Center, Dallas, TX, USA

David F. Penson
Department of Urologic Surgery, Vanderbilt University and VA Tennessee Valley Healthcare System, Nashville, TN, USA

Frédéric Pouliot
Institute of Urologic Oncology and Department of Urology, David Geffen School of Medicine, University of California, Los Angeles, CA, USA

Glenn M. Preminger
Comprehensive Kidney Stone Center, Division of Urologic Surgery, Duke University Medical Center, Durham, NC, USA

Puneeta Ramachandra
Division of Urology, University of Connecticut Health Center, Farmington, CT, USA

Jay D. Raman
Division of Urology, Penn State Milton S. Hershey Medical Center, Hershey, PA, USA

Amanda Beth Reed
Department of Urology, University of Texas Health Sciences Center at San Antonio, San Antonio, TX, USA

Kristin C. Reed
South Texas Veterans Health Care System, San Antonio, TX, USA

Monique J. Roobol
Erasmus University Medical Centre, Rotterdam, The Netherlands

Charles J. Rosser
Department of Urology, University of Florida, Gainesville, FL, USA

Edmund S. Sabanegh, Jr
Center for Reproductive Medicine, Glickman Urological and Kidney Institute, The Cleveland Clinic, Cleveland, OH, USA

Charles D. Scales, Jr
Division of Urology, Department of Surgery, Duke University Medical Center, Durham, NC, USA

Harriette Scarpero
Department of Urologic Surgery, Vanderbilt Medical Center, Nashville, TN, USA

Fritz H. Schröder
Erasmus University Medical Centre, Rotterdam, The Netherlands

Holger J. Schünemann
Department of Clinical Epidemiology and Biostatistics, McMaster University Health Sciences Centre, Hamilton, Ontario, Canada

Mark Shaw
Department of Radiation Oncology, University of Toronto, and the Radiation Medicine Program, Princess Margaret Hospital, Toronto, Canada

Mike D. Shelley
Cochrane Urological Cancers Unit, Velindre NHS Trust, Cardiff, UK

Elizabeth Soll
University of Michigan, Department of Urology, Division of Health Services Research, Ann Arbor, MI, USA

Mathew D. Sorensen
Department of Urology, University of Washington School of Medicine, Seattle, WA, USA

James Thomasch
Department of Urologic Surgery, Vanderbilt University Medical Center, Nashville, TN, USA

Timothy Y. Tseng
Comprehensive Kidney Stone Center, Division of Urologic Surgery, Duke University Medical Center, Durham, NC, USA

Przemyslaw W. Twardowski
City of Hope National Medical Center, Department of Medical Oncology and Therapeutics Research, City of Hope Comprehensive Cancer Center, Duarte, CA, USA

Pim J. van Leeuwen
Erasmus University Medical Centre, Rotterdam, The Netherlands

Bryan B. Voelzke
Department of Urology, Harborview Medical Center, Seattle, WA, USA

Padraig Warde
Department of Radiation Oncology, University of Toronto, and the Radiation Medicine Program, Princess Margaret Hospital, Toronto, Canada

Angela C. Webster
School of Public Health, University of Sydney, New South Wales, Australia

John T. Wei
University of Michigan, Department of Urology, Division of Health Services Research, Ann Arbor, MI, USA

Hunter Wessells
Department of Urology, University of Washington School of Medicine, Seattle, WA, USA

John S. Wiener
Departments of Surgery and Pediatrics, Duke Univesity Medical Center, Durham, NC, USA

Lawrence L. Yeung
Department of Urology, University of Florida, Gainesville, FL, USA

Preface

Evidence-based clinical practice has been defined in many different ways, but fundamentally relates to the use of systematically appraised evidence to guide clinical decision-making while incorporating the values, preferences and specific circumstances of an individual patient. This evidence may, in the future, become the critical determining factor in the development of comparative effectiveness as it applies to the field of urology. *Evidence-Based Urology* was conceptualized to address focused, clinical questions across all domains of our specialty to help urologists practice according to the current best evidence.

We have asked authors to identify the most relevant clinical questions in their sub-specialty, perform systematic literature searches, appraise the quality of available evidence using the GRADE framework, and make practical recommendations that reflect this evidence. We hope that the reader will find this text useful not only as a free-standing urology textbook, but as a valuable resource in their day-to-day practice.

We further hope that this text will assist readers to update their knowledge in specific content areas for their own continuous medical education by using the techniques employed in this text (formulating a clinically relevant question, systematic literature search and rating of the quality of evidence). Finally, our wish is that this text will stimulate further interest in evidence-based urology, thus promoting the best possible care to our patients.

Philipp Dahm MD, MHSc, FACS
University of Florida
Gainesville, Florida, USA

Roger R. Dmochowski MD
Vanderbilt University
Nashville, Tennessee, USA

Foreword

Evidence-based medicine (EBM) – or evidence-based surgery, or evidence-based urology (EBU) – is about solving clinical problems. In particular, EBU provides tools for using the medical and surgical literature to determine the benefits and risks of alternative patient management strategies, and to weigh those benefits and risks in the context of an individual patient's experiences, values and preferences.

The term evidence-based medicine first appeared in the medical literature in 1991; it rapidly became something of a mantra. EBM is sometimes perceived as a blinkered adherence to randomized trials, or a health-care managers' tool for controlling and constraining recalcitrant physicians. In fact, EBM and EBU involve informed and effective use of all types of evidence, but particularly evidence from the medical literature, in patient care.

EBM's evolution has included outward expansion. We now realize that optimal health care delivery must include evidence-based nursing, physiotherapy, occupational therapy, and podiatry – and specialization. We need evidence-based obstetrics, gynecology, internal medicine and surgery – and indeed, orthopedics, and neurosurgery. And of course, we need evidence-based urology.

Applying EBU to management decisions in individual patients involves use of a hierarchy of study design, with high-quality randomized trials showing definitive results directly applicable to an individual patient at the apex, to relying on physiological rationale or previous experience with a small number of similar patients near the bottom rung. Ideally, systematic reviews and meta-analyses summarize the highest quality available evidence. The hallmark of evidence-based practitioners is that, for particular clinical decisions, they know the strength of the evidence, and therefore the degree of uncertainty.

What is required to practice EBU? Practitioners must know how to frame a clinical quandary to facilitate use of the literature in its resolution. Evidence-based urologists must know how to search the literature efficiently to obtain the best available evidence bearing on their question, to evaluate the strength of the methods of the studies they find, extract the clinical message, apply it back to the patient, and store it for retrieval when faced with similar patients in the future.

Traditionally, neither medical schools nor postgraduate programs have taught these skills. Although this situation has changed dramatically in the last decade, the biggest influence on how trainees will practice is their clinical role models, few of whom are currently accomplished EBU practitioners. The situation is even more challenging for those looking to acquire the requisite skills after completing their clinical training.

This text primarily addresses the needs of both trainees and of this last group, practicing urologists. Appearing 20 years after the term EBM was coined, the text represents a landmark in a number of ways. It is the first comprehensive EBU text. The book represents a successful effort to comprehensively address the EBU-related learning needs of the urology community, and summarize the key areas of urological practice.

To achieve its goals of facilitating evidence-based urologic practice, the text begins with chapters that introduce the tools for evaluating the original urologic literature. Those interested in delving deeper into issues of how to evaluate the literature, and apply it to patient care, can consult a definitive text (see http://www.mcgraw-hillmedical.com/jama/).

The bulk of the current text, however, provides evidence summaries to guide each of the key common problems of urologic practice. Thorough and up to date at the time of writing, they provide a definitive guide to evidence-based urologic practice today. That evidence will, of course, change – and in some areas change quickly. Clinicians must therefore use *Evidence-Based Urology* not only as a text for the present, but as a guide for updating their knowledge in the future. That future will hopefully hold the advent of an evidence-based secondary journal similar to those that have been developed in other areas including *Evidence-based Mental Health*, *Evidence-based Nursing*, and the *ACP Journal Club* – which does the job for internal medicine – survey a large number of journals relevant to their area and choose individual studies and systematic reviews that meet both relevance and validity screening criteria. These journals present the results of these studies in structured abstracts that provide clinicians with the key information they need to judge their applicability to their own practices. Fame and fortune await the enterprising group who applies this methodology to produce evidence-based urology.

Whatever the future holds for the increasing efficiency of evidence-based practice, the current text provides an introduction to a system of clinical problem-solving that is becoming a pre-requisite for modern urologic practice.

Gordon Guyatt
BSc (Toronto), MD (McMaster),
MSc (McMaster) FRCPC
Professor, Department of Clinical
Epidemiology & Biostatistics
Joint Member, Department of Medicine
Member, CLARITY (Clinical Advances
through Research and Information Translation)

1 Searching for evidence

Jeanette Buckingham

John W. Scott Health Sciences Library, University of Alberta, Alberta, Canada

The shape of clinical literature

The mass of published literature now far exceeds our ability to cope with it as individuals; the evidence for practice is out there but in blinding volume and a bewildering array of formats and platforms. Experienced clinicians in the past have tended to choose one or two principal sources of information, often old friends like PubMed, a general journal like *BMJ* or the *New England Journal of Medicine*, plus two or three journals in their specialty – say, *Urology*, *BJU International* or *European Urology* – and stick with them. This is no longer sufficient to allow a practitioner to keep up with new relevant and applicable clinical research. However, in a very positive turn of events over the past decade, the geometrically growing mass of published clinical research has brought with it the development of resources to synthesize this new knowledge and present it in methodologically sound as well as extremely accessible formats. Armed with these resources and a few relatively simple techniques, it is indeed possible to find evidence for practice quickly and efficiently.

The three general classes of clinical information are (Box 1.1):

• *bibliographic databases* – indexes to published primary literature, usually journal articles

• *selected, often preappraised sources* – selections of high-impact primary clinical research, published as databases (such as EvidenceUpdates + or the Cochrane Central Registry of Controlled Trials) or as digest journals (*ACP Journal Club*, *Evidence-based Medicine*), which, searched electronically, become like small, select databases

• *synthesized sources* – including systematic reviews, practice guidelines, textbooks, and point-of-care resources;

Evidence-Based Urology. Edited by Philipp Dahm, Roger R. Dmochowski.
© 2010 Blackwell Publishing.

BOX 1.1 Sources of evidence for clinical practice

1. **Synthesized sources**
   a. Point-of-care resources
      i. *ACP PIER*
      ii. *Clinical Evidence*
      iii. *BMJ Point of Care*
      iv. *Dynamed*
   b. Textbooks and handbooks
      i. *ACP Medicine/ACS surgery*
      ii. *E-Medicine (via TRIP)* http://www.tripdatabase.com/
      iii. Other textbooks—many textbooks are on-line; some are in sets, such as STAT!Ref, MD Consult (includes *Campbell's Urology*), Books@OVID, Access Medicine--check textbooks for explicit references, and check the references for clinical research
   c. Practice guidelines
      i. *National Guideline Clearinghouse* http://www.guideline.gov/
      ii. *Clinical Knowledge Summaries* http://www.cks.library.nhs.uk/
      iii. Via *TRIP* http://www.tripdatabase.com/
      iv. American Urological Association Guidelines http://www.auanet.org/guidelines/
   d. Systematic reviews
      i. Cochrane Database of Systematic Reviews
      ii. DARE (Database of Abstracts of Reviews of Effects)
      iii. Medline/PubMed—search systematic reviews in clinical queries.
2. **Filtered sources**
   a. *Evidence-based Medicine*
   b. *BMJ Updates* + *http://bmjupdates.mcmaster.ca*
   c. Cochrane Central Registry of Controlled Trials
3. **Filtering unfiltered sources**
   a. Clinical Queries—MEDLINE (PubMed, Ovid—under "More limits")
   b. TRIP—one-stop shopping http://www.tripdatabase.com/ (TRIP Medline search uses "clinical queries" filters)
   c. Combine search statement with description of most appropriate study design
4. **Other therapeutic resources**
   a. *Medicines Complete* (*Martindales, Stockley's Drug Interactions*)
   b. *Natural Standard* (for herbal and other complementary and alternative therapies)

these gather and critically appraise primary clinical research articles and combine their information into a new entity, often with a focus on accessibility and clinical relevance.

The approach for finding evidence for practice is exactly opposite to that for conducting a literature search preparatory to conducting a literature review. In the case of the literature review, one conducts a thorough search of the appropriate bibliographic databases – Medline (whether via PubMed or some other search interface), EMBASE, Web of Science, Scopus, Biosis Previews, plus resources such as the Cochrane Library (to ensure one hasn't missed an important controlled trial or systematic review) or databases of clinical trials in progress, to ensure that all relevant studies have been found. If possible, one consults a research librarian to be sure that no stone has been left unturned. However, to find evidence to apply to clinical problems, the search begins with synthesized resources, progresses through selected, preappraised resources, and only moves into bibliographic databases if no satisfactory answer has been found in the first two resource classes. With a literature review, the search is exhaustive. With the search for applicable clinical evidence, it is acceptable to stop when a good answer has been found.

Some of the resources described are free; most are broadly available to those affiliated with medical societies or institutions or are available by individual subscription. New synthesized resources, point-of-care resources in particular, are emerging rapidly and established resources are continuously evolving. Understanding the elements of evidence-based practice will enable the practitioner to be an enlightened consumer of these resources.

A case to consider

Mr W, 63 years old and otherwise fit and healthy, has been referred to you with symptoms of benign prostatic hyperplasia (BPH) (frequency, nocturia, and slow flow). Digital rectal examination reveals an enlarged prostate gland, about 45 g, with no nodules. His postvoid is approximately 100 cc and he reports three documented urinary tract infections over the course of the last year. His serum creatinine and prostate-specific antigen (PSA) levels are normal.

He has been advised by his family physician that he may require surgery to resolve his condition. He is apprehensive about this and asks if there are medical interventions for the BPH that could be tried first. He has searched the web and has found information that saw palmetto may be an effective herbal remedy to improve his voiding symptoms.

What do you want? Asking a focused clinical question

The first two steps of the protocol of evidence-based practice (Assess, Ask, Acquire, Appraise, Apply) [1] involve *assessing* the situation – pulling out the salient features of a patient's presentation and history – and *asking* one or more questions that are both focused and answerable. Assessing the situation may require some background information about the condition itself – for example, "how does BPH promote voiding complaints?." To find primary research evidence to apply to the patient at hand, however, a focused, answerable question must be crafted. Asking a focused clinical question is a mental discipline that will also pay off enormously in effective searching and in finding good evidence to apply to practice.

Assigning a domain – therapy/prevention, diagnosis, prognosis, etiology/harm – is the essential first step in framing the question, because questions are asked differently, depending on the domain (Box 1.2). Often questions regarding a single case will fall into multiple domains. In this instance, separate focused questions for each relevant domain will result in clearer answers.

Once the domain has been established, the elements of the focused clinical question must be identified.
- *P* = Population. The patient's characteristics, including age, gender, and condition, plus other relevant clinical or medical history features.
- *I* = Intervention. What intervention are you considering using? In a diagnostic question, this becomes "what new test do I wish to try?." In a prognostic question, this equates to "prognostic factor" and in the etiology domain, this becomes "exposure."
- *C* = Comparison. In the therapy domain, this might be the standard of care or a placebo, where this is appropriate; in diagnosis, the comparison is always the "gold standard" diagnostic test; in the case of a causation/etiology question, this obviously might be "no exposure;" and in prognosis, this might be the lack of the relevant prognostic factor.
- *O* = Outcome. For therapy, what changes are you looking to accomplish in the patient's condition? Are they clinical changes, such as the reduction of the number of urinary tract infection (UTI) recurrences? Or are they surrogate, such as reduction in the size of the prostate? In diagnosis, how likely is the new test, in comparison with the gold standard, to predict or rule out the presence of a condition? In a prognostic question – often the most important for the patient – what is the expected disease progression? And in the etiology domain, how closely is this risk factor associated with the condition?
- *T* = Type of study. What study design will generate the best level of evidence with which to answer this question? This will vary from domain to domain, and also depending upon the subject itself.

BOX 1.2 The well-built clinical question (PICOT)

Therapy

Population (patient)

How would I describe a group of patients similar to mine? (condition, age, gender, etc.)

Intervention (medication, procedure, etc.)

Which main/new intervention am I considering?

Comparison

What is the alternative to compare with the intervention? (placebo, standard of care, etc.)

Outcome

What might I accomplish, measure, improve, or affect?

Type of study

What study design would provide the best level of evidence for this question?

Diagnosis

Population (patient)

What are the characteristics of the patients? What is the condition that may be present?

Intervention (diagnostic test)

Which diagnostic test am I considering?

Comparison

What is the diagnostic gold standard?

Outcome

How likely is the test to predict/rule out this condition?

Type of study

What study design would provide the best level of evidence for this question?

Prognosis

Population (patient)

How would I describe a cohort of patients similar to mine (stage of condition, age, gender, etc.)?

Intervention (prognostic factor)

Which main prognostic factor am I considering?

Comparison (optional)

What is the comparison group, if any?

Outcome

What disease progression can be expected?

Type of study

What study design would provide the best level of evidence for this question?

Harm/Causation/Etiology

Population (patient)

How would I describe a group of patients similar to mine?

Intervention (exposure, risk factor)

Which main exposure/risk factor am I considering?

Comparison

What is the main alternative to compare with the exposure?

Outcome

How is the incidence or prevalence of the condition in this group affected by this exposure?

Type of study

What study design would provide the best level of evidence for this question?

While the pinnacle of research quality is usually considered to be the double-blinded randomized controlled trial (RCT) or systematic reviews of such studies, blinding and randomization are not feasible for many kinds of investigations, particularly in surgery. Similarly, strong observational studies, specifically prospective cohort studies, are most appropriate for the prognosis domain. RCTs cannot be carried out for studies of diagnostic tests, because all subjects must receive both the gold standard test and the investigational test. For etiological studies, while RCTs are perhaps the ideal way of testing adverse drug reactions, they are ethically inappropriate for potentially harmful exposures, so case–control studies are perhaps the most appropriate. The key with study design is flexibility: the point is to find the best available evidence (as opposed to the best possible) that is relevant to the topic and applicable to the patient.

The points extracted into a PICOT structure may be framed into a question. In the case example, for instance, one question might be "In an otherwise healthy 63 year old with BPH (P), how effective is medical therapy (I), compared with surgery (C), in reducing lower urinary tract symptoms (O), as demonstrated in a randomized controlled trial or systematic review of randomized controlled trials (T)?."

Searching for clinical evidence: start with synthesized sources

The "new" evidence-based medicine looks first for sources that have synthesized the best available evidence. The first mental question that must be asked is, "How common is this situation and how likely am I to find an answer derived from the best evidence?" Synthesized resources may be point-of-care resources, practice guidelines, and systematic reviews. The more common a condition, the more likely it is that good evidence will be found here.

Systematic reviews

In systematic reviews, primary research on a topic is thoroughly searched, selected through explicit inclusion criteria, and critically appraised to provide a reliable overview of a topic. Data from the included studies may be pooled (meta-analysis) to produce a statistical summary of the studies' findings.

Systematic reviews have existed since the 1970s in other disciplines but came into their own for medicine in the 1990s, with the advent of the Cochrane Collaboration. The purpose of the Cochrane Collaboration is to facilitate knowledge transfer from research to practice, and their influence on medical publishing has certainly achieved that [2]. Cochrane review groups collaborate to produce the highest standard of systematic reviews of clinical research. Among other review groups, there is a Cochrane Prostatic Diseases and Urologic Cancers Group, a Cochrane Renal Group, and also a Cochrane Incontinence Group, all of them producing a substantial volume of high-quality systematic reviews. Although Cochrane reviews tend to be very long, quick clinically oriented information can be found either in the "plain language summary" or by going directly to the "forest plots" which provide graphic presentations of the data summaries (meta-analyses) contained in the review. (For a detailed description of Cochrane reviews and the work of the Cochrane Collaboration, see: www. cochrane.org/.) Previously, review articles were much relied upon for clinical information but were a mixed and often subjective bag. Cochrane systematic reviews implied an elaborate methodological protocol and became the quality benchmark for evidence for practice and for published reviews.

The Cochrane Library, which includes the Cochrane Database of Systematic Reviews, the Database of Abstracts of Reviews of Effects (DARE, an index with commentary of systematic reviews other than Cochrane reviews), the Central Registry of Controlled Trials, the Health Technology Assessment database and the National Health Service Economic Evaluation Database, is an excellent source of evidence for urologists. In the example, a search for "benign prostatic hyperplasia" in the Cochrane Library turned up a Cochrane review assessing the effectiveness of saw palmetto (*Serenoa repens*) for BPH [3], providing an answer for one of the patient's questions (Figure 1.1). On the broad topic of BPH, the Cochrane Library also produced a substantial number of Cochrane reviews, other published systematic reviews from DARE, clinical trials from Central, and useful studies from the Health Technology Assessment database and the NHS Economic Evaluations Database.

Point-of-care resources

Point-of-care information resources have been available as long as medicine has been practiced, traditionally taking the form of handbooks and textbooks. The key is to look for references to find where their information came from, whether those sources were grounded in primary research, and if so, whether that research is believable, important and applicable to your patients.

Point-of-care resources available now are very different from the traditional handbooks. They are elaborately produced, explicitly tied to the evidence, and designed for rapid, easy use by clinicians. The best of them incorporate aspects of systematic reviews into their methodology, requiring critical appraisal of the primary research they cite and discussion of the quality of evidence behind recommendations made.

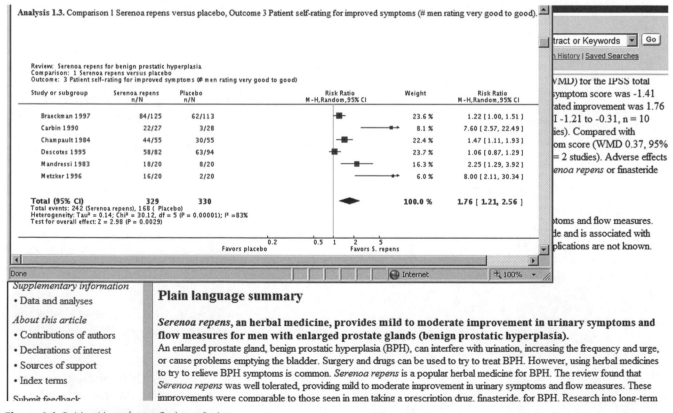

Figure 1.1 Quick evidence from a Cochrane Review.

BMJ Clinical Evidence (http://clinicalevidence.bmj.com/ceweb/index.jsp) is a point-of-care resource based in a detailed systematic review but presented in a very accessible format. Interventions are displayed in a simple tabular form, with gold medallions for effective therapies, red for ineffective or potentially harmful therapies, and white for therapies whose effectiveness is unknown (Figure 1.2). Additional information, such as causation, prevalence and incidence, diagnosis, and prognosis, is found beneath the "About this condition" tab; links are also provided to new and important articles from EvidenceUpdates + (see

below) and to practice guidelines. Although its coverage is limited to approximately 2000 conditions most commonly seen in primary practice, the content is reviewed every couple of years and is therefore both current and reliable. Clinical Evidence sections relevant to urology include Men's Health, Women's Health, and Kidney Disorders. A systematic review on BPH provides evidence for several of the questions posed by this case (effectiveness of alpha-blockers, surgery, and herbal remedies).

BMJ Point of Care (http://group.bmj.com/products/knowledge/bmj-point-of-care) (Figure 1.3) appeared in

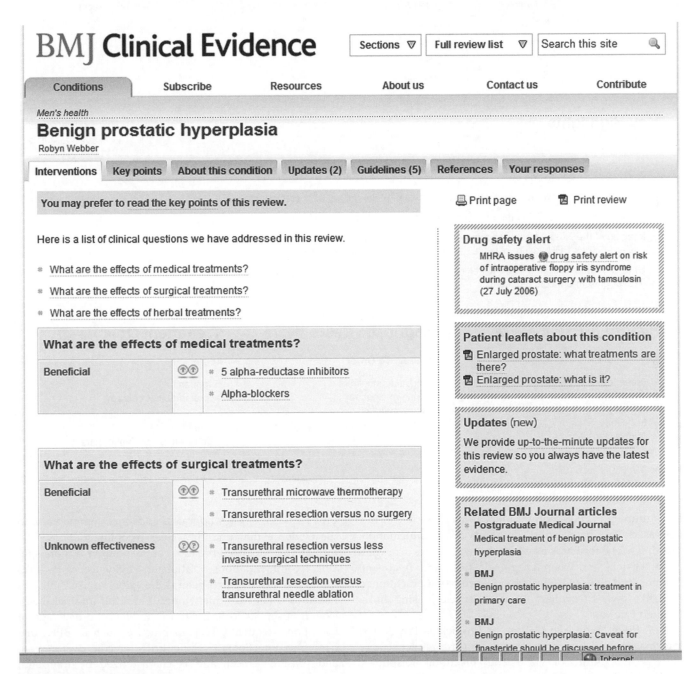

Figure 1.2 BMJ Clinical Evidence.

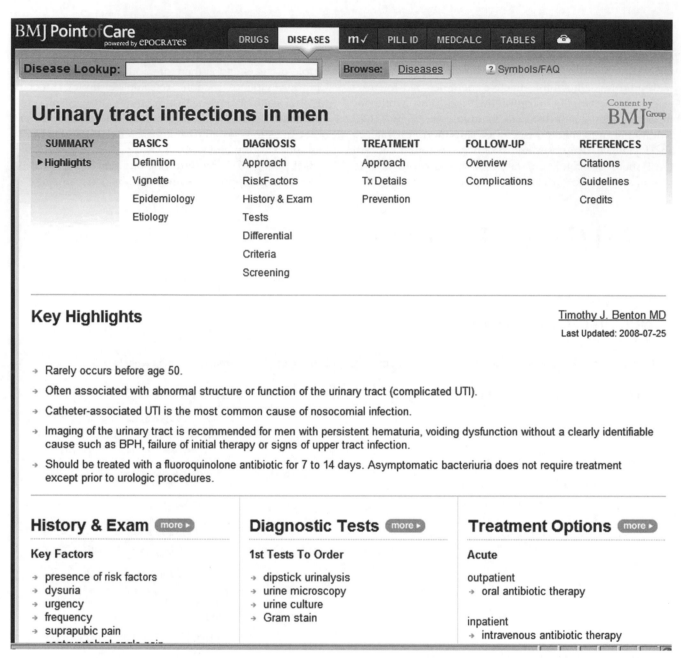

Figure 1.3 BMJ Point of Care.

the summer of 2008, combining Clinical Evidence, the US-based Epocrates, and detailed drug information resources. The format is user friendly, with topics arranged under History and Exam, Diagnostic Tests, and Treatment Options, and allows the curious evidence-based practitioner to drill down to primary research articles, using links through PubMed.

ACP PIER (American College of Physicians Physicians Information and Education Resource) (http://pier.acponline.org/index.html) or via StatRef Electronic Resources for Health Professionals (www.statref.com/) (Figure 1.4)

provides access, with appraisal and brief commentary, to the evidence that underlies clear recommendations. The format proceeds from broad recommendation > more specific recommendations > rationale > evidence, with links to the primary research behind the evidence. ACP PIER is not limited (as ACP might imply) to adult internal medicine. It is similar to BMJ Clinical Evidence in coverage of conditions frequently seen in practice, such as BPH, urinary tract infections, pyelonephritis, erectile dysfunction, and prostate cancer, and is characterized by thorough, explicit and succinctly presented evidence. For the case

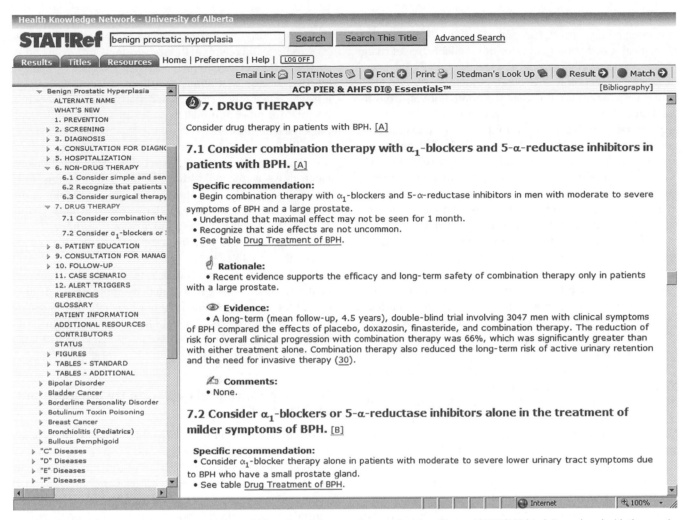

Figure 1.4 StatRef – benign prostatic hyperplasia. Available at: http://pier.acponline.org/physicians/diseases/d225/d225.html. Reproduced with the permission of the American College of Physicians, 2008.

used as an example here, the chapter on BPH provides excellent evidence to answer the questions posed. In addition, ACP PIER features at the beginning of the chapter new and important literature on the topic, continually updated, provides helpful tabular presentations for differential diagnosis and treatment, and includes links to professional association practice guidelines and patient information resources. The quality of evidence, critical appraisal of evidence included, and organization make this an excellent point of care resource that can only improve as new conditions are added.

DynaMed is another excellent evidence-based, peer-reviewed point-of-care resource, with somewhat broader coverage than Clinical Evidence and ACP PIER but with explicit links to the primary literature supporting statements and recommendations. The advantage of DynaMed is in more extensive coverage of causation and risk factors, complications and prognosis, while providing good outline

format approaches to history taking, physical examination, and diagnosis, prevention and treatment. The coverage for urology appears to be very good. It is available by subscription but can be obtained at no cost if one wishes to contribute chapters to the resource. Further information is available at DynaMed's website: www.ebscohost.com/dynamed/.

Practice guidelines

Practice guidelines focus on patient management and summarize current standard of care. The best guidelines are based explicitly on the best available clinical evidence, indicating the level of evidence supporting each recommendation and linking to the primary research on which the recommendation is based. The source and purpose of individual guidelines are important: are the guidelines produced by professional societies to promote optimum care or are they the product of healthcare providers like HMOs or insurers, where the aim might be cost-effectiveness in disease management. The American Urological Association guidelines are available free of charge at the Association's website: www.auanet.org/guidelines/. European Association of Urology guidelines are also available for members (or for a fee for nonmembers) from the association's website: www.uroweb.org/.

National Guideline Clearinghouse (www.guideline. gov/) is also available free as an initiative of the Agency for Healthcare Research and Quality (AHRQ). The National Guideline Clearinghouse has inclusion criteria: guidelines must have systematically developed recommendations or information that will assist health professionals in deciding on appropriate care, must be produced by public or private medical organizations, and must be supported by a systematic review of the literature. The full text of guideline must also be available, and it must have been produced or revised within the past 5 years. One particular bonus in searching the National Guideline Clearinghouse is that multiple guidelines on similar topics may be compared at all points, from purpose to recommendations.

Clinical Knowledge Summaries, sponsored by the National Health Service in the United Kingdom, provides excellent practice guidelines (www.cks.library.nhs.uk/ home). Under the broad topic of "urology" are several guidelines, including one on BPH and on lower UTIs in men, which would be highly useful in this case.

TRIP – Turning Research Into Practice (www.tripdatabase. com/index.html) – presents a quick way of searching for guidelines, as well as searching other resources on a topic. A search for "benign prostatic hyperplasia" on TRIP produced 12 North American, seven European, and two other practice guidelines, with functional links for access. Beyond providing an excellent route to practice guidelines, TRIP searches evidence-based practice digests of important journal articles (e.g. *Evidence Based Medicine*), searches for systematic reviews in both Cochrane and DARE, links to e-textbook articles, and simultaneously searches PubMed applying the quality filters for all four clinical query domains of Therapy, Diagnosis, Etiology, and Prognosis (this will be discussed below).

In addition, a PubMed search via TRIP (see below) may be limited by "practice guideline" as a publication type, to provide access to guidelines published in journals.

Textbooks and handbooks

Textbooks, particularly specialist textbooks like *Campbell's Urology*, have been a mainstay of clinical information throughout the history of medicine. Over the past decade, however, most of the standard medical textbooks have become available in an electronic format, which changes continuously (as opposed to the large paper volumes that appear in new editions every few years). Most electronic textbooks and sets are searchable simply by keywords. Electronic textbooks usually are grouped into collections, such as MD Consult (which includes *Campbell's Urology*), StatRef, Access Medicine, and Books@Ovid. These sets are available through professional associations, universities, hospitals or other administrative groups, and also through personal subscription.

NCBI Bookshelf (www.ncbi.nlm.nih.gov/sites/entrez? db=Books&itool=toolbar) (searchable) and FreeBooks4-Doctors(www.freebooks4doctors.com/) (searchable only by specialty, title, and language) are available at no cost. E-Medicine is an excellent free textbook, triple peer reviewed and with good urology content (www. emedicine.com/urology/index.shtml); it is most easily searchable via TRIP.

The key with all textbooks is to ensure that they are evidence based, as demonstrated by footnotes and bibliographies. With electronic textbooks, usually the notes are linked to the references, which in turn are linked to the PubMed record, allowing the reader to track back to the evidence underlying a statement.

Searching for clinical evidence: try preappraised sources next

In response to the volume of published clinical research and the need to extract the best and most important studies to inform practitioners, ACP Journal Club (www.acpjc. org/) emerged in 1991. ACP JC provides an expanded structured abstract of articles selected from core clinical journals by an editorial board, plus a thumbnail critical appraisal of the validity, importance, and applicability of the study, all usually in a single page. Evidence-based Medicine (http://ebm.bmj.com/) emerged shortly thereafter, based on ACP JC but expanding its subject coverage beyond internal medicine to include pediatrics, surgery, obstetrics, and other disciplines. Now both sources include ratings, applied by a panel of clinical experts, showing the relative importance and newsworthiness of each study, according to discipline. Both can be searched by keyword.

EvidenceUpdates + (http://plus.mcmaster.ca/Evidence Updates/) selects important articles from an array of 130 core journals, rates them for their importance and provides expanded structured abstracts but does not go the additional step of appraising the quality of the study. Evidence Updates + can be also searched by keyword.

The Cochrane Central Register of Controlled Trials (often known simply as "Central" – www.mrw.interscience.-wiley.com/cochrane/cochrane_clcentral_articles_fs.html), part of the Cochrane Library, consists of studies included in Cochrane Reviews, plus other controlled studies on the same topic, selected by the review teams. Unlike the other resources, studies included in Central are not limited to a core of English-language clinical journals. No critical appraisal is provided; simple inclusion in Central achieves a preappraised status for these papers.

The advantage of preappraised sources is that they remove the "noise" of minor or duplicative studies, case reports, and commentary found in the larger databases by providing highly selective small databases. All link to the full-text original article, usually via PubMed, so the clinician can review the study. All these resources provided good studies relevant to the case under consideration, and all would be appropriate for urologists (although ACP Journal Club would perhaps be more applicable to medical urological questions than to surgical questions).

Searching for clinical evidence: filtering unfiltered databases

Synthesized and preappraised sources may fail to answer questions in specialties like urology or urological surgery. Synthesized sources may carry a limited number of topics, usually only the most commonly seen; preappraised sources and systematic reviews are most frequently in the therapeutic domain or are RCTs or systematic reviews of RCTs, which are inappropriate for surgical, procedural, diagnostic or prognostic questions. In these cases, the large bibliographic databases of primary research evidence are the fall-back.

The most commonly used health sciences database in English-speaking medicine is Medline. Produced since 1966 by the US National Library of Medicine in Bethesda, MD, Medline is available through a wide variety of search engines, the best known of which is PubMed (www.ncbi.nlm.nih.gov/sites/entrez?db = PubMed). Medline currently indexes about 5200 US and international biomedical

and health sciences journals, and contains about 17 million references dating from 1950 to the present. Medline's great strength lies in its system of subject headings, known as MeSH, including subheadings and limits that allow the knowledgeable searcher to conduct a very precise search. Tutorials are available online to provide more detailed instruction in searching PubMed than is possible here (www.nlm.nih.gov/bsd/disted/pubmed.html).

The clinical queries function in Medline, available on PubMed and other platforms as well, injects quality filters (search strategies based largely on study designs) into a search statement. The clinical queries search strategies were developed by Haynes et al. of McMaster University; a detailed bibliography showing the derivation and validation of their filters is found at www.nlm.nih.gov/pubs/techbull/jf04/cq_info.html. The value added by searching with a quality filter is similar to that of preappraised sources: the removal of "noise" by extracting clinical trials from the vast sea of news, commentaries, case studies and general articles. Care must be taken, however, with topics that do not lend themselves to RCTs, masking or higher levels of study designs, because they will be lost when the quality filters for articles on therapy or prevention are applied.

The PICOT question described at the beginning of this chapter provides an excellent way of crafting a sound search strategy. Starting with the population (P) then adding intervention (I) and outcome (O), and finally the study design will enable the searcher to conduct a precise search and stay on target for answering the original question. An example of a search strategy for the question posed by this case is shown in Figure 1.5, to demonstrate how limits, clinical queries and subject searches for study designs can be used to improve the precision of a search. Employing the "therapy (specific)" clinical query filter resulted in a set of studies that were primarily medical

Search	Most Recent Queries	Time	Result
#10	Search (#8) AND (#7) Limits: **Core clinical journals**	13:38:36	6
#9	Search (#8) AND (#7)	13:37:31	50
#8	Search **cohort study**	13:37:06	704883
#7	Search (#6) AND (#4)	13:36:35	119
#6	Search **transurethral prostatectomy**	13:36:01	5290
#5	Search (#3) AND (randomized controlled trial[Publication Type] OR (randomized[Title/Abstract] AND controlled[Title/Abstract] AND trial[Title/Abstract])) Limits: **Male, Middle Aged + Aged: 45+ years**	13:31:52	36
#4	Search (#1) AND (#2) Limits: **Male, Middle Aged + Aged: 45+ years**	13:27:53	371
#3	Search (#1) AND (#2)	13:27:06	526
#2	Search **urinary tract infection**	13:26:32	43708
#1	Search **benign prostatic hyperplasia**	13:26:17	17413

Figure 1.5 PubMed/Medline search strategy.

treatments. Adding a surgical procedure to the original strategy (statement #3) produced a large number of case studies and general reviews but combining these results with an appropriate study design (cohort study) brought the number of postings down and produced a good set of references to clinical trials of transurethral resection of the prostate (TURP).

Other databases

Sometimes Medline does not produce the desired information, possibly because it does not index all journals. Alternative databases that are useful for urology are EMBASE, Scopus, and Web of Science. EMBASE principally indexes clinical medical journals; frequently it indexes journals not caught by Medline. Like Medline, EMBASE has a detailed subject heading thesaurus; recently, EMBASE has added Medline subject headings (MeSH) to its indexing, so that it may be possible on a search platform that includes both (such as OVID) to carry a search strategy from Medline to EMBASE.

Scopus and Web of Science are more general academic databases. They do not have controlled vocabularies, so topic searching must include as many synonyms as possible. Scopus indexes approximately 14,000 journals, almost three times as many as Medline, as well as book series and conference proceedings; moreover, Scopus searches international patents and the web, making it an excellent source of information about instruments, techniques and guidelines. Web of Science covers more than 10,000 journals, dating from 1900. Articles listed in Scopus and Web of Science are not analyzed by indexers and while this makes these indexes somewhat harder to search than Medline or EMBASE, it also means that newly published articles appear much more quickly. Of all the indexes, Scopus picks up new journals the fastest and provides possibly the best coverage of open-access electronic publications. A very thorough literature search, for a research project or grant proposal, would involve a detailed search of all four databases, and possibly others as well.

Backing up your search: citation searching

Both Scopus and Web of Science allow citation searching – tracking studies that have cited other studies. Aside from its use as a quick way to determine the relative importance of an article as shown by the number of times it has been cited since publication, citation searching allows one to find newer studies on a similar topic [4,5]. In this example, the evidence from ACP PIER for proceeding to surgical ablation as opposed to watchful waiting was a study conducted by Flanigan in 1998 [6]. Citation searching would permit one to search for references citing this paper: Web

of Science (August 2009) found 82 papers citing this study, including several published within the past 2 years describing therapeutic options for men diagnosed with BPH. On obscure or interdisciplinary topics, citation tracking is a very powerful search method.

Evidence that your patients can understand

In this information-rich time, your patients will be very interested in searching for information on their condition. They may well come to their appointment armed with studies and information that they have found for themselves on the web, as they seek to participate in their own treatment (as the gentleman in our case scenario has, in his information about saw palmetto).

A physician or the physician's clinic staff should be aware of reliable resources to which to guide patients, should they express an interest. ACP PIER recommends approaches a clinician might take to patient education for the condition at hand, plus links to sound patient information on the web (in this case, to the American Urological Association: Benign Prostatic Hyperplasia: a Patient's Guide (www.auanet. org/guidelines/patient_guides/bph_guide_2003.pdf). The American Academy of Family Physicians also provides excellent resources in lay language through its website; the Conditions A to Z section provides excellent patient information on BPH (http://familydoctor.org/online/ famdocen/home/men/prostate/148.html). The Cochrane Collaboration is particularly interested in getting research information out to patients, and to that end now provides a "plain language summary" with each review; these are available free at www.cochrane.org/reviews/.

Clinical Evidence provides links to useful patient information leaflets, that are in fact provided by BMJ Best Treatments (http://besttreatments.bmj.com/btuk/home. jsp). MedlinePlus (http://medlineplus.gov/), produced by the National Library of Medicine in Bethesda, MD, also provides sound medical information and trustworthy links for further investigation by patients.

Conclusion

Searching for evidence is actually relatively simple, thanks to new resources designed specifically for clinicians. It may be helpful to consult information specialists, such as experienced medical librarians or clinical informaticists, to advise on which of these resources might best fit your needs. Such professionals are themselves a resource, especially when you are stumped for evidence or are conducting an intensive literature search.

References

1. Straus SE. *Evidence-Based Medicine: how to practice and teach EBM*, 3rd edn. Edinburgh: Elsevier/Churchill Livingstone, 2005.
2. Grimshaw J. So what has the Cochrane Collaboration ever done for us? A report card on the first 10 years. CMAJ 2004;171(7):747-9.
3. Tacklind J, MacDonald R, Rutks I, Wilt TJ. *Serenoa repens* for benign prostatic hyperplasia. Cochrane Database Syst Rev 2009;2:CD001423.
4. Pao ML. Perusing the literature via citation links. Comput Biomed Res 1993;26(2):143-56.
5. Pao ML. Complementing Medline with citation searching. Academic Med 1992;67(8):550.
6. Flanigan RC, Reda DJ, Wasson JH, Anderson RJ, Abdellatif M, Bruskewitz RC. 5-year outcome of surgical resection and watchful waiting for men with moderately symptomatic benign prostatic hyperplasia: a Department of Veterans Affairs cooperative study. J Urol 1998;160(1):12-16, discussion 16-17.

2 Clinical trials in urology

Charles D. Scales, Jr[1] *and David F. Penson*[2]

[1]Division of Urology, Department of Surgery, Duke University Medical Center, Durham, NC, USA
[2]Department of Urologic Surgery, Vanderbilt University and VA Tennessee Valley Healthcare System, Nashville, TN, USA

Introduction

Evidence-based clinical practice has been defined as the "conscientious, explicit and judicious use of current best evidence in making decisions about the care of individual patients."[1,2]. Clinical decision making should combine patient preferences and values with the best available evidence when making treatment choices for individual patients [3]. Inherent in this philosophy of practice is that a hierarchy of evidence exists; certain study types provide higher quality evidence than others. This chapter will briefly outline the hierarchy of evidence for questions of therapy and identify the place of clinical trials within that hierarchy. Subsequently, the design and analytical elements of clinical trials which provide key safeguards against bias will be explained, followed by an overview of key principles for applying the results of clinical trials to practice.

The hierarchy of evidence

A central tenet of evidence-based practice is that a hierarchy of evidence exists. Among individual studies, the randomized controlled trial (RCT) provides the highest level of evidence, although ideally a meta-analysis of several RCTs will provide better estimates of treatment effects than a single RCT. Below the RCT in the hierarchy of evidence come cohort studies, which follow groups of patients through time. The key difference between cohort studies and RCTs is that patients are not randomly allocated to treatments in a cohort study. Cohort studies may be prospective – that is, patients are allocated into cohorts prior

to the occurrence of the primary outcomes. Alternatively, cohort studies may be retrospective, when the primary outcome has already occurred. RCTs comprise approximately 10% of the urology literature, while cohort studies comprise approximately 45% [4]. Below cohort studies are case–control studies, case series or reports, and finally expert opinion.

The hierarchy of evidence exists because individual study designs are inherently prone to *bias*, that is, systematic deviation from the truth. As opposed to random error, bias has a magnitude and a specific direction. Bias may serve to over- or underestimate treatment effects, and therefore lead to erroneous conclusions about the value of therapeutic interventions. RCTs sit at the top of the hierarchy of evidence because well-designed and executed RCTs contain the strongest methodological safeguards against bias. Study designs further down the hierarchy of evidence are subject to increasing potential for bias, and therefore constitute lower levels of evidence.

Randomized controlled trials are unique in the hierarchy of evidence, as participants in the trial are not selected for specific interventions but instead are allocated randomly to a specific therapy or control. With appropriate methodological safeguards, RCTs have the potential to provide the highest level of evidence for questions of therapy. For this reason, informed consumers of the urologic literature should understand how to appropriately interpret the results of a clinical trial [5]. RCTs form only a small proportion of published studies in the urologic literature, likely due to several barriers to the conducting of surgical RCTs [4], including the lack of equipoise among surgeons and patients regarding interventions and lack of expertise among urologists with respect to clinical research methodology [6]. In addition, new techniques inherently involve a learning curve; technical proficiency is a requisite for unbiased conduct of a RCT.

One potential method for overcoming technical proficiency barriers is the expertise-based RCT [7] in which the patient is randomized to an intervention conducted by an

Evidence-Based Urology. Edited by Philipp Dahm, Roger R. Dmochowski.
© 2010 Blackwell Publishing.

expert in the technique. For example, in a hypothetical trial of robot-assisted laparoscopic prostatectomy versus open retropubic prostatectomy, the surgery in each arm would be performed by an expert in that specific procedure, recognizing that it is difficult to separate the surgeon from the scalpel when evaluating surgical interventions. In addition, RCTs are not always feasible or ethical [8] and for these reasons, physicians must also incorporate results from observational studies (i.e. prospective cohort), while maintaining awareness of the increased potential for bias in observational designs.

Observational designs, such as cohort and case–control studies, have certain advantages over RCTs although at the significant limitation of greatly increased risk of bias. However, for certain questions, such as those of harm, observational designs may provide the only feasible means to examine rare adverse outcomes of an intervention. Cohort studies for harm may be most useful when randomization of the exposure is not possible, and may be more generalizable than RCTs [9]. Case–control studies can overcome long delays between exposure and outcome, as well as the need to accrue enormous sample sizes to identify rare events [9]. In addition, for questions of prognosis, prospective cohort designs comprise the highest level of evidence.

Clinical trial design elements: safeguarding against bias

Several elements of clinical trial design safeguard against the introduction of bias into the results of the treatment under evaluation. Overall, the objective of these design elements is to ensure that (on average) patients begin the trial with a similar prognosis and retain a similar prognosis (outside therapeutic effect) once the trial begins. The Consolidated Standards of Reporting Trials (CONSORT) statement provides a comprehensive list of reporting guidelines for clinical trials [10,11]. Included in the CONSORT statement are several design elements which provide important safeguards against bias in trial results. These include randomization, concealment, blinding, equal treatment of groups, and complete follow-up.

Randomization refers to the method by which patients are allocated to treatment arms within the trial. As the name implies, patients should be placed into treatment arms in a random, that is, not predictable, fashion. The purpose of randomization is to balance both *known* and *unknown* prognostic factors between treatment arms [3]. For example, in a trial of active surveillance versus radical prostatectomy for prostate cancer, it would be important for Gleason grade (among other factors) to be balanced between the active surveillance and radical prostatectomy

group. It would also be important to balance potentially unknown prognostic factors, such as co-morbid conditions, in such a trial, and randomization optimizes the balance of these conditions. It is important to realize that randomization is not always successful in balancing prognostic factors, particularly with smaller sample sizes. Thus, when interpreting the results of any trial, the reader should examine the balance of patient characteristics (often presented in the first table in the manuscript) between groups.

Equally important to maintaining an initial balance of prognostic factors is the concept of *concealment*. Concealment refers to the principle that study personnel should not be able to predict or control the assignment of the next patient to be enrolled in a trial [3]. This concept is important because it prevents selection, either conscious or unconscious, of subjects for specific treatment arms. Remote randomization, where investigators call to a centralized center to ascertain the assignment of a study subject, is a method frequently used to ensure concealment of randomization. Other methods, such as placing study arm assignments into sealed envelopes, may not always ensure concealment. For example, in a study of open versus laparoscopic appendectomy, concealment by sealed envelope was compromised when surgery occurred overnight, potentially introducing bias to the trials results [3,12]. Lack of concealment has empirically been associated with bias in study results [13-15]. Therefore, it is very important for the informed consumer of medical literature to be aware of whether randomization in a clinical trial was concealed, in order to ensure balance of prognostic factors in the study.

Once a trial is under way, the balance of prognostic factors remains important. Other design features of RCTs assist in maintaining the balance of prognostic factors through the progress and completion of the study. During the study, it is critically important, to the extent feasible, that several groups remain *blinded* to the treatment assignment for each study subject. These groups include patients, caregivers, data collectors, outcome assessors, and data analysts [3]. In this context, the frequently used terms "double blind" or "single blind" may be difficult to interpret, and should be avoided [16]. Patients should be blinded in order to minimize the influence of well-known placebo effects [17,18]. Caregivers, to the extent possible, should be blinded to the intervention to prevent differences in the delivery of the experimental or control treatment. In pharmacological trials, it is relatively straightforward to administer a placebo intervention which blinds both patients and caregivers. However, blinding of caregivers presents special challenges in surgical trials, as surgeons clearly would be aware of which specific surgical intervention a patient has undergone. This may be a potential source of bias, if a surgeon consciously or subconsciously favors one procedure over another [7]. One potential solution to this challenge is the concept introduced by Devereaux et al. [7] of "expertise-based" clinical trials, where a surgeon only performs one procedure in which he/she has special skill or experience. The comparison procedure would be performed by a different surgical expert. In this manner, potential bias from unblinded surgeons would be minimized.

Other groups within the study can feasibly be blinded, even when caregivers or patients cannot, which provides additional methodologic safeguards against the introduction of bias. Perhaps most importantly, adjudicators of outcomes should be blind to the treatment assignment, even if caregivers or patients cannot be feasibly blinded. Blinding of outcome adjudicators prevents differential interpretation of marginal results or variations in subject encouragement during performance tests, either of which could result in the introduction of bias [19]. For example, in a trial of laparoscopic versus open radical prostatectomy, assessors of continence and erectile function should ideally be blind to the treatment arm, to avoid unconscious introduction of bias on the part of the surgeon. In a similar fashion, data collectors should also be blinded to the treatment assignment of subjects. Finally, analysts should be blind to the study assignment in order to prevent introduction of bias in the analytic phase of the study.

In addition to blinding, two other design elements are important to maximize the balance of prognostic factors throughout the conduct of the trial. First, subjects in each study arm should be treated equally, aside from the intervention of interest, throughout the duration of the trial. For example, if subjects undergoing an intervention receive closer or more frequent follow-up than the control subjects, the potential for introduction of bias into the results exists. Therefore, study procedures should remain the same for participants in each arm of a trial. Second, follow-up of subjects should be complete. As more patients are lost to follow-up, the risk of biased results increases. If differences in follow-up rates exist between treatment arms, the risk of bias becomes very high. For example, consider a hypothetical trial of medical versus surgical therapy for benign prostatic hyperplasia. If patients undergoing surgical treatment do well and do not return for follow-up, then bias may be introduced to the surgical arm of the trial. Similarly, if subjects in the medical therapy arm do poorly and seek care elsewhere, this could also introduce bias into the results. An appropriate follow-up rate depends on a number of factors but loss to follow-up of less than 20% is generally considered acceptable [5]. Similar treatment of study subjects and ensuring complete follow-up will minimize introduction of bias during the conduct of the trial.

In summary, several key design elements help to minimize bias in the results of a RCT including randomization,

concealment, blinding, equal treatment, and complete follow-up. The informed consumer of the urology literature should look for these elements when assessing the validity of a clinical trial [5]. It is important to note that reporting of many of these trial elements in RCTs in the urology literature remains suboptimal [20] although lack of reporting of these key elements does not always imply absence of the design element during trial execution [21]. However, reporting remains the only assurance that key safeguards against bias are retained, and thus complete reporting of trial design is encouraged by widely accepted standards [10,11].

Clinical trial analysis elements: safeguarding against bias

In addition to design elements, a number of analytical principles are necessary to safeguard against biased or misleading results in RCTs. Several of these elements are identified in the CONSORT statement [10,11] and include appropriate sample size calculations, conducting analyses according to the intention-to-treat principle, reporting effect size and precision for primary and secondary outcomes, and accounting for the effects of subgroup analyses and multiple testing when interpreting trial results. Notably, randomized trials in the urologic literature are frequently deficient in the utilization or reporting of these key statistical elements [4,22,23]. Therefore, it is incumbent on the informed consumer of the urologic literature to critically appraise reports of randomized trials, with a close eye on use of key elements in the data analysis.

Perhaps the most important statistical element to consider when planning a randomized trial is the sample size necessary to detect a clinically meaningful difference in the primary outcome. Frequently referred to as a sample size or power calculation, this procedure takes into account the expected event rate in the trial arms, the expected variation in the event rate, and the minimum clinically relevant difference which the trial is expected to detect in order to arrive at the number of subjects needed to perform the study. Inadequate sample size (an underpowered study) can result in the appearance of no difference between groups, when in fact a clinically meaningful difference exists [24]. Underpowered clinical trials are scientifically unsound, are of questionable ethics, and may inhibit study of clinically important questions [23,24]. The reporting of sample size calculations in RCTs in the urology literature improved from 19% of studies in 1996 to 47% of studies in 2004 (odds ratio (OR) 2.36, 95% confidence interval (CI) 1.39–4.02, $p < 0.001$) [22]. Despite this improvement, however, Breau et al. demonstrated that among urologic randomized trials reporting no difference between treatment arms, fewer than one in three had sufficient power to detect a 25% difference in treatment effect [23].

Consumers of the urologic literature should therefore devote particular attention to the reporting of sample size calculations, especially when the outcome of the trial demonstrates no statistically significant difference between groups.

Another particularly important analytical element in the reporting of RCTs is the intention-to-treat principle. Briefly, this means assessing all patients in a clinical trial in the arm to which they were randomized, regardless of their adherence to or completion of therapy [3]. The intention-to-treat principle helps to avoid systematic error introduced by nonrandom loss of subjects to treatment or follow-up [25]. Investigators will often report an analysis of only adherent subjects, frequently termed a *per protocol analysis*. However, results of per protocol analyses are often misleading [3]. For example, in a RCT of clofibrate, a lipid-lowering agent, the mortality rate among patients with less than 80% adherence to medication was 24.6%, as compared with a mortality of 15.0% in adherent patients (p < 0.001) [26]. However, a similar risk difference in mortality (28.2% in low-adherence versus 15.1% in adherent patients) was noted in the placebo arm. Thus, the high-adherence groups were prognostically different, which would potentially lead to an erroneous conclusion had the intention-to-treat principle not been followed.

In the urology literature, only about one-third of randomized trials published in 1996 and 2004 reported an intention-to-treat analysis [22]. Even when authors use the term "intention-to-treat analysis," reports may not be complete and the term may be incorrectly applied [27,28]. Adherence to the intention-to-treat principle is empirically associated with overall methodological quality in clinical trials [27,28]. Thus, adherence to the intention-to-treat principle should be a point of emphasis for investigators and users of the urological literature.

Users of the urological literature are likely most interested in the results of clinical trials; that is, the effect of treatment with the intervention under study. Informative reporting of trial results includes a measure of contrast between the control and experimental arms, as well as some measure of the precision of the observed treatment effect [29]. The difference in outcomes (e.g. death, symptom score) between the experimental and control groups is typically referred to as the *effect size*. Effect size is frequently expressed as a risk ratio or odds ratio for categorical outcomes or a difference between means for continuous outcomes. It is important to recognize, however, that the results of a single RCT represent a *point estimate* of a given treatment effect, and the true effect size for all patients

with the target condition lies within a range of values, typically expressed as the *confidence interval*. For example, consider the results of a RCT of the long-term efficacy and safety of finasteride (PLESS trial) for the treatment of benign prostatic hyperplasia [30]. In this trial, the rate of urinary retention in the treatment arm was 7%, compared to 3% in the placebo arm, a relative risk reduction of 57%. The confidence interval for the relative risk reduction was 40–69%. One way to interpret the confidence interval is that if the trial were repeated 100 times, in 95 of those cases the treatment effect (relative risk reduction) would be between 40% and 69%. The reporting of effect size and precision is important for clinicians, as they provide both a measure of the expected treatment result and a plausible range of results with which to counsel patients. Therefore, effect size and precision should be considered one of the key statistical reporting elements for RCTs in the urological literature.

Another key statistical element to consider when interpreting trial results, particularly in trials where multiple endpoints or outcomes are reported, is the effect of multiple testing. Multiple testing typically involves comparing the control and experimental arms across several different clinical outcomes. Alternatively, conducting subgroup analyses (i.e. comparison within gender groups or within age groups) also constitutes multiple testing. This practice greatly increases the likelihood of false-positive results [29]. Analyses which are prespecified and account for the potential effects of multiple testing are more reliable than those inspired by the data [29]. It is frequently difficult to determine whether subgroup analyses are prespecified [31]. In addition, empirical evidence from comparison of trial protocols and reports suggests that selective reporting of outcomes is problematic in the medical literature [32]. Ideally, when subgroup analyses or multiple outcome analyses are conducted, corrections for the risk of false-positive findings should be employed (i.e. the Bonferroni correction). Uncorrected multiple testing is a significant problem in the urological literature: only 6% of RCTs reported in 2004 addressed the potential effects of multiple testing on results [22]. Therefore, consumers of the urologic literature should be aware of the potential for misleading trial results when safeguards against the effects of multiple testing are lacking.

Applying clinical trial results

Once the results of a clinical trial are deemed valid, they must be applied in practice. Generalizability (external validity) refers to the extent to which the findings of a study may be extended to other settings [29]. Patients treated in actual practice frequently differ from those in a clinical trial, and a decision as to the applicability of trial results must be made by the clinician. Frequently clinicians determine whether a compelling reason exists why the trial results should not apply to a given patient [33]. In addition, providers should assess whether patients can comply with the treatment, whether the intended intervention can be delivered adequately, and whether the benefits are worth the risks and costs [3]. These potential barriers to applicability of trial results frequently result in observable differences between the effect size of an intervention in a clinical trial (efficacy) and the effect of an intervention in practice (effectiveness). Therefore, clinicians must carefully weigh the risks, benefits, feasibility and costs when applying the results of clinical trials to individual patients.

Conclusion

Results of well-designed and executed RCTs provide the highest level of evidence for the practice of urology. Evidence suggests that the quality of reporting in urologic RCTs is at times suboptimal [20,22]. Therefore, the informed reader of the urological literature should be aware of the design and statistical elements which safeguard against bias and misleading results from trials. Ultimately, becoming an informed consumer of the urological literature should be the goal of every urologist aspiring to an evidence-based clinical practice.

References

1. Sackett DL, Rosenberg WM, Gray JA, Haynes RB, Richardson WS. Evidence based medicine: what it is and what it isn't. BMJ 1996;312:71-2.
2. Shaneyfelt T, Baum KD, Bell D, et al. Instruments for evaluating education in evidence-based practice: a systematic review. JAMA 2006;296:1116-27.
3. Guyatt G, Rennie D, Meade MO, Cook DJ. *Users' Guides to the Medical Literature: a manual for evidence-based clinical practice*, 2nd edn. New York: McGraw-Hill, 2008.
4. Scales CD Jr, Norris RD, Peterson BL, Preminger GM, Dahm P. Clinical research and statistical methods in the urology literature. J Urol 2005;174:1374-9.
5. Bajammal S, Dahm P, Scarpero HM, Orovan W, Bhandari M. How to use an article about therapy. J Urol 2008;180:1904-11.
6. McCulloch P, Taylor I, Sasako M, Lovett B, Griffin D. Randomised trials in surgery: problems and possible solutions. BMJ 2002;324:1448-51.
7. Devereaux PJ, Bhandari M, Clarke M, et al. Need for expertise based randomised controlled trials. BMJ 2005;330:88.
8. Smith GC, Pell JP. Parachute use to prevent death and major trauma related to gravitational challenge: systematic review of randomised controlled trials. BMJ 2003;327:1459-61.
9. Levine M, Ioannidis J, Haines T, Guyatt G. Harm (observational studies). In: Guyatt G, Rennie D, Meade MO, Cook DJ. *Users' Guides to the Medical Literature: a manual for evidence-based clinical practice*, 2nd edn. New York: McGraw-Hill, 2008.
10. Begg C, Cho M, Eastwood S, et al. Improving the quality of reporting of randomized controlled trials. The CONSORT statement. JAMA 1996;276:637-9.
11. Moher D, Schulz KF, Altman DG. The CONSORT statement: revised recommendations for improving the quality of reports of parallel-group randomised trials. Lancet 2001;357:1191-4.
12. Hansen JB, Smithers BM, Schache D, Wall DR, Miller BJ, Menzies BL. Laparoscopic versus open appendectomy: prospective randomized trial. World J Surg 1996;20:17-20, discussion 1.
13. Schulz KF, Chalmers I, Hayes RJ, Altman DG. Empirical evidence of bias. Dimensions of methodological quality associated with estimates of treatment effects in controlled trials. JAMA 1995;273:408-12.
14. Moher D, Pham B, Jones A, et al. Does quality of reports of randomised trials affect estimates of intervention efficacy reported in meta-analyses? Lancet 1998;352:609-13.
15. Balk EM, Bonis PA, Moskowitz H, et al. Correlation of quality measures with estimates of treatment effect in meta-analyses of randomized controlled trials. JAMA 2002;287:2973-82.
16. Devereaux PJ, Manns BJ, Ghali WA, et al. Physician interpretations and textbook definitions of blinding terminology in randomized controlled trials. JAMA 2001;285:2000-3.
17. Kaptchuk TJ. Powerful placebo: the dark side of the randomised controlled trial. Lancet 1998;351:1722-5.
18. McRae C, Cherin E, Yamazaki TG, et al. Effects of perceived treatment on quality of life and medical outcomes in a double-blind placebo surgery trial. Arch Gen Psychiatry 2004;61:412-20.
19. Guyatt GH, Pugsley SO, Sullivan MJ, et al. Effect of encouragement on walking test performance. Thorax 1984;39:818-22.
20. Scales CD Jr, Norris RD, Keitz SA, et al. A critical assessment of the quality of reporting of randomized, controlled trials in the urology literature. J Urol 2007;177:1090-5.
21. Huwiler-Muntener K, Juni P, Junker C, Egger M. Quality of reporting of randomized trials as a measure of methodologic quality. JAMA 2002;287:2801-4.
22. Scales CD Jr, Norris RD, Preminger GM, Vieweg J, Peterson BL, Dahm P. Evaluating the evidence: statistical methods in randomized controlled trials in the urological literature. J Urol 2008;180:1463-7.
23. Breau RH, Carnat TA, Gaboury I. Inadequate statistical power of negative clinical trials in urological literature. J Urol 2006;176:263-6.
24. Moher D, Dulberg CS, Wells GA. Statistical power, sample size, and their reporting in randomized controlled trials. JAMA 1994;272:122-4.
25. Lachin JL. Statistical considerations in the intent-to-treat principle. Control Clin Trials 2000;21:526.
26. (No authors listed) Influence of adherence to treatment and response of cholesterol on mortality in the coronary drug project. N Engl J Med 1980;303:1038-41.

27. Ruiz-Canela M, Martinez-Gonzalez MA, de Irala-Estevez J. Intention to treat analysis is related to methodological quality. BMJ 2000;320:1007-8.

28. Hollis S, Campbell F. What is meant by intention to treat analysis? Survey of published randomised controlled trials. BMJ 1999;319:670-4.

29. Altman DG, Schulz KF, Moher D, et al. The revised CONSORT statement for reporting randomized trials: explanation and elaboration. Ann Intern Med 2001;134:663-94.

30. McConnell JD, Bruskewitz R, Walsh P, et al. The effect of finasteride on the risk of acute urinary retention and the need for surgical treatment among men with benign prostatic hyperplasia. Finasteride Long-Term Efficacy and Safety Study Group. N Engl J Med 1998;338:557-63.

31. Assmann SF, Pocock SJ, Enos LE, Kasten LE. Subgroup analysis and other (mis)uses of baseline data in clinical trials. Lancet 2000;355:1064-9.

32. Chan AW, Hrobjartsson A, Haahr MT, Gotzsche PC, Altman DG. Empirical evidence for selective reporting of outcomes in randomized trials: comparison of protocols to published articles. JAMA 2004;291:2457-65.

33. Scales CD Jr, Preminger GM, Keitz SA, Dahm P. Evidence based clinical practice: a primer for urologists. J Urol 2007;178:775-82.

3

Conduct and interpretation of systematic reviews and meta-analyses in urology

Martha M. Faraday

Four Oaks, LLC; Keedysville, MD, USA

Systematic reviews and meta-analyses in context: a brief history of evidence-based medicine

Systematic reviews and meta-analyses have emerged as powerful tools to facilitate healthcare decision making by individual practitioners as well as by institutions and organizations. Their prominence is intimately tied to the momentum generated by the evidence-based medicine (EBM) movement. EBM has profoundly altered standards for evaluating and integrating research-derived information into clinical practice with its focus on processes that emphasize explicit, unbiased, and transparent consideration of available research evidence and its quality to formulate care decisions. It is in this context that systematic reviews and meta-analyses have come to prominence. It is instructive to briefly examine these roots.

Evidence-based medicine

The use of evidence to make treatment decisions has a history that goes back to antiquity and includes examples from the Bible as well as ancient Greek and Eastern writings [1]. The current EBM movement, therefore, is not a new phenomenon and is not a change in the essential nature of medicine; good doctors have always tried to incorporate the best available information to treat the individual patient before them (see Doherty [2] for excellent historical examples). Why, then, is there currently such explicit emphasis on the use of evidence in medical decision making? Multiple cultural forces have converged to spotlight evidence usage, with an emphasis on quantification of benefits versus harms and resource allocation.

Modern roots of EBM

The framework that became modern EBM has its foundation in the work of Archie Cochrane, David Sackett, and Walter O. Spitzer. At its core was a need articulated by governments to know whether healthcare services were beneficial to patients and to cease providing harmful or unproven services for reasons of both compassion and cost. Cochrane's *Effectiveness and Efficiency: random reflections on health services* was written in response to a request to evaluate the United Kingdom's National Health Service [3]. In this now classic work, Cochrane explicitly defined effectiveness of interventions, diagnostic tests, and screening procedures as the demonstration that the procedure does more good than harm, with the most convincing demonstration occurring in the context of a randomized controlled trial (RCT) [3,4].

The themes of effectiveness and evaluation were further pursued in the 1970s by Sackett and colleagues at McMaster University, Ontario, Canada, in the context of evaluating interventions to improve effectiveness of the Canadian national Medicare program [4,5]. Review and evaluation of evidence for preventive interventions in primary care also were occurring in Canada during this period, conducted by Walter O. Spitzer and the Task Force on the Periodic Health Examination [4]. As part of its deliberations, the Task Force explicitly graded evidence, with RCT evidence considered the most convincing, and tied level of evidence to strength of recommendation [6]. In the 1980s, the Cochrane Collaboration was formed based on efforts of Iain Chalmers at the University of Oxford and the McMaster group [7]. Its mission is to create and maintain a database of systematic reviews of healthcare with the goal of grounding healthcare in high-quality evidence.

Several additional medical, social, and cultural forces came together in the last part of the 20th century that changed the environment in which medicine is practiced and further sharpened the focus on evidence. Until the 1950s, medicine depended on expert opinion as the source of the best information. In the last half of the 20th century,

Evidence-Based Urology. Edited by Philipp Dahm, Roger R. Dmochowski.
© 2010 Blackwell Publishing.

however, major changes occurred. These included the emergence and widespread implementation of the RCT design with its emphasis on testing hypotheses (rather than gathering expert opinions) while minimizing bias with randomization and blinding procedures; a major shift in the physician–patient relationship away from paternalism and toward a collaborative partnership model; the birth of the internet and the emergence of widespread access to medical information; increased prevalence of chronic disease in an aging population; rising costs of healthcare and the interest of payers in supporting care known to be effective; substantial practice variation in many disease states; and the increasingly interdisciplinary nature of medicine itself. In particular, the volume, density, and complexity of the scientific literature have made it nearly impossible for the practicing clinician to remain up to date. Some estimates suggest that to remain current in general medicine, one would have to read and integrate into one's practice several thousand articles per year [8].

It is in this medical, social, and cultural context that systemic reviews and meta-analyses have emerged as major influences on healthcare decision making; when done well, these methodologies can provide unbiased synopses of the best evidence to guide decisions.

Conducting systematic reviews

Literature reviews versus systematic reviews

The peer-reviewed literature is filled with narrative review articles on every conceivable topic. To conduct a narrative literature review, authors select a topic of interest, conduct literature searches, examine the identified articles, decide upon articles to be included, and write a narrative synopsis. Decisions about article inclusion and exclusion, literature search terms, and search methods may or may not be specified. Review articles often reflect the taste and judgment of the authors in terms of what they view as valid scientific contributions. It is possible, therefore, to find review articles on the same topic that include different studies and come to different conclusions. The narrative synopsis also can be an unwieldy means of attempting to synthesize evidence when the number of articles is large.

Systematic reviews differ from literature reviews in a number of important ways. Simply put, a systematic review applies the scientific method to the concept of a literature review. That is, like a convincing experiment, the review is conducted in as unbiased a manner as possible using rigorous methodology that is transparent and replicable by outside parties. Because high-quality systematic reviews can provide an relatively unbiased overview of the research in a particular area, they may be used to describe the content and boundaries of existing evidence

in a given area; synthesize evidence; provide background for decision making by individual physicians, institutions or governments; and, by making clear what is not known, define research needs and determine where lack of evidence means that clinical judgment and experience are the primary determinants of care decisions.

Steps in performing a systematic review

To evaluate the quality of a systematic review, it is helpful to understand the steps involved in conducting one and how this process differs from the conduct of a simple literature review.

The question

A systematic review begins with a clearly defined, answerable, and relevant clinical question. The elements that compose the question set the literature search parameters and the study inclusion and exclusion criteria. The question must specify populations, interventions, outcomes, settings, and study designs to be considered.

The population of interest The population of interest is the group of individuals to whom the findings from the review will be generalized. It sets the literature search parameters for the samples of interest. The population may be broad – adult males and females of any age with a sporadic renal carcinoma regardless of how the tumor was treated. It also may be quite narrow – adult males within a specific age range who present with a particular stage of prostate cancer and who were treated with adjuvant radiotherapy after radical prostatectomy. The important criterion is that it is clearly defined so that studies which report on samples that do not match the target population are culled from the review. Authors will have to decide how to handle articles in which only part of the sample meets the selection criterion, particularly if findings are not broken out for the subgroup of interest. For example, authors may decide to reject all articles which contain any patients who are not of interest or they may decide to include articles if at least half of the patients are the sample of interest. The important point is to have a decision rule that is reported, applied consistently, and followed without exception.

Interventions or treatments of interest, including relevant comparison groups These decisions set additional literature search parameters that govern article inclusion and exclusion. These terms also may be narrow or broad. Authors may be interested in a single intervention performed in a specific way (i.e. radiofrequency ablation using a percutaneous approach) or in multiple treatments (i.e. all ablation therapies across modalities and approaches). They may only be interested in comparative outcomes between two treatments (i.e. local recurrence-free survival for laparoscopic partial nephrectomy vs open partial nephrectomy) or between a control group and a given treatment (i.e. interstitial cystitis global symptom improvement rates for placebo intravesical instillation vs active drug intravesical instillation). Authors will have to set decision rules for how to handle articles that do not completely meet the search criteria. For example, some articles may include additional treatment groups that are not of interest; often these articles are included and only the data of interest are reviewed.

Outcomes of interest These decisions set further inclusion and exclusion criteria. Authors must specify which outcomes they wish to evaluate. There are different philosophies regarding how to decide upon outcomes. Some authors focus on outcomes that are directly relevant to patients, such as survival or symptoms or quality of life. Others may focus on intermediate endpoints that are believed to be part of the causal chain that leads to a patient-relevant outcome but which does not constitute, in and of itself, a direct measure of patient welfare or improvement (i.e. PSA levels). In addition, depending on the field of study, the way in which the same outcome is quantified and reported may vary from article to article. For example, there are many measures of quality of life and it is not uncommon for study authors to create their own measures. When the outcome is of this type, the authors will have to decide *a priori* which measures are considered acceptable for the review purpose.

Intervention settings Systematic reviews ideally specify intervention settings (although many do not). Authors may be interested in all settings or only in high-volume clinical centers of excellence or only in community-based hospitals and practices. If authors do not specify settings of interest, then some attention should be paid in the review to whether or not setting is believed to influence outcomes. If the authors do not address this issue, then the reader should ponder this question (see below under Evaluating Systematic Reviews).

Study designs Study designs that will be considered also should be specified. The validity of various study designs to provide scientific evidence is typically conceptualized in a hierarchy. The hierarchy is derived from the theoretical certainty with which one can make causal attributions regarding the effects of an intervention on an outcome. In its simplest form, the hierarchy has two levels: randomized controlled trials (RCTs) and observational studies. The selection of study design should be informed by a balanced understanding of the strengths and weaknesses of these design types as well as by the nature of the question to be addressed. If authors do not specifically detail their rationale for study design selection, then the careful reader should consider whether the focus on a particular design is valid, given the question.

Randomized controlled trials. Randomized controlled trials are considered the gold-standard design to prove efficacy because, in theory, randomization of patients to treatment groups should protect against sources of bias and confounding and should ensure that patient groups are more or less equivalent at the beginning of the study – one important component of interpreting any change once the intervention begins. In nonrandomized trials that use samples of convenience, bias may be present in terms of selection (i.e. patients with more severe disease may end up assigned to one particular treatment group) or demographics (i.e. older patients may be clustered in one particular treatment group). Lack of equivalence between groups at study outset makes it difficult to know if any treatment effects are the result of the treatment or the result of initial differences between patient groups. The randomization in RCTs is intended to protect against this problem.

Blinding is another important component of RCTs. The strongest RCTs use a double-blind procedure in which neither clinicians nor patients know which treatment is being administered. Blinding is particularly important when the disorder under study is likely to manifest large placebo effects. Blinding is not always possible, however. For example, it is not possible to blind a surgeon to the type of surgery he or she is to perform or to blind a patient to the fact that she is to receive a pill rather than an intravesical treatment. In addition, some treatments have hallmark signs that are difficult to mask.

The use of placebo control groups is another strength of the RCT design. Placebo controls are critical in the study of disorders that tend to manifest substantial placebo effects. In disorders of this type, studies that use randomization and blinding but lack placebo controls (i.e. that compare a new treatment to an established treatment rather than to a regimen that is believed to have no efficacy) may not yield definitive evidence for the new treatment.

Randomized controlled trials have their weaknesses, however. An important evolution over the last several years has been growing appreciation that factors in addition to study design are potentially important components of evidence quality. For example, although RCTs are considered ideal for measuring efficacy, they do not provide certain types of information needed to make decisions in the context of individual patients or to make policy judgments that potentially affect large numbers of patients [9]. The very factors that give RCTs their strength (randomization, blinding, and intention-to-treat statistical procedures to limit bias; careful and generally narrow patient selection to limit within-group variability and maximize the detection of treatment effects; selection of highly qualified providers of care; comparison of treatments to placebo controls; and careful follow-up procedures to promote adherence) compromise generalizability [9]. Trial patients may differ from the typical patient in important ways such as the presence of co-morbidities or specific demographic variables such as ethnicity, gender or age.

Intention-to-treat procedures may underestimate both benefits and risks because adherence is not considered. Many patients may not be treated at large clinical centers by highly experienced practitioners. Patients and physicians may want to know how a new treatment compares to the usual treatment, not to placebo. The outcomes measured may be of limited relevance to the individual patient if they are clinical rather than patient focused, outcomes may be reported in a way that makes them difficult to interpret (i.e. collapsing certain types of side effects into one category), and follow-up may be too short to accurately capture long-term risks or rare events [9]. In addition, some types of interventions, such as surgeries, are more challenging to evaluate in a fully fledged RCT design because of the complexity of creating placebo or sham treatments or the ethical considerations of withholding treatment if it is believed that the treatment has real efficacy.

Observational studies. There are many types of observational studies; they are called "observational" because they lack assignment to treatment group via randomization (and therefore lack the protection against bias that randomization provides) and instead are made up of unblinded observations on a group or groups of patients that were assigned to treatments based on some criterion other than randomization. Often, the patients are samples of convenience (i.e. patients treated by a particular clinician or who come to a specific center). They may be retrospective (i.e. a chart review) or prospective. They may or may not have some type of control group but generally do not have a placebo control group.

The attribution of causality to an intervention evaluated in an observational study is problematic because of the lack of randomization, blinding, and placebo controls. The degree to which it is problematic depends on the disorder under study. For example, when objective indices of disease presence, progress, and remission exist, such as in renal cancer, the utility of observational studies may be high as long as other confounding factors are identified and acknowledged. For example, patients who underwent different types of surgical procedures for renal cancer may also have differed in age or tumor size. However, in disorders such as interstitial cystitis for which placebo effects are large and objective indices of improvement are lacking , the absence of placebo controls becomes a major interpretive challenge because it is not possible to determine the extent to which the treatment effect is partly or wholly accounted for by the placebo effect. For these kinds of questions, observational studies may suffer from serious deficits in validity and may have very limited value to assess efficacy of a given treatment.

Observational studies have their strengths, however, and in some circumstances can be used to fill in the deficits of RCTs. For example, observational studies typically study broader samples that can provide greater generalizability. They may be conducted by a greater variety of clinicians, allowing some understanding of how the community-based practitioner approaches particular diseases. They may provide longer-term follow-up data. They also often provide more information about low-probability adverse events than do RCTs because of the greater variety of patients and clinicians involved and the longer follow-up durations. For disorders that are likely to manifest substantial placebo effects, although efficacy may be problematic to evaluate in the context of observational studies, observational studies may be quite useful to ascertain adverse event rates.

Conducting literature searches

Authors should decide at the outset how literature searches will be conducted, including which databases will be used, the search terms, and the years of the search. If procedures in addition to electronic database searches are used, such as hand-searches of journals, searches for unpublished studies, queries to experts in the field or organizations (i.e. pharmaceutical companies), then these efforts also should be documented. For each search type, the authors should report the years of inclusion and how many studies were retrieved. For RCTs in particular, the Cochrane database is an excellent resource [10]. Trial registries such as www.TrialsCentral.org also can be valuable.

Applying study inclusion and exclusion criteria

The study inclusion and exclusion criteria set by decisions regarding the population, interventions, settings, outcomes, and study designs of interest are then applied. Ideally, more than one person should be involved in making these decisions and authors should decide before beginning on a procedure to be used if there are disagreements. Commonly used procedures are discussion until consensus is reached or arbitration by a third author who was not involved in the initial decisions. Authors should specify how many studies were excluded, how many produced disagreements, and the final decisions resulting from the disagreement resolution process.

Assessment of study quality

Assessment of study quality is generally performed at the time of data extraction. Typically, this is done only for RCTs and focuses on two sets of issues: the quality of randomization and blinding processes, and participant dropout rates. With regard to participant dropout rates, it is problematic if large proportions of individuals dropped out of the study. It is particularly troublesome if dropouts are concentrated primarily within one treatment group because the utility of randomization to create more or less equivalent groups at study outset is then undermined.

Data extraction and synthesis

Once the included articles are assembled, the process of data extraction is carried out. The information extracted from each article is determined by prior decisions made regarding the populations, interventions, settings, and outcomes of interest. Extracted information is entered on a paper or electronic form that has been structured to organize information in a way that best facilitates addressing the review questions. Independent extraction by two individuals is the best means of performing data extraction because not only is it more likely to ensure accuracy but the correspondence between them can be evaluated either qualitatively by examining the values or quantitatively by calculating a statistic that reflects interobserver agreement (i.e. the kappa statistic; see McGinn et al. [11]). Similar to the application of study inclusion and exclusion criteria, procedures for resolving discordant extractions when the source of the discord is not simply data entry error should be specified. Authors also should indicate what proportion of extractions were discordant.

Data are then synthesized qualitatively in the form of evidence tables. Evidence tables come in a variety of formats but have in common that they organize information in columns that typically specify the study author(s), year of publication, and country; relevant patient parameters (i.e. patient age, gender breakdown, ethnic breakdown, etc.); the number of groups and number of patients in each group; the intervention or treatment and any relevant procedural details; and the outcomes. Additional information also may be presented that is relevant to the question under study. The value of evidence tables is that they present key information from the included studies in the same format and in one place, facilitating the assessment of how each study fits within a group of similar studies as well as the evaluation of a group of similar studies. Evidence tables also may be organized in terms of the separate questions the review is intended to address. For example, it is common when multiple outcomes are considered that not every included study reports on every outcome. The evidence tables may be organized by outcome, with only the relevant studies contained in each table. Many systematic reviews conduct only qualitative synthesis. Some also conduct quantitative synthesis in the form of meta-analysis.

Meta-analysis

Meta-analysis is a statistical technique that allows data to be combined or pooled across studies. In the analysis of data from a single study, the individual data points are derived from individual patients and summarized in some way to facilitate the performance of parametric or nonparametric statistical tests. For t-tests or analyses of variance (ANOVA), for example, data for each group are typically expressed as means and standard deviations and comparisons are made to determine whether statistically significant differences are present. Meta-analysis is literally the "meta" version of this procedure. The word "meta" is used to indicate a concept which is an abstraction from another concept and often defined as a concept at a higher or more general level.

In meta-analysis, the individual data points are derived from individual studies rather than from individual patients and the various summary expressions reflect the group of studies rather than the group of patients. Just as familiar summary statistics can be used descriptively (i.e. the mean or median of a particular group) or analytically (i.e. to compare means or medians among two or more groups and determine whether statistically significant differences exist), meta-analysis can be used to summarize and describe a group of studies (i.e. the average cancer-specific survival rate for all laparoscopic partial nephrectomy studies) or to compare outcomes across groups of studies (i.e. determine whether statistically significant differences exist in cancer-specific survival for groups of studies that used different surgical procedures).

There are advantages and disadvantages to pooling information across studies. One important advantage is that meta-analysis can be used to detect small effects across a group of studies that individually lack enough statistical power to detect the effect. (Note that for the purpose of meta-analysis, whether an individual study finds a statistically significant difference is irrelevant.)

The concept of combining data from multiple sets of observations to achieve greater precision goes back to 17th-century astronomers who were aware that the error in any single set of observations by a single observer was likely to be high [12]. The use of the meta-analysis concept to assess medical information was first undertaken more than 100 years ago by the statistician Karl Pearson who combined studies on the efficacy of inoculations against enteric fever because he recognized that any single study did not have enough participants to demonstrate convincing efficacy [13].

The use of meta-analysis in this context can clarify whether there may be an advantage to a particular treatment that is not apparent on a study-by-study basis but is apparent when a group of studies is considered together. It also can help clarify whether it is worth doing another study on a particular topic. If a meta-analysis indicates that there is no significant treatment effect across of a group of well-conducted studies, then one might question whether the conduct of another study on the same topic merits the investment of time, effort, and money, and also weigh the ethical issues of conducting studies on treatments that the best combined evidence indicates do not work. Using the same framework, meta-analysis also can be used to understand the comparative efficacy of different treatments, resulting in two types of extremely useful clinical information: whether one treatment has better outcomes than another or whether treatments have equivalent outcomes and either one is appropriate.

There are important caveats to the use of meta-analysis, however. As with any type of statistical procedure, the output of the analysis is only as good as the information that goes into it. Studies should only be pooled or combined if they are similar enough on key characteristics that it makes good common sense to combine them. For example, one would not want to pool studies that used different types of surgical procedures to assess complication rates unless an excellent case can be made that the technical differences across surgeries are trivial and the procedures are similar on important issues such as operative time, blood loss, and hospital stay. Pooling also can be made invalid by more subtle differences among studies, such as differences in patient types and treatment settings.

The most common problem encountered in attempting to perform a meta-analysis is that heterogeneity of studies emerges. Heterogeneity means that studies chosen for pooling exhibit dissimilar or divergent findings. Heterogeneity is the meta-version of large amounts of variability observed within one treatment group in the context of an individual study. When highly variable responses occur in the context of one treatment group in which the individual patients were presumably treated similarly, variability suggests that patients had differential responses to the treatment, either because of attributes of the patients or because of variability in how the treatment was administered. In meta-analyses, heterogeneity indicates that there is variability across studies. This variability may be related to the patients or the procedures or the settings or other factors. Every effort should be made to determine the source of the divergence because if heterogeneity is substantial, doubts are raised that the studies should be pooled. If there is doubt that the studies should be pooled, then any conclusions that flow from combining studies also are suspect.

It is also important to recognize that mathematical precision is not the same as conceptual clarity. Almost any parameter can be mathematized. However, if measures of a given phenomenon are fundamentally weak measures – that is, they lack precision, they were poorly designed, poorly administered, etc. – then even the most carefully conducted meta-analysis will be weak. In addition, meta-analysis cannot correct for deficits in study design such as failures of randomization or blinding, patient selection bias, reporting bias, etc. Even the application of more sophisticated meta-analytical techniques such as meta-regression cannot correct for fundamental weaknesses of measurement and study quality. Mathematical manipulations are a poor substitute for carefully constructed measures and properly designed studies.

In addition, it is critical to understand the concept of statistical significance. At the level of the individual study, statistical significance is a function of three inter-related quantities: sample size or statistical power, the size of the differences between or among groups, and variability within groups. Of the three quantities, statistical significance is most heavily dependent on power. With 10,000 patients per group, almost any difference, including those that are extremely small, will be statistically significant regardless of whether the differences have any meaning. This situation is analogous to using a high-powered telescope to examine blades of grass – one can easily detect small differences in texture, height, and shade of green (regardless of whether they may meaningfully be related to the health of the grass). With 10 patients per group, statistically significant differences can only emerge if the difference between groups is extremely large and the variability within each group is small (i.e. the signal-to-noise ratio is high). This situation is analogous to examining the blades of grass from 10 feet away; extremely large differences will be obvious but small differences will not be detectable.

These principles also apply to meta-analysis. In meta-analysis, statistical power refers to the number of studies (rather than the number of patients) and variability refers to the divergence among studies for a given outcome (i.e. heterogeneity) rather than the divergence among patient responses. When the number of studies is large and variability among them is small, then it will be relatively easy to detect statistically significant effects. When the number of studies is small, statistically significant effects will only emerge if there is very little heterogeneity and/or the size of the differences between study types is large.

Therefore, statistical significance, because it is largely a function of power, may or may not equate to clinical significance. The careful reader should ignore p values and put the meta-analytic output into a meaningful clinical context. If procedure A has a 2% major urological complication rate and procedure B has a 2.6% complication rate, regardless of whether this difference is statistically significant, the key question is whether it is clinically significant. Similarly, a meta-analysis may indicate that recurrence-free survival rates of 95% for procedure A and 99% for procedure B were not statistically different. However, the reader should ponder whether these differences are clinically meaningful.

Evaluating systematic reviews

Standards have been promulgated for how systematic reviews and meta-analyses should be performed and reported (i.e. the QUOROM statement; see Moher et al. [14]). However, systematic reviews vary considerably in methodological quality [15-20] and methodological quality is the key to the validity of their conclusions. The reader should look for several features.

Detailed transparency of procedures

The hallmark of a well-performed systematic review is transparent fidelity to the principles of the scientific method. That is, the methods by which the review was performed should have accepted validity and be clearly described such that another group of authors could replicate the procedures and, presumably, the conclusions.

The question

The question or questions the review is intended to answer should be specified, including the populations, interventions, outcomes, settings, and study designs of interest. The question should be clinically relevant and unambiguous.

Literature searches and literature selection

All literature search parameters should be reported, including the databases used, whether additional techniques also were employed (i.e. hand-searching), the key words and years searched, and the total number of searches performed. The criteria for study inclusion and exclusion should be detailed and any decision rules used to deal with studies that did not neatly fall into included or excluded categories should be articulated. The authors should note who made inclusion/exclusion decisions and how disagreements were arbitrated. The total number of studies initially retrieved by the searches should be reported and the number of studies ultimately excluded should be indicated, including the reasons for exclusion.

Study quality assessment

One of the most common deficits in systematic reviews is the absence of study quality assessment [14-16]. The assumption that all studies are equivalent in validity is simply not tenable. Some form of study quality assessment should be incorporated if RCTs are involved. There is no single, accepted instrument for this purpose. Evidence indicates, however, that compromised randomization and blinding procedures in particular are associated with exaggerated treatment effects [21]; at a minimum, these processes should be evaluated. Dropout rates also should be noted, particularly if they differ across groups.

The importance of quality assessment for RCTs is that their position at the top of the evidence hierarchy depends on randomization and blinding having been carried out correctly and the treatment groups assembled by these procedures remaining relatively intact at the end of the study. If randomization procedures are not reported or appear to have been compromised (i.e. a proportion of patients did not receive the treatment to which they were

randomized), then doubts are raised that the advantages of randomization to make treatment groups comparable and control bias were fully realized. Similarly, if blinding procedures are not reported or if they have the potential to have been compromised, then it is possible that treatment effects are contaminated by clinician or patient knowledge about the treatments. Further, if participant dropout rates are high or higher in one treatment group than in another, then the advantages of correctly performed randomization and blinding may have been compromised. RCTs with deficits in these areas may lose their position at the top of the evidence hierarchy and be on a par with observational studies in terms of evidence quality. The authors should clearly indicate any RCTs that have procedural weaknesses and describe how this information was taken into account in the review and meta-analysis, if it was performed.

For observational studies, assessment of study quality is much more difficult and there are no universally accepted instruments or standards for this purpose. The best procedure is to apply an understanding of the strengths and weaknesses of observational studies in the context of the goal of the review. Specifically, authors should clearly indicate that they understand the weaknesses of observational studies in general and should note any particular problems that may be evident because of the nature of the question under study. For example, if the goal of the review is to assess treatment efficacy for a disorder suspected to manifest clinically meaningful placebo effects and all the available studies are observational (i.e. without placebo control groups), then the authors should discuss this issue, particularly if it is not readily resolvable. In contrast, if the disease state is one in which placebo effects are unlikely or nonexistent, then the authors should focus on the relevant weaknesses of observational studies in this context. If authors do attempt to rate the quality of observational studies, then they should describe the strengths and weaknesses of the instrument employed.

Evidence tables should be well organized with the relevant information reported in a consistent format. If information is not reported in a particular study, then its absence should be explicitly noted.

Meta-analysis

Variables and statistics

If a meta-analysis was performed as part of the systematic review, then several criteria should be met. Authors should clearly describe which variables they chose to meta-analyze, how these variables were quantified in the included articles, and the choice of meta-analysis statistic. The statistic used to express meta-analysis output depends on two issues: whether the data were categorical or continuous and the number of groups in the studies [22,23]. For categorical data in which the outcome is binary (i.e. patients are alive or dead), the effect size statistic for single-group studies is the mean proportion or mean event rate with a range from 0.0 to 1.0. When the proportions of interest cluster in the very low or very high end of the range (i.e. 0.2 or lower or 0.8 or higher), then the logit of the proportion or event rate is used; these quantities are difficult to interpret and are usually converted back to mean proportions or event rates when reported. When outcomes are binary and two groups are compared, the most common statistics are the odds ratio or relative risk ratio. For continuous measures, with single-group studies the mean is used if all studies reported the data using the same measurement scale (i.e. number of days in the hospital). For two-group studies when the variable of interest was measured in the same way (i.e. all studies used the same pain scale), the unstandardized mean difference is used. When different measures of the same phenomenon were used (studies used different types of pain scales), the standardized mean difference is used. Note that all these statistics can be reported for individual studies as well as in the form of a pooled effect size.

Confidence intervals

In all cases, a confidence interval (typically 95%) should be reported. The confidence interval can be thought of in several ways. For example, it is frequently used to understand the most likely values (i.e. approximately 95% of the time the measured variable should fall within the reported limits) that the measured variable will take on for the purpose of generalization. It also can be understood as a measure of estimate stability. If survival rates for a particular cancer treatment average 85% at 5 years but the confidence interval ranges from 62% to 97%, then the information provided by the mean survival rate may not be particularly valuable clinically (and, as an aside, suggests significant heterogeneity across studies that should have been investigated). The narrower the confidence interval, the more stable (or less variable) the estimate is considered. In general, wide confidence intervals are most likely when the number of studies in the analysis is small and/or when studies exhibit divergent findings.

Statistical models

A common omission in systematic reviews is the rationale for choice of statistical model for pooling data [24]. The choice of statistical model – fixed versus random effects – has several important conceptual and mathematical consequences and should be specified with a rationale provided for the choice. The models are underpinned by different assumptions [23]. The fixed effects model assumes that, in the abstract, there is one true effect, that similar studies all provide estimates of the one true effect, and that study-to-study variability constitutes error or noise. This model also assumes that error is less likely as sample size

increases; therefore, larger studies are assumed to provide better estimates of the true effect. Studies are weighted in the analysis using inverse variance, which is roughly proportional to sample size; larger studies receive more weight and have more influence on the pooled estimate of the effect.

In contrast, the random effects model assumes that, rather than one true effect, there is a distribution of true effects that varies from study to study because of factors known to differ across studies that legitimately influence outcomes. For example, among studies that all report on outcomes of laparoscopic partial nephrectomy, the fact that some surgeons are more experienced than others or that some reports are from high-volume centers and others are from low-volume centers might legitimately influence the treatment effect in a way that is not error. These factors may play a causal role and may also be present to different degrees across studies. Unlike the fixed effects model in which all study-to-study variability is assumed to constitute statistical noise, in the random effects model part of the study-to-study variability is assumed to represent legitimate variability that makes up the distribution of true effects. The remaining variability is considered error. Studies are weighted in the analysis using inverse variance but because each study is assumed to estimate one of a population of true effects and because the variability is partitioned differently, sample size has less impact on weighting.

As a practical matter, it is very difficult to meet the assumptions of the fixed effect model for most systematic reviews because it assumes that the pooled studies are identical in every important regard that could influence the true effect. For most systematic reviews, this assumption is unlikely to be met. However, this does not prevent it from being used frequently. One reason it may be used is a consequence of the way in which variance is handled in the two models: statistically significant differences are more likely to emerge with the fixed effects model. The exception is when study-to-study dispersion is minimal; in this circumstance the fixed and random effects models will provide identical estimates.

If authors chose to use this model, then they should provide a convincing rationale. In most circumstances, the random effects model is preferable and will provide more conservative and appropriate estimates.

Heterogeneity

Heterogeneity or variability among studies presumably of the same type should be assessed both quantitatively and qualitatively. Heterogeneity is common in meta-analyses [25] but the attempt to explain it is often missing [15,16,24]. Heterogeneity within intervention type is quantified by the I^2 statistic [26,27]. This statistic ranges from 0% (no heterogeneity) to 100% (substantial heterogeneity) and is a measure of the magnitude of heterogeneity among studies that used the same intervention. A p value also is typically reported for I^2 with nonsignificant values indicating that the level of heterogeneity is not of concern. Rules of thumb typically employed in interpreting I^2 are that values less than 20% are of no concern, values between 20% and 50% are of moderate concern, and values greater than 50% are of substantial concern.

It is important to remember, however, the same two caveats that apply to all statistical tests. First, the statistical test for heterogeneity is, like any other statistical test, dependent on statistical power for the detection of significant effects (i.e. the number of studies in the analysis). Second, the presence of statistically significant heterogeneity may or may not constitute clinically relevant heterogeneity. Further, the lack of statistical heterogeneity does not eliminate the possibility of clinically relevant heterogeneity. The reader should attend less to p values and more to the range of values reported and judge whether the variability is of concern in a clinical context.

Heterogeneity also should be assessed qualitatively. Typically, meta-analyzed data are displayed in graphics called forest plots (so named because they are intended to allow visualization of the overall "forest" while de-emphasizing the individual studies that make up the "trees"). When heterogeneity is minimal, the study symbols will line up more or less together. As heterogeneity increases, the study symbols will display more and more divergence. In the presence of heterogeneity, it is absolutely critical that authors search for an explanation. Common sources of heterogeneity are procedural differences across studies (e.g. drug dosage and timing, surgical technique), differences in patient-level variables across studies (e.g. patient age, gender or ethnic distributions, disease stage), clinical setting differences (e.g. high-volume vs low-volume centers) or other issues that render what appeared to be similar studies on the surface dissimilar when they are examined in more detail (e.g. large differences in follow-up). Authors should report explanations for heterogeneity that were explored and their conclusions. Sometimes it is not possible to determine the source of heterogeneity; in this circumstance, the lack of explanation after a rigorous search also should be reported.

Combining studies with different designs

If the systematic review includes both RCTs and observational studies, then the authors should indicate whether for any analysis the two design types were combined. In most circumstances, it is not appropriate to combine RCTs with observational studies because of the presumed advantages of the RCT design to provide higher-quality evidence. However, it may make sense to do this in specialized circumstances. For example, if the available RCTs are flawed (i.e. randomization or blinding was compromised), and believed to provide information essentially equivalent in value to observational designs, then it may be permissible. Authors should provide a rationale for doing so, however.

Publication bias

Publication bias refers to the tendency for studies that do not report significant findings to never be published (older nomenclature referred to this issue as the "file drawer problem"; see Rosenthal [28]). As a consequence, the systematic review may be inevitably biased even after using the highest quality procedures because it does not contain information from studies that never reached the public domain.

One of the most straightforward qualitative techniques for assessing publication bias is the funnel plot [22]. This type of graphic is a scatterplot in which the effect size from each study is plotted against a measure of its precision (typically 1/standard error). In the absence of publication bias, the plot should resemble a symmetrical inverted funnel with less precise (usually studies with smaller sample sizes) clustering near the bottom and more precise (usually studies with larger sample sizes) clustering near the top. In the presence of publication bias, the funnel shape will be asymmetrical, with small-n studies that reported small effect sizes missing from one side of the plot. The funnel plot can be evaluated visually for its integrity and/or statistically (i.e. with Egger's regression although Egger's regression may not be appropriate when effect measures are odds ratios; see Peters et al. [29]). The authors should describe whether they considered publication bias and how it was evaluated (i.e. graphically or statistically).

Interpretation

The interpretation section of systematic reviews is critically important. Ideally, it accomplishes three goals: it clearly summarizes the findings; it explicitly links the findings to the quality of evidence reviewed; and it places the findings into a clinically relevant context. In particular, the authors should describe the limitations and strengths of the evidence and indicate how any evidentiary weaknesses (i.e. problems with study quality, measures, lack of evidence, potential for publication bias) were taken into account in the review conclusions. If a meta-analysis was conducted and heterogeneity was detected, then this issue should be highlighted, particularly if it was not possible to explain the heterogeneity. The implications of the findings should be detailed and the relevance to clinical practice clearly articulated. It is as important to point out what cannot be concluded as to point out what can be concluded based on the available evidence.

Conflict of interest

Authors should fully disclose all possible conflicts of interest, particularly where financial or other important professional relationships are involved. Part of the context of the systematic review is the context of potential bias that arises from authors. If bias is suspected, then the validity and impact of the review are seriously undermined.

Authors can thoughtfully manage issues of conflict of interest at the beginning of the review process. Management should be done at two levels: the elimination or minimization of the real potential for bias and the management of perceptions that bias may have occurred. Ideally, individuals with significant vested interests (or the appearance of such interests) that the findings of a systematic review come to a particular conclusion should not be review authors. For example, if all or most of the authors have a significant financial relationship with a pharmaceutical firm that makes the drug that is the topic of the review, the potential for real and perceived bias is high. However, it may be the case that the individuals who are willing to do the substantial work involved in a systematic review have such interests and that is part of their motivation for conducting the review. In this case, strong, transparent, widely accepted processes are one means of reassuring readers that the potential for bias was controlled. In addition, balancing the author panel by using some individuals who do not have such interests and who are meaningfully involved in study inclusion/exclusion and interpretation of findings is helpful. Authors should consider this issue carefully as they begin the review process. Even the best-intentioned individuals cannot avoid the appearance of potential bias in certain circumstances. For example, if most authors benefit financially from the sale of a particular drug or piece of equipment that is the focus of the review and if the review conclusions are favorable for drug or equipment use, even if this is a valid conclusion, then it is reasonable for a reader to question the conclusions. Or, if the group of authors includes a well-known scientist and his or her protégés, one may wonder about how free and frank the discussion of interpretation may have been. For this reason, balancing authorships with some individuals who are free from the appearance of conflicts is helpful if it is not possible to eliminate problematic authorships entirely.

Conclusion

The practitioner seeking guidance for a care decision should keep the clinical context firmly in mind when using systematic reviews and meta-analyses. The extent to which the findings from a given review apply to a particular clinical situation depends on three sets of factors. The first has to do with the quality of the review and analyses – the focus of this chapter. The second has to do with how well the clinical perspective was reflected in the review and analysis process. The clinician reader should attend carefully to clinically relevant details regarding patients, interventions, and outcomes; one cannot assume that the authors necessarily had commonly encountered clinical issues in mind as they assembled the review. As Hopayian [30] points out, even when clinicians are involved in systematic reviews as authors, clinically important issues may be overlooked despite adherence to quality review procedures. The only antidote to this problem is an alert, clinically attuned reader. The third issue has to do with how well the review findings generalize to the clinician's patient – the final step in judgment before applying review findings to a specific patient. That is, were the patients, interventions, settings, and outcomes similar enough to the target patient to make generalization reasonable, assuming the review was well done and clinically informed? Even if there were some dissimilarities between the scenario covered by the review and the scenario faced by the clinician, good clinical common sense can serve as an excellent guide to determine whether these differences are important.

References

1. Claridge JA, Fabian TC. History and development of evidence-based medicine. World J Surg 2005;29:547-53.
2. Doherty S. History of evidence-based medicine. Oranges, chloride of lime and leeches: barriers to teaching old dogs new tricks. Emerg Med Australas 2005;17:314-21.
3. Cochrane AL. *Effectiveness and Efficiency. Random reflections on health services.* London: Nuffield Hospitals Trust, 1972.
4. Hill GB. Archie Cochrane and his legacy: an internal challenge to physicians' autonomy? J Clin Epidemiol 2000;53:1189-92.
5. Sackett DL, Baskin M (eds). *Health Care Evaluation.* Hamilton, Ontario: McMaster University, 1973.
6. Canadian Task Force on the Periodic Health Examination. The periodic health examination. CMAJ 1979;121:1193-254.
7. Chalmers I, Dickersin K, Chalmers TC. Getting to grips with Archie Cochrane's agenda. BMJ 1992;305:786-8.
8. Davidoff F, Haynes B, Sackett D, Smith R. Evidence-based medicine: a new journal to help doctors identify the information they need. BMJ 1995;310:1085-6.
9. Atkins D. Creating and synthesizing evidence with decision makers in mind: integrating evidence from clinical trials and other study designs. Med Care 2007;45(10 suppl 2):S16-S22.
10. Dickersin K, Manheimer E, Wieland S, et al., for the Central Development Group. Development of the Cochrane Collaboration's CENTRAL register of ontrolled clinical trials. Eval Health Prof 2002;25(1):38-64.
11. McGinn T, Wyer PC, Newman TB, Keitz S, Leipzig R, For GG. Tips for learners of evidence-based medicine: 3. Measures of observer variability (kappa statistic). CMAJ 2004;171:1369-73.
12. Plackett RL. Studies in the history of probability and statistics: VII. The principle of the arithmetic mean. Biometrika 1958;45:130-5.

13. Pearson K. Report on certain enteric fever inoculation statistics. BMJ 1904;3:1243-6.

14. Moher D, Cook DJ, Jadad AR, et al. Assessing the quality of reports of randomized trials: implications for the conduct of meta-analyses. Health Technol Assess 1999;3(12):i-iv, 1-98.

15. Petticrew M, Song F, Wilson P, Wright K. Quality-assessed reviews of health care interventions and the database of abstracts of reviews of effectiveness (DARE). Int J Technol Assess Health Care 1999;15(4):671-8.

16. Jadad AR, Moher M, Browman GP, et al. Systematic reviews and meta-analyses on treatment of asthma: critical evaluation. BMJ 2000;320:537-40.

17. Mulrow CD. The medical review article: state of the science. Ann Intern Med 1987;106(3);485-8.

18. McAlister FA, Clark HD, van Walraven C, et al. The medical review article revisited: has the science improved? Ann Intern Med 1999;131(12):947-51.

19. Olsen O, Middleton P, Ezzo J, et al. Quality of Cochrane reviews: assessment of sample from 1998. BMJ 2001;323:829-32.

20. Jadad AR, Cook DJ, Jones A, et al. Methodology and reports of systematic reviews and meta-analyses: a comparison of Cochrane reviews with articles published in paper-based journals. JAMA 1998;280(3):278-80.

21. Schulz KF, Chalmers I, Hayes RJ, Altman DG. Empirical evidence of bias: dimensions of methodological quality associated with estimates of treatment effects in controlled trials. JAMA 1995;273:408-12.

22. Sutton AJ, Abrams KR, Jones DR, Sheldon TA, Song F. *Methods for Meta-analysis in Medical Research*. Chichester: Wiley, 2000.

23. Lipsey MW, Wilson DB. *Practical Meta-Analyses*. Thousand Oaks, CA: Sage Publications, 2001.

24. Petitti DB. Approaches to heterogeneity in meta-analysis. Stat Med 2001;20(23):3625-33.

25. Engels EA, Schmid CH, Terrin N, Olkin I, Lau J. Heterogeneity and statistical significance in meta-analysis: an empirical study of 125 meta-analyses. Stat Med 2000;19:1707-28.

26. Hatala R, Keitz S, Wyer P, Guyatt G. Tips for learners of evidence-based medicine: 4. Assessing heterogeneity of primary studies in systematic reviews and whether to combine their results. CMAJ 2005;172:661-5.

27. Schoenfeld PS, Loftus EV Jr. Evidence-based medicine (EBM) in practice: understanding tests of heterogeneity in meta-analysis. Am J Gastroenterol 2005;100:1221-3.

28. Rosenthal R. The "file drawer problem" and tolerance for null results. Psych Bull 1979;86(3):638-41.

29. Peters JL, Sutton AJ, Jones DR, Abrams KR, Rushton L. Comparison of two methods to detect publication bias in meta-analysis. JAMA 2006;295(6):676-80.

30. Hopayian K. The need for caution in interpreting high quality systematic reviews. BMJ 2001;323:681-4.

4 Rating the quality of evidence and making recommendations

Philipp Dahm[1] and Holger J. Schünemann[2]

[1]Department of Urology, University of Florida, Gainesville, FL, USA
[2]Department of Clinical Epidemiology and Biostatistics, McMaster University Health Sciences Centre, Hamilton, Ontario, Canada

Introduction

Urologists require clinical expertise to integrate a patient's circumstances and values with the best available evidence to initiate decision making related to the medical and surgical treatment of their patients. Using "best evidence" implies that a hierarchy of evidence exists and that clinicians are more confident about decisions based on evidence that offers greater protection against bias and random error [1].

Protection against bias and greater confidence in decisions arise from high-quality research evidence. We can consider quality of evidence as a continuum that reflects the confidence in estimates of the magnitude of effect of alternative patient management interventions on the outcomes of interest. However, gradations of this continuum are useful for communication with practicing clinicians, providing useful summaries of what is known for specific clinical questions to aid interpretation of clinical research.

Aiding interpretation becomes increasingly important considering that much of clinicians' practice is guided by recommendations from experts summarized in clinical practice guidelines and textbooks such as this new book, *Evidence-Based Urology*. To integrate recommendations with their own clinical judgment, clinicians need to understand the basis for the clinical recommendations that experts offer them. A systematic approach to grading the quality of evidence and the resulting recommendations for clinicians thus represent an important step in providing evidence-based recommendations.

In this chapter we will describe the key features of "quality of evidence" and how we asked the authors of individual chapters to evaluate the available evidence and formulate

their recommendations using a pragmatic approach that, out of necessity, falls short of the full development of evidence-based guidelines. The approach that most authors used was based on the work of the Grading of Recommendations Assessment, Development and Evaluation (GRADE) Working Group [2-6]. Over 20 international organizations, including the World Health Organization, the American College of Physicians, the American College of Chest Physicians, the American Thoracic Society, the European Respiratory Society, UpToDate® and the Cochrane Collaboration, are now using the GRADE system.

Question formulation and recommendations in this book

The editors asked authors to ask clinical questions that are particularly relevant to urology practice using the framework of identifying the patient population(s), the intervention(s) examined (or exposure), alternative interventions (comparison) and the outcomes of interest [7]. Authors were further asked to identify relevant studies related to these questions or sets of questions. For example, in Chapter 30, the authors address the question whether asymptomatic patients with metastatic kidney cancer benefit from a cytoreductive debulking radical nephrectomy with regard to overall survival.

The authors were further asked to base the answers to their questions on evaluations of the scientific literature, in particular focusing on recent, methodologically rigorous systematic reviews of randomized controlled trials (RCTs) [8]. If authors could not identify a recent and rigorous systematic review, they were asked to search for RCTs and summarize the findings of these studies to answer their clinical questions. Only if RCTs did not answer the specific question (or did not provide information on a particular outcome) were observational studies included. Thus, the search studies we suggested focused on relevant

Evidence-Based Urology. Edited by Philipp Dahm, Roger R. Dmochowski.
© 2010 Blackwell Publishing.

systematic reviews or meta-analyses (a pooled statistical summary of relevant studies) followed by searches for randomized trials and observational studies if systematic reviews did not exist or did not include sufficient information to answer the questions posed.

Evaluating the quality of evidence and making recommendations

Many authors applied the GRADE system for evaluating the quality of evidence and presenting their recommendations. This approach begins with an initial assessment of the quality of evidence, followed by judgments about the direction (for or against) and strength of recommendations. Since clinicians are most interested in the best course of action, the GRADE system usually presents the strength of the recommendation first as strong (Grade 1) or weak (Grade 2), followed by the quality of the evidence as high (A), moderate (B), low (C) and very low (D). Authors of this book adopted a version of the grading system that combines the low and very low categories. Furthermore, the editors asked authors to phrase recommendations in a way that would express their strength. For strong (Grade 1) recommendations, many authors chose the words: "We recommend . . . (for or against a particular course of action)." For weak (Grade 2) recommendations, they

used: "We suggest . . . (using or not using)" what they believed to be an optimal management approach. They then indicated the methodological quality of the supporting evidence, labeling it as A (high quality), B (moderate quality) or C (low or very low quality). Thus, recommendations could fall into one of the following six categories: 1A, 1B, 1C, 2A, 2B, and 2C (Table 4.1).

The GRADE system suggests the use of the wording "we recommend" for strong (Grade 1) recommendations and "we suggest" for weak (Grade 2) recommendations. The categories of low and very low quality that GRADE includes in its four category system are collapsed here into a single category, resulting in three categories of quality of evidence.

Strength of the recommendation

In determining the strength of recommendations, the GRADE system focuses on the degree of confidence in the balance between desirable effects of an intervention on the one hand and undesirable effects on the other (see Table 4.1). Desirable effects or benefits include favorable health outcomes, decreased burden of treatment, and decreased resource use (usually measured as costs). Undesirable effects or downsides include rare major adverse events, common minor side effects, greater burden of treatment, and more resource consumption. We define burdens

Table 4.1 Grading recommendations

Grade of recommendation	Balance of desirable versus undesirable effects	Methodological quality of supporting evidence
Strong recommendation, high-quality evidence **1A**	Desirable effects clearly outweigh undesirable effects, or vice versa	Consistent evidence from randomized controlled trials without important limitations or exceptionally strong evidence from observational studies
Strong recommendation, moderate-quality evidence **1B**	Desirable effects clearly outweigh undesirable effects, or vice versa	Evidence from randomized controlled trials with important limitations (inconsistent results, methodological flaws, indirect or imprecise), or very strong evidence from observational studies
Strong recommendation, low- or very low-quality evidence **1C**	Desirable effects clearly outweigh undesirable effects, or vice versa	Evidence for at least one critical outcome from observational studies, case series, or from randomized controlled trials with serious flaws or indirect evidence
Weak recommendation, high-quality evidence **2A**	Desirable effects closely balanced with undesirable effects	Consistent evidence from randomized controlled trials without important limitations or exceptionally strong evidence from observational studies
Weak recommendation, moderate-quality evidence **2B**	Desirable effects closely balanced with undesirable effects	Evidence from randomized controlled trials with important limitations (inconsistent results, methodological flaws, indirect or imprecise), or very strong evidence from observational studies
Weak recommendation, low- or very low-quality evidence **2C**	Desirable effects closely balanced with undesirable effects	Evidence for at least one critical outcome from observational studies, case series, or from randomized controlled trials with serious flaws or indirect evidence

as the demands of adhering to a recommendation that patients or caregivers (e.g. family) may dislike, such as taking medication, need for inconvenient laboratory monitoring, repeated imaging studies or office visits. If desirable effects of an intervention outweigh undesirable effects, we recommend that clinicians offer the intervention to typical patients. The balance between desirable and undesirable effects, and the uncertainty associated with that balance, will determine the strength of recommendations.

Table 4.2 describes the factors GRADE relies on to determine the strength of recommendation. When chapter authors were confident that the desirable effects of adherence to a recommendation outweighed the undesirable effects or vice versa, they offered a strong recommendation. Such confidence usually requires evidence of high or moderate quality that provides precise estimates of both benefits and downsides, and their clear balance in favor of, or against, one of the management options. The authors offered a weak recommendation when low-quality evidence resulted in appreciable uncertainty about the magnitude of benefits and/or downsides or the benefits and downsides were finely balanced. We will describe the factors influencing the quality of evidence in subsequent sections of this chapter. Other reasons for not being confident in the balance between desirable and undesirable effects include: imprecise estimates of benefits or harms, uncertainty or variation in how different individuals value particular outcomes and thus their preferences regarding management alternatives, small benefits, or situations when benefits may not be worth the costs (including the costs of implementing the recommendation). Although the balance between desirable and undesirable effects, and thus the strength of a recommendation, is a continuum, the GRADE system classifies recommendations for or against an intervention into two categories: strong or weak. This is inevitably arbitrary. The GRADE Working Group believes that the simplicity and behavioral implications of this explicit grading outweigh the disadvantages.

Clinical decision making in the setting of weak recommendations remains a challenge. In such settings, urologists should have more detailed conversations with their patient than for strong recommendations, to explore the individual patient's values and to ensure that the ultimate decision is consistent with these. For highly motivated patients, decision aids that present patients with both benefits and downsides of therapy are likely to improve their understanding, reduce decision-making conflict, and may promote a decision most consistent with the patient's underlying values and preferences [9]. Thus, another way for clinicians to interpret strong recommendations is that they provide, for typical patients, a mandate for the clinician to provide a simple explanation of the intervention along with a suggestion that the patient will benefit from its use. Further elaboration will seldom be necessary. On the other hand, when clinicians face weak recommendations, they should more carefully consider the benefits, harms and burdens in the context of the patient before them, and ensure that the treatment decision is consistent with the patient's values and preferences. These situations arise when appreciable numbers of patients, because of variability in values and preferences, will make different choices.

As benefits and risks become more finely balanced or more uncertain, decisions to administer an effective therapy also become more cost sensitive. We have not asked authors to explicitly include cost in the recommendations, but cost will bear on the implementation of many recommendations in clinical practice [10].

Interpreting strong and weak recommendations

Table 4.3 shows suggested ways to interpret strong and weak recommendations. For decisions in which it is clear

Table 4.2 Determinants of strength of recommendation

Factors that influence the strength of a recommendation	Comment
Balance between desirable and undesirable effects	A strong recommendation is more likely as the difference between the desirable and undesirable consequences becomes larger. A weak recommendation is more likely as the net benefit becomes smaller and the certainty around that net benefit decreases
Quality of the evidence	A strong recommendation becomes more likely with higher quality of evidence
Values and preferences	A strong recommendation is more likely as the variability of or uncertainty about patient values and preferences decreases. A weak recommendation is more likely as the variability or uncertainty about patient values and preferences increases
Costs (resource allocation)	A weak recommendation is more likely as the incremental costs of an intervention (more resources consumed) increase

Table 4.3 Implications of strong and weak recommendations

Implications	Strong recommendation	Weak recommendation
For patients	Most individuals in this situation would want the recommended course of action and only a small proportion would not. Formal decision aids are not likely to be needed to help individuals make decisions consistent with their values and preferences	The majority of individuals in this situation would want the suggested course of action, but many would not
For clinicians	Most individuals should receive the intervention. Adherence to this recommendation according to the guideline could be used as a quality criterion or performance indicator	Recognize that different choices will be appropriate for different patients, and that you must help each patient arrive at a management decision consistent with her or his or her values and preferences. Decision aids can help indviduals to make decisions consistent with their values and preferences
For policy makers	The recommendation can be adapted as policy in most situations	Policy making will require substantial debate and involvement of many stakeholders

that benefits far outweigh downsides, or downsides far outweigh benefits, almost all patients will make the same choice and guideline developers can offer a strong recommendation.

Another important factor that affects the strength of a recommendation is the importance of a given outcome. For example, recommendations involving outcomes of high patient importance, i.e. outcomes to which patients assign greater values and preferences, will usually lead to stronger recommendations than those involving outcomes of lesser importance to the patient. For example, prophylactic antibiotics have been shown to be effective in preventing recurrent urinary tract infections (UTIs) in nonpregnant women. In fact, the number needed to treat (NNT), i.e. the number of women with recurrent UTIs who need to be exposed to prolonged antibiotics for one patient to gain a small but important reduction in the number of UTI recurrences, is only two patients [11]. In contrast, one might need to treat 100 patients with a history of myocardial infarction (MI) with agents such as aspirin (ASA), beta-blockers, angiotensin-converting enzyme (ACE) inhibitors or statins to extend one patient's life. Despite the much lower NNT to prevent one recurrent UTI, compared to preventing one MI, many women in that situation might choose to forego antibiotic prophylaxis, but take the agents that might prevent a future MI. This discrepancy may be explained by the differential value that patients assign to different outcomes. In consequence, the use of ASA would warrant a stronger recommendation.

Individualization of clinical decision making in the context of weak recommendations remains a challenge. Although clinicians always should consider patients' preferences and values, when they face weak recommendations they should consider more detailed conversations

with patients than for strong recommendations to ensure that the ultimate decision is consistent with the patient's values. For patients who are interested, a decision aid that presents patients with both benefits and downsides of therapy is likely to improve knowledge, decrease decision-making conflict, and may support a decision most consistent with patients' values and preferences [12,13]. Because of time constraints and because decision aids are not universally available, clinicians cannot use decision aids with all patients, and for strong recommendations, the use of decision aids is inefficient.

Other ways of interpreting strong and weak recommendations relate to performance or quality indicators. Strong recommendations are candidate performance indicators. For example, proposed quality indicators for prostate cancer such as those directed against the overuse of bone scans for the staging of low-risk patients or the use of adjuvant hormonal therapy in patients with high-risk disease undergoing external beam radiation are based on strong recommendations from existing guidelines [14]. For weak recommendations, performance could be measured by monitoring whether clinicians have discussed recommended actions with patients or their surrogates or carefully documented the evaluation of benefits and downsides in the patient's chart.

How methodological quality of the evidence contributes to strength of recommendation

In the GRADE system, evidence of the highest quality comes from one or more well-designed and well-executed

RCTs yielding consistent and directly applicable results. High-quality evidence can also come from well-performed observational studies yielding very large effects (defined as a relative risk reduction of at least 80%).

Randomized controlled trials with important methodological limitations and well-performed observational studies yielding large effects constitute the moderate quality category. Well-performed observational studies yielding modest effects and RCTs with very serious limitations will be rated as low-quality evidence. In the following paragraphs we describe the system of grading the methodological quality of evidence in more detail.

Factors that decrease the quality of evidence

Box 4.1 shows the limitations that may decrease the quality of evidence supporting a recommendation.

Limitation of methodology

Our confidence in recommendations decreases if studies suffer from major limitations that are likely to result in a biased assessment of the treatment effect. These methodological limitations include lack of blinding when subjective outcomes highly susceptible to bias are measured, failure to adhere to an intention-to-treat principle in the analysis of results, a large loss to follow-up or stopping the study early because of observed benefit.

For example, a systematic review has compared the efficacy of long-term antibiotic use versus placebo/no treatment to prevent recurrent UTIs in children [15]. Based on three RCTs, antibiotics compared to placebo/no treatment reduced the risk of recurrent UTI (relative risk (RR) 0.36, 95% confidence interval (CI) 0.16–0.77; risk difference (RD) –46%, 95% CI –59% to –33%). However, the method of allocation concealment in the three trials was inadequate, unclear and adequate, respectively. Allocation concealment protects randomization by preventing any individual involved in enrolling participants knowing or predicting the allocation sequence in advance, which might alter their behavior. In this example, lack of allocation concealment

raises the question as to whether the true treatment effect was overestimated. Therefore, guideline developers would formulate a weaker recommendation than they may have otherwise if allocation concealment in these trials was found to be adequate.

Inconsistent results (unexplained heterogeneity of results)

If studies yield widely differing estimates of the treatment effect (heterogeneity or variability in results) investigators should look for explanations for that heterogeneity. For example, interventions may have larger relative effects in sicker populations or when given in larger doses. When heterogeneity exists but investigators fail to identify a plausible explanation, the quality of evidence decreases. For example, a meta-analysis of 26 studies in children investigating the utility of a urine dipstick test to rule out the presence of infection showed major heterogeneity of diagnostic accuracy across studies, which could not be fully explained by differences in age or by differences in the definition of the criterion standard [16,17]. Many elements and differences in the process of urine collection and analysis, and in the selection of patients, may influence the presence of micro-organisms which can be detected by the dipstick, as well as the presence of substances that may give false results. The methodological quality of the studies might also be an important determinant of the reported accuracy and cause heterogeneity of the results. However, at present the lack of an adequate explanation for the heterogeneity of the dipstick accuracy remains an ongoing debate. This unexplained heterogeneity could lead guideline panelists to make a weaker recommendation.

Indirectness of evidence

In this situation, the question being addressed in the recommendation is quite different from the available evidence with regard to the population, intervention, comparison or outcome. Investigators may have undertaken studies in similar but not identical populations to those under consideration for a recommendation. For example, a RCT has demonstrated that local treatment in the form of radical prostatectomy is effective in reducing the risk of prostate cancer-specific death in patients with localized prostate cancer (PCA) when compared to watchful waiting [18,19]. After a median of 8 years, death rates from PCA were 8.6% versus 14%, which presents a relative risk reduction (RRR) of 40% (95% CI 8.2–61%) and a NNT of 18 (95% CI 10–101). The study was designed nearly 20 years ago, and in the meantime, prostate-specific antigen (PSA) screening and stage migration have changed the clinical picture of early prostate cancer. Also, watchful waiting has been replaced by active surveillance [20]. It is therefore unclear to what extent the results of this trial are applicable to today's patient population. This may raise concerns

---

BOX 4.1 Factors that may decrease the quality of evidence

- Limitations in the design and implementation suggesting high likelihood of bias
- Inconsistency of results (including problems with subgroup analyses)
- Indirectness of evidence (indirect population, intervention, control, outcomes)
- Imprecision of results (wide confidence intervals)
- High probability of publication bias

about indirectness of evidence to a guideline panel, which may lead to a downgrading of the level of evidence.

Imprecision

Imprecision exists if studies include few patients and few events and thus have wide confidence intervals, because of resulting uncertainty in the outcomes. For instance, one small trial investigated men who had undergone radical prostatectomy catheterized with antibiotic-impregnated catheter versus standard catheters and found a lower rate of asymptomatic bacteriuria in the antibiotic group at less than 1 week of catheterization (RR 0.36, 95% CI 0.18–0.73). One of 56 men in the antibiotic-impregnated group had a symptomatic UTI compared with six of 68 who had standard catheters (RR 0.20, 95% CI 0.03–1.63) [21]. While the results indicate a potentially large benefit, the results are not statistically significant and are still compatible with an increase in risk when using impregnated catheters.

Publication bias

The quality of evidence can be reduced if investigators fail to report outcomes (typically those that may be harmful or for which no effect was observed) or studies (typically those that show no effect) or if other reasons lead to results being withheld. Unfortunately, it is often necessary to make guesses about the likelihood of reporting bias. A prototypical situation that should elicit suspicion of reporting bias is when published evidence includes a number of small trials, all of which are industry funded [22]. For example, 14 trials of flavanoids in patients with hemorrhoids have shown apparent large benefits, but enrolled a total of only 1432 patients [23]. The heavy involvement of sponsors in most of these trials raises questions of whether unpublished trials suggesting no benefit exist. A particular body of evidence can suffer from more than one of these limitations, and the greater the limitations, the lower the quality of the evidence. One could imagine a situation in which several RCTs were available but all or virtually all of these limitations would be present, and in serious form, a very low quality of evidence would then result.

Factors that increase the quality of evidence

One of the strengths of the GRADE system is its recognition that observational studies can, in select cases, provide moderate or strong evidence [24]. While well-performed observational studies usually yield low-quality evidence, there may be particular circumstances in which the developers of guidance documents may classify such evidence as moderate or even high quality (Box 4.2).

Magnitude of the effect size

On rare occasions when methodologically strong observational studies yield large or very large and consistent

> **BOX 4.2** Factors that may increase the quality of evidence
>
> - Large magnitude of effect (direct evidence, RR >2 or RR <0.5 with no plausible confounders; very large with RR >5 or RR <0.2 and no threats to validity
> - All plausible confounding would reduce a demonstrated effect
> - Dose–response gradient

estimates of the magnitude of a treatment effect, we may be confident about the results. While the observational studies are likely to overestimate the true effect, a weak study design is unlikely to explain the entire benefit if the treatment effect is very large. Thus, despite reservations based on the observational study design, we are confident that the effect exists. Box 4.2 shows how the magnitude of the effect in these studies may move the assigned quality of evidence from low to moderate, or even to high quality. For example, the effectiveness of androgen ablation (e.g. orchidectomy or ketoconazole administration) in hormone-naive prostate cancer patients with impending spinal cord compression due to metastatic disease has never been evaluated in a RCT. However, treatment results in a large reduction in neurological symptoms and pain in the vast majority of patients [25]. In this setting, conducting a RCT may be considered unethical, and existing observational studies provide strong enough evidence to support a strong recommendation.

Direction of bias

On occasion, all plausible biases from observational studies may be working to underestimate an apparent treatment effect. For example, if only sicker patients receive an experimental intervention or exposure, yet they still fare better, it is likely that the actual intervention or exposure effect is larger than the data suggest. This will be a rare circumstance and only a few good examples exist. A rigorous systematic review of observational studies including a total of 38 million patients compared private for-profit versus private not-for-profit hospital care. The meta-analysis demonstrated higher death rates in the private for-profit hospitals [26]. The investigators postulated two likely sources of bias. The first was residual confounding with disease severity. It is likely that, if anything, patients in the not-for-profit hospitals were sicker than those in the for-profit hospitals. Thus, to the extent that residual confounding existed, it would bias results against the not-for-profit hospitals. The second likely bias was the possibility that higher numbers of patients with excellent private insurance coverage could lead to a hospital having more resources and a "spill-over" effect that would benefit those without such coverage. Since for-profit hospitals are likely to admit a larger proportion of such well-insured patients than not-for-profit hospitals, the bias is once again against the not-for-profit hospitals. Because the plausible biases would all diminish the demonstrated treatment effect, one might consider the evidence from these observational studies as moderate rather than low quality.

Dose–response gradient

The presence of a dose–response gradient may also increase our confidence in the findings of observational studies and thereby enhance the assigned quality of evidence. For example, our confidence in the results of observational studies that show an increased risk of bleeding in patients who have supratherapeutic anticoagulation levels is increased by the observation that there is a dose–response gradient between higher levels of the international normalized ratio (INR) and the increased risk of bleeding [24].

What to do when strength of evidence differs across outcomes?

In this book, authors provide a single rating of quality of evidence for every recommendation. Recommendations, however, depend on evidence regarding a variety of outcomes and it is possible that evidence quality may differ across those outcomes. For example, when RCT results are available, strength of evidence will often differ between efficacy and toxicity outcomes, usually between efficacy outcomes and cost, and almost always between efficacy outcomes and rare but serious adverse effects. The GRADE approach suggests explicit judgments about the importance of all outcomes by a guideline panel, including those that are considered harmful adverse events. This judgment requires assigning levels of importance to the outcomes. The GRADE approach asks the developers of guidance documents to decide whether outcomes are critical, important or not important for a recommendation. For example, a meta-analysis has compared tacrolimus to ciclosporin as primary immunosuppression in renal transplant patients [27]. At 1 year, tacrolimus patients suffered less acute rejection (RR 0.69, 95% CI 0.60–0.79) and less steroid-resistant rejection (RR 0.49, 95% CI 0.37–0.64), but more insulin-requiring diabetes mellitus (RR 1.86, 95% CI 1.11–3.09), as well as other side effects. In this scenario, the quality of evidence and strength of recommendation about the use of tacrolimus will depend on whether new-onset diabetes mellitus is judged as a critical adverse event or not.

Only critical outcomes influence the overall judgment about the quality of evidence and strength of a recommendation. Important outcomes can influence the strength (weak or strong) of a recommendation. For example, if harmful events are critical to decision making, guideline developers should rate the overall quality of evidence based on the lowest quality evidence of any critical outcome, including that of harm. For example, there is evidence from a systematic review and meta-analysis that estrogens are more effective in treating urinary incontinence in women when compared to placebo [28]. Subjective impression of cure was higher amongst those treated with estrogen for all categories of incontinence (36/101, 36% versus 20/96, 21%; RR for cure 1.61, 95% CI 1.04–2.49). However, there was little evidence from the trials after estrogen treatment had finished and none about long-term effects.

Consideration of potential risk of endometrial and breast cancer after long-term use will impact on the strength of recommendation that guideline developers make, especially in women with an intact uterus. If one ignores toxicity, one might rate the quality of evidence as high. If, however, one considers the potential long-term risk of malignancy as crucial, the uncertainty about impact of treatment increases. If editors look for observational studies to estimate steroid toxicity, the quality of the evidence about toxicity is likely to be low and this may be the most appropriate rating for the overall quality of evidence. Alternatively, they may seek randomized trials of steroids in other conditions, and face limitations of directness. They may then conclude that the evidence regarding long-term toxicity, and the overall quality of the evidence, is moderate. On the other hand, if most outcomes are of higher quality than a few others, but across all outcomes there is an indication either that the benefits outweigh the risks and burdens, or vice versa, authors may decide to base the overall quality of evidence on those of the critical outcomes of higher quality and consider the other outcomes important but not critical. Thus, guideline panels should consider whether toxicity endpoints are critical to the decision regarding the optimal management strategy. If they are, they should consider the strength of evidence regarding those endpoints, and make a final rating about strength of evidence accordingly. Outcomes that are neither critical nor important do not influence the overall quality of evidence or the strength of a recommendation.

Interpreting recommendations

Practicing urologists, third-party payers, institutional review committees, and the courts should not construe recommendations in this book as absolute. Generally, anything other than a 1A recommendation indicates that the chapter authors acknowledge that other interpretations of the evidence, and other clinical policies, may be reasonable and appropriate. Even Grade 1A recommendations will not apply to all patients in all circumstances and following Grade 1A recommendations will at times not serve the best interests of patients with atypical values or preferences, or whose risks differ markedly from the usual patient.

Conclusion

The strength of any recommendation for practice depends on two factors: the trade-off between desirable factors and undesirable factors (risks, burdens and cost) and our confidence in estimates of those effects. The GRADE framework, with the minor modifications adopted by the authors of this book, classifies the trade-off between desirable and undesirable effects in two categories:

1 in which the trade-off is clear enough that most patients, despite differences in values, would make the same choice; and

2 in which the trade-off is less clear, and individual patient values will likely lead to different choices.

Three categories of methodological strength exist:

A, high-quality evidence, usually from RCTs

B, randomized trials with important limitations or observational studies with large effects; and

C, usually from observational studies.

The framework summarized in Table 4.1 therefore generates recommendations from the very strong (1A: desirable and undesirable effects clear, methods high quality) to the very weak (2C: desirable and undesirable effects questionable, methods are of low quality). Clinicians must use their judgment when using the recommendations, considering both local and individual patient circumstances and patient values, to help patients make individual decisions. In general, however, urologists should place progressively greater weight on expert recommendations as they move from 2C to 1A.

References

1. Scales CD Jr, Preminger GM, Keitz SA, Dahm P. Evidence based clinical practice: a primer for urologists. J Urol 2007;178(3 pt 1): 775-82.

2. Guyatt GH, Oxman AD, Vist GE, et al. GRADE: an emerging consensus on rating quality of evidence and strength of recommendations. BMJ 2008:336:924-6.

3. Guyatt GH, Oxman AD, Kunz R, et al. What is "quality of evidence" and why is it important to clinicians? BMJ 2008:336:995-8.

4. Guyatt GH, Oxman AD, Kunz R, et al. Going from evidence to recommendations. BMJ 2008: 336:1049-51.

5. Guyatt G, Vist G, Falck-Ytter Y, Kunz R, Magrini N, Schunemann H. An emerging consensus on grading recommendations? ACP J Club 2006:144:A8-9.

6. Dahm P, Guyatt G, Wiechmann BC, Schunemann H. Developing a common approach for clinical practice guidelines and recommendations in urology. American Urological Association Annual Meeting 2008, Orlando, FL.

7. Krupski TL, Dahm P, Fesperman SF, Schardt CM. How to perform a literature search. J Urol 2008:179:1264-70.

8. Tseng TY, Dahm P, Poolman RW, Preminger GM, Canales BJ, Montori VM. How to use a systematic literature review and meta-analysis. J Urol 2008:180:1249-56.

9. Murray E, Davis H, Tai SS, Coulter A, Gray A, Haines A. Randomised controlled trial of an interactive multimedia decision aid on benign prostatic hypertrophy in primary care. BMJ 2001:323:493-6.

10. Guyatt GH, Oxman AD, Kunz R, et al. Incorporating considerations of resources use into grading recommendations. BMJ 2008:336:1170-3.

11. Albert X, Huertas I, Pereiro, II, Sanfelix J, Gosalbes V, Perrota C. Antibiotics for preventing recurrent urinary tract infection in non-pregnant women. Cochrane Database Syst Rev 2004;3: CD001209.

12. O'Connor AM, Stacey D, Entwistle V, et al. Decision aids for people facing health treatment or screening decisions. Cochrane Database Syst Rev 2003;2:CD001431.

13. Canfield SE, Dahm P, Evidence Based Urology Working Group. Evidence-based urology in practice: incorporating patient values in evidence-based clinical decision making. BJU Int 2009: Oct 10 (Epub ahead of print).

14. Miller DC, Saigal CS. Quality of care indicators for prostate cancer: progress toward consensus. Urol Oncol 2009:27:427-34.

15. Williams GJ, Lee A, Craig JC. Long-term antibiotics for preventing recurrent urinary tract infection in children. Cochrane Database Syst Rev 2001;4:CD001534.

16. Gorelick MH, Shaw KN. Screening tests for urinary tract infection in children: a meta-analysis. Pediatrics 1999:104:e54.

17. Deville WL, Yzermans JC, van Duijn NP, Bezemer PD, van der Windt DA, Bouter LM. The urine dipstick test useful to rule out infections. A meta-analysis of the accuracy. BMC Urol 2004: 4:4.

18. Bill-Axelson A, Holmberg L, Ruutu M, et al. Radical prostatectomy versus watchful waiting in early prostate cancer. N Engl J Med 2005:352:1977-84.

19. Bill-Axelson A, Holmberg L, Filen F, et al. Radical prostatectomy versus watchful waiting in localized prostate cancer: the Scandinavian Prostate Cancer Group-4 randomized trial. J Natl Cancer Inst 2008;100(16):1144-54.

20. Munro AJ. Radical prostatectomy reduced death and progression more than watchful waiting in early prostate cancer. ACP J Club 2005:143:57.

21. Brosnahan J, Jull A, Tracy C. Types of urethral catheters for management of short-term voiding problems in hospitalised adults. Cochrane Database Syst Rev 2004;1:CD004013.

22. Bhandari M, Busse JW, Jackowski D, et al. Association between industry funding and statistically significant pro-industry findings in medical and surgical randomized trials. CMAJ 2004:170:477-80.

23. Alonso-Coello P, Zhou Q, Martinez-Zapata MJ, et al. Meta-analysis of flavonoids for the treatment of haemorrhoids. Br J Surg 2006:93:909-20.

24. Levine MN, Raskob G, Beyth RJ, Kearon C, Schulman S. Hemorrhagic complications of anticoagulant treatment: the Seventh ACCP Conference on Antithrombotic and Thrombolytic Therapy. Chest 2004:126:287S-310S.

25. Flynn DF, Shipley WU. Management of spinal cord compression secondary to metastatic prostatic carcinoma. Urol Clin North Am 1991:18:145-52.

26. Devereaux PJ, Choi PT, Lacchetti C, et al. A systematic review and meta-analysis of studies comparing mortality rates of private for-profit and private not-for-profit hospitals. CMAJ 2002:166:1399-406.

27. Webster A, Woodroffe RC, Taylor RS, Chapman JR, Craig JC. Tacrolimus versus cyclosporin as primary immunosuppression for kidney transplant recipients. Cochrane Database Syst Rev 2005;4:CD003961.

28. Moehrer B, Hextall A, Jackson S. Oestrogens for urinary incontinence in women. Cochrane Database Syst Rev 2003;2: CD001405.

5 Evidence-based guidelines in urology

Susan L. Norris

Department of Medical Informatics and Clinical Epidemoiology, Oregon Health and Science University, Portland, OR, USA

Introduction

"Decisions about the care of individual patients should be based on the conscientious, explicit, and judicious use of the current best evidence on the effectiveness of clinical services," according to the Institute of Medicine (IOM) 2008 report entitled *Knowing What Works in Healthcare* [1]. Clinical practice guidelines are systematically developed statements to assist practitioner and patient decisions about appropriate healthcare for specific clinical circumstances [2] and are based on an unbiased synthesis of the best available evidence.

Clinical practice guidelines are an important tool for achieving optimal patient care. Since the emergence of the concept of evidence-based medicine [3], healthcare providers have sought ways to synthesize evidence into formats and products that are both valid and readily implemented into routine practice. Rigorously developed, high-quality (i.e. trusted) practice guidelines have the potential to promote the use of effective clinical services, decrease undesirable practice variation, reduce the use of services that are of minimal or questionable value, increase the use of effective but underused services, and target services to populations most likely to benefit [1]. Guidelines do not supplant the clinical judgment of physicians, rather they provide guidance based on the best available evidence.

Clinical practice guidelines have been used by healthcare providers for decades; perhaps some of the earliest were published by the American Academy of Pediatrics [4]. The Canadian Task Force on the Periodic Health Examination was established in 1976, followed by the US Preventive Services Task Force in 1984, both with the goal of generating evidence-based recommendations on preventive

services. Since these early works, the generation of practice guidelines has become epidemic: there are 2452 guidelines contained in the National Guideline Clearinghouse (NGCH) (www.guideline.gov/) (as of September 2009), a comprehensive database of international, evidence-based clinical practice guidelines and related documents in the public domain.

Evidence demonstrating improvement in clinical outcomes attributed to the use of practice guidelines is sparse. This situation may be due in part to difficulty achieving high-quality randomized studies examining this question as confounders, co-interventions and temporal changes in care all exist in practice settings, and blinding of providers and patients and follow-up intervals sufficient to demonstrate changes in long-term health outcomes are all difficult to achieve. Existing studies largely focus on process measures in observational studies [5-10].

Quality of clinical practice guidelines

Clinical practice guidelines can influence a large number of healthcare providers and patients [8] so their quality is critically important. The quality of practice guidelines refers to the confidence that the potential biases of guidelines development have been addressed adequately, recommendations are both internally and externally valid, and the guidelines are feasible for practice [11]. High-quality guidelines are valid (unbiased), reproducible, clinically applicable to the populations of interest, flexible, clearly presented, developed through a multidisciplinary process, reviewed on a regular schedule, and well documented [1].

The quality of practice guidelines depends on the quality and rigor of each of the steps performed in formulating the guidelines: crafting of the key clinical questions to be addressed in the guidelines, identification of studies for inclusion, assessment of the quality of individual studies, synthesis of the body of evidence and assessment of its quality, and the formulation of recommendations or practice guidelines. The process of generating and assessing high-quality systematic reviews is addressed in Chapter 3 and discussion of the linkage between the body of evidence and recommendations is presented in Chapter 4.

There are a number of published instruments available to assess the quality of practice guidelines. One of the most widely used instruments is the Appraisal of Guidelines Research and Evaluation (AGREE) Instrument [11] which provides a framework for assessing the quality of clinical practice guidelines, taking into account the benefits, harms, and costs of the guideline recommendations, as well as issues of the feasibility of implementation. This instrument is largely based on theoretical assumptions as empirical data are lacking [11]. It was, however, developed by a multinational group, is widely used by organizations that use the products of other guideline groups (including the World Health Organization), and has been validated [12,13]. The AGREE Instrument encompasses six domains: scope and purpose, stakeholder involvement, rigor of development, clarity and presentation, applicability, and editorial independence, and includes 23 questions in total. An overall assessment is then made as to whether the appraiser would recommend these guidelines for use in practice.

Although AGREE is a very useful instrument for assessing practice guideline quality, it may not encompass all aspects of quality that are relevant to guideline developers. Nuckols and colleagues [14] found that even guidelines that were rigorously developed, as measured with the AGREE Instrument, frequently omitted common clinical situations and contained content rated by experts to be of "uncertain validity." Another guideline team also noted that high-scoring guidelines with the AGREE instrument may still be problematic with respect to applicability of the available studies to general populations of interest [15].

The quality of clinical practice guidelines has not been extensively studied, but the available literature suggests that guidelines are frequently suboptimal because of flaws in their development, inadequacies in the evidence underlying the guidelines or both [15-20].

Development of clinical practice guidelines

Clinical practice guidelines and the recommendations contained therein are distinct from, but should usually be based on, systematic reviews of the clinical questions addressed in the guidelines. High-quality systematic revi-ews provide an exhaustive, unbiased synthesis of the available evidence (see Chapter 3). Guidelines present recommendations about which approaches should or should not be taken in specific clinical circumstances based on the evidence identified in the systematic review. There are thus two separate junctures where guideline developers must provide a transparent, reliable, and valid assessment: quality or grade of the body of evidence identified in the systematic review process which reflects the level of confidence that if a recommendation is followed, the anticipated outcome will occur; and second, assessment of the strength of recommendations, which takes into account the balance of benefits and harms and the importance of adhering to the recommendations [21].

The criteria for an optimal system for assessing the quality of a body of evidence and linking that evidence to practice guidelines or recommendations include [21]:
• the separation of grades of recommendation from the quality of the evidence
• simplicity and transparency
• a sufficient number of (but not too many) categories for quality of the body of evidence
• an explicit methodology
• levels of evidence that can vary across different outcomes.

In the past, the strength of evidence was combined with strength of recommendation in the formulation of recommendations in practice guidelines, and the strength of evidence was based only on a hierarchy of study design. The science has moved away from this overly simplistic model, as different types of study designs are optimal for different questions; hierarchies and definitions of levels of evidence vary across guideline groups; and this approach can lead to anomalous conclusions [22].

A large number of different approaches has been used to link a body of evidence to clinical practice recommendations; in fact, a 2002 review identified more than 50 systems for grading a body of evidence [23] and many more have been developed since. These include the Grading of Recommendations, Assessment, Development, and Evaluation (GRADE) approach [24], discussed in detail in Chapter 4. GRADE provides a framework for assessing the quality of a body of evidence (based on the underlying systematic reviews) and for the formulation of recommendations [24].

The process of generating evidence-based recommendations from a high-quality systematic review is a complex one, as even when there is consensus on the body of evidence, clinical experts formulating recommendations may disagree on the specific recommendations for clinical practice. Recommendations depend on an assessment of the balance of benefits and harms, which are often presented in different metrics that are difficult to compare. Value systems are important in weighing benefits and harms, and these vary across healthcare providers and patients, and physicians' perceptions may not be an accurate reflection of patient values and priorities. In addition, decision making by expert panel members may depend on their unique training and experiences, as well as on resource constraints and existing infrastructures in their local setting.

Clinical practice guidelines in urology

A number of urological, obstetric and gynecological, internal medicine, radiologic, pediatric, and governmental organizations have published practice guidelines on urological topics. These include topics related to diagnosis, prevention, screening or treatment. The NGCH provides a compendium of current guidelines which can be readily searched by topic, diagnosis, organization producing the guideline, and intended user of the guideline. Of a total of 2452 guidelines, 170 are categorized as specifically related to urology, with additional guidelines relevant to urologists found in obstetrics and gynecology, pediatric, and other categories. Organizations producing urology-related guidelines include the European Association of Urologists, the American Urological Association, National Institute for Health and Clinical Excellence, the Scottish Intercollegiate Guidelines Network, American College of Obstetricians and Gynecologists, and many other organizations.

The purpose of the NGCH is to give healthcare providers, health plans, and health care delivery systems access to objective, detailed information on practice guidelines in order to further their dissemination, implementation, and use [25]. Started in 1998, the NGCH is an initiative of the Agency for Healthcare Research and Quality (AHRQ), is readily searchable, and contains structured abstracts (summaries) of each guideline, links to the full text of the guideline, when available, and the means to readily compare and contrast guidelines on related topics.

A clinical practice guideline must meet all the following criteria to be included in the NGCH [26].
• The guideline contains systematically developed statements that include recommendations, strategies or other information that assists healthcare practitioners and patients in specific clinical circumstances.
• The guideline was produced under the auspices of a relevant professional organization or association or by a public or private organization.
• Collaborating documentation can be produced and verified that a systematic literature search and review of existing scientific evidence published in peer-reviewed journals was performed during guideline development.
• The guideline is in English.
• The guideline is current (less than 5 years since development or revisions).

Several critical evaluations of practice guidelines in urology have been published recently. Aus and colleagues [27] evaluated the methods used to produce the European Association of Urology (EAU) guidelines using the AGREE instrument. These authors concluded that the EAU guidelines scored "acceptably well" but noted several weaknesses: lack of broad stakeholder involvement (including patients); no discussion of potential organizational barriers or cost implications; the guidelines were "evidence-based medicine light" with the retrieval of only recent randomized controlled trials and meta-analyses; and no external peer review.

In a similar, contemporaneous work, Dahm and colleagues [28] examined guidelines in the NGCH produced by a number of organizations for the management of localized prostate cancer. These authors noted disparate recommendations across guidelines which they attributed to different methodologies for guideline development. They also noted a paucity of high-level evidence upon which to develop evidence-based practice guidelines.

Issues in practice guideline development and use

There are a number of important potential issues relevant to practice guideline development and use by clinicians, which the urologist should keep in mind as she or he evaluates and implements practice guidelines. Three of these issues will be discussed briefly: sources of potential bias in guidelines generation, including conflict of interest by guideline developers; the generation of practice guidelines when evidence is lacking or is of poor quality; and the applicability of practice guidelines to specific clinical scenarios.

Sources of bias in clinical practice guidelines

There are a multitude of potential sources of bias in the formulation of clinical practice guidelines, which may be introduced at the level of the primary studies, the systematic reviews of the primary studies or the translation of the body of evidence (i.e. the systematic review) into practice guidelines. Bias almost always results in an overestimation of benefit and an underestimation of harm [29] and therefore biased practice guidelines can have profound implications for healthcare and ultimately patient outcomes.

The assessment of the potential for bias at the individual study level is achieved using validated tools such as the Risk of Bias instrument for randomized controlled trials used by the Cochrane Collaboration [30] and instruments recommended by the UK Health Technology Assessment programme in a 2003 review [31]. The assessment of bias and quality in systematic reviews is discussed in Chapter 3.

The formulation of recommendations and practice guidelines from systematic reviews can also be subject to bias.

Using formalized systems for translating evidence into guidelines (as discussed in Chapter 4) will help to minimize bias at this stage of guideline development. Even with the use of standardized, explicit, and transparent approaches, however, guideline development can be subject to bias because of the specialty composition of the guideline development panel. Specialists and generalist physicians, other healthcare providers, consumers of healthcare, payers, and policy makers all have different experiences and motivations which can have bearings on practice guideline content. As a result, the Institute of Medicine recommends that guideline panels have multispecialty, patient, and methodologic representation [1].

Conflict of interest is an important potential source of bias in the development of practice guidelines. Much attention has focused recently on the frequency and types of conflict of interest and its impact on basic biomedical and clinical research can be profound. This was highlighted by the tragic death in 1999 of a participant in an industry-sponsored trial where investigators and the academic institutions held significant financial stakes [32]. Conflict of interest is a critical issue in the development of practice guidelines, as guidelines are designed to be widely used, to impact healthcare provider practice, to have economic implications, and to ultimately improve patient outcomes.

A conflict of interest is a set of conditions in which professional judgment concerning a primary interest (such as the health and well-being of a patient or the validity of research) is unduly influenced by a secondary interest [33]. The secondary interests may be financial or nonfinancial. The influence of secondary interests can occur at many different steps in the process of clinical research: conception of the study question [34], design and conduct of the study, selection of outcomes for reporting in publications, formulation of study conclusions, and decisions on whether to publish a study or not [35].

Industry funding has been associated with outcomes favorable to the sponsor. In a systematic review, Bekelman and colleagues [36] examined the extent, impact, and management of financial conflict of interest in biomedical research. These authors noted a positive relationship between financial ties and pro-industry conclusions in all 11 studies that examined this association. Numerous other studies have also found positive associations between the industry affiliations of study authors and outcomes or conclusions favorable to the sponsor [37-39].

Although financial interests are often the most obvious, nonfinancial interests are increasingly recognized and can be powerful motivators for researchers, systematic reviewers, and guideline authors. Nonfinancial interests include the advancement of medical science, as well as benefits from publication and the acquisition of research funding. These interests are appropriate in themselves, but may conflict with the interests of research subjects and patients [40].

In addition to study-level influences, conflict of interest can occur with the production of systematic reviews and clinical practice guidelines. A number of examples of the potential effects of conflict of interest on clinical practice guideline development have come to light over the last 15 years [41-43]. Perhaps the most dramatic example occurred in 1995 when the House of Representatives voted to effectively stop funding the Agency for Health Care Policy and Research (AHCPR, now the Agency for Healthcare Research and Quality) because orthopedic surgeons lobbied House members, objecting to the largely conservative management strategies put forth in the AHCPR's guidelines on the treatment of acute back pain [44]. More recently, the Connecticut Attorney General challenged the Infectious Diseases Society of America's 2006 guidelines on Lyme disease [45]. The Attorney General's investigation revealed that important conflicts of interest were not disclosed by guideline panel members, and that there were multiple flaws in their guideline process. A new guideline panel and review were mandated.

There is a paucity of literature on the effects of conflicts of interest on systematic reviews and clinical practice guideline development. *Nature* published results of a survey conducted on guidelines in the NGCH in 2004 [46]. Of more than 200 guidelines, only 90 contained information on individual authors' conflicts of interest, and of those, only 31 were free of industry influence. Of the 685 total disclosures, 65% claimed no conflict of interest and 35% reported some kind of conflict. More than one-third of guideline panels included at least one member who gave seminars on behalf of a relevant drug company. The author of this commentary expressed concern that guideline authors may under-report conflict of interest and reported that the Center for Science in the Public Interest examined the disclosure statements on randomly chosen blood pressure guidelines, and found that several authors did not report research funding that they had obtained [46].

Generation of practice guidelines when evidence is lacking or of poor quality

Frequently the evidence base is of poor quality or nonexistent, providing a major challenge for practice guideline developers. Guideline groups deal with this issue differently. On one hand, the US Preventive Services Task Force uses the assessment of "insufficient evidence" when the data are insufficient upon which to make an evidence-based decision on the balance of benefits and harms [47,48]. A number of recent Preventive Task Force statements are so rated, including the 2008 assessment of the evidence on screening men less than 75 years of age for prostate cancer [49].

On the other hand, guideline developers may feel compelled to generate guidelines when data are insufficient. The American College of Cardiology and the American Heart Association [18] recently examined the evidence base for their joint clinical practice guidelines and only 11% of recommendations were classified as being based on level A evidence (based on multiple randomized trials or meta-analyses), while 48% were based on level C evidence (based on expert opinion, case studies or standards of care). Only 19% of Class I recommendations (for which there is evidence and/or general agreement that a given procedure or treatment is useful and effective) were based on level A evidence. The authors note that because of this paucity of adequate evidence, "expert opinion remains a dominant driver of clinical practice" [18]. Expert opinion is unavoidable if guideline developers wish to present recommendations in the absence of high-quality evidence, but it should be clear which recommendations in a guideline are evidence based and which are not [1].

There are few data on the quality of the evidence base for practice guidelines in urology. As noted above, Dahm and colleagues identified few high-quality trials and observational studies supporting practice guidelines focused on localized prostate cancer [28]. Other authors have noted deficits in the quality and reporting of urologic studies, including both trials [50,51] and observational studies [52].

Lack of an adequate evidence base can occur for any clinical question, but several specific types of questions are particularly notorious for having a paucity of evidence. Data are frequently deficient on important subpopulations based on racial or ethnic characteristics or age subgroups such as older adults. Head-to-head trials (i.e. direct comparisons) may not be available, particularly with comparators which represent usual care or current standard treatments; often the only available data are placebo-controlled trials. Trials may focus on benefits and not harms, with high-quality, longer-term observational data unavailable. Studies may focus on intermediate or surrogate outcomes such as urinary peak flow, and not on outcomes important to patients such as symptoms and quality of life.

Randomized controlled trials examining the efficacy of an intervention have limitations as compared to effectiveness studies for applicability to broad populations and common clinical scenarios. Randomized trials, however, may not be available for many surgical interventions where randomization may be difficult to implement and techniques to minimize risk of bias, such as blinding of the patient and healthcare provider to specific interventions, may not be possible.

Applicability of practice guidelines to specific clinical scenarios

The applicability of a practice guideline to a specific population or patient is critical to the validity and usefulness of a recommendation or guideline. Applicability of a practice guideline is the extent to which the guideline will produce the outcomes achieved in the body of evidence in the relevant population or patient. The terms applicability, generalizability, and external validity are inter-related. Applicability, however, is a relative term and refers to a specific context (usually a patient and setting) in which the guideline is being used. It is the *applicability* of a recommendation or guideline to a specific patient in the clinical setting which is of most interest to the practicing physician. While some authors and systems for grading quality of studies and bodies of evidence include applicability in an assessment of quality (either of a study or of a body of evidence), recent recommendations suggest that quality and applicability be assessed separately, as the latter is a contextual issue, while quality is not [53].

Not unlike assessment of the quality of a body of evidence, there are a number of published scoring systems for assessing applicability [54-56]. There are no data, however, validating any scoring system, so it is not possible to recommend one applicability scoring system over others. The clinician is thus faced with the difficult decision as to if and how a practice guideline applies to a specific patient or population in the clinical setting. The factors that affect applicability differ across types of interventions (e.g. surgical procedures versus pharmacotherapy) and outcomes (e.g. benefits versus harms) [53].

An example of a study with potentially limited applicability is an efficacy trial of a new drug therapy, where the study population was highly selected (no co-morbidities, demonstrated adherence, and persons with adverse events related to treatment were excluded during a trial run-in period), the intervention optimally delivered, the comparator a placebo (rather than another active drug or standard treatment), and the outcome a physiologic measure (e.g. urinary peak flow) and not a health outcome (e.g. symptoms). If the body of evidence upon which the practice guideline was based is formulated almost entirely from such efficacy studies, the recommendations may have limited applicability to the average patient seen in the urologist's office.

It is only recently, as GRADE and other systems for assessing the quality of evidence have been developed, disseminated, and implemented, that practice guidelines have included statements on potential applicability to subpopulations and settings. In the absence of specific guidance in the practice guidelines, the clinician needs to assess on his or her own the applicability of the guidelines to each specific clinical scenario. Potential threats to applicability can be considered in terms of the PICOTS framework: Population, Intervention, Comparator, Outcome, Timing, and Setting [53]. For example, if there is evidence that a drug treatment effect may relate to race/ethnicity, does the practice guideline present specific recommendations on that subpopulation? How might the patient's nonadherence to a treatment regime affect outcomes? What is the patient's relative value system with respect to weighting benefits (improved urinary flow symptoms) against harms (adverse effects on sexual function)? Every clinical recommendation should take into account the clinical context, using the best available synthesis of the evidence, along with each individual patient's values and preferences.

Acknowledgments

The author currently receives funding from the American Urological Association and the American College of Chest Physicians for the preparation of clinical practice guidelines. The author has been a member of the GRADE Working Group since 2002 and has received support from the Agency for Healthcare Quality and Research to attend one GRADE meeting.

The author received no funding for the preparation of this manuscript.

References

1. Institute of Medicine. *Knowing What Works in Health Care: a roadmap for the nation.* Washington, DC: National Academies Press, 2008.
2. Institute of Medicine. *Clinical Practice Guidelines: directions for a new program.* Washington, DC: National Academies Press, 1990.
3. Evidence-Based Medicine Working Group. Evidence-based medicine. A new approach to teaching the practice of medicine. JAMA 1992;268(17):2420-5.
4. American Academy of Pediatrics. History of the Red Book, 2007. Available from: http://aapredbook.aappublications.org/about/.
5. Peterson E, Roe M, Mulgund J, et al. Association between hospital process performance and outcomes among patients with acute coronary syndromes. JAMA 2006;295(16):1912.
6. Peterson E, Shah B, Parsons L, et al. Trends in quality of care for patients with acute myocardial infarction in the National Registry of Myocardial Infarction from 1990 to 2006. Am Heart J 2008;156(6):1045.
7. Rogers W, Frederick P, Stoehr E, et al. Trends in presenting characteristics and hospital mortality among patients with ST elevation and non-ST elevation myocardial infarction in the National Registry of Myocardial Infarction from 1990 to 2006. Am Heart J 2008;156(6):1026.
8. Woolf SH, Grol R, Hutchinson A, Eccles M, Grimshaw J. Clinical guidelines: potential benefits, limitations, and harms of clinical guidelines. BMJ 1999;318(7182):527-30.
9. Davis DA, Taylor-Vaisey A. Translating guidelines into practice. A systematic review of theoretic concepts, practical experience and research evidence in the adoption of clinical practice guidelines. CMAJ 1997;157(4):408-16.
10. Grimshaw J, Eccles M, Thomas R, et al. Toward evidence-based quality improvement. Evidence (and its limitations) of the effectiveness of guideline dissemination and implementation strategies 1966–1998. J Gen Intern Med 2006;21(suppl 2): S14-20.
11. AGREE Collaboration. The Appraisal of Guidelines for Research & Evaluation (AGREE) Instrument. 2001. Available from: www.agreecollaboration.org.
12. Graham ID, Calder LA, Hebert PC, Carter AO, Tetroe JM. A comparison of clinical practice guideline appraisal instruments. Int J Technol Assess Health Care 2000;16(4):1024-38.
13. Sudlow M, Thomson R. Clinical guidelines: quantity without quality. Qual Health Care 1997;6(2):60-1.
14. Nuckols TK, Lim YW, Wynn BO, et al. Rigorous development does not ensure that guidelines are acceptable to a panel of knowledgeable providers. J Gen Intern Med 2008;23(1):37-44.
15. McAlister FA, van Diepen S, Padwal RS, et al. How evidence-based are the recommendations in evidence-based guidelines? PLoS Med 2007;4(8):e250.
16. Shaneyfelt TM, Mayo-Smith MF, Rothwangl J. Are guidelines following guidelines? The methodological quality of clinical practice guidelines in the peer-reviewed medical literature. JAMA;281(20):1900-5.
17. Burgers JS, Cluzeau FA, Hanna SE, et al. Characteristics of high-quality guidelines: evaluation of 86 clinical guidelines developed in ten European countries and Canada. Int J Technol Assess Health Care 2003;19(1):148-57.
18. Tricoci P, Allen JM, Kramer JM, et al. Scientific evidence underlying the ACC/AHA clinical practice guidelines. JAMA 2009;301(8):831-41.
19. Harpole LH, Kelley MJ, Schreiber G, et al. Assessment of the scope and quality of clinical practice guidelines in lung cancer. Chest 2003;123(1 suppl):7S-20S.
20. Fretheim A, Williams JW Jr, Oxman AD, et al. The relation between methods and recommendations in clinical practice guidelines for hypertension and hyperlipidemia. J Fam Pract 2002;51(11):963-8.
21. Guyatt G, Gutterman D, Baumann MH, et al. Grading strength of recommendations and quality of evidence in clinical guidelines: report from an American College of Chest Physicians Task Force. Chest 2006;129(1):174-81.
22. Glasziou P, Vandenbroucke JP, Chalmers I. Assessing the quality of research. BMJ 2004;328(7430):39-41.
23. West S, King V, Carey TS, et al. Systems to rate the strength of scientific evidence. Evid Rep Technol Assess 2002;47:1-11.
24. Guyatt GH, Oxman AD, Vist GE, et al. GRADE: an emerging consensus on rating quality of evidence and strength of recommendations. BMJ 2008;336(7650):924-6.
25. National Guideline Clearinghouse. Available from: www.guideline.gov/about/about.aspx.
26. Department of Health and Human Services, Agency for Health Care Policy and Research. Invitation to submit guidelines to the National Guideline Clearinghouse. Fed Regist 1998;63(70):18027.
27. Aus G, Chapple C, Hanus T, et al. The European Association of Urology (EAU) guidelines methodology: a critical evaluation. Eur Urol 2008 Jul 14 (Epub ahead of print).

28. Dahm P, Yeung L, Chang S, Cookson M. A critical review of clinical practice guidelines for the management of clinically localized prostate cancer. J Urol 2008;180:10.

29. Laupacis A. On bias and transparency in the development of influential recommendations. CMAJ 2006;174(3):335-6.

30. Higgins JP, Sally G (eds). Cochrane Handbook for Systematic Reviews of Interventions. Chichester: Wiley-Blackwell, 2008.

31. Deeks JD, d'Amico R, Sowden AJ, et al. Evaluating non-randomised intervention studies. Health Technol Assess 2003;7(27).

32. Weiss R, Nelson D. Teen dies undergoing experimental gene therapy. Washington Post 1999 Dec 8;Sect. A1, A10.

33. Thompson DF. Geography of U.S. biomedical publications, 1990 to 1997. N Engl J Med 1999;340(10):817-18.

34. Hill KP, Ross JS, Egilman DS, Krumholz HM. The ADVANTAGE seeding trial: a review of internal documents. Ann Intern Med 2008;149(4):251-8.

35. Boyd EA, Bero LA. Improving the use of research evidence in guideline development: 4. Managing conflicts of interests. Health Res Policy Syst 2006;4:16.

36. Bekelman JE, Li Y, Gross CP. Scope and impact of financial conflicts of interest in biomedical research: a systematic review. JAMA 2003;289(4):454-65.

37. Lexchin J, Bero LA, Djulbegovic B, Clark O. Pharmaceutical industry sponsorship and research outcome and quality: systematic review. BMJ 2003;326(7400):1167-70.

38. Stelfox HT, Chua G, O'Rourke K, Detsky AS. Conflict of interest in the debate over calcium-channel antagonists. N Engl J Med 1998;338(2):101-6.

39. Als-Nielsen B, Chen W, Gluud C, Kjaergard LL. Association of funding and conclusions in randomized drug trials: a reflection of treatment effect or adverse events? JAMA 2003;290(7):921-8.

40. Levinsky NG, Levinsky NG. Nonfinancial conflicts of interest in research. N Engl J Med 2002;347(10):759-61.

41. Coyne DW. Influence of industry on renal guideline development. Clin J Am Soc Nephrol 2007;2(1):3-7.

42. Eichacker PQ, Natanson C, Danner RL. Separating practice guidelines from pharmaceutical marketing. Crit Care Med 2007;35(12):2877-8

43. Strippoli GF, Tognoni G, Navaneethan SD, Nicolucci A, Craig JC. Haemoglobin targets: we were wrong, time to move on. Lancet 2007;369(9559):346-50.

44. Deyo RA, Psaty BM, Simon G, Wagner EH, Omenn GS. The messenger under attack – intimidation of researchers by special-interest groups. N Engl J Med 1997;336(16):1176-80.

45. Connecticut Attorney General's Office. Attorney General's investigation reveals flawed Lyme disease guideline process, IDSA agrees to reassess guidelines, install independent arbiter. Available from: www.ct.gov/AG/cwp/view.asp?a = 2795&q = 414284&pp = 12&n = 1.

46. Taylor R, Giles J. Cash interests taint drug advice. Nature 2005;437(7062):1070-1.

47. Barton M, Miller T, Wolff T, et al. How to read the new recommendation statement: methods update from the U.S. Preventive Services Task Force. Ann Intern Med 2007; 147(2):123-7.

48. Sawaya G, Guirguis-Blake J, LeFevre M, Harris R, Petitti D. Update on the methods of the U.S. Preventive Services Task Force: estimating certainty and magnitude of net benefit. Ann Intern Med 2007;147(12):871-5.

49. Lin K, Lipsitz R, Miller T, Janakiraman S. Benefits and harms of prostate-specific antigen screening for prostate cancer: an evidence update for the U.S. Preventive Services Task Force. Ann Intern Med 2008;149:9.

50. Scales CJ, Norris R, Keitz S, et al. A critical assessment of the quality of reporting of randomized, controlled trials in the urology literature. J Urol 2007;177(3):1090-4.

51. Scales CJ, Norris R, Peterson B, Preminger G, Dahm P. Clinical research and statistical methods in the urology literature. J Urol 2005;174(4 pt 1):1374-9.

52. Tseng T, Breau R, Fesperman S, Vieweg J, Dahm G. Evaluating the evidence: the methodological and reporting quality of comparative observational studies of surgical interventions in urological publication. BJU Int 2008;103:6.

53. Agency for healthcare Quality and Research. *Methods Reference Guide for Effectiveness and Comparative Effectiveness Reviews*, Version 1.0. Available from: http://effectivehealthcare.ahrq.gov/repFiles/2007_10DraftMethodsGuide.pdf.

54. Bornhoft G, Maxion-Bergemann S, Wolf U, et al. Checklist for the qualitative evaluation of clinical studies with particular focus on external validity and model validity. BMC Med Res Methodol 2006;6:56.

55. Glasgow RE, Green L, Klesges LM, et al. External validity: we need to do more. Ann Behav Med 2006;31(1):4.

56. Rothwell P. External validity of randomised controlled trials: to whom do the results of this trial apply? Lancet 2005;365(9453):12.

6 Understanding concepts related to health economics in urology

Yair Lotan

Department of Urology, University of Texas Southwestern Medical Center at Dallas, TX, USA

Introduction

With national healthcare expenditures reaching record levels, medical decision making is increasingly affected by economic concerns [1]. While urologists often view cost as a secondary or tertiary issue in the care of a patient, the impact of economics on the day-to-day practice of urology is increasing. Financial issues affect the availability of new technologies in the hospital and outpatient settings, development of medications by companies, willingness of patients to take medications based on cost and the personal income of urologists. The main issue in economics involves the choices made between different options based on the scarcity of resources. The current healthcare environment is one in which institutions and healthcare plans face limited budgets which need to be utilized in the most efficient manner. Thus, choices must be made regarding different treatments, taking into consideration both efficacy and cost. Such cost-utility or cost-effectiveness analyses will play a greater role as the costs of new treatments and drugs increase and the margin of benefit decreases. There will be a growing need to identify the best use of resources, especially in the presence of competing risks, benefits and costs.

In order for urologists to optimize their care of patients, there is a need to understand the economic factors that affect their ability to practice medicine. In this chapter we will review the concepts that form the foundation of health economics and try to apply them from a urologic perspective.

Evidence-Based Urology. Edited by Philipp Dahm, Roger R. Dmochowski.
© 2010 Blackwell Publishing.

Economic parameters

There are several issues that apply to all economic analyses. These include the perspective of the analysis, outcomes using cost versus charge, and discounting.

The importance of perspective

Cost analyses can be constructed in different ways based on the factors included in the analysis. In order to determine which costs to include in an analysis, one needs to determine the perspective of the payer. In the US healthcare system, there are three "payer" perspectives: society, the hospital, and the patient.

The perspective of the patient is the most difficult and subjective to evaluate as it depends on the patient's individual insurance, deductible level and employment status. In the US, many employers are the primary source of health insurance. A patient with insurance or financial independence may be more likely to seek medical care rather than delay care until it is urgent. The level of drug benefits and co-pay may affect a patient's willingness to initiate medical management and/or remain compliant with medications which are relatively expensive. Patients without insurance may delay their care and are less likely to purchase costly medications. In countries where medical care is freely available to all citizens, this issue may have less impact on patient decision making.

The hospital's perspective is usually the easiest to measure because most of the resources utilized can be itemized and accounted. The hospital costs include the resources required to perform a procedure and immediate postoperative care. Hospitals have costs which are individualized to the patient, including the cost of the resources used in surgery (equipment, supplies), medications, room and board, nursing, etc. There are also the general costs such as hospital administration and amortization of capital equipment. In evaluating the cost-effectiveness of surgical approaches, for example, the cost of capital equipment can play a significant role. A hospital usually does not receive additional payment for robotic prostatectomy but has to pay for the robot and its maintenance [2,3]. Similarly, the outlays for a shock-wave lithotripter and a ureteroscope are significantly different while treatment outcomes may be very similar.

An important consideration when evaluating costs from the hospital's perspective is that budgets within hospitals are often divided into different departments. Some areas may be financially profitable while other areas may lose money for certain procedures. Thus, the costs associated with obtaining new equipment or maintaining current equipment must be viewed in relation to the entire hospital rather than considering the impact on one budget, such as that of the operating room. Some procedures may be associated with decreased length of stay, but may also have higher operating room supply costs (e.g. laparoscopic procedures such as nephrectomy and retroperitoneal lymphadenectomy). Hospital administrations must therefore take a broader look at the financial implications of new technologies as they affect different cost centers in different ways.

The perspective of society involves both direct and indirect costs. As Medicare plays a large role in financing healthcare in the US, a significant percentage of direct costs affects the overall national healthcare budget. Costs borne by private insurance companies are also passed on to employers and participants through higher premiums. Society is also influenced by loss of work productivity that results during an illness and recovery. These indirect costs can be difficult to measure but can represent a significant loss of gross national revenue. Other indirect costs include those incurred by caregivers who lose productivity. Furthermore, there are quality of life issues and morbidities that can have significant costs for the rest of a patient's life. For example, a patient with incontinence and impotence after prostatectomy will incur life-long costs not immediately accounted for by his hospital and immediate postoperative care. Likewise, a patient who has renal insufficiency after nephrectomy may incur significant costs that are a direct outcome of kidney cancer but not accounted for by evaluating the cost of the nephrectomy from a hospital perspective.

Cost versus charge

Evaluating the literature regarding health economics can be confusing because of the interchangeable use of the terms *cost* and *charge*. The charge of a service, procedure or medication incorporates the cost of an item, indirect costs and profit margins. Discerning between analyses that use cost data as opposed to charge data is critical because there are significant differences in how these values are

derived and their accuracy in reflecting true resource utilization. Many published evaluations use charge figures provided by the hospital system because they are often easier to obtain [4]. The disadvantage of using charge data is that they do not reflect the true resource allocation as they account for profit margins. There are several confounding factors involving use of charge data. Different departments in a hospital use different cost-to-charge ratios such that the radiology department may charge twice as much as the cost for an x-ray but the pharmacy may charge four times as much for a medication. Another consideration is the fact that most hospitals do not get paid the actual amount that they charge due to Medicare set rates and insurance contracts. The reimbursement varies per hospital and geographic location such that comparing costs is a more uniform means of evaluating differences between treatment or management options.

Unfortunately, even the use of costs can bring variability. The true cost of a procedure depends on utilization. For example, if one pays $1 million for a robot and uses the procedure 10 times per year then that cost is distributed over those 10 patients. However, if one uses the robot 100 times per year then the cost is 10-fold lower per patient [2]. This is true for use of any capital equipment such as computed tomography, shock-wave lithotripters, laboratory equipment, etc. It is also true for hospital beds since the costs of nursing and building the hospital are fixed, so the increased utilization of the facilities of the hospital, such as the emergency room or beds, will affect the per-unit cost of patient care.

There are also problems with the accurate assessment of the cost of capital equipment. Items such as a robot, laparoscopic ultrasound, camera and televisions are usually paid for from operating room capital budgets and amortized over many years. Depreciation costs and usage per case can then only be estimated. Conversely, costs of disposable equipment and medications can be established with more accuracy but are still influenced by the vendor contract which varies based on the volume of purchase.

While cost analyses result in a more accurate estimation of resource utilization than analyses using charge data, it is important to understand where the data upon which the cost analyses were obtained. Furthermore, when comparing cost within an institution or country, there is need to understand that the conclusions may not be accurate in other economic settings or with other cost assumptions [5].

Discounting

In many analyses, there is a time component so that outcomes occur in the future. This applies to many cancer-related analyses in which the main outcome such as survival occurs at a different time point from the initial treatment. In order to compare future costs with current costs, the concept of discounting needs to be utilized [6]. Discounting is necessary when the experience of the patient in the near term is valued more than future costs and health outcomes [7,8]. It is necessary because people in general prefer benefits today rather than next year. For example, $1 today is worth more to an individual than the same $1 next year. Most cost analyses apply a yearly discounting rate around 3% to future costs and future years of life [8,9]. This is based on typical annual inflation rates of 0–5% in the US.

Most cost analyses in urology involve comparison of costs associated with procedures or techniques but discounting is very important for cost-effectiveness analyses evaluating screening or chemoprevention where the initial costs are high but benefits may take a long time to materialize [10,11].

Costs in economic evaluation

In cost analyses, it is important to determine how to obtain the costs used in the analysis. The costs are determined by the resources used and the value of the resources. They are typically recorded on a per-patient basis. While costs used to be categorized as direct and indirect, this has led to confusion regarding categorization of indirect costs [12]. Classification of costs as health service related and non-healthcare related is utilized for better categorization.

Health service costs

Health service costs include the direct costs of the treatment, general illness costs, trial costs and future costs. Direct costs include any inpatient and outpatient costs associated with an illness or treatment. These include any cost associated with treatment including room and board, any laboratory tests or imaging, medications use as well as use of capital equipment and overheads such as nursing.

General illness includes any related diseases that are diagnosed while being treated for the primary diagnosis. If someone diagnoses high blood pressure or skin cancer during prostate cancer screening then there are additional costs incurred that would not have been included if the patient had not undergone screening. If these diagnoses are related to the primary diagnosis then their costs should be included.

Trial costs are only relevant if a patient is involved in a clinical protocol and has additional tests or visits that are specific to the protocol. If tests performed are part of standard practice then they are not added specifically to the trial arm but if they are unique to a protocol then they need to be accounted for.

Future costs include those that are specifically related to treatment [13]. Future costs may include cost of future

treatment for diseases specifically related to the initial therapy or illnesses that are unrelated but occur because of added life-years which result from treatment. There is no consensus on the need to include all costs in every cost-effectiveness analysis but some rationale should be used for including or excluding certain costs. In some instances, it makes sense to include costs such as morbidities related to treatment. In an analysis of quality of life-years saved after prostatectomy or prostate cancer screening, it is logical to include the loss of quality of life in patients who suffer from incontinence or impotence [11]. On the other hand, if a screening policy saves a patient from dying of prostate cancer early, it is not clear whether the cost of having pneumonia or a heart attack in the latter part of his life should be included in determining the cost-effectiveness of screening.

Nonhealthcare costs

Nonhealth service costs are those not directly related to the treatment of a disease. This includes those costs incurred by social services provided to the patient and loss of productivity to society by either the patient or caregivers. There are also patient-related costs such as out-of-pocket expenses and travel [14].

Economic analyses

The purpose of economic analyses is to try to address a particular question. This is most useful when there is a discrepancy between economic aspects (i.e. cost) and effectiveness. Effectiveness is a critical issue in economic evaluations because of the fixed nature of resources. If there were unlimited resources then one would always choose the most effective treatment or approach to a problem. The crux of economic analyses is that there is a trade-off between a less costly approach and a less effective approach.

Effectiveness is typically measured in terms of direct outcomes, such as survival, or as utilities. Utilities may reflect preferences of patients or society. Values are assigned to various health states on a scale ranging from 0 (dead) to 1 (perfect health). A common utility is quality of life which can be measured using validated questionnaires. There are general health questionnaires such as the SF-36 which is composed of 36 items relating to eight dimensions of well-being: physical functioning, role limitation caused by physical health problems, bodily pain, general health perception, energy/fatigue, social functioning, role limitation caused by emotional problems, and emotional well-being [15]. These types of questionnaires are useful for evaluating chronic conditions such as nephrolithiasis

[16,17]. There are several validated questionnaires specific to urological practice. One of the most commonly used is the AUA Symptom Score Index [18]. In studies evaluating outcomes that are affected by quality of life measures such as quality-adjusted life-years (QALYs) saved, these types of validated questionnaires are critical. For example, in determining the cost-effectiveness of chemoprevention or screening QALYs, the use of prostate-specific questionnaires is needed to determine the impact of treatments and age on related symptoms such as voiding [19], potency, and continence [11,20,21]. Validated questionnaires can be used to assign a utility value to living with certain conditions, including different states of cancer [22,23]. Patients with cancer, even those who are "cured," have a lower quality of life than if they had never had to worry about cancer in the first place.

In order to perform a cost analysis, one needs to determine the cost of different approaches and the measured outcome of the different approaches. The cost-effectiveness ratio is the difference between costs (cost 1–cost 2) and the difference in outcome (effect 1–effect 2). The increase in cost between approaches is known as the incremental cost and the increase in outcome is the incremental utility, whether it is survival or QALYs, etc. As noted above, if time is a factor, such as in Markov models, then both cost and effect need to be discounted.

There are several different types of economic analyses that vary by the type of information used and the question that is being asked. Cost-effectiveness (CE) analyses assume a limited financial resource and attempt to find the most efficient way to spend a certain budget. These types of analyses are only necessary if there is a difference in outcome and difference in cost. If the cost is the same then the most effective outcome is preferred. If the outcome is equivalent then the analysis is a cost-minimization analysis (see below). CE analyses are primarily helpful when there are many variables and the outcome is not clearly obvious. For example, in the case of chemoprevention for prostate cancer, the primary endpoint of the Prostate Cancer Prevention Trial was a reduction in cancer prevalence [24]. However, a more important question is whether chemoprevention saves lives and is it cost-effective? Since the cost per life-year saved was not part of the trial design, it can only be extrapolated using a CE analysis. In this study, finasteride resulted in a reduction of cancer and subsequent survival advantage but at a cost of medication to many subjects who never had cancer and treatment to patients who may not have an increase in survival. In order to determine the CE ratio, a Markov model estimating the survival advantage of finasteride (incremental life-years) and cost of chemoprevention (incremental cost) can be designed to determine the cost-effectiveness of chemoprevention [25]. One advantage of models is the ability to utilize sensitivity analyses which can allow evaluation of outcomes with varying assumptions. Thus if there is a variable cost, one can determine the CE ratio under different circumstances.

Cost-utility analyses are essentially CE analyses which compare effects using different utilities such as QALYs. Cost-minimization analyses are those in which the benefits of different approaches are deemed to be equivalent and the goal is to find the least costly approach. This would be the case in determining the least expensive way to remove a kidney (open vs laparoscopic) on the assumption that the oncological outcomes are identical [26]. On the other hand, if there is concern that the outcomes may be different qualitatively then one should consider performing a CE analysis, assuming a difference in effect. Thus if, when comparing radical to partial nephrectomy, one wants to take into consideration a small difference in recurrence rates, then one would evaluate the difference in cost and difference in outcome.

Conclusion

Financial considerations play a major role in healthcare decisions both directly and indirectly. As new technologies and medications are introduced there will be an increased scrutiny into the likely benefit of these treatments. At the same time, any decision to incorporate these new approaches into management of disease will also include an attempt to evaluate the likely financial impact. Cost analyses will help in this type of decision making whether at the patient, hospital or societal level. For urologists, it will be important to understand the concepts that underlie such decision making.

References

1. Cowan CA, Lazenby HC, Martin AB, et al. National health expenditures, 1998. Health Care Financ Rev 1999;21(2):165-210.
2. Lotan Y, Cadeddu JA, Gettman MT. The new economics of radical prostatectomy: cost comparison of open, laparoscopic and robot assisted techniques. J Urol 2004;172(4 pt 1):1431-5.
3. Anderson JK, Murdock A, Cadeddu JA, Lotan Y. Cost comparison of laparoscopic versus radical retropubic prostatectomy. Urology 2005;66(3):557-60.
4. Dunn MD, McDougall EM, Clayman RV. Laparoscopic radical nephrectomy. J Endourol 2000;14(10):849-55; discussion 855-7.
5. Lotan Y, Cadeddu JA, Pearle MS. International comparison of cost effectiveness of medical management strategies for nephrolithiasis. Urol Res 2005;33(3):223-30.
6. Cairns J. *Discounting in Economic Evaluation. Economic evaluation in health care: merging theory with practice.* Oxford: Oxford University Press, 2001.
7. Fleming C, Wasson JH, Albertsen PC, Barry MJ, Wennberg JE. A decision analysis of alternative treatment strategies for

clinically localized prostate cancer. Prostate Patient Outcomes Research Team. JAMA 1993;269(20):2650-8.

8. Gold M, Siegel J, Russell L, et al. *Cost Effectiveness in Health and Medicine*. New York: Oxford University Press, 1996.

9. Siegel JE, Torrance GW, Russell LB, Luce BR, Weinstein MC, Gold MR. Guidelines for pharmacoeconomic studies. Recommendations from the Panel on Cost Effectiveness in Health and Medicine. Pharmacoeconomics 1997;11(2):159-68.

10. Lotan Y, Svatek RS, Sagalowsky AI. Should we screen for bladder cancer in a high-risk population? A cost per life-year saved analysis. Cancer 2006;107(5):982-90.

11. Svatek RS, Lee JJ, Roehrborn CG, Lippman SM, Lotan Y. Cost-effectiveness of prostate cancer chemoprevention: a quality of life-years analysis. Cancer 2008;112(5):1058-65.

12. Johnston K, Buxton MJ, Jones DR, Fitzpatrick R. Assessing the costs of healthcare technologies in clinical trials. Health Technol Assess 1999;3(6):1-76.

13. Meltzer D. Accounting for future costs in medical cost-effectiveness analysis. J Health Econ 1997;16(1):33-64.

14. Secker-Walker RH, Vacek PM, Hooper GJ, Plante DA, Detsky AS. Screening for breast cancer: time, travel, and out-of-pocket expenses. J Natl Cancer Inst 1999;91(8):702-8.

15. McHorney CA, Ware JE Jr, Raczek AE. The MOS 36-Item Short-Form Health Survey (SF-36): II. Psychometric and clinical tests of validity in measuring physical and mental health constructs. Med Care 1993;31(3):247-63.

16. Penniston KL, Nakada SY. Health related quality of life differs between male and female stone formers. J Urol 2007;178(6):2435-40; discussion 2440.

17. Bensalah K, Tuncel A, Gupta A, Raman JD, Pearle MS, Lotan Y. Determinants of quality of life for patients with kidney stones. J Urol 2008;179(6):2238-43; discussion 2243.

18. Barry MJ, Fowler FJ Jr, O'Leary MP, et al. The American Urological Association symptom index for benign prostatic hyperplasia. The Measurement Committee of the American Urological Association. J Urol 1992;148(5):1549-57; discussion 1564.

19. Stewart ST, Lenert L, Bhatnagar V, Kaplan RM. Utilities for prostate cancer health states in men aged 60 and older. Med Care 2005;43(4):347-55.

20. Krahn M, Ritvo P, Irvine J, et al. Patient and community preferences for outcomes in prostate cancer: implications for clinical policy. Med Care 2003;41(1):153-64.

21. Litwin MS, Hays RD, Fink A, Ganz PA, Leake B, Brook RH. The UCLA Prostate Cancer Index: development, reliability, and validity of a health-related quality of life measure. Med Care 1998;36(7):1002-12.

22. Mittmann N, Trakas K, Risebrough N, Liu BA. Utility scores for chronic conditions in a community-dwelling population. Pharmacoeconomics 1999;15(4):369-76.

23. Ritvo P, Irvine J, Naglie G, et al. Reliability and validity of the PORPUS, a combined psychometric and utility-based quality-of-life instrument for prostate cancer. J Clin Epidemiol 2005;58(5):466-74.

24. Thompson IM, Goodman PJ, Tangen CM, et al. The influence of finasteride on the development of prostate cancer. N Engl J Med 2003;349(3):215-24.

25. Svatek RS, Lee JJ, Roehrborn CG, Lippman SM, Lotan Y. The cost of prostate cancer chemoprevention: a decision analysis model. Cancer Epidemiol Biomarkers Prev 2006;15(8):1485-9.

26. Lotan Y, Gettman MT, Roehrborn CG, Pearle MS, Cadeddu JA. Cost comparison for laparoscopic nephrectomy and open nephrectomy: analysis of individual parameters. Urology 2002;59(6):821-5.

7 Antibiotic prophylaxis in urological surgery

Philipp Dahm, Ngoc-Bich Le and Susan F. Fesperman
Department of Urology, University of Florida, Gainesville, FL, USA

Introduction

Antimicrobial prophylaxis is defined as the periprocedural systemic administration of an antimicrobial agent intended to reduce the risk of surgical site infection as well as secondary systemic infections [1]. Surgical site infections are a major contributor to patient injury, mortality, and healthcare costs and represent the focus of major national and international quality improvement projects. The prophylactic agent should be effective against the organisms that are characteristic of the operative site but should only be recommended when the potential benefit outweighs the risks and anticipated costs. In this chapter, we will systematically review the evidence for or against the use of prophylactic antibiotics in four commonly performed urological procedures.

Methods

The methods used in this chapter follow those developed by the GRADE Working Group [2-4]. We formulated four focused clinical questions which directed comprehensive literature searches for high-quality systematic reviews as well as relevant individual randomized controlled trials. Only studies comparing at least one treatment arm to a placebo or nontreatment control arm were included. Observational studies were not considered. Outcome variables were rated as critical, important or not important according to their importance to clinical decision making [5]. These ratings were consistent for all four clinical questions. The prevention of sepsis was considered a critical outcome according to GRADE. The prevention of fever, a new onset of unspecific urinary tract symptoms and positive urine cultures were rated as important yet not critical outcomes for clinical decision making. Expected side effects of short-term antibiotic prophylaxis were also considered as important yet not critical to decision making in this setting.

Study information was abstracted by a single reviewer and entered into RevMan. The quality of evidence informing each clinical question was rated on an outcome-specific basis as high, moderate, low or very low according to GRADE [2]. Dimensions of evidence quality considered were study limitations (appropriate randomization, allocation concealment, blinding, completeness of follow-up, intention-to-treat analysis and stopping early for benefit), inconsistency, indirectness, imprecision and publication bias. These steps were performed independently by two reviewers; disagreements were resolved by discussion and arbitration by a third reviewer. We performed formal meta-analyses and generated forest plots when appropriate while formally assessing for heterogeneity and publication bias. The information from RevMan was subsequently transferred into GRADEPRO and used to generate evidence profiles in the standard GRADE format.

Based on the outcomes deemed critical to clinical decision making, the quality of evidence was determined across outcomes. Recommendations were then formulated as either strong or weak (conditional), either for or against a given intervention. These recommendations were based on judgments about the balance of desirable and undesirable effects, the quality of evidence, the degree of certainty with which patients' values and preferences were known and the anticipated costs of the intervention.

Clinical question 7.1

In patients undergoing ureteroscopy for ureteral stones, does antibiotic prophylaxis decrease the incidence of infectious complications when compared to no prophylaxis?

Evidence-Based Urology. Edited by Philipp Dahm, Roger R. Dmochowski.
© 2010 Blackwell Publishing.

Literature search

We conducted a systematic literature search in PubMed (1966–2009) using the search terms "antibiotic prophylaxis," "antimicrobial prophylaxis" and "ureteroscopy." The search was limited to randomized controlled trials and systematic reviews in English, Spanish, German and French language with a human population.

The evidence

Two eligible randomized controlled trials were identified. A study by Fourcade et al. randomized 120 patients undergoing ureteroscopy for ureteral stones to cefotaxime 1 g IV versus placebo [6]. Interpretation of this study was made difficult by the inclusion of a subset of patients undergoing percutaneous nephrolithotripsy that were not reported separately. A second, more recent study by Knopf et al. randomized 113 patients to 250 mg levofloxacin versus placebo [7].

The available evidence is summarized in Table 7.1. A statistically significant benefit for the use of antibiotics in this setting was only documented for the incidence of positive cultures (Figure 7.1) which was reduced from 16% (15/94) to 3.3% (3/90), reflecting a relative risk (RR) of 0.22 (95% confidence interval (CI) 0.07–0.71). The underlying quality of evidence was low with downgrading for study limitations as well as imprecision. Meanwhile, the rate of antibiotic-related side effects was low (1.7%) to mild in severity.

Clinical implications

Based on low-quality evidence, we make a conditional recommendation for the use of prophylactic antibiotics to prevent infectious complications in patients undergoing uncomplicated ureteroscopy for stone disease. The use of prophylactic antibiotics was not associated with a statically significant reduction of any adverse patient-important outcomes, although it reduced the rate of positive urine cultures, thereby indirectly supporting the use of antibiotics.

Clinical question 7.2

In patients undergoing shock-wave lithotripsy for the treatment of renal and ureteral calculi, does antibiotic prophylaxis decrease the incidence of infectious complications when compared to no prophylaxis?

Literature search

We conducted a systematic literature search in PubMed (1966–2009) using the search terms "antibiotic prophylaxis," "antimicrobial prophylaxis" and "shock-wave lithotripsy." The search was limited to randomized controlled trials and systematic reviews in English, Spanish, German and French language with a human population.

The evidence

We identified a total of six randomized controlled trials addressing this clinical question [8-13]. All studies had methodological limitations as well as low event rates which led to downgrading to low- or very low-quality evidence for all relevant outcomes (Table 7.2). A single study by Pettersson & Tiselius [13] addressed the prevention of sepsis, which did not demonstrate a statistically significant benefit, but also failed to exclude a potentially beneficial effect (Figure 7.2). All six studies addressed a reduction of febrile episodes with a calculated RR of 0.12 (95% CI 0.03–0.46; Figure 7.3) [8-13]. Antibiotic prophylaxis given to 1000 patients would therefore result in 46 fewer (95% CI 28 fewer to 50 fewer) patients with fever. However, no significant effect on the prevention of infection-associated lower urinary tract symptoms was demonstrated, nor was the number of positive urinary cultures significantly reduced (Figure 7.4). None of the studies addressed the incidence of side effects related to antibiotic prophylaxis.

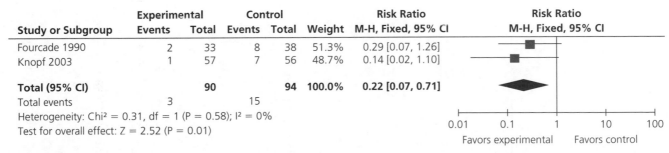

Study or Subgroup	Experimental Events	Total	Control Events	Total	Weight	Risk Ratio M-H, Fixed, 95% CI	Risk Ratio M-H, Fixed, 95% CI
Fourcade 1990	2	33	8	38	51.3%	0.29 [0.07, 1.26]	
Knopf 2003	1	57	7	56	48.7%	0.14 [0.02, 1.10]	
Total (95% CI)		**90**		**94**	**100.0%**	**0.22 [0.07, 0.71]**	
Total events	3		15				

Heterogeneity: Chi² = 0.31, df = 1 (P = 0.58); I² = 0%
Test for overall effect: Z = 2.52 (P = 0.01)

Figure 7.1 Forest plot comparing antibiotic prophylaxis versus no antibiotic prophylaxis in patients undergoing ureteroscopy to prevent postoperative positive urine cultures.

Table 7.1 GRADE evidence profile for Clinical Question 7.1: Should antibiotic prophylaxis versus no antibiotic prophylaxis be used in patients undergoing ureteroscopy?

Quality assessment							Summary of findings				Quality	Importance
							No of patients		Effect			
No of studies	Design	Limitations	Inconsistency	Indirectness	Imprecision	Other considerations	Antibiotic prophylaxis versus no antibiotic prophylaxis	Control	Relative (95% CI)	Absolute		
Sepsis												
0[1]	no evidence available					none	0/0 (0%)	0/0 (0%)	not estimable	not estimable		CRITICAL
Fever												
1	randomized trials	serious[2]	no serious inconsistency[3]	no serious indirectness[4]	serious[5,6]	none	9/60 (15%)	12/60 (20%)	RR 0.75 (0.34 to 1.65)	50 fewer per 1000 (from 132 fewer to 130 more)	⊕⊕OO LOW	IMPORTANT
Lower urinary tract symptoms												
2	randomized trials	very serious[7]	no serious inconsistency[8]	no serious indirectness[4]	serious[5,6]	none	0/117 (0%)	2/116 (1.7%)	RR 0.2 (0.01 to 4.08)	14 fewer per 1000 (from 17 fewer to 53 more)	⊕OOO VERY LOW	IMPORTANT
Postoperative bacteriuria												
2	randomized trials	serious[9]	no serious inconsistency	no serious indirectness	serious[5]	none	3/90 (3.3%)	15/94 (16%)	RR 0.22 (0.07 to 0.71)	124 fewer per 1000 (from 46 fewer to 148 fewer)	⊕⊕OO LOW	IMPORTANT
Side effects												
2	randomized trials	very serious[7,10]	no serious inconsistency[8]	no serious indirectness[4]	serious[5,6]	none	2/117 (1.7%)	0/116 (0%)	RR 5 (0.25 to 102)	0 more per 1000 (from 0 fewer to 0 more)	⊕OOO VERY LOW	IMPORTANT

[1] This outcome was not addressed by the included studies
[2] No mention of allocation concealment; double-blind objective outcome; no mention of intention-to-treat (ITT); adequate follow-up
[3] Not applicable
[4] The data of one study are from both percutaneous nephrolithotomy and ureterorenoscopy procedures; data of ureterorenoscopy alone were not available for that study
[5] Small number of events
[6] The 95% CI includes both negligible effect and appreciable benefit or appreciable harm
[7] No mention of allocation concealment; no mention of blinding or double-blind for subjective outcome; no mention of ITT; one study with inadequate follow-up
[8] Not applicable; only one study with events reported
[9] No mention of allocation concealment; no mention of blinding or double-blind for objective outcome; no mention of ITT; one study with inadequate follow-up
[10] Only the treatment groups were followed for this outcome; data values are 0 events for control groups by default

Table 7.2 GRADE evidence profile for Clinical Question 7.2: Should antibiotic prophylaxis versus no antibiotic prophylaxis be used in patients undergoing shock-wave lithotripsy?

No of studies	Design	Limitations	Inconsistency	Indirectness	Imprecision	Other considerations	Antibiotic prophylaxis versus no prophylaxis in shock-wave lithotripsy (short-term)	Control	Relative (95% CI)	Absolute	Quality	Importance
							No of patients		**Effect**			
Sepsis												
1	randomized trials	serious[1,2]	no serious inconsistency[3]	no serious indirectness	serious[4,5]	none	1/104 (1%)	0/45 (0%)	RR 1.31 (0.05 to 31.66)	0 more per 1000 (from 0 fewer to 0 more)	⊕⊕OO LOW	CRITICAL
Fever												
6	randomized trials	serious[6,7]	no serious inconsistency	no serious indirectness[8]	serious[4]	none	2/553 (0.4%)	19/365 (5.2%)	RR 0.12 (0.03 to 0.46)	46 fewer per 1000 (from 28 fewer to 50 fewer)	⊕⊕OO LOW	IMPORTANT
Lower urinary tract symptoms												
2	randomized trials	very serious[7,9,10]	no serious inconsistency[3,11]	no serious indirectness	serious[4,5]	none	63/310 (20.3%)	13/178 (7.3%)	RR 0.99 (0.63 to 1.55)	1 fewer per 1000 (from 27 fewer to 40 more)	⊕OOO VERY LOW	IMPORTANT
Positive urine culture (any definition)												
6	randomized trials	serious[6,7]	serious[12]	no serious indirectness	serious[4,5]	none	39/553 (7.1%)	22/365 (6%)	RR 0.65 (0.36 to 1.17)	21 fewer per 1000 (from 39 fewer to 10 more)	⊕OOO VERY LOW	IMPORTANT

(Continued on p. 54)

53

Table 7.2 (Continued)

Quality assessment							Summary of findings					Importance
							No of patients		Effect		Quality	
No of studies	Design	Limitations	Inconsistency	Indirectness	Imprecision	Other considerations	Antibiotic prophylaxis versus no prophylaxis in shock-wave lithotripsy (short-term)	Control	Relative (95% CI)	Absolute		
Side effects												
0[13]	no evidence available					none	0/0 (0%)	0/0 (0%)	not pooled	not pooled		IMPORTANT

[1] No mention of allocation concealment, lack of blinding but objective outcome, no mention of ITT, exact follow-up counts not provided

[2] Out of six included studies, only one reported on this outcome

[3] Not applicable

[4] Small number of events

[5] The 95% CI includes both negligible effect and appreciable benefit or appreciable harm

[6] No mention of allocation concealment, lack of blinding or only placebo used (objective outcome), no mention of ITT

[7] One study stopped early at interim analysis

[8] Two studies do not provide data on fever alone; rather, fever is grouped with other signs of infection

[9] No mention of allocation concealment, lack of blinding or only placebo used (subjective outcome), no mention of ITT

[10] Out of six included studies, only two reported on this outcome

[11] One study had no events

[12] I-squared value is 56%

[13] Out of six included studies, none reported on this outcome

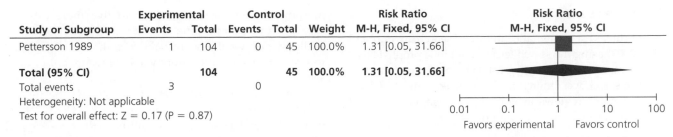

Figure 7.2 Forest plot comparing antibiotic prophylaxis versus no antibiotic prophylaxis for the prevention of sepsis in patients undergoing shock-wave lithotripsy.

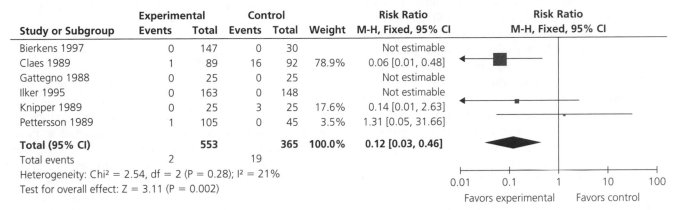

Figure 7.3 Forest plot comparing antibiotic prophylaxis versus no antibiotic prophylaxis for the prevention of fever in patients undergoing shock-wave lithotripsy.

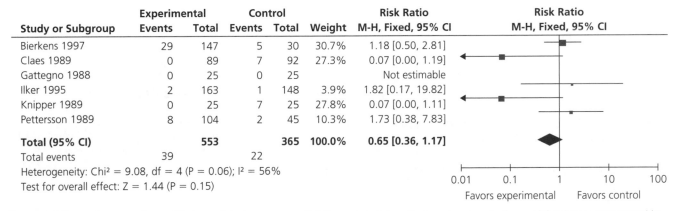

Figure 7.4 Forest plot comparing antibiotic prophylaxis versus no antibiotic prophylaxis in patients undergoing shock-wave lithotripsy to prevent positive urine cultures.

Clinical implications

Based on the current best evidence, antibiotic prophylaxis is strongly recommended in patients undergoing shock-wave lithotripsy. This recommendation is based on low-quality evidence for a clinically important rate of reduction in the incidence of fever as a patient-important outcome. We assumed that the benefits of antibiotic prophylaxis clearly outweighed the risks, that there was relatively little variability with regard to relevant patients' values and preferences related to the question of antibiotic prophylaxis, and that the costs of antibiotic prophylaxis were low.

Clinical question 7.3

In patients undergoing transrectal biopsy of the prostate, does antibiotic prophylaxis decrease the incidence of infectious complications when compared to no prophylaxis?

Literature search

We conducted a systematic literature search in PubMed (1966–2009) using the search terms "antibiotic prophylaxis," "antimicrobial prophylaxis," prostate biopsy" and "transrectal." The search was limited to randomized controlled trials and systematic reviews in English, Spanish, German and French language with a human population.

The evidence

Six randomized controlled trials met eligibility criteria and were included in the evidence profile (Table 7.3) [14-19]. All studies had important methodological limitations across different outcomes with regard to allocation concealment, blinding, intention-to-treat analysis and completeness of follow-up and were therefore downgraded.

Two randomized controlled trials with a total of 504 patients reported the therapeutic effectiveness of antibiotics to prevent symptoms of sepsis [16,18]. Studies for this outcome provided low-quality evidence. Seven of 254 (2.8%) patients receiving no antibiotics and 1 of 250 patients (0.4%) in the treatment group developed sepsis, corresponding to a RR of 0.21 (95% CI 0.04–1.17; Figure 7.5). In absolute terms, antibiotic treatment of 1000 patients undergoing prostate biopsy would be expected to result

in somewhere between 26 fewer to five more cases of sepsis, with a point estimate of 22 fewer cases. Therefore, while suggestive of a beneficial effect, these studies failed to prove that antibiotic prophylaxis prevents episodes of sepsis.

Meanwhile, antibiotic therapy appeared effective at reducing episodes of fever (RR 0.48, 95% CI 0.27–0.86; Figure 7.6) and positive urine cultures (RR 0.31, 95% CI 0.2–0.48; Figure 7.7) but not the incidence of infection-related lower urinary tract symptoms (RR 0.72, 95% CI 0.39–1.34). Only a single study reported antibiotic prophylaxis-related side-effects in 4.3% of patients, all of which were mild (Figure 7.8).

Clinical implications

Despite the availability of only low-quality evidence in aggregate, we strongly recommend that men undergoing prostate biopsy should receive prophylactic antibiotics. Although there is no convincing evidence that antibiotic prophylaxis in the average-risk patient prevents rare episodes of sepsis, it is effective at reducing episodes of fever as a patient-important outcome as well as reducing the incidence of postbiopsy positive urinary cultures. While poorly reported in these studies, other studies on the adverse effects of the short-term courses of antibiotics used

Study or Subgroup	Experimental Events	Total	Control Events	Total	Weight	Risk Ratio M-H, Fixed, 95% CI	Risk Ratio M-H, Fixed, 95% CI
Crawford 1982	1	23	3	25	39.1%	0.36 [0.04, 3.24]	
Kapoor 1998	0	227	4	229	60.9%	0.11 [0.01, 2.07]	
Total (95% CI)		**250**		**94**	**100.0%**	**0.21 [0.04, 1.17]**	
Total events	3		15				
Heterogeneity: Chi² = 0.42, df = 1 (P = 0.52); I² = 0%							
Test for overall effect: Z = 1.78 (P = 0.07)							

Figure 7.5 Forest plot comparing antibiotic prophylaxis versus no antibiotic prophylaxis for the prevention of sepsis in patients undergoing transrectal prostate biopsy.

Study or Subgroup	Experimental Events	Total	Control Events	Total	Weight	Risk Ratio M-H, Fixed, 95% CI	Risk Ratio M-H, Fixed, 95% CI
Aron 2000	4	156	5	75	24.8%	0.38 [0.11, 1.39]	
Brown 1981	5	10	3	9	11.6%	1.50 [0.49, 4.56]	
Crawford 1982	4	23	12	25	42.3%	0.36 [0.14, 0.97]	
Melekos 1990	2	22	5	16	21.3%	0.29 [0.06, 1.31]	
Total (95% CI)		**211**		**125**	**100.0%**	**0.48 [0.27, 0.86]**	
Total events	15		25				
Heterogeneity: Chi² = 4.86, df = 3 (P = 0.18); I² = 38%							
Test for overall effect: Z = 2.50 (P = 0.01)							

Figure 7.6 Forest plot comparing antibiotic prophylaxis versus no antibiotic prophylaxis for the prevention of fever in patients undergoing transrectal prostate biopsy.

Table 7.3 GRADE evidence profile for Clinical Question 7.3: Should antibiotic prophylaxis versus no antibiotic prophylaxis be used in patients undergoing TRUS biopsy?

Quality assessment							Summary of findings				Quality	Importance
							No of patients		Effect			
No of studies	Design	Limitations	Inconsistency	Indirectness	Imprecision	Other considerations	Antibiotic prophylaxis versus no antibiotic prophylaxis (short term)	Control	Relative (95% CI)	Absolute		
Sepsis												
2	randomized trials	serious[1,2]	no serious inconsistency	no serious indirectness	serious[3,4]	none	1/250 (0.4%)	7/254 (2.8%)	RR 0.21 (0.04 to 1.17)	22 fewer per 1000 (from 26 fewer to 5 more)	⊕⊕⊕OO LOW	CRITICAL
Fever												
4	randomized trials	serious[5]	no serious inconsistency	no serious indirectness	serious[4]	none	15/211 (7.1%)	25/125 (20%)	RR 0.48 (0.27 to 0.86)	104 fewer per 1000 (from 28 fewer to 146 fewer)	⊕⊕⊕OO LOW	IMPORTANT
Lower urinary tract symptoms												
1	randomized trials	very serious[6,7,8]	no serious inconsistency[9]	no serious indirectness	serious[4,10]	none	21/156 (13.5%)	14/75 (18.7%)	RR 0.72 (0.39 to 1.34)	52 fewer per 1000 (from 114 fewer to 63 more)	⊕OOO VERY LOW	IMPORTANT
Positive urine culture												
6	randomized trials	serious[11]	no serious inconsistency	no serious indirectness	serious[4]	none	28/539 (5.2%)	59/390 (15.1%)	RR 0.31 (0.2 to 0.48)	104 fewer per 1000 (from 79 fewer to 121 fewer)	⊕⊕OO LOW	IMPORTANT

(Continued on p. 58)

Table 7.3 (Continued)

No of studies	Design	Limitations	Inconsistency	Indirectness	Imprecision	Other considerations	Antibiotic prophylaxis versus no antibiotic prophylaxis (short term)	Control	Relative (95% CI)	Absolute	Quality	Importance
							Summary of findings					
							No of patients		Effect			
1	randomized trials	very serious[7,12]	no serious inconsistency[9]	no serious indirectness	very serious[4,10]	none	1/23 (4.3%)	0/25 (0%)	RR 3.25 (0.14 to 76.01)	0 more per 1000 (from 0 fewer to 0 more)	⊕◯◯◯ VERY LOW	IMPORTANT

[1] No mention of allocation concealment, double-blind studies do not indicate who is blinded but objective outcomes, one study performed ITT analysis, follow-up numbers are unclear
[2] Unclear whether sepsis was defined in same way across studies
[3] The 95% CI includes both negligible effect and appreciable benefit
[4] Small number of events
[5] No mention of allocation concealment, exact follow-up counts not provided, no mention of ITT, incomplete blinding but objective outcome
[6] No mention of allocation concealment, exact follow-up count not provided, no mention of ITT, only patients blinded for subjective outcome
[7] Out of six included studies, only one reported on this outcome
[8] This study only reported lower urinary tract symptom events in the absence of detectable infection
[9] Not applicable
[10] The 95% CI includes both negligible effect and appreciable harm or appreciable benefit
[11] No mention of allocation concealment, exact follow-up counts not provided, in all but one study no mention of ITT, incomplete blinding or no mention of blinding but objective outcome
[12] No mention of allocation concealment, double blind but does not specify who is blinded for subjective outcome, no mention of ITT, follow-up numbers not reported

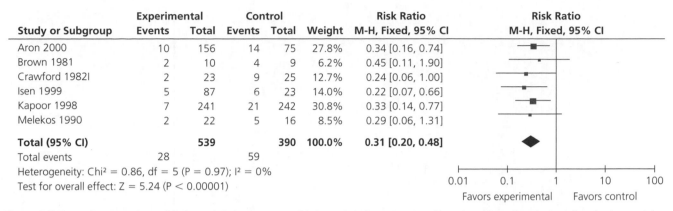

Study or Subgroup	Experimental Events	Experimental Total	Control Events	Control Total	Weight	Risk Ratio M-H, Fixed, 95% CI
Aron 2000	10	156	14	75	27.8%	0.34 [0.16, 0.74]
Brown 1981	2	10	4	9	6.2%	0.45 [0.11, 1.90]
Crawford 1982I	2	23	9	25	12.7%	0.24 [0.06, 1.00]
Isen 1999	5	87	6	23	14.0%	0.22 [0.07, 0.66]
Kapoor 1998	7	241	21	242	30.8%	0.33 [0.14, 0.77]
Melekos 1990	2	22	5	16	8.5%	0.29 [0.06, 1.31]
Total (95% CI)		**539**		**390**	**100.0%**	**0.31 [0.20, 0.48]**
Total events	28		59			

Heterogeneity: Chi² = 0.86, df = 5 (P = 0.97); I² = 0%
Test for overall effect: Z = 5.24 (P < 0.00001)

Figure 7.7 Forest plot comparing antibiotic prophylaxis versus no antibiotic prophylaxis to prevent positive urine cultures in patients undergoing transrectal prostate biopsy.

Study or Subgroup	Experimental Events	Experimental Total	Control Events	Control Total	Weight	Risk Ratio M-H, Fixed, 95% CI
Crawford 1982	1	23	0	25	100.0%	3.25 [0.14, 76.01]
Total (95% CI)		**23**		**25**	**100.0%**	**3.25 [0.14, 76.01]**
Total events	1		0			

Heterogeneity: Not applicable
Test for overall effect: Z = 0.73 (P = 0.46)

Figure 7.8 Forest plot comparing reported side effects in patients receiving antibiotic prophylaxis versus no antibiotic prophylaxis prior to undergoing transrectal prostate biopsy.

for antibiotic prophylaxis in this setting would suggest that these are rare and mild in severity. Therefore, the ratio of potential benefit to harm favors the use of prophylactic antibiotics.

Clinical question 7.4

In patients undergoing transurethral resection of the prostate, does antibiotic prophylaxis decrease the incidence of infectious complications when compared to no prophylaxis?

Literature search

We conducted a systematic literature search in PubMed (1966–2009) using the search terms "antibiotic prophylaxis," "antimicrobial prophylaxis," "transurethral resection" and "prostate." The search was limited to randomized controlled trials and systematic reviews in English, Spanish, German and French language with a human population.

The evidence

We identified a total of 39 relevant RCTs from 1976 to 2007 [20-56]. Six studies addressed the incidence of septic episodes, 17 studies that of procedure-related fever and 39 studies that of positive urine cultures following TURP. The quality of evidence for these outcomes was low, very low and moderate, respectively (Table 7.4).

Prophylactic antibiotics were associated with an approximately 50% relative risk reduction (RR 0.51, 95% CI 0.27–0.96; Figure 7.9) for septic episode as well as 2% absolute risk reduction (number needed to treat (NNT) = 50). The rate of febrile episodes was 0.64 (95% CI 0.55–0.75; Figure 7.10). Lastly, the rate of positive urine cultures was approximately one-third (RR 0.37, 95% CI 0.32–0.41; Figure 7.11) in the antibiotic-treated group compared to the control group with an absolute risk reduction of 21.0% (NNT = 5). None of these studies reported data on adverse events.

Clinical implications

Based on the available evidence, we make a strong recommendation for the use of prophylactic antibiotics in patients undergoing TURP based on, in aggregate, low-quality evidence. This recommendation considers the consistent benefit of prophylactic antibiotics across critical and important outcomes, as well as the fact that the adverse events associated with these agents are relatively

Table 7.4 GRADE evidence profile for Clinical Question 7.4: Should antibiotic prophylaxis versus no antibiotic prophylaxis be used in patients undergoing TURP?

Quality assessment							Summary of findings				Quality	Importance
							No of patients		Effect			
No of studies	Design	Limitations	Inconsistency	Indirectness	Imprecision	Other considerations	Short Term	Control	Relative (95% CI)	Absolute		
Sepsis												
6	randomized trials	serious[1]	no serious inconsistency	no serious indirectness	serious[2]	none	14/995 (1.4%)	23/671 (3.4%)	RR 0.51 (0.27 to 0.96)	17 fewer per 1000 (from 1 fewer to 25 fewer)	⊕⊕OO LOW	CRITICAL
Fever												
17	randomized trials	serious[1]	serious[3]	no serious indirectness	no serious imprecision	reporting bias[4]	197/1645 (12%)	245/1109 (22.1%)	RR 0.64 (0.55 to 0.75)	80 fewer per 1000 (from 55 fewer to 99 fewer)	⊕OOO VERY LOW	IMPORTANT
Positive urine culture												
39	randomized trials	serious[1]	no serious inconsistency	no serious indirectness	no serious imprecision	none	368/2900 (12.7%)	763/2265 (33.7%)	RR 0.37 (0.32 to 0.41)	212 fewer per 1000 (from 199 fewer to 229 fewer)	⊕⊕⊕O MODERATE	IMPORTANT

[1] Most studies have inadequate allocation concealment, lack of blinding but objective outcome, no mention of ITT, and inadequate or unclear follow-up
[2] Small number of events
[3] I-squared value is 61%; some studies have little to no overlap of 95% confidence intervals
[4] Not all studies fall within bounds of funnel plot; funnel plot asymmetrical

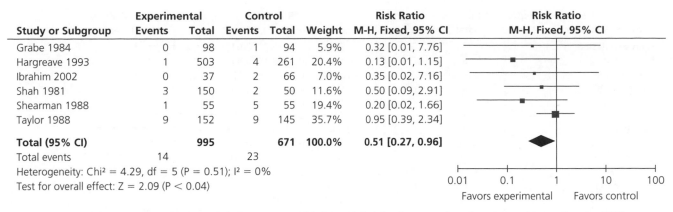

Study or Subgroup	Experimental Events	Experimental Total	Control Events	Control Total	Weight	Risk Ratio M-H, Fixed, 95% CI
Grabe 1984	0	98	1	94	5.9%	0.32 [0.01, 7.76]
Hargreave 1993	1	503	4	261	20.4%	0.13 [0.01, 1.15]
Ibrahim 2002	0	37	2	66	7.0%	0.35 [0.02, 7.16]
Shah 1981	3	150	2	50	11.6%	0.50 [0.09, 2.91]
Shearman 1988	1	55	5	55	19.4%	0.20 [0.02, 1.66]
Taylor 1988	9	152	9	145	35.7%	0.95 [0.39, 2.34]
Total (95% CI)		**995**		**671**	**100.0%**	**0.51 [0.27, 0.96]**
Total events	14		23			

Heterogeneity: Chi² = 4.29, df = 5 (P = 0.51); I² = 0%
Test for overall effect: Z = 2.09 (P < 0.04)

Figure 7.9 Forest plot comparing antibiotic prophylaxis versus no antibiotic prophylaxis for the prevention of sepsis in patients undergoing TURP.

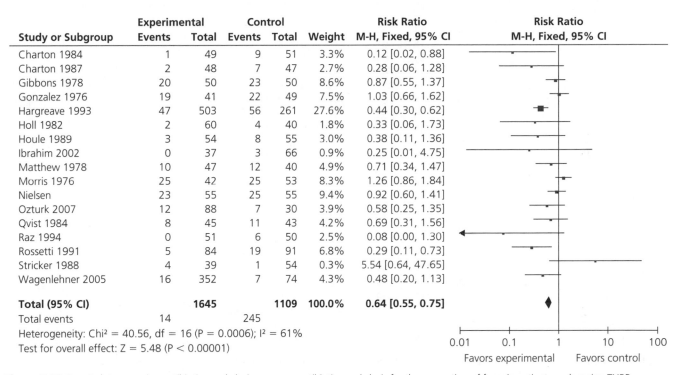

Study or Subgroup	Experimental Events	Experimental Total	Control Events	Control Total	Weight	Risk Ratio M-H, Fixed, 95% CI
Charton 1984	1	49	9	51	3.3%	0.12 [0.02, 0.88]
Charton 1987	2	48	7	47	2.7%	0.28 [0.06, 1.28]
Gibbons 1978	20	50	23	50	8.6%	0.87 [0.55, 1.37]
Gonzalez 1976	19	41	22	49	7.5%	1.03 [0.66, 1.62]
Hargreave 1993	47	503	56	261	27.6%	0.44 [0.30, 0.62]
Holl 1982	2	60	4	40	1.8%	0.33 [0.06, 1.73]
Houle 1989	3	54	8	55	3.0%	0.38 [0.11, 1.36]
Ibrahim 2002	0	37	3	66	0.9%	0.25 [0.01, 4.75]
Matthew 1978	10	47	12	40	4.9%	0.71 [0.34, 1.47]
Morris 1976	25	42	25	53	8.3%	1.26 [0.86, 1.84]
Nielsen	23	55	25	55	9.4%	0.92 [0.60, 1.41]
Ozturk 2007	12	88	7	30	3.9%	0.58 [0.25, 1.35]
Qvist 1984	8	45	11	43	4.2%	0.69 [0.31, 1.56]
Raz 1994	0	51	6	50	2.5%	0.08 [0.00, 1.30]
Rossetti 1991	5	84	19	91	6.8%	0.29 [0.11, 0.73]
Stricker 1988	4	39	1	54	0.3%	5.54 [0.64, 47.65]
Wagenlehner 2005	16	352	7	74	4.3%	0.48 [0.20, 1.13]
Total (95% CI)		**1645**		**1109**	**100.0%**	**0.64 [0.55, 0.75]**
Total events	14		245			

Heterogeneity: Chi² = 40.56, df = 16 (P = 0.0006); I² = 61%
Test for overall effect: Z = 5.48 (P < 0.00001)

Figure 7.10 Forest plot comparing antibiotic prophylaxis versus no antibiotic prophylaxis for the prevention of fever in patients undergoing TURP.

uncommon and mild, and the associated costs of antibiotic prophylaxis are relatively low.

Implications for research

This chapter provides a systematic review of the current best evidence for the use of prophylactic antibiotics for four commonly performed urological procedures. The particular questions that were addressed were selected based on information obtained from the recently published Best Practice Policy Statement by the American Urological Association indicating the presence of at least

one randomized controlled trial that would potentially provide high-quality evidence to guide clinical decision making [1]. While this was indeed the case, the methodological quality of these studies was largely poor, thereby providing only low- or very low-quality evidence for the majority of outcomes. At the same time, adverse event reporting was scarce.

Meanwhile, this chapter leaves unaddressed many critical questions with regard to the use of prophylactic antibiotics in other settings, and does not provide guidance about the optimal type of antibiotic, its timing or dosage. Findings of this chapter therefore underscore the critical need for more randomized controlled trials of high methodological quality

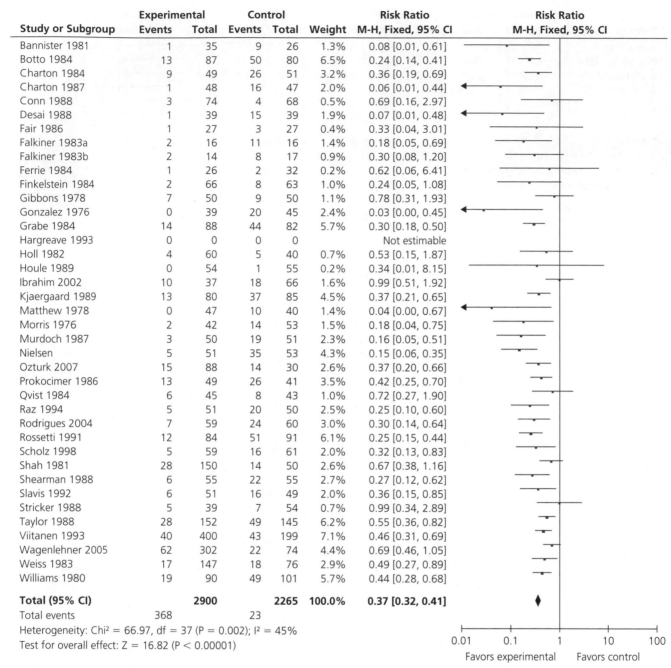

Study or Subgroup	Experimental Events	Total	Control Events	Total	Weight	Risk Ratio M-H, Fixed, 95% CI
Bannister 1981	1	35	9	26	1.3%	0.08 [0.01, 0.61]
Botto 1984	13	87	50	80	6.5%	0.24 [0.14, 0.41]
Charton 1984	9	49	26	51	3.2%	0.36 [0.19, 0.69]
Charton 1987	1	48	16	47	2.0%	0.06 [0.01, 0.44]
Conn 1988	3	74	4	68	0.5%	0.69 [0.16, 2.97]
Desai 1988	1	39	15	39	1.9%	0.07 [0.01, 0.48]
Fair 1986	1	27	3	27	0.4%	0.33 [0.04, 3.01]
Falkiner 1983a	2	16	11	16	1.4%	0.18 [0.05, 0.69]
Falkiner 1983b	2	14	8	17	0.9%	0.30 [0.08, 1.20]
Ferrie 1984	1	26	2	32	0.2%	0.62 [0.06, 6.41]
Finkelstein 1984	2	66	8	63	1.0%	0.24 [0.05, 1.08]
Gibbons 1978	7	50	9	50	1.1%	0.78 [0.31, 1.93]
Gonzalez 1976	0	39	20	45	2.4%	0.03 [0.00, 0.45]
Grabe 1984	14	88	44	82	5.7%	0.30 [0.18, 0.50]
Hargreave 1993	0	0	0	0		Not estimable
Holl 1982	4	60	5	40	0.7%	0.53 [0.15, 1.87]
Houle 1989	0	54	1	55	0.2%	0.34 [0.01, 8.15]
Ibrahim 2002	10	37	18	66	1.6%	0.99 [0.51, 1.92]
Kjaergaard 1989	13	80	37	85	4.5%	0.37 [0.21, 0.65]
Matthew 1978	0	47	10	40	1.4%	0.04 [0.00, 0.67]
Morris 1976	2	42	14	53	1.5%	0.18 [0.04, 0.75]
Murdoch 1987	3	50	19	51	2.3%	0.16 [0.05, 0.51]
Nielsen	5	51	35	53	4.3%	0.15 [0.06, 0.35]
Ozturk 2007	15	88	14	30	2.6%	0.37 [0.20, 0.66]
Prokocimer 1986	13	49	26	41	3.5%	0.42 [0.25, 0.70]
Qvist 1984	6	45	8	43	1.0%	0.72 [0.27, 1.90]
Raz 1994	5	51	20	50	2.5%	0.25 [0.10, 0.60]
Rodrigues 2004	7	59	24	60	3.0%	0.30 [0.14, 0.64]
Rossetti 1991	12	84	51	91	6.1%	0.25 [0.15, 0.44]
Scholz 1998	5	59	16	61	2.0%	0.32 [0.13, 0.83]
Shah 1981	28	150	14	50	2.6%	0.67 [0.38, 1.16]
Shearman 1988	6	55	22	55	2.7%	0.27 [0.12, 0.62]
Slavis 1992	6	51	16	49	2.0%	0.36 [0.15, 0.85]
Stricker 1988	5	39	7	54	0.7%	0.99 [0.34, 2.89]
Taylor 1988	28	152	49	145	6.2%	0.55 [0.36, 0.82]
Viitanen 1993	40	400	43	199	7.1%	0.46 [0.31, 0.69]
Wagenlehner 2005	62	302	22	74	4.4%	0.69 [0.46, 1.05]
Weiss 1983	17	147	18	76	2.9%	0.49 [0.27, 0.89]
Williams 1980	19	90	49	101	5.7%	0.44 [0.28, 0.68]
Total (95% CI)		**2900**		**2265**	**100.0%**	**0.37 [0.32, 0.41]**
Total events	368		23			

Heterogeneity: Chi² = 66.97, df = 37 (P = 0.002); I² = 45%
Test for overall effect: Z = 16.82 (P < 0.00001)

Figure 7.11 Forest plot comparing antibiotic prophylaxis versus no antibiotic prophylaxis to prevent positive urine cultures in patients undergoing TURP.

in this arena which should subsequently be transparently reported with similar emphasis on reporting of both benefit and harm. Consideration of the necessary resource allocation and comparative effectiveness analyses is also expected to be a point of major emphasis in the future. A more widespread recognition of the principles of evidence-based clinical practice in the urological community appears to be a critical step to spur this development.

References

1. Wolf JS Jr, Bennett CJ, Dmochowski RR, Hollenbeck BK, Pearle MS, Schaeffer AJ. Best practice policy statement on urologic surgery antimicrobial prophylaxis. J Urol 2008;179(4):1379-90.
2. Guyatt GH, Oxman AD, Kunz R, Vist GE, Falck-Ytter Y, Schunemann HJ. What is "quality of evidence" and why is it important to clinicians? BMJ (Clin Res) 2008;336(7651):995-8.

3. Guyatt G, Vist G, Falck-Ytter Y, Kunz R, Magrini N, Schunemann H. An emerging consensus on grading recommendations? ACP J Club 2006;144(1):A8-9.

4. Guyatt GH, Oxman AD, Vist GE, et al. GRADE: an emerging consensus on rating quality of evidence and strength of recommendations. BMJ (Clin Res) 2008;336(7650):924-6.

5. Guyatt GH, Oxman AD, Kunz R, et al. Going from evidence to recommendations. BMJ (Clin Res) 2008;336(7652):1049-51.

6. Fourcade RO, the Cefotaxime Cooperative Group. Antibiotic prophylaxis with cefotaxime in endoscopic extraction of upper urinary tract stones: a randomized study. J Antimicrob Chemother 1990;26(suppl A):77-83.

7. Knopf HJ, Graff HJ, Schulze H. Perioperative antibiotic prophylaxis in ureteroscopic stone removal. ur Urol 2003;44(1):115-18.

8. Bierkens A, Hendrikx A, Ezz el Din K, et al. The value of antibiotic prophylaxis during extracorporeal shock wave lithotripsy in the prevention of urinary tract infections in patients with urine proven sterile prior to treatment. Eur Urol 1997;31(1):30-5.

9. Claes H, Vandeursen R, Baert L. Amoxycillin/clavulanate prophylaxis for extracorporeal shock wave lithotripsy – a comparative study. J Antimicrob Chemother 1989;24(suppl B):217-20.

10. Gattegno B, Sicard F, Alcaidinho D, Arnaud E, Thibault P. Extracorporeal lithotripsy and prophylactic antibiotic therapy. Ann Urol 1988;22(2):101-2.

11. Ílker Y, Türkerí LN, Korten V, Tarcan T, Akdas A. Antimicrobial prophylaxis in management of urinary tract stones by extracorporeal shock-wave lithotripsy: is it necessary? Urology 1995;46(2):165-7.

12. Knipper A, Bohle A, Pensel J, Hofstetter A. Antibiotic prophylaxis with enoxacin in extracorporeal shockwave lithotripsy. Infection 1989;17(suppl 1):S37-8.

13. Pettersson B, Tiselius H. Are prophylactic antibiotics necessary during extracorporeal shockwave lithotripsy? BJU 1989;63(5):449-52.

14. Aron M, Rajeev TP, Gupta NP. Antibiotic prophylaxis for transrectal needle biopsy of the prostate: a randomized controlled study. BJU Int 2000;85(6):682-5.

15. Brown R, Warner JJ, Turner B, et al. Bacteremia and bacteriuria after transrectal prostatic biopsy. Urology 1981;18(2):145-8.

16. Crawford ED, Haynes AL Jr, Story MW, Borden TA. Prevention of urinary tract infection and sepsis following transrectal prostatic biopsy. J Urol 1982;127(3):449-51.

17. Isen K, Küpeli B, Sinik Z, Sözen S, Bozkirli I. Antibiotic prophylaxis for transrectal biopsy of the prostate: a prospective randomized study of the prophylactic use of single dose oral fluoroquinolone versus trimethoprim-sulfamethoxazole. Int Urol Nephrol 1999;31(4):491-5.

18. Kapoor D, Klimberg I, Malek G, et al. Single-dose oral ciproflaxcin versus placebo for prophylaxis during transrectal prostate biopsy. Urology 1998;52(4):552-8.

19. Melekos M, Asbach H, Giannoulis S, Perimenis P, Barbalias G. Aspects concerning posterior urethral valves. Int Urol Nephrol 1989;21(1):57-62.

20. Bannister G, Arkell DG, Menday AP. Prostatectomy and prophylaxis. J Antimicrob Chemother 1981;7(2):209-10.

21. Botto H, Richard F, Mathieu F, Perreau A, Camey M. Short-term prophylaxis with cefotaxime in prostatic surgery. J Antimicrob Chemother 1984;14(suppl B):231-5.

22. Charton M, Dosne B, Escovar P, Kopf A, Brisset JM. Single-dose prophylactic treatment of urinary tract infections after transurethral prostatectomy. Presse Med 1984;13:545-8.

23. Charton M, Vallancien G, Veillon B, Brisset J. Antibiotic prophylaxis of urinary tract infection after transurethral resection of the prostate: a randomized study. J Urol 1987;138(1):87-9.

24. Desai K, Abrams P, White L. A double-blind comparative trial of short-term orally administered enoxacin in the prevention of urinary infection after elective transurethral prostatectomy: a clinical and pharmacokinetic study. J Urol 1988;139(6):1232-4.

25. Fair W. Perioperative use of carbenicillin in transurethral resection of prostate. Urology 1986;27(2 suppl):15-18.

26. Falkiner F, Ma P, Murphy D, Cafferkey M, Gillespie W. Antimicrobial agents for the prevention of urinary tract infection in transurethral surgery. J Urol 1983;129(4):766-8.

27. Ferrie B, Scott R. Prophylactic cefuroxime in transurethral resection. Urologic Res 1984;12(6):279-81.

28. Finkelstein L, Arsht D, Manfrey S, Childs S. Ceftriaxone in the prevention of postoperative infection in patients undergoing transurethral resection of the prostate. Am J Surg 1984;148(4A):19-21.

29. Gibbons R, Stark R, Correa RJ, Cummings K, Mason J. The prophylactic use – or misuse – of antibiotics in transurethral prostatectomy. J Urol 1978;119(3):381-3.

30. Gonzalez R, Wright R, Blackard C. Prophylactic antibiotics in transurethral prostatectomy. J Urol 1976;116(2):203-5.

31. Grabe M, Forsgren A, Hellsten S. The effect of a short antibiotic course in transurethral prostatic resection. Scand J Urol Nephrol 1984;18(1):37-42.

32. Hargreave T, Botto H, Rikken G, et al. European collaborative study of antibiotic prophylaxis for transurethral resection of the prostate. Eur Urol 1993;23(4):437-43.

33. Holl W, Rous S. Is antibiotic prophylaxis worthwhile in patients with transurethral resection of prostate? Urology 1982;19(1):43-6.

34. Houle A, Mokhless I, Sarto N, Elhilali M. Perioperative antibiotic prophylaxis for transurethral resection of the prostate: is it justifiable? J Urol 1989;142(2 pt 1):317-19.

35. Ibrahim AI, Rashid M. Comparison of local povidone-iodine antisepsis with parenteral antibacterial prophylaxis for prevention of infective complications of TURP: a prospective randomized controlled study. Eur Urol 2002;41(3):250-6.

36. Kjaergaard B, Petersen E, Lauridsen K, Petersen A. Prophylactic one-dose treatment with clindamycin and gentamicin in transurethral prostatic resection. A double-blind placebo controlled study. Scand J Urol Nephrol 1989;23(2):109-13.

37. Matthew A, Gonzalez R, Jeffords D, Pinto M. Prevention of bacteriuria after transurethral prostatectomy with nitrofurantoin macrocrystals. J Urol 1978;120(4):442-3.

38. Morris MJ, Golovsky D, Guinness MD, Maher PO. The value of prophylactic antibiotics in transurethral prostatic resection: a controlled trial, with observations on the origin of postoperative infection. BJU 1976;48(6):479-84.

39. Murdoch DA, Badenoch DF, Gatchalian ER. Oral ciprofloxacin as prophylaxis in transurethral resection of the prostate. BJU 1987;60(2):153-6.

40. Nielsen O, Maigaard S, Frimodt-Møller N, Madsen P. Prophylactic antibiotics in transurethral prostatectomy. J Urol 1981;126(1):60-2.

41. Ozturk M, Koca O, Kaya C, Karaman MI. A prospective randomized and placebo-controlled study for the evaluation of antibiotic prophylaxis in transurethral resection of the prostate. Urologia Int 2007;79(1):37-40.

42. Prokocimer P, Quazza M, Gibert C, et al. Short-term prophylactic antibiotics in patients undergoing prostatectomy: report of a double-blind randomized trial with 2 intravenous doses of cefotaxime. J Urol 1986;135(1):60-4.

43. Qvist N, Christiansen H, Ehlers D. Prophylactic antibiotics in transurethral prostatectomy. Urologic Res 1984;12(6):275-7.

44. Raz R, Almog D, Elhanan G, Shental J. The use of ceftriaxone in the prevention of urinary tract infection in patients undergoing transurethral resection of the prostate (TUR-P). Infection 1994;22(5):347-9.

45. Rocca Rossetti S, Boccafoschi C, Pellegrini A, et al. Aztreonam monotherapy as prophylaxis in transurethral resection of the prostate: a multicenter study. Rev Infect Dis 1991;13(suppl 7):S626-8.

46. Rodrigues P, Hering F, Meller A, Campagnari JC, d'Império M. A randomized and prospective study on the value of antibiotic prophylaxis administration in transurethral resection of the prostate. Sao Paulo Med J 2004;122:4-7.

47. Scholz M, Luftenegger W, Harmuth H, Wolf D, Höltl W. Single-dose antibiotic prophylaxis in transurethral resection of the prostate: a prospective randomized trial. BJU 1998;81(6):827-9.

48. Shah PJ, Williams G, Chaudary M. Short-term antibiotic prophylaxis and prostatectomy. BJU 1981;53(4):339-43.

49. Shearman CP, Silverman SH, Johnson M, et al. Single dose, oral antibiotic cover for transurethral prostatectomy. BJU 1988;62(5):434-8.

50. Slavis S, Miller J, Golji H, Dunshee C. Comparison of single-dose antibiotic prophylaxis in uncomplicated transurethral resection of the prostate. J Urol 1992;147(5):1303-6.

51. Stricker PD, Grant AB. Relative value of antibiotics and catheter care in the prevention of urinary tract infection after transurethral prostatic resection. BJU 1988;61(6):494-7.

52. Taylor E, Lindsay G. Antibiotic prophylaxis in transurethral resection of the prostate with reference to the influence of preoperative catheterization. J Hosp Infect 1988;12(2):75-83.

53. Viitanen J, Talja M, Jussila E, et al. Randomized controlled study of chemoprophylaxis in transurethral prostatectomy. J Urol 1993;150(5 pt 2):1715-17.

54. Wagenlehner FME, Wagenlehner C, Schinzel S, Naber KG. Prospective, randomized, multicentric, open, comparative study on the efficacy of a prophylactic single dose of 500 mg levofloxacin versus 1920 mg trimethoprim/sulfamethoxazole versus a control group in patients undergoing TUR of the prostate. Eur Urol 2005;47(4):549-56.

55. Weiss J, Wein A, Jacobs J, Hanno P. Use of nitrofurantoin macrocrystals after transurethral prostatectomy. J Urol 1983;130(3):479-80.

56. Williams M, Hole D, Murdoch W, Ogden A, Hargreave T. 48-hour cephradine and post-prostatectomy bacteriuria. J Urol 1980;52:311-15.

8

Venous thromboembolism: risks and prophylaxis in urological surgery

Melissa R. Kaufman and Roger R. Dmochowski

Department of Urologic Surgery, Vanderbilt University, Nashville, TN, USA

Introduction

Contemporary management of the urological surgery patient incorporates perioperative appreciation of the possibility for thromboembolic complications. Venous thromboembolism (VTE) and the sequelae of pulmonary embolism (PE) continue to be one of the most critical nonsurgical morbidities for urological procedures. The magnitude of the issue is staggering, with approximately 10% of hospital deaths attributed to PE [1,2]. The true incidence of such potentially life-threatening complications from VTE and PE is prone to underestimation as these issues frequently manifest following hospital discharge [3].

Vast numbers of randomized clinical trials have provided sound evidence that primary thromboprophylaxis reduces VTE and PE [4]. However, the optimal prophylaxis for urological interventions, whether mechanical or pharmacological, as well as the duration of the treatment remains a largely unanswered question. Indeed, only one randomized controlled trial (RCT) has emerged in the urology literature specifically addressing thromboprophylaxis [5].

The incidence of silent VTE is unknown, as are the long-term repercussions of this seemingly occult condition, but estimates suggest a prevalence of asymptomatic DVT of 15–40% following urological surgery for patients without prophylaxis [4]. For symptomatic VTE, rates are highly dependent on the type of surgical intervention, as will be discussed individually in the following sections. In general, symptomatic VTE in urological surgery patients is estimated to occur at procedure-dependent rates between 1% and 5% [4].

A wide variety of factors are known to influence VTE formation from both the medical and surgical perspective.

These VTE risk factors are generally agreed to be cumulative [6]. Thrombosis is usually focused in the deep veins of the leg (deep vein thrombosis, DVT) including the iliac, femoral, and popliteal veins. Pelvic veins are particularly at risk for thrombosis during many urological surgeries. Thrombosis may also occur for the urological surgery patient in the operating room simply from the venous stasis caused by immobilization and paralysis.

With recognition of the heightened risk in the surgical patient, the American College of Chest Physicians (ACCP) has created extensive guidelines detailing pharmacological and mechanical strategies for prevention of VTE [4]. The ACCP performed a comprehensive review of available medical literature to define evidence-based guidelines for VTE prophylaxis with specific recommendations for urological surgery. Recently, the American Urological Association (AUA) guidelines panel has published the AUA best practice policy statement with risk-stratified recommendations presented in Table 8.1 [7]. This practice statement integrates available evidence from the urological and surgical literature into treatment strategies for pharmacological and mechanical prophylaxis for each category of urological surgery, with the predominant focus being patient risk stratification. The AUA recommends that once the patient's risk profile regarding co-morbidities is identified, the urologist must then determine the specific risk category to which the proposed procedure belongs. In this context, according to the AUA classification, minor surgery is defined as a procedure with a relatively short operating time in which the patient is rapidly ambulatory. This chapter incorporates many of these best practice recommendations to develop strategies for perioperative management to diminish the risk for VTE and PE.

In creating guidelines and recommendations for clinical practice, numerous methods of grading evidence exist with no global consensus regarding method. This multiplicity of grading strategies, despite the best intentions of involved researchers, may actually create confusion for clinicians attempting to make point-of-care decisions. Ideally,

Evidence-Based Urology. Edited by Philipp Dahm, Roger R. Dmochowski.
© 2010 Blackwell Publishing.

Table 8.1 Venous thromboembolism prophylaxis recommendations

Patient risk stratification	Description	Prophylactic treatments
Low risk	Minor surgery in patient <40 years with no additional risk factors	No prophylaxis other than early ambulation
Moderate risk	Minor surgery in patients with additional risk factors Surgery in patients aged 40–60 years with no additional risk factors	LDUH 5000 units every 12 hours subcutaneous OR LMWH 40 mg subcutaneous daily OR Mechanical prophylaxis if risk of bleeding is high
High risk	Surgery in patients >60 years Surgery in patients aged 40–60 years with additional risk factors	LDUH 5000 units every 12 hours subcutaneous OR LMWH 40 mg subcutaneous daily OR Mechanical prophylaxis if risk of bleeding is high
Highest risk	Surgery in patients with multiple risk factors (ex age >40 years, cancer, prior VTE)	LMWH 40 mg subcutaneous daily AND adjuvant mechanical prophylaxis OR LMWH 5000 units every 8 hours subcutaneous AND adjuvant mechanical prophylaxis

quality evidence should be defined by a set of factors that have been described by the Grading of Recommendations Assessment, Development and Evaluation (GRADE) Working Group [8-13]. These definitions of quality evidence incorporate several factors including study limitations, consistency of results, directness of the evidence, precision, publication bias, factors that might increase quality of evidence, large magnitude of effect, plausible confounding factors, and any dose–response gradient. The GRADE system culminates with evidence categorized in a binary fashion as *strong* or *weak* (alternatively termed *conditional*). With regard to utilizing these criteria to create a body of evidence, unfortunately only a single RCT on the critical topic of VTE that meets these standards has been published in the urological literature in the past 20 years [5]. Indeed, even the AUA Best Practice Statement on prevention of DVT remarks that due to the lack of robust data, an evidence table could not be developed [7]. Therefore, much of the data upon which recommendations for urological surgery are based have either been derived from other surgical

disciplines, somewhat limiting their usefulness or emanate from less rigorous types of analyses.

The grade of data and recommendations for VTE prophylaxis as outlined in the ACCP review have been extensively defined in several versions [14]. Briefly, evidence was graded for the recommendations on a scale from 1A to 2C. In this mode of evidence stratification, evidence earning a grade of 1A–C demonstrates clear clarity of risk/benefit and is generally regarded as providing a strong recommendation for implementation in practice. For the clinical questions discussed in this chapter, the individual grades of evidence as assigned by the ACCP as well as the GRADE score, along with an explanation as applied to the particular urological surgery, are outlined.

Even with prophylaxis against thrombosis, events will occur. This has become of increasing concern as federal regulatory agencies are now mandating hospital-wide reforms to prevent VTE, placing the individual practitioner at jeopardy. Many physicians will themselves be graded on the incidence of VTE and PE in their patients, with scant regard for the complexity of the population that may be seen at tertiary care centers or the extenuating factors driving an alternative choice to prophylaxis. If there is a generally accepted protocol at the hospital for VTE prophylaxis, documentation should reflect for each individual patient any deviations in protocol. In addition to utility as a quality metric by the hospital, the use or failure in use of VTE prophylaxis has transformed into a medicolegal issue of substantial importance. Risk assessment must be carried out for each individual patient and treatment options tailored. However, in the age of computerized order entry, often integrated with hospital policy and evidence-based guidelines, decision trees must be overridden by the physician to obtain alternative prophylaxis regimes. Several newer agents are also changing the landscape of VTE prophylaxis, although with every new therapy costs escalate and must be compared against standard regimens with known efficacy and minimal expense.

Modalities of VTE prophylaxis to be discussed include the most commonly employed mechanical and pharmacological agents with robust studies available. With regard to mechanical methods of thromboprophylaxis, early ambulation, graduated compression stockings (GCS) and intermittent pneumatic compression (IPC) devices are the most frequently utilized modalities to reduce venous stasis in the lower extremities. In addition to ease of use and often decreased cost when compared to select pharmaceutical agents, mechanical devices do not increase the risk of hemorrhage. Despite several studies that demonstrate a decreased risk of DVT with mechanical prophylaxis, no studies have reported that these methods diminish the risk of PE or death [4].

For the urologist, a major concern with pharmacological prophylaxis is the risk of postoperative bleeding complications [15,16]. This delicate risk/benefit ratio must be assessed on a case-by-case basis. The majority of contemporary pharmacological prophylaxis is performed with low-dose unfractionated heparin (LDUH) [17], low molecular weight heparin (LMWH) [18] or the activated coagulation factor X inhibitor fondaparinux [19]. Of particular importance for the urological surgery patient is caution regarding use of LMWH and fondaparinux in the setting of renal impairment as their accumulation may potentiate bleeding [4].

Search strategy and study selection criteria

Relevant studies were identified by electronic database query, restricted to English-language literature, of Medline via PubMed to retrieve available articles that described both primary studies and consensus opinions on appropriate aspects of VTE in the surgical patient. Search terms included venous thromboembolism, DVT, and prophylaxis in combination with urology or surgery. Select references were additionally obtained directly from the source material including the ACCP guidelines [4] and the AUA Best Practice Policy Statement on prevention of DVT [7].

Venous thromboembolism prophylaxis for urological surgical procedures

Clinical question 8.1

Should patients undergoing transurethral endoscopic procedures have VTE prophylaxis?

Literature search

Early studies estimated rates of DVT after transurethral prostate resection to be as high as 20% [20]. However, according to more recent large-scale retrospective analysis, the risk of venous thromboembolic disease in patients undergoing transurethral procedures is actually substantially lower [21-23]. In a series including over 58,000 endoscopic procedures from the California Patient Discharge Data Set, the majority of which were transurethral resection of the prostate (TURP), the incidence of symptomatic VTE was 0.3% [22]. Typically, endoscopic procedures are not extended and the patient is generally managed on an outpatient basis, factors contributing to the lower risk profile. Indeed, for general surgical procedures,

the overall risk for low-acuity patients undergoing day surgery is consistently small [24]. The majority of the urological literature regarding VTE and transurethral procedures involves conventional TURP and was published in the remote past [7]. Due to the advent of new technologies which have substantially altered the surgical therapy for TURP and other endoscopic interventions, these series are of historical interest only with limited utility in modern analysis. Indeed, several contemporary technologies can be safely performed in patients on active anticoagulation with warfarin or platelet inhibition agents [25]. When reviewing older series, one must also consider advances in perioperative anesthesia allowing shorter operative times as well as nursing developments which routinely promote protective behaviors such as early ambulation.

Conflicting data have emerged regarding the risk of postoperative hemorrhage in patients undergoing TURP treated with pharmacological prophylaxis, again with the majority of data being mainly historical in context [7]. None of these series incorporates contemporary medical management with 5-alpha reductase inhibitors, use of which often precedes surgical intervention, which may reduce vascular density with a concomitant decrease in hemorrhagic complications [26,27].

Outcomes and recommendations

With reported rates in sizeable series in the range of 0.2–0.3%, the incidence of VTE for selected transurethral procedures is quite low. For the majority of transurethral procedures in patients deemed low risk with regard to co-morbid factors, VTE prophylaxis may be accomplished with early ambulation. Use of mechanical or pharmacological agents for VTE prophylaxis should be reserved for patients with factors producing increased thrombotic risk (Grade 2C).

Clinical question 8.2

Should patients undergoing pelvic reconstructive and/or incontinence procedures have VTE prophylaxis?

Literature search

Most studies on benign pelvic reconstructive procedures emanate from the gynecology literature and report DVT rates of up to 14% in the absence of prophylaxis [28]. The ACCP reports that the risks of this population are similar to those seen in the general surgical population in the absence of gynecological malignancy [4]. Additionally complicating guidelines on the use of thromboprophylaxis for pelvic reconstruction is the vast array of procedures encompassed by the term. Risks of endoscopic or limited transvaginal cases such as mid-urethral slings confer a very different profile from complex transvaginal prolapse or open abdominal fistula repair or sacrocolpopexy [7].

Outcomes and recommendations

Both the ACCP and the AUA concur that for low-risk patients undergoing brief procedures, prophylaxis may be accomplished with early mobilization. For moderate-risk patients undergoing more complex procedures, mechanical or pharmacological agents should be employed. And unless there is a substantial bleeding risk, combination therapy is recommended for high-risk patients undergoing complicated interventions (Grade 2C).

Clinical question 8.3

Should patients undergoing urological laparoscopy, including robotically assisted procedures, receive VTE prophylaxis?

Literature search

Since the widespread use of laparoscopy, in particular robotic-assisted procedures, is a relatively recent advent in urology, evidence-based guidelines for thromboprophylaxis have been developed mainly from the general surgical literature. Obvious limitations exist with this extrapolation, so a recent multi-institutional retrospective review was conducted to assess the rates of symptomatic DVT and PE following robotic-assisted laparoscopic prostatectomy [29]. In this cohort of almost 6000 patients, the rate of symptomatic DVT was very low, at 0.5%. Factors associated with VTE in this population of laparoscopic prostatectomy patients were prior DVT, current tobacco use, larger prostate volume, patient re-exploration, longer operative time, and longer hospital stay. All patients in the study utilized mechanical prophylaxis with GCS or IPC to the lower limbs. Patients in this series treated with heparin prophylaxis had significantly increased intraoperative estimated blood loss, longer hospital stay, higher transfusion rates, and higher reoperation rates.

Outcomes and recommendations

The ACCP found sparse data regarding laparoscopic urological procedures and concluded that it could not make specific recommendations for this group. The AUA guidelines agree that with few trials available to

drive therapeutic interventions, for most laparoscopic procedures only mechanical thromboembolic prophylaxis is recommended. For those patients with additional thromboembolic risk factors, use of one or more of the following is recommended: LDUH, LMWH, IPC or GCS. Additional data specifically addressing urological laparoscopy found increased hemorrhagic complications associated with use of fractionated heparin without a reduction of thrombotic complications compared with sequential compression devices [30] (Grade 2C).

Clinical question 8.4

Should patients undergoing open urological surgery receive DVT prophylaxis?

Literature search

The population at highest risk for thromboembolic disease are patients undergoing major open urological procedures [7]. These individuals often have multiple co-morbid conditions, including malignancy, which dramatically increases the risk for postoperative thrombotic events [31]. Indeed, VTE is the most common cause of death following urological cancer surgery [32]. Urologists may be reluctant to employ thromboprophylaxis consistently as several studies have demonstrated that anticoagulation in the context of pelvic surgery, particularly prostatectomy with lymphadenectomy, increases the risk of prolonged lymphatic drainage and lymphocele formation [33-35]. Alternatively, other prospective studies of men undergoing radical prostatectomy with pelvic lymphadenectomy have failed to find an association between heparin administration and either lymphocele or transfusion [36].

Outcomes and recommendations

The AUA Best Practice policy indicates that at least mechanical prophylaxis should be utilized for all patients undergoing open urological procedures. However, in particularly high-risk groups such as patients undergoing radical cystectomy, combination measures are suggested.

From the ACCP guidelines, data deemed Grade 1A indicate that the magnitude of benefits, risks, burdens, and costs are certain and RCTs generated consistent results. The Grade 1A data recommend the routine use of thromboprophylaxis for all patients undergoing major urological surgery. Grade 1B data indicate that the magnitude of benefits, risks, burdens, and costs are certain; however, RCTs generated inconsistent results. These data indicate that for patients undergoing major urological surgery, thromboprophylaxis may be accomplished with the use of LDUH 2–3 times daily or GCS and/or IPC. **Grade 1C** data are derived from observational studies and provide intermediate-strength recommendations which may change when stronger evidence is available. This grade of data indicates that, for patients undergoing major urological surgery, thromboprophylaxis using a LMWH, fondaparinux or combination therapy is recommended. Many patients undergoing open urological procedures are at substantial risk of postoperative hemorrhage. For these patients, the ACCP and AUA recommend the optimal use of mechanical thromboprophylaxis until the bleeding risk decreases, at which time pharmacological therapies can be employed (**Grade 1A**).

Clinical question 8.5

What are the risk factors for DVT, including procedures?

Literature search

Risk factors generally accepted for development of thromboembolic disease encompass mechanical factors promoting venous stasis, various co-morbid medical conditions, patient age, pharmaceutical therapies, specificities of the surgical intervention, as well as a prior history of DVT [4]. For select urological and orthopedic procedures, the duration of anesthesia may contribute significantly to the incidence of VTE, even when controlling for multiple co-variate factors [32,37]. This may be secondary to not only venous stasis from a supine, immobile position but additionally the effect of increased venous capacitance from the vasodilatory effect of the anesthetic agents [38].

Outcomes and recommendations

As presented in Table 8.1 and extensively outlined in the recent Best Practice statement on prevention of DVT in urological surgery patients, the AUA has stratified patients according to individual risk groups that accommodate many of the predisposing factors for development of VTE. This risk assessment model is additionally embraced by the ACCP to promote a simplified stratification scheme that can rapidly assign risk and implement appropriate prophylaxis [4] (**Grade 2C**).

Clinical question 8.6

What is the optimal method and duration of DVT prophylaxis?

Literature search

Enduring controversy exists concerning the optimal duration of thromboembolic therapy when administered for VTE prophylaxis [4]. With even extensive urological surgeries such as radical prostatectomy enjoying minimal inpatient hospitalization, the persistent risks of VTE manifesting after discharge become pronounced. Studies have indeed suggested that patients remain in a hypercoagulable state for up to a month following surgery [3]. Continuation of anticoagulant therapy following hospital discharge is often determined at the level of the individual patient with special consideration given to patient history, age, and mobility [39]. A recent meta-analysis revealed that prolonged prophylaxis (4 weeks post discharge) with LMWH significantly reduces the risk of symptomatic VTE in patients undergoing major abdominal or pelvic surgery (14.3% vs 6.1%) [3]. In this study, no difference was discovered between groups with regard to either bleeding or mortality. In contrast, another systematic review which utilized the identical studies and employed the aforementioned GRADE system determined that for cancer patients undergoing abdominal or pelvic surgery, no high-quality evidence supported use of extended-duration LMWH for perioperative thromboprophylaxis [40].

Outcomes and recommendations

In the absence of studies reporting on long-term benefit for extended-duration pharmacological prophylaxis specifically in the urological surgery patient, decisions must be accomplished on an individualized basis. The ACCP does recommend that for selected high-risk general and gynecological surgery patients, including some who have undergone major cancer surgery or have previously had VTE, continuing thromboprophylaxis after hospital discharge with LMWH for up to 28 days should be considered (**Grade 2A**).

Conclusion

Venous thromboembolism continues to represent a crucial public health concern with associated morbidity, mortality, and expenditure. Therefore, adherence to methods of prophylaxis for urological surgery patients is an agenda that should merit high priority. Difficulties involving implementation of large-scale RCTs for VTE prophylaxis in the urology patient are enormous, including the estimated need for unrealistic sample sizes to detect a fractional relative risk [29]. However, careful attention to determining the grades of evidence in the literature may dispel some currently promoted therapies that have a tenuous basis in high-level evidence.

Recommendations

Risk stratification for potential thromboembolic disease must be accomplished for every patient prior to each urological intervention. For low-risk individuals undergoing limited procedures, early ambulation may be sufficient. However, as the risk of both patient co-morbidities and interventions increases, mechanical and often pharmacological interventions should be routinely employed to reduce postoperative complications of DVT and PE. Creation of clinical care algorithms and pathways for use of VTE prophylaxis is encouraged to increase compliance and optimize patient safety.

References

1. Lindblad B, Eriksson A, Bergqvist D. Autopsy-verified pulmonary embolism in a surgical department: analysis of the period from 1951 to 1988. Br J Surg 1991;78:849-52.
2. Sandler DA, Martin JF. Autopsy proven pulmonary embolism in hospital patients: are we detecting enough deep vein thrombosis? J R Soc Med 1989;82:203-5.
3. Rasmussen MS, Jorgensen LN, Wille-Jorgensen P. Prolonged thromboprophylaxis with low molecular weight heparin for abdominal or pelvic surgery. Cochrane Database Syst Rev 2009;1: CD004318.
4. Geerts WH, Bergqvist D, Pineo GF, et al. Prevention of venous thromboembolism: American College of Chest Physicians Evidence-Based Clinical Practice Guidelines (8th edition). Chest 2008;133:381S-453S.
5. Soderdahl DW, Henderson SR, Hansberry KL. A comparison of intermittent pneumatic compression of the calf and whole leg in preventing deep venous thrombosis in urological surgery. J Urol 1997;157:1774-6.
6. Rosendaal FR. Venous thrombosis: a multicausal disease. Lancet 1999;353:1167-73.
7. Forrest JB, Clemens JQ, Finamore P, et al. AUA Best Practice Statement for the prevention of deep vein thrombosis in patients undergoing urologic surgery. J Urol 2009;181:1170-7.
8. Jaeschke R, Guyatt GH, Dellinger P, et al. Use of GRADE grid to reach decisions on clinical practice guidelines when consensus is elusive. BMJ 2008;337:a744.
9. Guyatt GH, Oxman AD, Kunz R, et al. Going from evidence to recommendations. BMJ 2008;336:1049-51.
10. Guyatt GH, Oxman AD, Kunz R, et al. Incorporating considerations of resources use into grading recommendations. BMJ 2008;336:1170-3.
11. Guyatt GH, Oxman AD, Kunz R, Vist GE, Falck-Ytter Y, Schunemann HJ. What is "quality of evidence" and why is it important to clinicians? BMJ 2008;336:995-8.
12. Guyatt GH, Oxman AD, Vist GE, et al. GRADE: an emerging consensus on rating quality of evidence and strength of recommendations. BMJ 2008;336:924-6.
13. Schunemann HJ, Oxman AD, Brozek J, et al. Grading quality of evidence and strength of recommendations for diagnostic tests and strategies. BMJ 2008;336:1106-10.
14. Guyatt G, Schunemann HJ, Cook D, Jaeschke R, Pauker S. Applying the grades of recommendation for antithrombotic and thrombolytic therapy: the Seventh ACCP Conference on Antithrombotic and Thrombolytic Therapy. Chest 2004;126:179S-87S.
15. Leonardi MJ, McGory ML, Ko CY. The rate of bleeding complications after pharmacologic deep venous thrombosis prophylaxis: a systematic review of 33 randomized controlled trials. Arch Surg 2006;141:790-7, discussion 7-9.
16. Goldhaber SZ. Prevention of Pulmonary Embolism in Patients Undergoing Urologic Surgery. AUA Update Series. Boston: Brigham and Women's Hospital, 2004.
17. (No authors listed) Prevention of fatal postoperative pulmonary embolism by low doses of heparin. An international multicentre trial. Lancet 1975;2:45-51.
18. Weitz JI. Low-molecular-weight heparins. N Engl J Med 1997;337:688-98.
19. Buller HR, Davidson BL, Decousus H, et al. Subcutaneous fondaparinux versus intravenous unfractionated heparin in the initial treatment of pulmonary embolism. N Engl J Med 2003;349:1695-702.
20. Moser KM. Thromboembolic disease in the patient undergoing urologic surgery. Urol Clin North Am 1983;10:101-8.
21. Collins R, Scrimgeour A, Yusuf S, Peto R. Reduction in fatal pulmonary embolism and venous thrombosis by perioperative administration of subcutaneous heparin. Overview of results of randomized trials in general, orthopedic, and urologic surgery. N Engl J Med 1988;318:1162-73.
22. White RH, Zhou H, Romano PS. Incidence of symptomatic venous thromboembolism after different elective or urgent surgical procedures. Thromb Haemost 2003;90:446-55.
23. Neal DE. The National Prostatectomy Audit. Br J Urol 1997;79(suppl 2):69-75.
24. Ahonen J. Day surgery and thromboembolic complications: time for structured assessment and prophylaxis. Curr Opin Anaesthesiol 2007;20:535-9.
25. Descazeaud A, Robert G, Azzousi AR, et al. Laser treatment of benign prostatic hyperplasia in patients on oral anticoagulant therapy: a review. BJU Int 2009;103:1162-5.
26. Pareek G, Shevchuk M, Armenakas NA, et al. The effect of finasteride on the expression of vascular endothelial growth factor and microvessel density: a possible mechanism for decreased prostatic bleeding in treated patients. J Urol 2003;169:20-3.
27. Donohue JF, Sharma H, Abraham R, Natalwala S, Thomas DR, Foster MC. Transurethral prostate resection and bleeding: a randomized, placebo controlled trial of role of finasteride for decreasing operative blood loss. J Urol 2002;168:2024-6.
28. Nicolaides AN, Breddin HK, Fareed J, et al. Prevention of venous thromboembolism. International Consensus Statement. Guidelines compiled in accordance with the scientific evidence. Int Angiol 2001;20:1-37.
29. Secin FP, Jiborn T, Bjartell AS, et al. Multi-institutional study of symptomatic deep venous thrombosis and pulmonary embolism in prostate cancer patients undergoing laparoscopic or robot-assisted laparoscopic radical prostatectomy. Eur Urol 2008;53:134-45.
30. Montgomery JS, Wolf JS Jr. Venous thrombosis prophylaxis for urological laparoscopy: fractionated heparin versus sequential compression devices. J Urol 2005;173:1623-6.

31. Heit JA, O'Fallon WM, Petterson TM, et al. Relative impact of risk factors for deep vein thrombosis and pulmonary embolism: a population-based study. Arch Intern Med 2002;162: 1245-8.

32. Scarpa RM, Carrieri G, Gussoni G, et al. Clinically overt venous thromboembolism after urologic cancer surgery: results from the @RISTOS Study. Eur Urol 2007;51:130-5, discussion 6.

33. Jessie BC, Marshall FF. Pharmacological prophylaxis of venous thromboembolism in contemporary radical retropubic prostatectomy: does concomitant pelvic lymphadenectomy matter? Int J Urol 2008;15:951-6.

34. Koch MO, Jr JS. Low molecular weight heparin and radical prostatectomy: a prospective analysis of safety and side effects. Prostate Cancer Prostatic Dis 1997;1:101-4.

35. Bigg SW, Catalona WJ. Prophylactic mini-dose heparin in patients undergoing radical retropubic prostatectomy. A prospective trial. Urology 1992;39:309-13.

36. Sieber PR, Rommel FM, Agusta VE, et al. Is heparin contraindicated in pelvic lymphadenectomy and radical prostatectomy? J Urol 1997;158:869-71.

37. Jaffer AK, Barsoum WK, Krebs V, Hurbanek JG, Morra N, Brotman DJ. Duration of anesthesia and venous thromboembolism after hip and knee arthroplasty. Mayo Clin Proc 2005;80:732-8.

38. Lindstrom B, Ahlman H, Jonsson O, Stenqvist O. Influence of anaesthesia on blood flow to the calves during surgery. Acta Anaesthesiol Scand 1984;28:201-3.

39. Bergqvist D, Agnelli G, Cohen AT, et al. Duration of prophylaxis against venous thromboembolism with enoxaparin after surgery for cancer. N Engl J Med 2002;346:975-80.

40. Akl EA, Terrenato I, Barba M, Sperati F, Muti P, Schunemann HJ. Extended perioperative thromboprophylaxis in patients with cancer. A systematic review. Thromb Haemost 2008;100:1176-80.

9 Prophylaxis and treatment of urinary tract infections in adults

S.L. Matheson,[1] Philip Masson,[2] Angela C. Webster[3] and Jonathan C. Craig[3]

[1]Centre for Kidney Research, The Children's Hospital at Westmead, Westmead, New South Wales, Australia
[2]Department of Renal Medicine, Royal Infirmary of Edinburgh, Edinburgh, Scotland
[3]School of Public Health, University of Sydney, New South Wales, Australia

Introduction

Urinary tract infections (UTIs) are defined as the presence of more than 100,000 bacterial colony-forming units per milliliter (cfu/mL) of urine. Associated signs and symptoms include frequency, dysuria, urgency, cloudy urine, lower back pain, fevers, hematuria and pyuria (urine white cell count greater than 10,000/mL). Encompassing a triad of cystitis, urethral syndrome and pyelonephritis, UTIs are one of the most common medical conditions requiring outpatient treatment, with complications resulting in significant morbidity, mortality and financial cost, the latter estimated at $1.6 billion/annum to the US economy alone [1].

Those particularly at risk include infants, pregnant women, the elderly (particularly those in extended care facilities), and patients who are immunosuppressed, have spinal cord injuries, indwelling urinary catheters, diabetes, multiple sclerosis or other underlying neurological or urological anatomical abnormalities. The aim of this chapter is to identify, report and evaluate the evidence to answer common clinical dilemmas in prophylaxis and treatment of urinary tract infections in adults.

Management options

Probiotics/antiseptics

Cranberries have been used widely for the prevention and treatment of UTIs for several decades. Ninety percent water, cranberries also contain mallic acid, citric acid, quinic acid, fructose and glucose. Although controversial, it is proposed that fructose and proacanthocyanidins inhibit adherence of type 1 and a-galactose-specific fimbriated *Escherichia coli* to the uroepithelial cell lining of the bladder. Urinary acidification with vitamin C is also proposed, but a lack of evidence for its ability to significantly alter urinary pH as well as concerns regarding the risk of calcium oxalate stone formation have limited its widespread use.

Pharmaceutical

Prescription of antibiotics for preventing and treating UTIs is the most commonly used strategy. Additionally, manipulation of co-medications prescribed for co-morbidity may be beneficial, as sedatives, narcotic analgesics and anticholinergic drugs may contribute to urinary retention and so exacerbate symptoms and interfere with treatment of UTIs. Use of alpha-adrenergic blocking agents in appropriately screened men over 50 years old may also prove advantageous in reducing urinary retention caused by prostatism.

Methods of systematic literature review

Five common clinical dilemmas were identified and framed into clinical questions. To identify best evidence to answer each question, we sought related systematic reviews of randomized controlled trials (RCT) and any additional RCTs in the published literature. The Cochrane Library and Medline were searched for relevant publications, limited to English-language articles. Sensitive search strategies were devised to answer each question, by combining medical subject headings (MeSH) with text words for UTI, including "urinary tract infection," "bacteriuria" and "pyuria." Terms specific to each question were then added (detailed with each question below). Each search strategy was then limited using terms to identify systematic reviews, meta-analyses and RCT. Search results were then screened, and all systematic reviews of RCTs that addressed each question were included, along with any RCTs

Evidence-Based Urology. Edited by Philipp Dahm, Roger R. Dmochowski.
© 2010 Blackwell Publishing.

published subsequently that also addressed the question. In addition, reference lists of all literature identified for inclusion were also screened to locate any potentially additional relevant publications, to detect either those excluded from the identified systematic reviews but still relevant to our questions or those not found by the database searches.

Once literature was identified, data for outcomes relevant to each question were abstracted and summarized, including details of methodological quality and quantative outcome data. To generate a recommendation from the evidence we had assembled, details of the evidence and its relation to each question were summarized using the Grading of Recommendations, Assessment, Development and Evaluation Working Group (GRADE) system (www.gradeworkinggroup.org/) noting the quality, consistency, directness and other issues of the evidence [2].

Clinical question 9.1

For people with a history of UTI, does the ingestion of cranberries or cranberry products reduce the frequency of subsequent UTI?

Literature search

Search terms included: "beverages," "fruit," "cranberries," "*Vaccinium macrocarpon*," "*Vaccinium oxycoccus*," "*Vaccinium vitis-idaea*."

Evidence

We included three systematic reviews of RCTs and quasi-RCTs [3-5]. One review also included nonrandomized trials (Table 9.1) [5]. No additional RCTs were identified that were not already included in the reviews. Two of the reviews had broad inclusion criteria [3,4] while the third was restricted to trials involving institutionalized elderly people [5]. Most of the RCTs included in the three reviews evaluated the effectiveness of either cranberry juice/cocktail or capsules versus placebo.

Results

One systematic review included meta-analysis of four RCTs evaluating 665 patients, concluding that cranberry products significantly reduced the incidence of UTI by 34% at 12 months compared with no treatment or placebo (relative risk (RR) 0.66, 95% confidence interval (CI) 0.47–0.92), particularly amongst women with recurrent UTI (Table 9.2) [4]. The primary outcome of UTI was variably defined and included symptomatic UTI, symptoms plus single organism growth $> 10^4$ cfu/mL or $> 100,000$ cfu/mL or detection

of asymptomatic or symptomatic bacteriuria $> 10^6$ cfu/mL on monthly urine culture. The reduction in experiencing at least one symptomatic UTI was more marked amongst participants with a history of recurrent UTI and for women with uncomplicated UTI, with a 39% reduction (RR 0.61, 95% CI 0.40–0.91). For elderly men and women, and participants with urinary catheters (intermittent or indwelling), there was no significant difference in incidence of symptomatic UTI. Six additional RCTs were identified in the review but not included in the meta-analysis because of methodological issues or lack of available data to contribute to the data synthesis. Of these, one cross-over RCT reported significant reduction in symptomatic UTI episodes amongst the group of sexually active 18–45-year-old nonpregnant women treated with cranberry product (six UTI cranberry group versus 15 UTI placebo group, N 19, p < 0.05), whilst a quasi-RCT reported a 58% reduction in rate of asymptomatic UTI amongst cranberry-treated elderly women (N 971 urine samples or 0.42, CI 0.23–0.76, p = 0.004). The remaining two systematic reviews identified no further contributory trials or data [3,5].

Grade profile

Quality
The 10 RCTs evaluated in the Jepson systematic review were of variable quality: of the four combined for meta-analysis, three were double blinded, three had adequate allocation concealment, and two reported results by intention to treat (ITT; Table 9.3) [4]. Only two RCTS that were not included in the meta-analysis reported significant results. One of these used unclear methods of allocation, was cross-over in design and did not analyze results by ITT, whilst the other used quasi-randomization, was double blinded but did not use ITT analysis.

Consistency
Trials varied in duration (from 4 weeks to 1 year of active treatment), population (from sexually active women to patients 1 year post spinal cord injury), and dosage (30–300 mL/day cranberry juice or cranberry capsules containing unquantified concentration of active cranberry product). Despite these differences, estimates of treatment effect were similar amongst synthesized trials, with no significant heterogeneity observed among population subgroups.

Precision
Estimates of effect were statistically significant for women with uncomplicated recurrent UTI and elderly women (narrower CI: 0.40–0.91 and 0.23–0.76 respectively), but less certain for elderly men and women combined (CI 0.21–1.22) and for patients with neuropathic bladders (CI 0.51–2.21), with small population size in this latter group (N 48).

Table 9.1 Summary of evidence identified to address clinical questions of prevention and treatment of UTI in adults: population studied and interventions investigated

Study ID	Study participants	Interventions*	Description
Question 1: For people with a history of UTI, does the ingestion of cranberries or cranberry products reduce the frequency of subsequent UTI?			
Griffiths 2003	Prevention of UTI in all patient populations	Cranberries vs no treatment or standard treatment	Overview of 7 systematic reviews and 1 RCT, no meta-analysis
Jepson 2008	Women with a history of recurrent UTI. Elderly men and women and people with either indwelling urinary catheters or intermittent catheterization. 2 RCTs included children	Cranberry juice or capsules vs placebo or no treatment	Systematic review of 10 randomized and quasi-randomized RCTs. Data from 4 were synthesized in meta-analysis
Regal 2006	Institutionalized elderly men and women	Cranberry juice vs none or placebo	Systematic review including 2 RCTs, 1 quasi- and 2 nonrandomized trials, no meta-analysis
Question 2: For people with a history of UTI, do prophylactic antibiotics reduce the frequency of subsequent infection?			
Albert 2004	Nonpregnant women over 14 yrs with a history of min 2 uncomplicated UTIs in the previous year	Various antibiotics vs placebo, 6–12 months treatment duration	Systematic review with meta-analysis of 11 RCTs
Regal 2006	Institutionalized elderly men and women	Various antibiotics vs none	Systematic review including 5 RCTs of short-term treatment, 1 RCTs for long-term treatment, no meta-analysis
Smaill 2007	Pregnant women with asymptomatic bacteriuria	Any antibiotic vs placebo or no treatment	Systematic review with meta-analysis of 11 RCTs
Question 3: For people with UTI, which class of antibiotic is most effective for treating the infection?			
Vazquez 2006	Pregnant women with symptomatic UTI	1 RCT – cephazolin vs ampicillin + gentamicin, and ceftriaxone vs ampicillin + gentamicin , 1 RCT – ampicillin vs nitrofurantoin, 1 RCT – fosfomicin vs ceftibuten	Systematic review, no meta-analysis
Arredondo-Garcia 2004	Premenopausal women over 18 yrs with a clinical diagnosis of acute uncomplicated cystitis	3 days ciprofloxacin vs 7 days trimethoprim-sulfamethoxazole vs 7 days norfloxacin	1 RCT
Bailey 1983	People with symptomatic and asymptomatic UTI	5 days augmentin vs 5 days co-trimoxazole	1 RCT
Bayrak 2007	Women in the second trimester of pregnancy with asymptomatic UTI	Single dose fosfomycin vs 5 days cefuroxime	1 RCT
Buckwold 1982	Women with symptomatic cystitis	Differing doses of sulfisoxazole vs differing doses of trimethoprim-sulfamethoxazole	1 RCT
Fancourt 1984	Inpatients with symptomatic UTI	7 days augmentin vs 7 days co-trimoxazole	1 RCT
Hill 1985	Elderly patients with uncomplicated UTI	10 days norfloxacin vs 10 days amoxicillin	1 RCT
Pedler 1985	Pregnant women with asymptomatic UTI	7 days amoxicillin vs 7 days cephalexin	1 RCT
Pontzer 1983	Nonpregnant women with symptomatic UTI	1 IM dose cephonicid vs 7 days amoxicillin	1 RCT
Minassian 1998	Nonpregnant women 18–65 years with uncomplicated lower symptomatic and asymptomatic UTI	Single-dose fosfomycin vs 5 days trimethoprim	1 RCT
Neu 1990	Nonpregnant women 18–65 years with uncomplicated lower symptomatic and asymptomatic UTI	Single-dose fosfomycin vs amoxicillin	1 RCT
Zinner 1990	Pregnant women with asymptomatic UTI	Single dose fosfomycin vs 7 days pipemidic acid	1 RCT

Study ID	Study participants	Interventions*	Description
Question 4: For people with UTI, what duration of antibiotic therapy is optimal?			
Lutters 2002	Elderly people with uncomplicated UTI	Short course (3–6 days) vs long course (7–14 days), single dose vs short and long course	Systematic review with meta-analysis, 15 RCTs
Milo 2005	Women with uncomplicated UTI	Short course (<3 days) vs long course (7–10 days). 19 RCTs tested the same antibiotic for different durations and 14 tested different antibiotics for different durations	Systematic review with meta-analysis, 33 RCTs
Vazquez 2006	Pregnant women with symptomatic UTI	Single- vs multiple-dose gentamicin	Systematic review, 1 RCT for this comparison, no meta-analysis
Villar 2000	Pregnant women with asymptomatic UTI	Single dose vs short course (4–7 days)	Systematic review with meta-analysis, 10 RCTs
Adelson 1992	Pregnant women with symptomatic and asymptomatic UTI	Single dose vs 10 days ampicillin	1 RCT
Arredondo-Garcia 2004	Premenopausal women over 18 yrs with a clinical diagnosis of acute uncomplicated cystitis	3 days ciprofloxacin vs 7 days trimethoprim-sulfamethoxazole vs 7 days norfloxacin	1 RCT
Bayrak 2007	Women in the second trimester of pregnancy with asymptomatic UTI	Single-dose fosfomycin vs 5 days cefuroxime	1 RCT
Dow 2004	Patients with spinal cord injury and acute UTI	3 days ciprofloxacin plus 11 days placebo vs 14 days ciprofloxacin	1 RCT
Fihn 1988	Women with symptomatic UTI	Single dose + placebo vs 10 days trimethoprim-sulfamethoxazole	1 RCT
Leelarasamee 1995	Women with symptomatic UTI	Single dose vs 3 days pefloxacin	1 RCT
Peterson 2008	Men and women ≥18 years with a diagnosis of either complicated UTI or acute pyelonephritis	5 days levofloxacin vs 10 days ciprofloxacin	1 RCT
Pontzer 1983	Nonpregnant women with symptomatic UTI	Single-dose cephonicid vs 7 days amoxicillin	1 RCT
Minassian 1998	Nonpregnant women 18–65 years with uncomplicated symptomatic and asymptomatic UTI	Single-dose fosfomycin vs 5 days trimethoprim	1 RCT
Richard 2002/ Naber 2004	Women with symptomatic uncomplicated UTI	Single-dose gatifloxacin vs 3 days gatifloxacin vs 3 days ciprofloxin	1 RCT
Schultz 1984	Women with symptomatic acute lower UTI	Single dose vs 10 days trimethoprim-sulfamethoxozole	1 RCT
Ulleryd 2003	Men with presumptive diagnosis of febrile UTI	Ciprofloxacin 2 weeks vs 4 weeks	1 RCT
Zinner 1990	Pregnant women with asymptomatic UTI	Single-dose fosfomycin vs 7 days pipemidic acid	1 RCT
Question 5: For people with UTI, which route of administration is more effective?			
Pohl 2007	Mostly women, some children with symptomatic UTI	6 RCTs switch (parenteral IV or IM then oral) vs 4–14 days parenteral, 5 RCT oral vs 10–14 days switch, 2 RCTs single parenteral plus oral vs switch, both 10 days, 1 RCT oral vs parenteral both 7 days, 1 RCT single IM plus oral vs oral	Systematic review with meta-analysis, 15 RCTs
Vazquez 2006	Pregnant women with symptomatic UTI	1 RCT compared IV followed by oral vs IV, 1 RCT IM ceftriaxone vs IV ampicillin + gentamicin, 1 RCT IM ceftriaxone vs IV cephazolin	Systematic review of 3 RCTs, no meta-analysis
Cherubin 1986	Hospitalized patients with complicated UTI	Parenteral therapy vs oral norfloxacin	1 RCT
Pontzer 1983	Nonpregnant women with symptomatic UTI	Single-dose IM cephonicid vs 7 days oral amoxicillin	1 RCT

*IM, intramuscular; IV, intravenous; RCT, randomized controlled trial; UTI, urinary tract infection; vs, versus

Table 9.2 Summary of evidence of effects of interventions for prevention and treatment of UTI in adults

Study ID	Outcomes relevant to clinical question*	Results
Question 1: For people with a history of UTI, does the ingestion of cranberries or cranberry products reduce the frequency of subsequent UTI?		
Griffiths 2003	Symptomatic and asymptomatic UTI	No additional meta-analysis
Jepson 2008	Symptomatic and asymptomatic UTI	Fewer symptomatic UTIs at 12 months (4 RCTs, N 665, RR 0.66, 95% CI 0.47–0.92, p=0.01, + 1 cross-over RCT, N 19, p<0.005), results most marked for women with a history of recurrent UTI and sexually active women
	Side effects	Reduced bacteriuria in elderly women (1 quasi/cross-over RCT, N 192 or 0.42, 95% CI 0.23–0.76, p=0.004) No significant differences for side effects (no data provided)
Regal 2006	Symptomatic and asymptomatic UTI	No additional meta-analysis
Question 2: For people with a history of UTI, do prophylactic antibiotics reduce the frequency of subsequent infection?		
Albert 2004	Symptomatic, asymptomatic UTI	Fewer asymptomatic UTIs during antibiotic prophylaxis vs placebo (11 RCTs, N 372, RR 0.21, 95% CI 0.13–0.34, p<0.00001). No significant differences after prophylaxis ceased (RR 0.82, 95% CI 0.44–1.53) Fewer symptomatic UTIs during antibiotic prophylaxis vs placebo (7 RCTs, N 257, RR 0.15, 95% CI 0.08–0.28, p<0.00001). No studies assessed symptomatic UTI after prophylaxis ceased
	Side effects	No significant differences in severe side effects (11 RCTs, N 420, RR 1.58, 95% CI 0.47–5.28), mild side effects reported more frequently for antibiotic group (RR 1.78, 95% CI 1.06–3.00)
Regal 2006	Symptomatic and asymptomatic UTI	No additional meta-analysis
Smaill 2007	Pyelonephritis Birthweight	Reduced pyelonephritis for antibiotic group (11 RCTs, N 1955, RR 0.23, 95% CI 0.13–0.41, p<0.00001) Reduced low birthweight (<2500 g) for antibiotic group (7 RCTs, N 1502, RR 0.66, 95% CI 0.49–0.89, p=0.006)
Question 3: For people with UTI, which class of antibiotic is most effective for treating the infection?		
Vazquez 2006	Symptomatic and asymptomatic UTI Recurrence	No significant differences observed for any comparison, cephazolin vs ampicillin + gentamicin (symptomatic and asymptomatic UTI: N 120 or 1.26, 95% CI 0.28–5.77; recurrence: N 107 or 1.56, 95% CI 0.34–7.19) Ceftriaxone vs ampicillin + gentamicin (symptomatic and asymptomatic UTI: N 121 or 3.29, 95% CI 0.55–19.58; recurrence: N 109 or 1.10, 95% CI 0.21–5.68) Ampicillin vs nitrofurantoin (symptomatic and asymptomatic UTI: N 86 or 0.79, 95% CI 0.21–2.93; recurrence: N 86 or 1.58, 95% CI 0.50–4.96) Fosfomicin vs ceftibuten (symptomatic and asymptomatic UTI: N 41 or 2.22, 95% CI 0.19–26.63)
Arredondo-Garcia 2004	Symptomatic and asymptomatic UTI	No significant differences in symptomatic UTI at 5–9 days post treatment (3 days ciprofloxacin 88.7% vs 7 days trimethoprim-sulfamethoxazole 86.4% vs 7 days norfloxacin 84.1%) or asymptomatic UTI at 5–9 days post treatment (91.8%, 85.2% and 86.9% respectively)
Bailey 1983	Asymptomatic UTI Side effects	Fewer asymptomatic UTIs with augmentin vs co-trimoxazole, favoring co-trimoxazole (83% vs 100%, p=0.039). No differences in side effects (no data)
Bayrak 2007	Asymptomatic UTI Side effects	No significant differences in asymptomatic UTI (single-dose fosfomycin 93.2% vs 5 days cefuroxime 95%) No differences in side effects (no data)
Buckwold 1982	Symptomatic and asymptomatic UTI	No significant differences in symptomatic or asymptomatic UTI (no data)
Fancourt 1984	Symptomatic and asymptomatic UTI Side effects	No significant differences in symptomatic UTI (augmentin 96% vs co-trimoxazole 85%) or asymptomatic UTI (augmentin 100% vs co-trimoxazole 88%). Augmentin achieved clinical cure faster (mean 3.2 days vs mean 4.7 days, p = 0.0004)
Hill 1985	Asymptomatic UTI Reinfection	Norfloxacin shows advantage over amoxicillin, although no statistical tests were run (asymptomatic UTI cure: norfloxacin 88%, vs amoxicillin 85%; reinfection: norfloxacin 18% vs amoxicillin 46%)
Pedler 1985	Asymptomatic UTI Side effects	No significant differences in asymptomatic cure (2 weeks: amoxicillin 77% vs cephalexin 74%; 6 weeks: amoxicillin 76% vs cephalexin 60%) or side effects at 2 weeks (amoxicillin 46% vs cephalexin 43%)
Pontzer 1983	Symptomatic and asymptomatic UTI Reinfection	No significant differences in symptomatic and asymptomatic cure (single-dose cefonicid 90% vs 7 days amoxicillin 89%), reinfection (single-dose cefonicid 11% vs 7 days amoxicillin 6%)

Study ID	Outcomes relevant to clinical question*	Results
Minassian 1998	Asymptomatic UTI Recurrence Reinfection	No significant differences day 7–9 bacteriological cure (single-dose fosfomycin 83% vs 5 days trimethoprim 83.3%), day 28 reinfection (single-dose fosfomycin 0.04% vs 5 days trimethoprim 0%), day 28 recurrence (single-dose fosfomycin 0.06% vs 5 days trimethoprim 0.03%)
Neu 1990	Symptomatic and asymptomatic UTI Recurrence Reinfection Side effects	Fewer persistent UTIs for fosfomycin vs amoxicillin (p<0.02) No significant differences for cure (fosfomycin 81.2% vs amoxicillin 71.8%), recurrence (fosfomycin 12.5% vs amoxicillin 7.6%), reinfection (fosfomycin 5% vs amoxicillin 10%) or side effects (fosfomycin 8.7% vs amoxicillin 11.5%)
Zinner 1990	Symptomatic and asymptomatic UTI Recurrence	No significant differences for dysuria cure (single-dose fosfomycin 97% vs 7 days pipemidic acid 91%), urinary frequency (single-dose fosfomycin 79% vs 7 days pipemidic acid 80%), bacteriological cure at 3–5 days (single-dose fosfomycin 96% vs 7 days pipemidic acid 94%), at 10–15 days (single-dose fosfomycin 95% vs 7 days pipemidic acid 91%), at 25–30 days (single-dose fosfomycin 93% vs 7 days pipemidic acid 90%), recurrence at 10–15 days (both 2%), at 25–30 days (both 3%)

Question 4: For people with UTI, which duration of antibiotic therapy is optimal?

Study ID	Outcomes relevant to clinical question*	Results
Lutters 2002	Symptomatic UTI Reinfection Any adverse events	Fewer persistent symptomatic UTIs for short course vs single dose up to 2 weeks post treatment (5 RCTs, N 356, RR 2.01, 95% CI 1.05–3.84, p=0.034), but not over 2 weeks (3 RCTs, N 95, RR 1.18, 95% CI 0.59–2.32). No significant difference in reinfection rate although results favor short course over long term (1 RCT, N 74, RR 2.81, 95% CI 0.91–9.79)
		Fewer persistent symptomatic UTIs for long course vs single dose up to 2 weeks post treatment (6 RCTs, N 628, RR 1.93, CI 1.01–3.70, p=0.047) but not over 2 weeks (3 RCTs, N 95, RR 1.28, 95% CI 0.89–1.84). No differences in adverse events (3 RCTs, N 595, RR 0.80, 95% CI 0.45–1.41)
		No significant differences in short vs long course (short-term 3 RCTs, N 431, RR 0.85, CI 0.29–2.47, long-term 3 RCTs, N 470, RR 0.85, 95% CI 0.54–1.32). No differences in reinfection rates (long-term, 2 RCTs, N 405, RR 1.30, 95% CI 0.42–4.01) or adverse events (1 RCT, N 223, RR 0.87, 95% CI 0.26–2.93). Two RCTs comparing same antibiotic across trial arms reported no difference for persistent UTI at short- (N 208, RR 1.00, 95% CI 0.12–8.57) or long-term follow-up (N 247, RR 1.18, 95% CI 0.50–2.81). Clinical failure was not significantly different in either short- (5 RCTs, N 395, RR 0.98, 95% CI 0.62–1.54) or long-term follow-up (1 RCT, N 223, RR 0.75, 95% CI 0.49–1.33)
		No differences in any outcome, single vs short/long course when short/long course data combined
Milo 2005	Symptomatic and asymptomatic UTI Pyelonephritis Any adverse events	No differences in symptomatic UTI within 2–15 days from the end of treatment for 3 days vs 5 to 10 days (24 RCTs, N 8752, RR 1.06, 95% CI 0.88–1.28) or within 4–10 weeks from the end of treatment (8 RCTs, N 3141, RR 1.09, 95% CI 0.94–1.27). Subgroup analyses showed similar results for trials testing the same antibiotic across groups and those testing different antibiotics across groups
		Fewer asymptomatic UTIs for the 5–10 group within 2–15 days from the end of treatment for 3 days vs 5–10 days (31 RCTs, N 5368, RR 1.19, 95% CI 0.98–1.44, p=0.08) and within 4–10 weeks from end of treatment (18 RCTs, N 3715, RR 1.31, 95% CI 1.08–1.60, p=0.006). Subgroup analyses showed this held only for trials testing same antibiotic in trial arms (2–15 days from end of treatment, 18 RCTs, N 3146, RR 1.37, 95% CI 1.07–1.74, p=0.01, 4–10 weeks 13 RCTs, N 2502, RR 1.43, 95% CI 1.19–1.73, p=0.0002). No significant differences for trials testing different antibiotics (2–15 days post treatment, 13 RCTs, N 2222, RR 0.96, 95% CI 0.68–1.35, p=0.80, 4–10 weeks, 5 RCTs, N 1213, RR 1.13, 95% CI 0.73–1.77)
		No significant differences for the development of pyelonephritis (5 RCTs, N 582, RR 3.04, 95% CI 0.32–28.93) or adverse events (29 RCTs, N 7617, RR 0.83, 95% CI 0.74–0.93)
Vazquez 2006	Symptomatic and asymptomatic UTI	No significant differences for asymptomatic and asymptomatic UTI for single vs multiple dose gentamicin (1 RCT, N 106 or 0.24, 95% CI 0.01–5.17)
Villar 2000	Recurrent asymptomatic UTI Pyelonephritis Side effects	No significant differences for single dose vs short course for "no cure" rates (10 RCTs, N 568, RR 1.25, 95% CI 0.93–1.67), recurrent asymptomatic UTI (7 RCTs, N 336, RR 1.14, 95% CI 0.77–1.67), pyelonephritis (2 RCTs, N 102, RR 3.09, 95% CI 0.54–17.55). For trials assessing the same antibiotic for different durations, no significant differences observed for "no cure" (6 RCTs, N 353, RR1.22, 95% CI 0.84–1.76), recurrence (6 RCTs, N 353, RR 1.08, 95% CI 0.70–1.66) or pyelonephritis (2 RCTs, N 102, RR 3.09, 95% CI 0.54–17.55). Fewer mild side effects for single dose (9 RCTs, N 507, RR 0.52, 95% CI 0.32–0.85, p=0.009)
Adelson 1992	Symptomatic and asymptomatic UTI Reinfection	Fewer symptomatic and asymptomatic UTI for multiple dose vs single dose (67.3% vs 57.1%, no p value)

(Continued on p. 78)

Table 9.2 (Continued)

Study ID	Outcomes relevant to clinical question*	Results
Arredondo-Garcia 2004	Symptomatic and asymptomatic UTI	No significant differences in symptomatic cure at 5–9 days post treatment, (3 days ciprofloxacin 88.7% vs 7 days trimethoprim-sulfamethoxazole 86.4% vs 7 days norfloxacin 84.1%) or for bacteriological cure at 5–9 days (91.8%, 85.2% and 86.9% respectively) or at 4–6 weeks (symptomatic cure, 83.5%, 81.5% and 82.2% respectively), bacterial cure (83.5%, 81.5%, 81.3%)
Bayrak 2007	Asymptomatic UTI Side effects	No significant differences in asymptomatic UTI cure (single-dose fosfomycin 93.2% vs 5 days cefuroxime) or side effects (no data)
Dow 2004	Symptomatic and asymptomatic UTI Recurrence Reinfection	Greater microbiological and symptomatic cure in 14-day group by 3 weeks (microbiological 100% vs 67%, RR 2.50, 95% CI 1.78–3.51, p=0.001, symptomatic 100% vs 83%, RR 2.20, 95% CI 1.65–2.94, p=0.05) and by 6 weeks (microbiological 93% v 73%, RR 2.09, 95% CI 1.38–3.18, p=0.010, symptomatic 100% vs 77%, RR 2.30, 95% CI 1.69–3.13, p=0.01)
Fihn 1988	Symptomatic and asymptomatic UTI Recurrence Side effects	No significant differences in symptomatic and asymptomatic UTI at 3 days (single dose 86% vs 10 day 91%), at 13 days (single dose 68% vs 10 day 79%, p=0.07) or 42 days (no data) No differences or subgroup with clinical diagnosis (N 216) for symptomatic and asymptomatic UTI at 3 days (single dose 89% vs 10 day 92%), 13 days (single dose 68% vs 10 day 77%) or 42 days (single dose 55% vs 10 day 60%) Fewer recurrences among subgroup with clinical diagnosis in the 10-day group at 13 days (N 216, 5% vs 24%, 95% CI 10–28, p=0.0002), not significant at 42 days (21% vs 32%, p=0.07) More side effects in 10-day group (25% vs 12%, p=0.009)
Leelarasamee 1995	Symptomatic and asymptomatic UTI Side effects	No significant differences observed in symptomatic, asymptomatic UTI and side effects
Peterson 2008	Symptomatic and asymptomatic UTI Side effects	No significant differences observed in asymptomatic cure at end of therapy (5 day 79.8% vs 10 day 77.5%, difference 2.3, 95% CI –8.8 to 4.1), symptomatic cure (5 day 82.6% vs 10 day 78.5%, difference 4.1, 95% CI –10.4 to 2.1) or side effects (5 day 35.5% vs 10 day 33%, 95% CI –7.9% to 3.3%) or at post therapy asymptomatic UTI (5 day 79.8% vs 10 day 79.8%. difference 0, 95% CI –6.3 to 6.3), symptomatic cure (5 day 81.1% vs 10 day 80.1%, difference –0.9, 95% CI –7.2 to 5.3)
Pontzer 1983	Symptomatic and asymptomatic UTI Reinfection Side effects	No significant difference in symptomatic and asymptomatic UTI cure (single-dose cefonicid 90% vs 7 days amoxicillin 89%), reinfection (single-dose cefonicid 11% vs 7 days amoxicillin 6%) or side effects (no data)
Minassian 1998	Asymptomatic UTI Recurrence Reinfection	No significant differences at 7–9 days for asymptomatic cure (single-dose fosfomycin 83% vs 5 days trimethoprim 83.3%), at 28 days for reinfection (single-dose fosfomycin 0.04% vs 5 days trimethoprim 0%) or recurrence (single-dose fosfomycin 0.06% vs 5 days trimethoprim 0.03%)
Richard 2002 / Naber 2004	Symptomatic and asymptomatic UTI Side effects	No significant differences for asymptomatic UTI cure (single-dose gatifloxacin 90%, 3-day gatifloxacin 95% and 3-day ciprofloxacin 89%) or clinical cure (single-dose gatifloxacin 93%, 3-day gatifloxacin 95% and 3-day ciprofloxacin 93%). No significant differences in sustained clinical cure 29–42 days post treatment (90%, 88% and 92%) or for side effects (no data)
Schultz 1984	Symptomatic and asymptomatic UTI Reinfection Side effects	Fewer relapses in the multiple-dose therapy group (0.03% vs 15% chi square test, p=<0.02) and fewer mild side effects in the single-dose group (25% vs 41% chi square test, p=<0.05). No differences in reinfection (22% both groups)
Ulleryd 2003	Symptomatic and asymptomatic UTI Side effects	No significant differences in asymptomatic cure at 2 weeks post treatment (2-week treatment group 89% vs 4-week group 97%, 95% CI for difference –3 to 19%) or at 1 year post treatment (2-week group 59% vs 4-week group 76%, 95% CI –5 to 39%) or for clinical cure at 2 weeks post treatment (2-week treatment group 92% vs 4-week group 97% , 95% CI –5 to 15%) and at 1 year post treatment (2-week group 72 vs 4-week group 82%, 95% CI –10 to 30%). Significantly more patients in the 4-week group reported mild side effects (37% vs 12%, p=0.008)
Zinner 1990	Symptomatic and asymptomatic UTI Recurrence	No significant differences in dysuria cure (single-dose fosfomycin 97% vs 7 days pipemidic acid 91%), urinary frequency (single-dose fosfomycin 79% vs 7 days pipemidic acid 80%), bacteriological cure at 3–5 days (single-dose fosfomycin 96% vs 7 days pipemidic acid 94%), at 10–15 days (single-dose fosfomycin 95% vs 7 days pipemidic acid 91%), at 25–30 days (single-dose fosfomycin 93% vs 7 days pipemidic acid 90%), recurrence at 10–15 days (both 2%,) at 25–30 days (both 3%)

Study ID	Outcomes relevant to clinical question*	Results
Question 5: For people with UTI, which route of administration is more effective?		
Pohl 2007	Symptomatic and asymptomatic UTI Re infection Recurrence Adverse events	More asymptomatic UTI cure for parenteral vs oral at the end of 7 days of therapy (1 RCT, N 38, RR 1.38, 95% CI 1.04–1.84) and after 4 weeks (RR 2.00, 95% CI 1.26–3.17) No significant differences for switch vs parenteral at end of treatment for asymptomatic (2 RCTs, N 76, RR 1.11, 95% CI 0.90–1.36) or symptomatic cure (2 RCTs, N 137, RR 1.01, 95% CI 0.94–1.10) or for both combined (4 RCTs, N 294, RR 0.99, 95% CI 0.93–1.06) or after an interval (3 RCTs, N 219, RR 0.99, 95% CI 0.86–1.13). No significant differences in reinfection at end of therapy (1 RCT, N 72, RR 1.00, 95% CI 0.15–6.72) or after an interval (4 RCTs, N 239, RR 0.76, 95% CI 0.30–1.90) or recurrence after an interval (3 RCTs, N 203, RR 2.79, 95% CI 0.30–25.67) or adverse events (4 RCTs, N 292, RR 0.85, 95% CI 0.19–3.83). Heterogeneity for the outcome adverse events was explored via subgroup analyses with pediatric studies having an RR of 0.67 (95% CI 0.30–1.53, I² 0%) and adult studies having an RR of 0.85 (95% CI 0.19–3.83) No significant differences for oral vs switch during treatment for asymptomatic or symptomatic cure (3 RCTs, N 599, RR 1.04, 95% CI 0.97–1.12), at end of therapy (1 RCT, N 54, RR 0.94, 95% CI 0.78–1.13) or after an interval (3 RCTs, N 493, RR 0.97, 95% CI 0.93–1.01). No differences in reinfection after an interval (2 RCTs, N 341, RR 0.64, 95% CI 0.29–1.42), recurrence after an interval (1 RCT, N 54, RR 5.77, 95% CI 0.29–114.79) or adverse events (2 RCTs, N 506, RR 0.96, 95% CI 0.06–15.02) No significant differences for single-shot plus oral vs switch during treatment for symptomatic cure (2 RCTs, N 225, RR 0.93, 95% CI 0.85–1.02), asymptomatic cure after therapy (1 RCT, N 110, RR 0.96, 95% CI 0.79–1.16) or adverse events (2 RCTs, N 225, RR 4.00, 95% CI 0.46–34.75) No significant differences for single-shot plus oral vs oral during treatment for symptomatic and asymptomatic cure (1 RCT, N 69, RR 4.00, 95% CI 0.46–34.75) or for adverse events (1 RCT, N 69, RR 1.37, 95% CI 0.33–5.68)
Vazquez 2006	Symptomatic and asymptomatic UTI Recurrence	No significant differences for IV plus oral vs IV in symptomatic and asymptomatic cure (1 RCT, N 67 or 2.43, 95% CI 0.46–12.90) or for recurrence (1 RCT, N 67 or 1.81, 95% CI 0.45–7.31) No significant differences for IM ceftriaxone vs IV ampicillin + gentamicin in symptomatic and asymptomatic UTI cure (N 121 or 3.29, 95% CI 0.55–19.58), recurrence (N 109 or 1.10, 95% CI 0.21–5.68) No significant differences for IM ceftriaxone vs IV cephazolin in symptomatic and asymptomatic UTI cure (N 117 or 2.84, 95% CI 0.39–20.70), recurrence (N 102 or 0.71, 95% CI 0.15–3.26)
Cherubin 1986	Symptomatic and asymptomatic UTI Side effects	No significant differences in parenteral therapy vs oral norfloxacin (100% vs 87.5%)
Pontzer 1983	Symptomatic and asymptomatic UTI Reinfection Side effects	No significant differences in symptomatic and asymptomatic UTI cure (early follow-up: single-dose IM cefonicid 90% vs 7 days amoxicillin 89%; late follow-up: 89% v 93%) or reinfection (single-dose IM cefonicid 11% vs 7 days amoxicillin 6%) or side effects (no data, reported fewer side effects in IM group)

* Symptomatic and asymptomatic UTI (bacteriuria) is defined as clinical and/or bacteriological cure, reinfection is defined as reinfection of a different bacterial strain, recurrence is defined as recurrence of the same bacterial strain

Directness

All trials examined direct, unconfounded comparisons of cranberry product versus placebo or no treatment. Direct evidence for all sub-populations of interest was included.

Other considerations

Dropout rates differed markedly among trials, and reasons for this were not clear.

Recommendations

For women with recurrent UTI, we propose a strong recommendation (**Grade 1A**) that daily intake of cranberry juice or capsules can reduce the incidence of symptomatic UTI compared to no cranberry product (see Table 9.3) based on consistent, direct, high-quality and precise evidence.

A conditional recommendation (**Grade 2B**) supports the role of cranberry product in reducing the incidence of

Table 9.3 Grade profile of identified evidence for clinical questions

Study ID	Design	Quality	Consistency	Directness	Precision	Other	Overall
Question 1: For people with a history of UTI, does the ingestion of cranberries or cranberry products reduce the frequency of recurrence?							
Griffiths 2003	Systematic overview	RCTs mostly low quality (implied randomization, unclear allocation concealment methods, most not blinded)	Consistent – no measure of heterogeneity	Direct comparisons for cranberry products (juice, capsules) vs none. Direct evidence for women and elderly people. Indirect for other populations	No meta-analysis	High number of dropouts, reporting bias may be evident	Strong recommendation for women
Jepson 2008	Cochrane review	3/4 synthesized studies had adequate randomization and allocation concealment and were double blind, 2 ITT analysis. 2 studies not synthesized reported significant results, 1 of sexually active women – cross-over, unclear methods, blinded, not ITT. The other of elderly women, quasi-randomized, not blinded and not ITT	Consistent, no significant heterogeneity	Direct comparisons for cranberry products (juice, capsules) vs none. Direct evidence for women and elderly people for outcomes and time periods reported. Indirect for other populations	Precise for women, less precise for elderly men and women	Considerable variation in dropout rates, some due to cranberry product intolerance	Conditional recommendation for elderly women
Regal 2006	Systematic review	1 RCT with adequate randomization and allocation concealment and double blind, 1 RCT with implied randomization and double blind, 1 quasi-random, nonblind and 2 nonrandomized, nonblind	Consistent, no measure of heterogeneity	Direct comparisons for cranberry products (juice, capsules) vs none. Direct for elderly men and women. Indirect for other populations	No meta-analysis		
Question 2: For people with a history of UTI, do prophylactic antibiotics reduce the frequency of subsequent infection?							
Albert 2004	Cochrane review	11/11 RCTs implied randomization, 10 were double blinded	Consistent evidence	Direct for the particular antibiotic, dose and duration in each RCT vs placebo/none. Direct for nonpregnant women for outcomes and time periods reported. Indirect for other populations. Different antibiotics in each arm, dose and duration a possible confounder for synthesized data	Precise for nonpregnant women		Strong recommendation for nonpregnant women during the prophylactic period only
Regal 2006	Systematic review, no meta-analysis	Unclear reporting of RCT quality	Consistent results across RCTs (no measure of heterogeneity)	Direct for elderly people. Direct for particular antibiotic, dose and duration in each RCT vs placebo/none. Indirect for other populations	No meta-analysis		Conditional recommendation for pregnant women for prevention of pyelonephritis
Smaill 2007	Cochrane review	7/11 RCTs implied randomization, 4 had inadequate randomization, 3 double blinded	Inconsistent results, significant heterogeneity partly explained by study quality	Direct for particular antibiotic, dose and duration in each RCT vs placebo/none. Direct for pregnant women for outcomes and time periods reported. Indirect for other populations. Different antibiotics in each arm, dose and duration a possible confounder for synthesized data	Precise for pregnant women	Precise results for lower incidence of birthweight <2500 g	

Question 3: For people with UTI, which class of antibiotic is most effective for treating the infection?

Vazquez 2006	Cochrane review	2 RCTs had adequate randomization and allocation concealment, 1 unclear	Judgment not possible as data not synthesized*	Direct for class of antibiotic tested in each RCT. Direct for route of administration (oral) and duration. Direct for pregnant women for outcomes and time periods reported. Indirect for other populations	Small samples	No recommendation favoring one drug class over another is possible
Arredondo-Garcia 2004	RCT	Implied randomization, open label, not ITT	Judgment not possible	Direct for ampicillin plus probenecid vs ampicillin. Direct for premenopausal women for outcomes and time periods reported. Indirect for other populations	Large sample (N 455)	
Bailey 1983	RCT	Implied randomization, not ITT, unsure if blinded	Inconsistent with other RCTs with same class comparison (Fancourt)	Direct for augmentin vs co-trimoxazole. Indirect for population – small RCT, all populations included	Small sample (N 52), CI not reported	Conflicting evidence
Bayrak 2007	RCT	Adequate randomization and allocation concealment, blinded allocation only	Judgment not possible	Direct for fosfomycin vs cefuroxime. Direct for women for outcomes and time periods reported. Indirect for other populations	Moderate sample (N 90), CI not reported	
Buckwold 1982	RCT	Implied randomization, blinding unclear	Judgment not possible	Direct for sulfisoxazole vs trimethoprim-sulfamethoxazole. Direct for women for outcomes and time periods reported. Indirect for other populations	Moderate sample (N 117), CI not reported	
Fancourt 1984	RCT	Implied randomization, single blind	Inconsistent with other RCTs making same class comparison (Bailey)	Direct for augmentin vs co-trimoxazole. Direct for inpatients for outcomes and time periods reported. Indirect for other populations	Small sample (N 52), CI not reported	Conflicting evidence
Hill 1985	RCT	Implied randomization, no mention of blinding	Judgment not possible	Direct for norfloxacin vs amoxicillin. Direct for elderly people for outcomes and time periods reported. Indirect for other populations	Small sample (N 37), CI not reported	No statistical tests were run so stated advantage for norfloxacin over amoxicillin is not confirmed
Pedler 1985	RCT	Implied randomization, single blind	Judgment not possible	Direct for amoxicillin vs cephalexin. Direct for pregnant women for outcomes and time periods reported. Indirect for other populations	Small sample (N 58)	
Pontzer 1983	RCT	Implied randomization, no mention of blinding	Judgment not possible	Direct for nonpregnant women. Direct for cephonicid vs amoxicillin. Indirect for other populations	Small sample (N 39)	

(Continued on p. 82)

Table 9.3 (Continued)

Study ID	Design	Quality	Consistency	Directness	Precision	Other	Overall
Minassian 1998	RCT	Implied randomization, no mention of blinding	Judgment not possible	Direct for fosfomycin vs trimethoprim. Direct for nonpregnant women for outcomes and time periods reported. Indirect for other populations	Large sample (N 547)		
Neu 1990	RCT	Implied randomization, no mention of blinding	Judgment not possible	Direct for fosfomycin vs amoxicillin. Direct for nonpregnant women for outcomes and time periods reported. Indirect for other populations	Moderate sample (N 158)	Only one of four relevant outcomes showed advantage for fosfomycin over amoxicillin	
Zinner 1990	RCT	Implied randomization, unsure if ITT or blinded	Judgment not possible	Direct for fosfomycin trometamol vs pipemidic acid. Direct for pregnant women for outcomes and time periods reported. Indirect for other populations	Moderate sample (N 153)		
Question 4: For people with UTI, which duration of antibiotic therapy is optimal?							
Lutters 2002	Cochrane review	5/15 RCTs had adequate randomization and allocation concealment, 9 implied randomization, 1 inadequate, 3 double blind	Consistent	Direct for short- vs long-course antibiotics. Direct for elderly people for outcomes and time periods reported. Indirect for other populations. Type of antibiotic in each RCT arm a possible confounder in RCTs that vary antibiotic type between trial arms	Large samples, wide CI	Most evidence is based on lower quality RCTs	Strong recommendation for longer term (10 day) for women and patients with spinal cord injury and acute UTI Conditional recommendation for short or long course treatment over single dose for elderly people
Milo 2005	Cochrane review	12/33 RCTs had adequate randomization and allocation concealment, remainder implied randomization, 9 double blind, 3 used ITT analysis	Consistent	Direct for short course vs long course. Direct for women for outcomes and time periods reported. Indirect for other populations and type of antibiotic in each RCT arm a possible confounder in RCTs that vary antibiotic type between trial arms	Large samples	Based on evidence from good-quality RCT	
Vazquez 2006	Cochrane review	1 RCT with adequate randomization and allocation concealment	Consistent	Direct for single vs multiple doses. Direct for pregnant women for outcomes and time periods reported. Indirect for other populations.	Moderate sample (N 106)		

Study	Type	Quality	Consistency	Directness	Sample	Comments
Villar 2000	Cochrane review	1/10 RCTs had adequate randomization and allocation concealment, 5 implied randomization, 4 inadequate or unclear, none were blinded	Consistent	Direct for single dose vs short course. Direct for pregnant women for outcomes and time periods reported. Indirect for other populations and type of antibiotic in each RCT arm a possible confounder in RCTs that vary antibiotic type between trial arms	Large samples	Inconsistent, moderate quality evidence of fewer mild side effects for single dose
Adelson 1992	RCT	Implied randomization and adequate allocation concealment, unclear if ITT or blind	Consistent	Direct for single dose vs 10 days. Direct for pregnant women for outcomes and time periods reported. Indirect for other populations	Moderate size sample (N 202), no CI reported	No statistical tests were reported so stated advantage for 10-day treatment over single dose is not confirmed
Arredondo-Garcia 2004	RCT	Implied randomization, open label, not ITT	Consistent	Direct for 3 day vs 7 days. Direct for premenopausal women for outcomes and time periods reported. Indirect for other populations	Large sample (N 455)	
Bayrak 2007	RCT	Adequate randomization and allocation concealment, blinded allocation only	Consistent	Direct for single dose vs 5 days. Direct for women for outcomes and time periods reported. Indirect for other populations	Small sample (N 84)	
Dow 2004	RCT	Adequate randomization and allocation concealment, double blinded, ITT	Consistent	Direct for 3 days vs 14 days. Direct for patients with spinal cord injury for outcomes and time periods reported. Indirect for other populations	Small sample (N 60)	
Fihn 1988	RCT	Implied randomization, double blind	Consistent	Direct for single dose vs 10 day. Direct for women for outcomes and time periods reported. Indirect for other populations	Large sample (N 255)	
Leelarasmee 1995	RCT	Implied randomization, single blind	Consistent	Direct for single dose vs 3 days. Direct for women for outcomes and time periods reported. Indirect for other populations	Small sample (N 87)	
Peterson 2008	RCT	Implied randomization, double blind	Consistent	Direct for 5 days vs 10 days. Direct for men and women (large sample) for outcomes and time periods reported. Indirect for other populations	Large sample (N 1093)	
Pontzer 1983	RCT	Implied randomization, no mention of blinding	Consistent	Direct for single IM dose vs 7 days. Direct for nonpregnant women for outcomes and time periods reported. Indirect for other populations	Small sample (N 39)	
Minassian 1998	RCT	Implied randomization, no mention of blinding	Consistent	Direct for single oral dose vs 5 days. Direct for nonpregnant women for outcomes and time periods reported. Indirect for other populations	Large sample (N 547)	

(Continued on p. 84)

Table 9.3 (Continued)

Study ID	Design	Quality	Consistency	Directness	Precision	Other	Overall
Richard 2002 Naber 2004	RCT	Implied blinded randomization, unclear participant/clinician blinded	Consistent	Direct for single oral vs 3 day. Direct for women for outcomes and time periods reported. Indirect for other populations	Large sample (N 1102)		
Schultz 1984	RCT	Adequate blind randomization, unclear participant/clinician blinded, not ITT	Consistent	Direct comparison for single dose vs 10 day same antibiotic. Direct for women for outcomes and time periods reported. Indirect for other populations	Moderate sample (N 200)		
Ulleryd 2003	RCT	Adequate randomization, open label	Consistent	Direct for 2 vs 4 weeks. Direct for men for outcomes and time periods reported. Indirect for other populations	Moderate size sample (N 114)		
Zinner 1990	RCT	Implied randomization, unsure if ITT or blinded	Consistent antibiotics	Direct for single dose vs 7 days. Direct for pregnant women for outcomes and time periods reported. Indirect for other populations	Moderate size sample (N 153)		
Question 5: For people with UTI, which route of administration is more effective?							
Pohl 2007	Cochrane review	8/15 RCTs had adequate randomization and allocation concealment, 6 had outcome assessors blind, 3 reported ITT	Consistent, heterogeneity explored through subgroup analysis of age	Direct for parenteral vs oral, although varying durations a possible confounder. Direct for women for outcomes and time periods reported. Indirect for other populations. Duration of treatment a possible confounding factor	Small sample (N 38) for RCT reporting differences	The RCT had unclear methods	Strong recommendation for IV or IM over oral therapy for adults with acute pyelonephritis
Vazquez 2006	Cochrane review	2/3 RCTs with adequate randomization and allocation concealment	Consistent	Direct for IV vs IV and IM vs IV. Direct for pregnant women. Indirect for other populations and type of antibiotics varied among RCTs	Small samples	No data could be synthesized	
Cherubin 1986	RCT	Implied randomization	Consistent	Direct for parenteral vs oral. Direct for hospitalized patients. Indirect for other populations	Small sample (N 28)		
Pontzer 1983	RCT	Implied randomization	Consistent	Direct for IM vs oral. Direct for nonpregnant women. Indirect for other populations	Small sample (N 39)		

CI, confidence interval; ITT, intention to treat; IM, intramuscularly; IV, intravenously; RCT, randomized controlled trial.

asymptomatic bacteriuria in elderly women. This is based on less precise evidence from one RCT and evidence from one quasi-RCT

The unresolved issue in applying these results in clinical practice is that the minimally effective dose of cranberry product remains unclear.

Clinical question 9.2

For people with a history of UTI, do prophylactic antibiotics reduce the frequency of subsequent infection?

Literature search

The following search terms were used: "antibiotic prophylaxis," "antibiotics," "urinary anti-infective agents."

Evidence

Three systematic reviews assessed prophylactic antibiotics versus placebo or no treatment for preventing UTI (see Table 9.1) [5-7]. Again, no additional RCTs were identified. Active prophylaxis agents investigated included a range of antibiotic classes, and members of those classes, with a variety of dosages, dosing schedules and durations of treatment. The outcome reported in reviews and contributing RCTs varied, and defined UTI as either microbiological UTI (culture of more than 100,000 cfu/mL) or clinical recurrence. The three reviews examined prophylactic antibiotic use in three different patient populations; one review included 10 RCTs of antibiotics versus placebo, in nonpregnant women with a history of at least two uncomplicated UTIs in the previous year [6]. Another included only pregnant women with asymptomatic bacteriuria, which affects 5–10% of pregnancies and can lead to acute pyelonephritis in up to 30% of mothers if left untreated [7]. The third review included only institutionalized elderly people [5].

Results

For nonpregnant women with a history of two or more uncomplicated UTIs within the previous year, results were synthesised from 11 trials comparing any antibiotic prophylaxis regimen of at least 6 months' duration versus placebo (see Table 9.2) [6]. During the active treatment phase, antibiotics significantly reduced the risk of microbiological recurrence by 79% (N 372, RR 0.21, CI 0.13–0.34), and clinical recurrence by 85% (N 257, RR 0.15, CI 0.08–0.28). Microbiological recurrence was defined as recurrence of a positive urine culture of $> 10^6$ cfu/mL with isolation of a responsible agent not necessarily the same as that causing original infection or pyuria ($> 10,000$ cfu/mL) plus

symptoms. No significant advantage was seen amongst the antibiotic-treated group once prophylactic treatment had ceased. Antibiotic-treated subjects were 58% (N 420, RR 1.58, CI 0.47–5.28) more likely to describe severe side effects (defined as those requiring withdrawal of treatment) and 78% (RR 1.78, CI 1.06–3.00) more likely to describe mild side effects (defined as not requiring withdrawal of treatment) than those on placebo.

For pregnant women, comparing antibiotic prophylaxis versus placebo, synthesis of 11 RCTs (1955 women) showed a 77% reduction in incidence of pyelonephritis with antibiotics (RR 0.23, CI 0.13–0.41, p < 0.00001) [7]. Among contributing trials, the duration of prophylaxis varied from a single dose to continuation of antibiotics to 6 weeks post partum.

The third systematic review examined the use of prophylactic antibiotics in elderly patients resident in extended care facilities, but did not include a meta-analysis [5]. This review identified five RCTs examining the role of prophylactic antibiotics in patients with indwelling urinary catheters, and concluded that there was a potential role for antibiotics in reducing rates of UTI amongst those with short-duration urinary catheters (3–14 days), on the basis of reduced rates of bacteriuria in three trials. One RCT included patients requiring perioperative indwelling urinary catheters and described a reduction in incidence of bacteriuria from 63% in placebo-treated to 15% in the antibiotic prophylaxis group of patients post gynecological surgery (N 105). Another RCT included in the review saw 8% of treated patients develop UTI versus 26% in the placebo group of 200 patients undergoing a range of abdominal, orthopedic and gynecological interventions, whilst another RCT found statistically significant benefit in patients undergoing abdominal surgery (N 429, 23% incidence UTI in placebo versus 9% incidence in antibiotic group), but not amongst those having vaginal surgery (N 86, UTI 23% treated versus 21% control).

Grade profile

Quality

The review of nonpregnant women included 11 trials with implied randomization although method of allocation concealment was not adequately reported in any, and so was judged unclear by review authors, but 10 of the 11 were double blinded (see Table 9.3) [6]. For pregnant women, the review identified 11 RCTs that reported development of pyelonephritis, which was the only preventive outcome [7]. Of these, none clearly reported method of allocation concealment, four were quasi-randomized, three were described as double blind and an additional five employed placebo. The review of preventive management strategies for UTI in extended care facilities did not systematically report the methodological quality of the five RCTs of catheterized patients [5].

Consistency

Among RCTs of nonpregnant women, there was no heterogeneity of results demonstrated (I^2 0%) [6]. For pregnant women, magnitude of treatment effect was inconsistent among trials (I^2 64% for pyelonephritis), though direction of effect was consistent [7]. This may be explained by study quality. The systematic review of elderly patients enrolled a cohort of catheterized patients, varying from incontinent stroke patients to surgical candidates requiring short-term perioperative catheterization [5]. Results across trials were consistent, though no measure of heterogeneity was reported.

Precision

For nonpregnant women, precise data derive from large sample sizes and narrow confidence ranges of 0.13–0.34 (microbiological recurrence) and 0.008–0.28 (clinical recurrence) for risk reduction during active prophylaxis. For pregnant women, estimates of effect were also precise, with reduction in incidence of pyelonephritis (CI 0.13–0.41). The review of elderly patients provided no meta-analysis, with sparse data and no reporting of confidence intervals for individual RCTs, making assessment of precision impossible.

Directness

In all three systematic reviews, trials made direct comparison of antibiotic therapy versus placebo. Different antibiotics of varying doses and routes of administration were used, with active prophylactic periods varying between single dose and 12 months. The evidence is direct for each population tested, pregnant and nonpregnant women and elderly people and indirect for other populations.

Other

A significant reduction in the incidence of low birthweight babies was seen amongst antibiotic-treated pregnant women (RR 0.66, CI 0.49–0.89, I^2 28%, p = 0.006).

Recommendation

For nonpregnant women, we propose a strong recommendation (Grade 1A) that prophylactic antibiotics reduce the risk of symptomatic and asymptomatic UTI, with only mild side effects observed (nausea, diarrhea and candidiasis) in those taking prophylactic antibiotics. This treatment advantage can be expected only during the period when antibiotics are being administered.

Amongst pregnant women with asymptomatic bacteriuria we suggest a conditional recommendation (Grade 2B) based on moderate-quality evidence supporting antibiotic prophylaxis in reducing the frequency of pyelonephritis. This recommendation is less strong because evidence is from moderate-quality RCT, with some inconsistency of findings.

Patients with catheters indwelling for more than 14 days have not been shown to benefit from antibiotic prophylaxis, although there is low-quality evidence from several RCTs of benefit in those requiring shorter duration catheterization. No recommendation for antibiotics in catheterized elderly patients is supported.

Clinical question 9.3

For people with UTI, which class of antibiotic is most effective for treating the infection?

Literature search

The following search terms were included: "antibiotics," "anti-infective agents," "quinolones," "beta-lactams," "trimethoprim-sulfamethoxazole," "nitrofurantoin."

Evidence

The search identified one relevant systematic review of RCTs in pregnant women with symptomatic UTI (see Table 9.1) [8]. This review included nine trials, but only three RCTs compared different antibiotic classes and reported outcomes of interest. Interventions were varied across trials, so there was no meta-analysis. The search also identified an additional 11 RCTs that were not included in the review, which investigated a variety of patient populations [9-19]. Seven of these RCTs were limited to female patients; three looked at asymptomatic bacteriuria in pregnant women [14,18,19], two examined nonpregnant women aged 18–65 with symptomatic and asymptomatic UTI [12,13], two looked specifically at nonpregnant women with symptomatic UTI [9,15] and another RCT included only premenopausal women with a clinical diagnosis of acute uncomplicated cystitis [16]. The remaining three RCTs included men and women; one looked at male and nonpregnant females aged 16–75 with symptomatic and asymptomatic UTI [17], another recruited inpatients of either sex without age restriction [10] and the final RCT included only elderly noncatheterized patients [11].

Results

The systematic review defined "cure" as symptomatic relief and/or urine clearance by laboratory test [8]. In one study with 120 participants, intravenous (IV) first-generation cephalosporin (cefazolin) appeared no more effective than combined IV penicillin/aminoglycoside at altering cure rate (94% versus 95% or 1.26, CI 0.28–5.77) or incidence of recurrent infections (5.3% versus 8% respectively or 1.56, CI 0.34–7.19; see Table 9.2). Similarly, ceftriaxone versus IV ampicillin and gentamicin showed no difference in cure rate (OR 3.29, CI 0.55–19.58) or recurrent infection (OR 1.10, CI 0.21–5.68). There was no difference demonstrated comparing either oral penicillin (ampicillin) alone with oral nitrofurantoin (cure rate 87% versus 90% or 0.79, CI 0.21–2.93, recurrence rate 19% versus 13% or 1.58, CI 0.50–4.96) or oral fosfomicin with the third-generation cephalosporin oral ceftibuten (cure rate 95% versus 90% or 2.22, CI 0.19–26.63).

Second-generation fluroquinolones (3 days ciprofloxacin 250 mg bd, 7 days norfloxacin 400 mg bd) were compared with 7 days of the sulfonamide co-trimoxazole (160/800 mg) in an RCT of 455 women with uncomplicated UTI [16]. Participants showed no significant differences in rates of clinical and bacteriological resolution of UTI at early follow-up 5–9 days after treatment (cure rates ciprofloxacin 88.7% versus norfloxacin 84.1% versus co-trimoxazole 86.4%, and bacteriological cure rates ciprofloxacin 88.7% versus norfloxacin 86.4% versus co-trimoxazole 85.2%). Another trial recruiting nonpregnant women compared a single intra-muscular dose of the second-generation cephalosporin cefonicid with 7 days of oral amoxicillin [15]. Cure rates were 90% versus 89%, with infection rates 11% versus 6%. Amongst nonpregnant women with symptomatic and asymptomatic UTI, single-dose fosfomycin was compared with trimethoprim (5 days) [12] and with single-dose amoxicillin [13]. There was no difference in cure rate (83% versus 83.3%) or 28-day reinfection rate (0.04% versus 0%) or recurrence rate (0.06% versus 0.03%) in the comparison of fosfomycin with trimethoprim. For single-dose fosfomycin versus single-dose amoxicillin, there were fewer persistent UTI for fosfomycin (p < 0.02) but no difference in cure rate (81.2% versus 71.8%), recurrence (12.5% versus 7.6%), reinfection (5% versus 10%) or side effects (8.7% versus 11.5%) [13].

From one small RCT of 37 elderly men and women with uncomplicated UTI, norfloxacin appeared to show advantage over amoxicillin in reducing reinfection rate (18% versus 46%), though no difference in cure rate for symptomatic or asymptomatic UTI (88% versus 85%) at 2 weeks post treatment and no statistical tests were reported [11].

Co-trimoxazole and co-amoxiclav (clavulinic acid-amoxicillin) were compared head to head in two RCTs including both men and women [10,17]. One reported a significantly higher cure rate with co-trimoxazole (N 52, 100% versus 83%, p = 0.039) [17]. The other found similar cure rates for co-amoxiclav and co-trimoxazole for symptomatic UTI (96% versus 85%) and asymptomatic UTI (100% versus 88% respectively), although time to clinical cure, defined as resolution of signs and symptoms, was faster in the co-amoxiclav group (3.2 days versus 4.7 days, p = 0.0004) [10].

In a study of 153 pregnant women with asymptomatic bacteriuria, no difference in clinical or microbiological cure rate was reported between single-dose fosfomycin and conventional 7-day therapy with the quinolone pipemidic acid (cure rates 96% versus 94%) [19]. Another study of women in the second trimester of pregnancy reported no difference in eradicating bacteriuria between those treated with single-dose fosfomycin or 5 days of cefuroxime (cure rate 93.2% versus 95%, N 80) [18]. Similarly, pregnant women with asymptomatic UTI treated with amoxicillin or cephalexin showed no difference in cure rate at 2 weeks (77% and 74% respectively) or in side effects (46% vs 43%) [14].

Grade profile

Quality

The systematic review included three RCTs of direct head-to-head antibiotic class comparisons, each trial testing different combinations of antibiotic classes (see Table 9.3) [4]. Of these, two used adequate randomization and concealment and one was unclear. Of the other four additional RCTs describing significant outcomes, the RCT comparing co-trimoxazole with co-amoxiclav implied randomization, was not clearly blinded and did not report analysis by ITT [17]. The other RCT making the same comparison also implied randomization and was single blind [10]. The comparison of fosfomycin versus amoxicillin implied randomization and was not clearly blinded [13] nor was the RCT comparing norfloxacin with amoxicillin [11].

Consistency

Consistency was limited given the diverse populations investigated, with multiple drug class comparisons being made, and the diverse definitions used to report varying outcomes. No meta-analysis was possible in the systematic review.

Precision

Precision in treatment estimates was limited by the small sample size of contributing trials within the systematic review, where no meta-analysis was possible, and for the additional trials. The individual RCTs comparing co-trimoxazole with co-amoxiclav both enrolled only 52 patients, and reported no confidence intervals [10,17]. Similarly, the sample size of the other RCT comparing norfloxacin with amoxicillin is small and no confidence intervals are reported (N 37) [11] and in the comparison of fosfomycin with amoxicillin, only a moderate sample size was studied (N 158), and results were mixed [13].

Directness

Within the review, RCTs used the same routes of administration across trial arms, and most RCTs used comparable durations of treatment. The additional RCTs all made direct drug class comparisons. Population comparisons were direct, targeting particular populations in three of the four RCTs [10,11,13] and one small RCT included all populations, which may have confounded results [17].

Recommendation

No recommendation favoring one drug class over another is possible (see Table 9.3). Larger, better designed and reported RCTs of class effectiveness would help to guide antibiotic choice in UTI. Clinicians should be guided by the sensitivity patterns of locally identified uropathogens to select the initial empiric antibiotic and change antibiotics based upon the resistance pattern of the identified uropathogen for affected patients.

Clinical question 9.4

For people with UTI, what duration of antibiotic therapy is optimal?

Literature search

The following search terms were included: "antibiotics," "anti-infective agents," "short/long-term," "duration."

Evidence

The search identified four systematic reviews and 13 additional RCTs (see Table 9.1). One systematic review [20] and seven additional RCTs [12,15,16, 21-24] enrolled women with uncomplicated UTI. Two systematic reviews [8, 25] and three additional RCTs investigated pregnant women [18,19,26]. One systematic review exclusively enrolled elderly women (> 65 years old) with uncomplicated UTI [27]. One RCT looked at both men and women with uncomplicated UTI or acute pyelonephritis [28]. Men were exclusively considered in one RCT [29] whilst patients with spinal cord injuries were the subject of another [30]. Some RCTs evaluated different durations of the same antibiotic, in unconfounded comparison, and others compared different antibiotics and different durations of treatment.

Results

For nonpregnant women, 32 RCTs of 18–65-year-old women with uncomplicated UTI were identified (N 9605), although not all RCTs reported outcomes of interest (see Table 9.2) [20]. Trials were synthesized comparing short course (3 days) with longer courses (5–10 days), with subgroup analysis of RCTs using different antibiotics across each arm, and those using the same antibiotics in each arm. Outcome measures were defined as short- or long-term failure (within 2 or 8 weeks) for symptomatic or bacteriological criteria (positive urine culture).

Overall, short-term symptomatic failure was not significantly different between short and longer course groups (24 trials, N 8752, RR 1.06, CI 0.88–1.28). In the 14 RCTs using the same antibiotic in each arm, the RR was 1.15, CI 0.95–1.39, whilst for the 10 trials using different antibiotics across trial arms, the RR was 0.90, CI 0.62–1.29. Long-term symptomatic failure was reported by eight trials, and showed no significant difference (N 3141, RR 1.09, CI 0.94–1.27). Short-term bacteriological failure (30 RCTs, N 5368) showed no difference for either treatment duration, with RR 1.19, CI 0.98–1.44. The 18 trials comparing the same antibiotic showed a significantly improved bacteriological cure in the longer duration course (N 3146, RR 1.37, CI 1.07–1.74, p = 0.01); this finding was not evident in the trials using different agents in each arm (13 RCTs, N 2222, RR 0.96, CI 0.68–1.35). Overall, long-term bacteriological failure was significantly higher in the short-duration group than the longer treatment arm (18 trials, N 3715, RR 1.31, CI 1.08–1.60, p = 0.006).

Subgroup analysis showed this to hold true for trials with the same drug in each allocation arm (13 RCTs, N 2502, RR 1.43, CI 1.19–1.73, p = 0.0002), with no difference seen when different drugs were used (5 RCTs, N 1213, RR 1.13, CI 0.73–1.77).

Two of the remaining seven RCTs are discussed in relation to class of antibiotic earlier in this chapter [12,15]. An additional RCT looking at nonpregnant women (< 65 years) compared three antibiotic regimens: short course (3 days) ciprofloxacin with longer course (7 days) co-trimoxazole or norfloxacin, with no significant difference in symptomatic cure at early follow-up (5–9 days post treatment, 88.7%, 86.4% and 84.1% respectively) or late follow-up (4–6 weeks post treatment, 83.5%, 81.5%, and 82.2% respectively) [16]. Bacterial cure rate was also no different at either early (91.8%, 85.2%, 86.9%) or late (83.5%, 81.5%, 81.3%) follow-up. Another RCT randomized 136 nonpregnant women with uncomplicated laboratory-proven UTI to either single dose or 10 days of co-trimoxazole, with significantly lower clinical relapse rates with longer treatment (respectively 14% versus 3%, p < 0.02) [24]. Single dose versus 10 days of oral co-trimoxazole was also compared in another RCT of 255 young women with symptomatic UTI [21]. Although differences favored the 10-day dose, none reached statistical significance for cure rate at 3 (single dose 86%, 10 days 91%, p = 0.07) or 13 days (single dose 68%, 10 days 79%, p = 0.07) post treatment. Amongst those with bacteriologically documented UTI (N 216), recurrence was significantly lower in the longer duration group at 13-day follow-up (5% vs 24%, p = 0.0002). Significantly more side effects were reported in the longer duration treatment group (25% vs 12%, p = 0.009). One additional RCT compared single-dose and 3-day fluoroquinolone treatment in women with uncomplicated UTI [23,31]. Single-dose gatifloxacin was compared with 3 days of either gatifloxacin or ciprofloxacin in a study enrolling 1334 women. Bacteriological cure rates of 90%, 95% and 89% respectively were reported, with clinical cure rates of 93%, 95% and 93% at "test of cure" follow-up (5–9 days post treatment). Sustained clinical cure, defined as symptomatic cure 29–42 days post treatment, also revealed no significant differences (90%, 88% and 92%). Finally, one small RCT compared singe dose with 3 days pefloxacin in women with symptomatic UTI and reported no significant differences for symptomatic or asymptomatic UTI or side effects [22].

For pregnant women with symptomatic UTI in pregnancy, one systematic review compared single versus multiple doses of gentamicin, finding no significant difference in cure rate (1 RCT, N 106 or 0.24, CI 0.01–5.17) [8]. Another review evaluated 568 women with asymptomatic bacteriuria in 10 RCTs, comparing 1-day with 7-day treatment [25]. "No cure" was not different between groups (RR 1.25, CI 0.93–1.67) in RCTs comparing different durations of different antibiotics. Incidence of recurrent bacteriuria was similar between groups (7 RCTs, N 336, RR 1.14, CI 0.77–1.67). These findings did not change when considering only the six trials comparing different durations of the same antibiotics, with no significant differences in "no cure" (RR 1.22, CI 0.84–1.76) or recurrent bacteriuria (RR 1.08, CI 0.70–1.66) being seen. Rates of pyelonephritis were similar for short- and long-duration treatment arms (5/52 versus 1/48). Two of the remaining three RCTs are discussed in relation to class of antibiotic earlier in the chapter [18,19]. The other RCT reported a significantly higher cure rate in longer (10 days) treatment versus single dose (67.3% vs 57.1%) in 200 women with symptomatic and asymptomatic bacteriuria [26].

For women over 65 years old, one systematic review evaluated 15 RCTs of 1644 elderly women [27]. Five RCTs compared single-dose versus short-course (3–6 days) treatment. Persistent UTI was less common in the short-course group up to 2 weeks post treatment (N 356, RR 2.01, CI 1.05–3.54, p = 0.034). This advantage was not sustained in the longer term (> 2 weeks), although fewer trials reported this outcome (3 RCTs, N 95, RR 1.18, CI 0.59–2.32). Six RCTs compared single-dose with long-course treatment (7–14 days), finding a significant decrease in persistent UTI for long-course compared to single-dose therapy at short-term (N 628, RR 1.93, CI 1.01–3.70, p = 0.047) but not long-term follow-up (3 RCTs, N 96, RR 1.28, CI 0.89–1.84). Six RCTs compared short-course with long-course treatments. Persistent UTI at short- and long-term follow-up was not significantly different in either group (3 RCTs, N 431, short-term RR 0.85, CI 0.29–2.47, and long-term RR 0.85, CI 0.54–1.32). Two trials compared the same antibiotic across trial arms, again with no difference for persistent UTI at short-term (N 208, RR 1.00, CI 0.12–8.57) or long-term follow-up (N 247, RR 1.18, CI 0.50–2.81). Clinical failure was not significantly different in either short-term (5 RCTs, N 395, RR 0.98, CI 0.62–1.54) or long-term follow-up (1 RCT, N 223, RR 0.75, CI 0.49–1.33).

Men and women with complicated UTI were randomized in one RCT comparing short-course levofloxacin (5 days) with longer course ciprofloxacin (10 days) [28]. At the end of the study, microbiological eradication rates were comparable, at 79.8% and 77.5% respectively (CI for difference –8.8% to 4.1%), and clinical cure rates of 82.6% and 78.5% (CI for difference –7.4 to 4.2%). One RCT exclusively included men with febrile UTI, receiving short- (2 weeks) or long-course (4 weeks) ciprofloxacin [29]. Short-term bacteriological and clinical cure rates (N 14, 89% versus 97%, CI –3 to 19%, and 92% versus 97%, CI –5% to 15% respectively) were not significantly different.

For people with spinal cord injuries, one RCT compared short (3 days) versus longer (14 days) ciprofloxacin treatment for acute UTI, and concluded that longer therapy provided significantly better long-term (6 weeks) microbiological (93% vs 73%, CI 1.38–3.18, p = 0.01) and symptomatic cure (100% vs 77%, CI 1.69–3.13, p = 0.01) [30].

Grade profile

Quality

For women with uncomplicated UTI, the systematic review included 12 of 33 RCTs with adequate randomization and allocation concealment, the remainder using unclear allocation methods (see Table 9.3). Three trials analyzed by ITT, and only nine were double blinded. The additional two RCTs reported adequate allocation concealment but neither analyzed by ITT [21,24]. One was double blind [24] but blinding was unclear in the other [21].

For pregnant women, the review of 10 RCTs judged randomization and allocation concealment adequate in only one RCT, and unclear in the remainder; in no trials were participants blinded [25]. The additional RCT enrolling pregnant women with symptomatic and asymptomatic bacteriuria implied randomization and used adequate concealment but it was unclear whether it was blinded or analyzed by ITT [26].

The systematic review enrolling elderly people included five RCTs with adequate randomization and allocation concealment, nine with unclear allocation, and one inadequate [27]. Only three trials were double blinded.

Patients with spinal cord injuries were considered in one RCT reporting good methodological quality, with adequate randomization and allocation concealment, blinding and ITT analysis [30]. The RCT enrolling men reported adequate allocation concealment, but was not blinded [29].

Consistency

Results in all three reviews and five RCTs reporting significant effects demonstrated consistent effects within and across populations, and across outcomes for advantages of longer term treatments.

Precision

Outcomes for women with uncomplicated UTI gave precise estimates of effect, with data from large numbers of combined RCT synthesized in the review with narrow confidence intervals [20]. Both the additional RCTs studying women had large samples sizes (N 255 and N 200) [21,24]. Similarly precise outcome estimates applied for pregnant women, including CI of 0.32–0.85 for side effects [25]. The review of elderly patients gave less precise estimates from fewer RCTs (5 RCTs, N 356), with wider confidence intervals for all significant outcomes [27]. In the RCT of spinal cord-injured patients with UTI, precision was limited by small sample size (N 60) [30] whilst the RCT of men was moderately sized and reported narrow confidence intervals [29].

Directness

For women, the systematic review gave direct comparisons of short- versus long-course antibiotics in a specific population, but the antibiotics investigated varied widely among trials [20]. The other evidence, provided by two additional RCTs in women, made direct population, duration and antibiotic comparisons [21,24]. Direct comparisons of single-dose versus short-course treatment in a direct population of pregnant women was made in both the review and additional RCTs of pregnant women [25].

Evidence for the elderly was direct with exclusive enrollment of the elderly in contributing RCTs, although antibiotics varied among studies and duration of therapy was defined by a range, with "short" course varying between 3 to 6 days, and "long" course from 7 to 14 days [27]. The RCT of patients with spinal cord injuries [30] and the one that exclusively enrolled men both made direct population, duration and antibiotic comparisons [29].

Recommendations

Among nonpregnant women with symptomatic and asymptomatic uncomplicated UTI, we propose a strong recommendation (Grade 1B) that long-course antibiotics are better than 3-day or single-dose courses in effecting bacteriological cure of UTI. This recommendation is based on evidence of moderate quality, with consistent, precise and direct findings, and also holds for patients with spinal cord injury and acute UTI, where long-course antibiotics (14 days) are more effective at treating both symptomatic and asymptomatic UTI than short course.

For the elderly with uncomplicated UTI, we suggest a conditional recommendation (Grade 2B) that both short- and long-course antibiotics are more effective than a single dose in reducing symptomatic UTI for up to 2 weeks post treatment, but not after 2 weeks post treatment (although it is expected that the risk of late recurrence is due to predisposing causes for recurrent UTI and not related to acute treatment). This recommendation is downgraded from strong as although evidence is of high quality, some RCTs used indirect comparisons of different antibiotics, and duration of benefit is only seen up to 2 weeks post treatment.

For pregnant women and for people with complicated UTI, the same benefit was not demonstrated.

Clinical question 9.5

For people with UTI treated with antibiotics, which route of administration is more effective?

Literature search

The following search terms were used: "antibiotics," "anti-infective agents," "oral," "intravenous," "parenteral," "administration."

Evidence

The search identified two relevant systematic reviews. One review examined mode of administration of antibiotics for severe UTI and included 15 RCTs [32]. Participants in the 15 RCTs were exclusively women and children, with one RCT including pregnant women, and nine RCTs including women and children with symptomatic UTI (see Table 9.1). For the trials including children with adult women, the results for adults alone could not be separated, and so we quote these combined results. The second review examined treatment of pregnant women with UTI, and included nine RCTs, two of which investigated route of administration of antibiotics, and so were relevant to our question [8]. Duration of therapy and class of antibiotics varied among individual RCTs included in the systematic reviews. We also identified two additional RCTs which addressed our question and were not part of either systematic review; one included male and female hospitalized patients with complicated UTI [33], the other evaluated nonpregnant women with symptomatic UTI [15].

Results

The review specifically addressing mode of administration of antibiotics reported outcome measures of cure rates (clinical, microbiological and combined), reinfection rate (new pathogen in urine), relapse rate (initial pathogen in urine) and adverse effects (see Table 9.2) [32]. Six studies of 373 patients compared "switch" therapy, defined as initial parenteral administration (more than one dose delivered via either intramuscular or intravenous route) followed by oral therapy, versus continued parenteral therapy. Clinical cure rate (2 RCTs, N 137, RR 1.01, CI 0.94–1.10), reinfection rates at end of therapy (1 RCT, N 72, RR 1.00, CI 0.15–6.72) and after an interval (4 RCTs, N 239, RR 0.76, CI 0.30–1.90) were not significantly different between switch and continued parenteral administration, and no significant difference was seen for any other outcomes. Switch versus oral therapy was evaluated in five RCTs (N 1040). At end of therapy (1 RCT, N 54, RR 0.94, CI 0.78–1.13), and after an interval (3 RCTs, N 493, RR 0.97, CI 0.93–1.01), no significant differences were seen for clinical and bacteriological and clinical cure. Single-shot versus oral therapy (1 RCT, N 69) showed no significant difference for any outcome (clinical and bacteriological cure, RR 0.97, CI 0.81–1.17). One RCT of 38 adult patients with pyelonephritis comparing oral versus parenteral administration reported a 38% higher bacteriological cure rate at the end of 7 days of therapy in the IM/IV group (RR 1.38, CI 1.04–1.84), increasing by 4 weeks after treatment (RR 2.00, CI 1.26–3.17) compared with those receiving oral therapy.

The review of UTI treatment in pregnancy included two RCTs of pregnant women with symptomatic UTI which compared route of administration, making three comparisons [8]. One compared IV plus oral versus IV administration alone, and showed no significant differences in cure rates of 94% and 87% (N 67 or 2.43, CI 0.46–12.90), and recurrent infection rates of 17% and 10% respectively (N 67 or 1.81, CI 0.45–7.31). The other trial had two head-to-head comparisons: IM ceftriaxone versus IV ampicillin and gentamicin, also with no significant differences in cure rates of 94% in each group (N 121 or 3.29, CI 0.55–19.58) and recurrence of 6% and 5% (N 121 or 1.10, CI 0.21–5.68) respectively; and IM ceftriaxone versus IV cephazolin, with cure rates of 98% and 95% (N 117 or 2.84, CI 0.39–20.70), and recurrence rates of 6% and 8% respectively (N 117 or 0.71, CI 0.15–3.26). No significant difference of any outcomes was seen for varying routes of antibiotic administration.

One additional RCT in nonpregnant women over 18 years old with symptomatic UTI compared single-dose IM cefonicid with 7-day oral amoxicillin, reporting no significant differences between cure rates at early (90% vs 89%) and late (89% vs 93%) follow-up [15]. The other additional RCT compared parenteral therapy with a range of unspecified antibiotics with oral norfloxacin for an unspecified length of time, reporting cure rates, again at an unclear time point, of 100% vs 87.5% (N 28) [33].

Grade profile

Quality
Eight of 15 RCTs in the review of nonpregnant women used adequate allocation concealment, six used blinded outcome assessors, and three reported by ITT analysis (see Table 9.3) [32]. The RCTs favoring parenteral administration over oral for acute pyelonephritis had unclear allocation concealment, did not describe blinding or clearly perform ITT analysis. The two RCTs included in the systematic review of pregnant women used adequate allocation concealment, though no detail of ITT analysis or blinding was provided [8].

Consistency
Results among trials for UTI outcomes were consistent. For adverse events in RCTs of nonpregnant women and children (minor, mainly gastrointestinal upset), moderate heterogeneity was seen among trials comparing switch with parenteral therapy (4 RCTs, N 292, RR 0.85, CI 0.19–3.83, I^2 44.8%), with subgroup analysis suggesting that this might be explained by age – pediatric studies had an RR of 0.67 (CI 0.30–1.53, I^2 0%) and adult studies an RR of 0.85 (CI 0.19–3.83).

Precision
In the studies of pregnant women, sample sizes were small and consequently confidence intervals were large for all outcomes. Amongst nonpregnant women, the trial reporting significant benefit of parenteral administration compared to the oral route included only 38 patients but gave a precise estimate, with narrow confidence intervals, for bacteriological cure rate at 7 days (CI 1.04–1.84) and 4 weeks (CI 1.26–3.17).

Directness
Evidence made direct comparisons of varying route of administration, but trials investigated different antibiotics and for varying durations, which when synthesized gave confounded comparisons.

Other
No data could be combined for meta-analysis for outcomes relevant to pregnant women, with individual trials being underpowered to report any significant effect.

Recommendation

For patients with pyelonephritis, we propose a strong recommendation (**Grade 1C**) based on evidence from one small RCT, that intravenous or intramuscular administration routes are better than oral for improving rates of bacteriological cure in adult patients with acute pyelonephritis. This RCT investigated direct comparison with precise results, but did not report methodology in detail.

Implications for practice

Prophylaxis

Cranberry products are effective at reducing the incidence of UTI in women with recurrent symptomatic UTI, with equivocal evidence for prevention of asymptomatic bacteriuria in elderly women. Their use in patients with neuropathic bladder is not supported by evidence. Large dropout rates in RCTs suggests that poor compliance may limit widespread use.

Prophylactic antibiotics are effective during administration in reducing symptomatic and asymptomatic UTI in nonpregnant women but are associated with increased incidence of mild side effects. Prophylactic antibiotics are also effective at reducing incidence of pyelonephritis in pregnant women. The effect of such a treatment strategy on local bacterial resistance patterns has not been established.

Treatment

Current literature does not provide evidence for determining optimal antibiotic class for either treatment or prophylaxis of UTI. The choice of optimum antibiotic is best guided by local resistance patterns, adverse events, and economic considerations. In patients with uncomplicated symptomatic or asymptomatic UTI, short or long courses are more effective in reducing recurrence than regimens using a single dose, but pregnant women appear to derive no benefit from more prolonged courses of antibiotics and experience significantly more side effects than with a single dose. Route of drug administration does not appear to significantly affect clinical outcomes, other than for patients with pyelonephritis in whom the IM or IV route is preferable.

Implications for research

This evidence summary has provided guidance on prophylaxis and treatment of UTI in adults, but has also highlighted areas where future research might further inform treatment recommendations. UTI may recur so for prophylactic interventions, RCTs with longer study duration would provide useful additional evidence. The effective dosage of cranberry product to prevent UTI is unknown, and further research to establish optimum dosage, and to investigate dropout rate and possible poor tolerability of cranberry juice would inform treatment recommendations. There is currently no evidence for optimal duration or dosages of different prophylactic antibiotics, nor is there any longer-term assessment of postprophylaxis benefit or harm. Unconfounded direct comparisons of the same antibiotic for different treatment durations would provide evidence that is not confounded by antibiotic efficacy, and longer term follow-up would clarify potential harms, such as development of antibiotic resistance in subsequent UTI. Antibiotic class comparisons comparing similar routes and durations of treatment would also inform treatment recommendations.

References

1. Foxman P, Brown P. Epidemiology of urinary tract infections: transmission and risk factors, incidence, and costs. Infect Dis Clin North Am 2003;17(2):227-41.
2. GRADE Working Group. Grading quality of evidence and strength of recommendations. BMJ 2004;328(7454):1490.
3. Griffiths P. The role of cranberry juice in the treatment of urinary tract infections. Br J Commun Nurs 2003;8(12):557-61.
4. Jepson RG, Craig JC. Cranberries for preventing urinary tract infections. Cochrane Database Syst Rev 2008;1:CD001321.
5. Regal RE, Pham CQ, Bostwick TR. Urinary tract infections in extended care facilities: preventive management strategies. Consult Pharm 2006;21(5):400-9.
6. Albert X, Huertas I, Pereiro II, et al. Antibiotics for preventing recurrent urinary tract infection in non-pregnant women. Cochrane Database Syst Rev 2004;3:CD001209.
7. Smaill F, Vazquez JC.Antibiotics for asymptomatic bacteriuria in pregnancy. Cochrane Database Syst Rev 2007;2: CD000490.
8. Vazquez JC,Villar J. Treatments for symptomatic urinary tract infections during pregnancy. Cochrane Database Syst Rev 2003;4:CD002256.
9. Buckwold F, Ludwig P,Harding GK, et al. Therapy for acute cystitis in adult women. Randomized comparison of single-dose sulfisoxazole vs trimethoprim-sulfamethoxazole. JAMA 1982;247(13):1839-42.
10. Fancourt GJ, Matts SG, Mitchell CJ. Augmentin (amoxicillin-clavulanic acid) compared with co-trimoxazole in urinary tract infections. BMJ (Clin Res) 1984;289(6437):82-3.
11. Hill S, Yeates M, Pathy J, Morgan JR. A controlled trial of norfloxacin and amoxicillin in the treatment of uncomplicated urinary tract infection in the elderly. J Antimicrob Chemother 1985;15(4):505-6.
12. Minassian MA, Lewis DA, Chattopadhyay D, et al. A comparison between single-dose fosfomycin trometamol (Monuril) and a 5-day course of trimethoprim in the treatment of uncomplicated lower urinary tract infection in women. Int J Antimicrob Agents 1998;10(1):39-47.
13. Neu H. Fosfomycin trometamol versus amoxicillin – single-dose multicenter study of urinary tract infections. Chemotherapy 1990;36(suppl 1):19-23.
14. Pedler SJ, Bint AJ. Comparative study of amoxicillin-clavulanic acid and cephalexin in the treatment of bacteriuria during pregnancy. Antimicrob Agents Chemother 1985;27(4):508-10.
15. Pontzer RE, Krieger RE, Boscia JA, et al. Single-dose cefonicid therapy for urinary tract infections. Antimicrob Agents Chemother 1983;23(6):814-16.
16. Arredondo-Garcia JL, Figueroa-Damian R, Rosas A, et al. Comparison of short-term treatment regimen of ciprofloxacin versus long-term treatment regimens of trimethoprim/sulfamethoxazole or norfloxacin for uncomplicated lower urinary tract infections: a randomized, multicentre, open-label, prospective study. J Antimicrob Chemother 2004;54(4):840-3.
17. Bailey RR, Bishop V, Peddie B, et al. Comparison of augmentin with co-trimoxazole for treatment of uncomplicated urinary tract infections. NZ Med J 1983;96(744):970-2.

18. Bayrak O, Cimentepe E, Inegol I, et al. Is single-dose fosfomycin trometamol a good alternative for asymptomatic bacteriuria in the second trimester of pregnancy? Int Urogynecol J 2007;18(5):525-9.

19. Zinner S. Fosfomycin trometamol versus pipemidic acid in the treatment of bacteriuria in pregnancy. Chemotherapy 1990;36(suppl 1):50-2.

20. Milo G, Katchman EA, Paul M, et al. Duration of antibacterial treatment for uncomplicated urinary tract infection in women. Cochrane Database Syst Rev 2005;2:CD004682.

21. Fihn S, Johnson C, Roberts PL, Running K, Stamm WE. Trimethoprim-sulfamethoxazole for acute dysuria in women: a single-dose or 10-day course. A double-blind, randomized trial. Ann Intern Med 1988;108(3):350-7.

22. Leelarasamee AL, Leelarasamee I. Comparative efficacies of oral pefloxacin in uncomplicated cystitis. Single dose or 3-day therapy. Drugs 1995;49(suppl 2):365-7.

23. Richard GA, Matthew CP, Kirstein JM, et al. Single-dose fluoroquinolone therapy of acute uncomplicated urinary tract infection in women: results from a randomized, double-blind, multicenter trial comparing single-dose to 3-day fluoroquinolone regimens. Urology 2002;59(3):334-9.

24. Schultz HJ, McCaffrey LA, Keys TF, Nobrega FT. Acute cystitis: a prospective study of laboratory tests and duration of therapy. Mayo Clin Proc 1984;59(6):391-7.

25. Villar J, Lydon-Rochelle MT, Gulmezoglu AM, Roganti A. Duration of treatment for asymptomatic bacteriuria during pregnancy. Cochrane Database Syst Rev 2000;2:CD000491.

26. Adelson MD, Graves WL, Osborne NG. Treatment of urinary infections in pregnancy using single versus 10-day dosing. J Nat Med Assoc 1992;84(1):73-5.

27. Lutters M Vogt N. Antibiotic duration for treating uncomplicated, symptomatic lower urinary tract infections in elderly women. Cochrane Database Syst Rev 2002;3:CD001535.

28. Peterson J, Kaul S, Khashab M, et al. A double-blind, randomized comparison of levofloxacin 750 mg once-daily for five days with ciprofloxacin 400/500 mg twice-daily for 10 days for the treatment of complicated urinary tract infections and acute pyelonephritis. Urology 2008;71(1):17-22.

29. Ulleryd P, Sandberg T. Ciprofloxacin for 2 or 4 weeks in the treatment of febrile urinary tract infection in men: a randomized trial with a 1 year follow-up. Scand J Infect Dis 2003;35(1):34-9.

30. Dow G, Rao P, Harding G, et al. A prospective, randomized trial of 3 or 14 days of ciprofloxacin treatment for acute urinary tract infection in patients with spinal cord injury. Clin Infect Dis 2004;39(5):658-64.

31. Naber KG, Allin DM, Clarysse L, et al. Gatifloxacin 400 mg as a single shot or 200 mg once daily for 3 days is as effective as ciprofloxacin 250 mg twice daily for the treatment of patients with uncomplicated urinary tract infections. Int J Antimicrob Agents 2004;23(6):596-605.

32. Pohl A. Modes of administration of antibiotics for symptomatic severe urinary tract infections. Cochrane Database Syst Rev 2007;4:CD003237.

33. Cherubin CS, Stilwell S. Norfloxacin versus parenteral therapy in the treatment of complicated urinary tract infections and resistant organisms. Scand J Infect Dis 1986;48(suppl):32-7.

10 Medical management of benign prostatic hyperplasia

John M. Hollingsworth, Elizabeth Soll and John T. Wei

University of Michigan, Department of Urology, Division of Health Services Research,
Ann Arbor, MI, USA

Clinical question 10.1

Is combination medical therapy (i.e. use of an alpha-1-adrenergic-antagonist plus a 5-alpha-reductase inhibitor) more efficacious than monotherapy with either drug class?

Background

While surgery was historically the mainstay of benign prostatic hyperplasia (BPH) care, the preferred initial treatment for the majority of men with symptomatic BPH today is either with an alpha-1-adrenergic antagonist, a 5-alpha-reductase inhibitor or a combination of both. Indeed, a recent American Urological Association (AUA) Gallup survey revealed that 88% of urologists recommended alpha-1-adrenergic antagonists for the initial care of men with moderate lower urinary tract symptoms (LUTS) and evidence of prostate enlargement [1].

High-level evidence supports the use of such medical therapies. Several short to moderate-term studies demonstrated the ability of alpha-1-adrenergic antagonists to both relieve symptoms and improve urinary flow rates [2-5]. Long-term trial data showed that the 5-alpha-reductase inhibitor finasteride not only ameliorated symptoms but also halted disease progression [6]. Adrenergic antagonists reduce smooth muscle tone in the prostate and bladder neck, whereas 5-alpha-reductase inhibitors reduce prostate volume through induction of epithelial atrophy. Given that the effects of these two medication classes are mediated by different mechanisms, investigators hypothesized an additive effect of using the combination of an alpha-1-adrenergic antagonist and a 5-alpha-reductase inhibitor.

Literature search

The English-language literature was searched for human studies relating to combination medical therapy using the Medline database from 1993, the year that the US Food and Drug Administration approved the first alpha-1-adrenergic-antagonist for BPH treatment, to 2008. The search was conducted by exploding the following MeSH terms: "combination therapy and benign prostatic hyperplasia." Only randomized controlled trials comparing combination medical therapy with placebo or an active control were eligible for inclusion in this systematic review. Initially, 117 citations were identified in the database search. Articles were reviewed from 16 pertinent abstracts. Those excluded were nonresearch reports (e.g. editorials and commentaries), studies on the wrong topic (e.g. trials involving different interventions and observational studies) and studies without report of clinical outcome. To judge the clinical trial quality, a numerical score between 0 and 5 (0 being the weakest and 5 being the strongest) was assigned according to the validated scale reported by Jadad et al. [7].

The evidence

The literature search yielded four randomized controlled trials that were reviewed in detail (Table 10.1). The first was the 52-week, multicenter Veterans Affairs Cooperative study, which randomized 1229 men aged 45–80 years to receive placebo, terazosin, finasteride or the combination of both drugs [8]. Eligibility criteria included a mean AUA Symptom Index score of at least 8 and a mean peak urinary flow rate of 4–15 mL per second. Among the 1007 men who completed the study, the authors found that while the terazosin and combination therapy groups had similar symptomatic relief (mean changes from baseline in symptom scores were decreases of 6.1 and 6.2 points, respectively) and improved peak urinary flow rates (mean changes were increases of 2.7 and 3.2 mL per second, respectively) compared to the placebo and finasteride groups, the combination

Evidence-Based Urology. Edited by Philipp Dahm, Roger R. Dmochowski.
© 2010 Blackwell Publishing.

Table 10.1 Randomized clinical trials comparing combination medical therapy to placebo or an active control

Authors	Intervention	Number randomized	Number completed	Therapy duration	Results	Adverse events
Roehrborn et al. [13] (CombAT)	Treatment 1: tamsulosin (0.4 mg daily) Treatment 2: dutasteride (0.5 mg daily) Treatment 3: combination of both drugs	Treatment 1 = 1611 Treatment 2 = 1623 Treatment 3 = 1610	Treatment 1 = 1254 Treatment 2 = 1301 Treatment 3 = 1267	2 years	1. Treatment 3 resulted in a significantly greater improvement in symptom scores compared to Treatments 1 and 2 2. There was a significantly greater improvement from baseline peak urinary flow rates for Treatment 3 compared to Treatments 1 and 2	Treatment 1 = 136 Treatment 2 = 108 Treatment 3 = 154
McConnell et al. [10] (MTOPS)	Treatment 1: doxazosin (8 mg daily) Treatment 2: finasteride (5 mg daily) Treatment 3: combination of both drugs	Treatment 1 = 756 Treatment 2 = 768 Treatment 3 = 786 Placebo = 737	Treatment 1 = 582 Treatment 2 = 565 Treatment 3 = 598 Placebo = 534	6 years	1. Treatments 1, 2, and 3 significantly reduced the risk of overall clinical progression compared to placebo 2. The reduction in risk associated with Treatment 3 was significantly greater than that associated with Treatments 1 or 2 3. The risks of urinary retention and need for surgery were significantly reduced by Treatments 2 and 3	Treatment 1 = 22.22* Treatment 2 = 17.37* Treatment 3 = 28.51* Placebo = 14.25*
Kirby et al. [9] (PREDICT)	Treatment 1: doxazosin (4–8 mg daily) Treatment 2: finasteride (5 mg daily) Treatment 3: combination of both drugs	Treatment 1 = 275 Treatment 2 = 264 Treatment 3 = 286 Placebo = 270	Treatment 1 = 250 Treatment 2 = 239 Treatment 3 = 265 Placebo = 253	1 year	1. Treatments 1 and 3 produced significant improvements in total symptom scores compared to Treatment 2 and placebo 2. Treatments 1 and 3 produced significant improvements in peak urinary flow rates compared to Treatment 2 and Placebo 3. Treatment 3 provided no further benefit to that achieved by Treatment 1	Treatment 1 = 32 Treatment 2 = 34 Treatment 3 = 35 Placebo = 30
Lepor et al. [8] (VA Co-operative)	Treatment 1: terazosin (10 mg daily) Treatment 2: finasteride (5 mg daily) Treatment 3: combination of both drugs	Treatment 1 = 305 Treatment 2 = 310 Treatment 3 = 309 Placebo = 305	Treatment 1 = 256 Treatment 2 = 243 Treatment 3 = 254 Placebo 254	1 year	1. Symptom scores were significantly lower than baseline for Treatments 1 and 3 2. Symptom scores were significantly lower for Treatments 1 and 3 than for Treatment 2 and Placebo 3. Mean peak urinary flow rates were significantly higher for Treatments 1 and 3 than for Treatment 2 and Placebo 4. Treatment 3 was no more efficacious than Treatment 1	Treatment 1 = 18 Treatment 2 = 15 Treatment 3 = 24 Placebo = 5

CombAT, combination of Avodart® and tamsulosin; MTOPS, medical therapy of prostatic symptoms; PREDICT, Prospective European Doxazosin and Combination Therapy; VA, Veterans Affairs
*Rate/100 person-years of follow-up

of terazosin and finasteride offered no additional benefit over terazosin alone with respect to those outcomes.

The Prospective European Doxazosin and Combination Therapy trial followed [9]. This 52-week, multicenter study randomized 1095 men aged 50–80 years to treatment with doxazosin, finasteride, doxazosin plus finasteride or placebo. Patients with a total International Prostate Symptom Score (IPSS) of at least 12 and a mean peak urinary flow rate between 5 and 15 mL per second were eligible for inclusion.

Although only 771 subjects (71%) completed the study, the discontinuations were evenly distributed amongst all four groups. Compared with the placebo and finasteride monotherapy groups, both the doxazosin and doxazosin plus finasteride groups experienced similar and statistically significant improvements from baseline in urinary flow rates (mean increases of 3.6 and 3.8 mL per second, respectively) and IPSS (mean decreases of 8.3 and 8.5 points, respectively). However, no statistically significant difference was demonstrated between the doxazosin and doxazosin plus finasteride groups.

The preceding two 52-week trials primarily assessed longitudinal changes in urinary symptom scores and flow rates. The Medical Therapy of Prostatic Symptoms trial (MTOPS) was conducted in order to examine the long-term effect of combination medical therapy on risk of clinical progression [10]. This 6-year, multicenter study randomized 3047 men aged 50 years and older to receive placebo, doxazosin, finasteride or combination medical therapy of doxazosin plus finasteride. Over a mean follow-up of 4.5 years, combination medical therapy significantly reduced the risk of overall clinical progression by 66% when compared with placebo. This reduction in risk was significantly greater than that associated with doxazosin or finasteride alone. Of note, approximately 78% of the primary outcome events took the form of improvement in AUA symptom scores. Further, doxazosin, finasteride and combination medical therapy each resulted in significant improvement in AUA symptom scores (median changes were decreases of 6.0, 5.0 and 7.0 points, respectively), with combination medical therapy superior to either monotherapy alone. Subsequent *post hoc* analysis of these data suggested that larger prostate volume was a strong predictor of benefit from combination medical therapy, and the risk of clinical progression amongst prostate volumes less than 25 mL was not statistically different between combination medical therapy and either monotherapy alone [11].

To further address the role of combination medical therapy for men with larger prostate glands, the Combination of Avodart® and Tamsulosin trial was conceived [12]. This 4-year, multicenter trial randomized 4844 men 50 years and older to receive dutasteride and tamsulosin-matched placebo, tamsulosin and dutasteride-matched placebo or combination medical therapy. Men with prostate volumes of 30 mL or greater and a total IPSS of at least 12 were eligible for inclusion. The investigators recently reported the results of a preplanned 2-year interim analysis. Combination medical therapy was associated with a significantly greater decrease from baseline in symptom score compared with dutasteride (at month 3) and tamsulosin group (at month 9)

alone [13]. Moreover, increases in peak urinary flow rates from baseline were significantly greater for combination medical therapy when compared with either monotherapy.

Comment

The reviewed trials of combination medical therapy are of substantially high quality (Table 10.2). In accordance with the Grading of Recommendations, Assessment, Development, and Evaluation (GRADE) Working Group statement [14], the published data provide strong support for long-term combined use of doxazosin and finasteride to reduce the risk of BPH progression (1A recommendation). And, in men with large glands (volumes greater than 30 mL), there is strong evidence to suggest that combined use of tamsulosin and dutasteride provides added symptom amelioration compared with either therapy alone. It remains uncertain whether there is a "class effect" (i.e. ability to generalize these findings to other pharmacotherapies within the same classes).

Clinical question 10.2

Is there a role for antimuscarinic agents in the treatment of male LUTS associated with BPH?

Background

Overactive bladder syndrome, characterized by urinary urgency and increased day and night-time micturition frequency [15], may co-exist with bladder outlet obstruction caused by BPH or may be secondary to the obstruction itself [16]. When the former situation occurs, treatments targeted at the prostate exclusively may not relieve overactive bladder symptoms [17]. In the latter scenario, some men will not respond to antimuscarinics alone. This is the rationale behind combining antimuscarinic agents with alpha-1-adrenergic antagonists for the management of men with overactive bladder and other LUTS.

Table 10.2 Study quality assessment using Jadad scores for combination medical therapy trials

Study	Study described as randomized?	Method used to generate the sequence of randomization described?	Described as double blind?	Was the method of double blinding described and appropriate?	Description of withdrawals and dropouts?	Jadad score [7]
Roehrborn et al. [13]	Yes	Yes	Yes	Yes	Yes	5
McConnell et al. [10]	Yes	Yes	Yes	Yes	Yes	5
Kirby et al. [9]	Yes	Yes	Yes	Yes	Yes	5
Lepor et al. [8]	Yes	Yes	Yes	Yes	Yes	5

Literature search

The English-language literature was searched for human studies relating to antimuscarinic therapy for the treatment of male LUTS associated with BPH using the Medline database from 1998, the year that tolterodine earned US Food and Drug Administration approval, to 2008. The search was conducted by exploding and combining the following MeSH terms: "muscarinic antagonists and benign prostatic hyperplasia," "adrenergic alpha-antagonists and benign prostatic hyperplasia," "muscarinic antagonists and luts," and "adrenergic alpha-antagonists and luts." Only randomized controlled trials comparing combination medical therapy, with antimuscarinics and adrenergic alpha-antagonists, with placebo or an active control were eligible for inclusion in this systematic review. Initially, 63 citations were identified in the electronic database search. Articles excluded were nonresearch reports (e.g. editorials and commentaries), studies on the wrong topic (e.g. trials involving different interventions and observational studies) or studies which did not include clinical outcomes. To judge quality of the clinical trials, a numerical score between 0 and 5 (0 being the weakest and 5 being the strongest) was assigned according to the validated scale reported by Jadad et al. [7].

The evidence

The literature search yielded six randomized controlled trials that were reviewed in detail (Table 10.3). First, in terms of safety, there exists the theoretical risk that the inhibitory effect of antimuscarinics could aggravate the voiding difficulties of men with concomitant bladder outlet obstruction, causing acute urinary retention. These concerns were echoed by a recent, multicenter Japanese study [18]. In total, 101 men with clinically diagnosed BPH and storage symptoms were randomized to receive the alpha-1-adrenergic antagonist naftopidil or naftopidil plus the anticholinergic agent propiverine hydrochloride for 12 weeks. After completing treatment, the median postvoid residual was significantly higher in the combination group compared with the naftopidil monotherapy group (45.0 versus 13.5 mL) but there were no cases of acute urinary retention. In that same year, results were also reported from a multicenter, double-blind trial that randomized 222 men 40 years and older with confirmed overactive bladder and bladder outlet obstruction to receive tolterodine or placebo for 12 weeks [19]. This study found that the mean change from baseline postvoid residual urine was significantly greater with tolterodine than placebo (49 versus 16 mL) although the clinical significance of this difference was uncertain. There were no significant between-group differences in the incidence of adverse events. Moreover, urinary retention was only reported for one subject who had been treated with placebo.

With respect to efficacy, several small clinical trials demonstrated the benefit of combining an antimuscarinic agent with an alpha-1-adrenergic-antagonist compared to use of an alpha-1-adrenergic antagonist agent alone. Athanasopoulos and colleagues randomized 50 consecutive men with urodynamically demonstrated bladder outlet obstruction and detrusor overactivity to receive tamsulosin versus tamsulosin plus tolterodine [20]. At 3-month assessment only those receiving the combination of tamsulosin and tolterodine reported significant improvement in quality of life scores (mean improvement from baseline of 102.6 points). Comparisons of urodynamic parameters before and after treatment revealed statistically significant differences for both groups favoring the combination of tamsulosin and tolterodine over monotherapy. The incidence of dropouts due to side effects was low amongst both groups. Two years later, Lee et al. reported the results of their multicenter trial in which 228 men aged 50–80 years with overactive bladder and urodynamically validated bladder outlet obstruction were randomized to receive doxazosin or doxazosin plus the antimuscarinic propiverine hydrochloride for 8 weeks [21]. At study completion, a more pronounced improvement in storage symptoms was detected amongst those treated with the combination of doxazosin plus propiverine compared with doxazosin alone. Specifically, greater rates were observed in the combination therapy group for urinary frequency (23.5% versus 14.3%), average micturition volume (32.3% versus 19.2%) and storage (41.3% versus 32.6%) when compared with monotherapy. In addition, those treated with the combination of doxazosin plus propiverine reported significantly higher satisfaction with overall treatment compared to those receiving doxazosin alone. Discontinuation and adverse event rates were similar between the combination and monotherapy groups.

In contrast to two prior studies with inclusion criteria based on urodynamic parameters, Yang et al. conducted an active-control trial, in which inclusion was based primarily on urinary symptoms, increasing its generalizability [22]. In total, 69 men with irritative LUTS associated with BPH were randomized into two groups, one receiving terazosin and the other terazosin plus tolterodine. After 6 weeks of treatment, the combination therapy group experienced a significantly greater reduction from baseline in mean IPSS scores compared with the terazosin group. Although no between-group differences were detected, both groups experienced increases in peak urinary flow rates and decreases in postvoid residuals.

The only placebo-controlled, randomized trial comparing combined use of an antimuscarinic and an alpha-1-adrenergic antagonist to either therapy alone was performed by Kaplan et al. [23]. In total, 879 men at least 40 years old were randomized to receive 12 weeks of placebo, extended-release (ER) tolterodine, tamsulosin or tolterodine ER plus

Table 10.3 Randomized clinical trials comparing an antimuscarinic agent (alone or combined with an alpha-1-adrenergic antagonist) to placebo or an active control

Authors	Intervention	Number randomized	Number completed	Therapy duration	Results	Adverse events
Yang et al. [22]	Treatment 1: terazosin (2 mg daily) Treatment 2: terazosin plus tolterodine (2 mg twice daily)	Treatment 1 = 36 Treatment 2 = 33	Treatment 1 = 36 Treatment 2 = 33	6 weeks	1. Symptom scores were significantly improved in both groups after treatment, but the reduction with Treatment 2 was significantly greater 2. Differences in peak urinary flow rates and residual urines were noted from baseline values in both groups, but the between-group differences were not significant	Treatment 1 = 1 Treatment 2 = 6
Kaplan et al. [23]	Treatment 1: tolterodine ER (4 mg daily) Treatment 2: tamsulosin (0.4 mg daily) Treatment 3: combination of both drugs	Treatment 1 = 210 Treatment 2 = 209 Treatment 3 = 217 Placebo = 215	Treatment 1 = 189 Treatment 2 = 186 Treatment 3 = 191 Placebo = 188	12 weeks	1. Patients receiving Treatment 3 compared with placebo experienced significant reductions in urge incontinence, urgency episodes, micturitions per 24 hours, and night-time micturitions 2. Patients receiving Treatment 3 had significant improvements on the symptom scores compared to those receiving placebo	Treatment 1 = 43 Treatment 2 = 60 Treatment 3 = 106 Placebo = 37
Abrams et al. [19]	Tolterodine (2 mg twice daily)	Treatment = 150 Placebo = 72	Treatment = 133 Placebo = 60	12 weeks	1. There were significant differences in the volume to first detrusor contraction and maximum cystometric capacity in patients treated with tolterodine versus placebo 2. There were no significant differences between groups in the incidence of adverse events	Treatment = 5 Placebo = 9
Maruyama et al. [18]	Treatment 1: naftopidil (25–75 mg daily) Treatment 2: naftopidil plus propiverine hydrochloride (10–20 mg daily)	Treatment 1 = 53 Treatment 2 = 48	Treatment 1 = 44 Treatment 2 = 36	12 weeks	1. Median post-therapy residual urine volume was significantly worse for patients receiving Treatment 2 versus Treatment 1 2. The ratio of patients with increased residual urine volume was significantly higher for Treatment 2 versus Treatment 1	Treatment 1 = 2 Treatment 2 = 3
Lee et al. [21]	Treatment 1: doxazosin (4 mg daily) Treatment 2: doxazosin plus propiverine hydrochloride (20 mg daily)	Treatment 1 = 69 Treatment 2 = 142	Treatment 1 = 67 Treatment 2 = 131	8 weeks	1. Compared to Treatment 1, improvement rates with regard to urinary frequency, average micturition volume, urgency, and symptom score were more significant with Treatment 2 2. Patient satisfaction rates were significantly higher with Treatment 2 versus Treatment 1	Treatment 1 = 1 Treatment 2 = 7
Athanasopoulos et al. [20]	Treatment 1: tamsulosin (0.4 mg daily) Treatment 2: tamsulosin plus tolterodine (2 mg twice daily)	Treatment 1 = 25 Treatment 2 = 25	Treatment 1 = 24 Treatment 2 = 22	3 months	1. There was a statistically significant improvement in quality of life score among patients receiving Treatment 2 2. There were statistically significant improvements in urodynamic parameters for those patients receiving Treatment 2	Treatment 1 = 1 Treatment 2 = 3

ER, extended release

tamsulosin. The primary efficacy endpoint was perception of treatment benefit. Secondary efficacy measures included changes from baseline in urge urinary incontinence episodes per 24 hours, total micturitions per 24 hours and micturitions per night. Although neither group receiving monotherapy reported a significantly greater treatment benefit compared with placebo, significantly more subjects (80%) receiving tolterodine ER plus tamsulosin reported treatment benefit by week 12 compared with 62% receiving placebo. What is more, subjects in the tolterodine ER plus tamsulosin group experienced significant reductions in all overactive bladder symptoms compared with the placebo group. The combination of tolterodine ER and tamsulosin was well tolerated, and the incidence of urinary retention was low (0.4%).

Comment

The reviewed trials of antimuscarinic therapy for treatment of overactive bladder and BPH are of mixed quality, two high and four moderate (Table 10.4). In accordance with the GRADE Working Group statement [14], the published data provide strong support for short-term safety and efficacy of tamsulosin plus tolterodine ER for LUTS associated with BPH (1B recommendation). Long-term data are still needed. Given the variety of antimuscarinic agents available, the optimal combination and regimen has yet to be determined.

Clinical question 10.3

Are there contemporary data demonstrating an efficacy of saw palmetto for symptomatic BPH?

Background

Treatment of BPH with phytotherapy was described as early as the 15th century BCE [24]. Widely used in Europe

for BPH symptom relief [25-28], plant extracts offer an alternative to pharmaceutical agents and the related side effects. Indeed, the popularity of phytotherapy is growing in the US, with an estimated 1% of American adults reporting use of extracts of the *Serenoa repens* fruit [29], one of the most extensively studied herbal remedies for BPH. Acting through multiple mechanisms, including modulation of human 5-alpha-reductase [30], the active ingredient from the *Serenoa repens* berry is thought to be the lipid/sterol extract saw palmetto. A high-profile systematic review and meta-analysis of the available literature published in the late 1990s by Wilt et al. suggested that saw palmetto extracts improved LUTS and urinary flow measures [31]. However, the effect sizes reported in the pooled studies were small, partially due to small sample sizes and relatively short study durations. As such, the authors fell short of giving saw palmetto extracts unequivocal endorsement for the management of BPH.

Literature search

The English-language literature was searched for human studies relating to saw palmetto for the treatment of BPH using the Medline database from 1999, the year after the Wilt et al. meta-analysis [31], to 2008. The search was conducted by exploding the following MeSH terms: "phytotherapy," "plant extracts" and "Serenoa," each combined with "benign prostatic hyperplasia." Only randomized controlled trials comparing an oral preparation of the saw palmetto extract to placebo or an active control were included in this systematic review. Initially, 38, 24 and 49 citations respectively were identified in the electronic database search. Articles excluded were nonresearch reports (e.g. editorials and commentaries), studies on the wrong topic (e.g. trials involving different interventions and observational studies) or studies without report of clinical outcomes (e.g. those examining enzyme or tissue effects). Studies which examined use of a saw palmetto extract in combination with

Table 10.4 Study quality assessment using Jadad scores for antimuscarinic therapy trials

Study	Study described as randomized?	Method used to generate the sequence of randomization described?	Described as double blind?	Was the method of double blinding described and appropriate?	Description of withdrawals and dropouts?	Jadad score [7]
Yang et al. [22]	Yes	Yes	No	No	Yes	3
Kaplan et al. [23]	Yes	Yes	Yes	Yes	Yes	5
Abrams et al. [19]	Yes	Yes	Yes	Yes	Yes	5
Maruyama et al. [18]	Yes	Yes	No	No	Yes	3
Lee et al. [21]	Yes	No	Yes	No	Yes	3
Athanasopoulos et al. [20]	Yes	Yes	No	No	Yes	3

other phytotherapeutic agents (e.g. roots of the stinging nettle) were also excluded. To judge the quality of the clinical trials, a numerical score between 0 and 5 (0 being the weakest and 5 being the strongest) was assigned according to the validated scale reported by Jadad et al. [7].

The evidence

The literature search yielded four randomized controlled trials that were reviewed in detail (Table 10.5). The first was reported by Marks and colleagues, in which 44 men from a single general urology practice in metropolitan Los Angeles were randomized to receive a saw palmetto herbal blend versus placebo [32]. Following a 1-month placebo lead-in, subjects were treated and followed for 6 months. Throughout the study and at completion, a variety of clinical parameters were assessed including IPSS, urinary flow rate and postvoid residual urine. A slight decrease in symptom scores (mean changes were decreases of 3.05 points for the placebo group and 5.58 points for the saw palmetto group) and a slight increase in urinary flow rates (mean changes were increases of 0.58 and 2.65 mL per second, respectively) were noted for subjects in both groups. While these changes were slightly greater in the saw palmetto group, the differences were not statistically significant. Overall, the saw palmetto extract was well tolerated and no adverse events were noted.

Two years later, Debruyne et al. published the results of an equivalency trial, comparing Permixon® (one trade name for the *Serenoa repens* lipid/sterol extract) with tamsulosin [33]. In this multicenter trial, 704 men were randomized to one of the two treatment arms and followed for 1 year. Eligibility criteria included an IPSS of at least 10 and a peak urinary flow rate between 5 and 15 mL per second. After study completion, IPSS decreased by 4.4 in both groups. No differences were noted between groups for either the irritative or obstructive IPSS domains. In addition, peak urinary flow rates increased similarly in both treatment groups. The treatments were well tolerated with only a similarly small number of subjects discontinuing therapy from each group. Given these data, the authors concluded that Permixon and tamsulosin were clinically equivalent. However, in the absence of a placebo arm, the investigators were unable to comment on the efficacy of Permixon.

In 2003, an Australian group reported the results of a single-institution clinical trial in which 100 men with symptomatic BPH were randomized to receive *Serenoa repens* extract versus placebo [34]. Men with at least three symptoms related to BPH (e.g. frequency of micturition, nocturia, hesitancy, poor force of stream, etc.) were eligible for participation. After 12 weeks of treatment, mean IPSS scores and improvements in peak urinary flow rates were not significantly different between the treatment and control groups. A subsequent long-term, multicenter

Table 10.5 Randomized clinical trials comparing saw palmetto extract to placebo or an active control

Authors	Intervention	Number randomized	Number completed	Therapy duration	Results	Adverse events
Bent et al. [35]	Saw palmetto extract (160 mg twice daily)	Treatment = 112 Placebo = 113	Treatment = 102 Placebo = 104	1 year	1. Both treatment and placebo groups had similar small decreases in their mean symptom scores 2. There was no significant difference between treatment and placebo groups in the change in peak urinary flow rates	Treatment = 8 Placebo = 18
Willetts et al. [34]	*Serenoa repens* extract (320 mg daily)	Treatment = 50 Placebo = 50	Treatment = 46 Placebo = 47	12 weeks	1. There was no significant difference in the decrease in symptom scores over time between the treatment and placebo groups 2. There was no significant difference between treatment and placebo groups in peak urinary flow rates after the trial	Treatment = 4 Placebo = 3
Debruyne et al. [33]	Treatment 1: Permixon (320 mg daily) Treatment 2: tamsulosin (0.4 mg daily)	Treatment 1 = 340 Treatment 2 = 345	Treatment 1 = 296 Treatment 2 = 298	1 year	1. Improvements in symptom scores were similar between Treatments 1 and 2 2. Increases in urinary flow rates were similar between Treatments 1 and 2	Treatment 1 = 28 Treatment 2 = 30
Marks et al. [32]	Saw palmetto herbal blend (320 mg daily)	Treatment = 21 Placebo = 23	Treatment = 20 Placebo = 23	6 months	Both treatment and placebo groups had similar small improvements in clinical parameters from baseline	Treatment = 0 Placebo = 0

Table 10.6 Study quality assessment using Jadad scores for saw palmetto trials

Study	Study described as randomized?	Method used to generate the sequence of randomization described?	Described as double blind?	Was the method of double blinding described and appropriate?	Description of withdrawals and dropouts?	Jadad score [7]
Bent et al. [35]	Yes	Yes	Yes	Yes	Yes	5
Willetts et al. [34]	Yes	Yes	Yes	Yes	Yes	5
Debruyne et al. [33]	Yes	No	Yes	No	Yes	3
Marks et al. [32]	Yes	Yes	Yes	Yes	Yes	5

trial confirmed those results [35]. In total, 225 men with moderate-to-severe BPH symptoms, based on the AUA Symptom Index score, were randomized to receive saw palmetto extract versus placebo. After 12 months of treatment both groups had small decreases in symptom scores, but those differences were insignificant over time between groups. In addition, peak urinary flow rates did not differ between the treatment and placebo groups at any time during the study period. These data led the authors to conclude that saw palmetto did not improve LUTS caused by BPH.

Comment

The majority of reviewed trials of saw palmetto therapy for symptomatic BPH are of high quality (Table 10.6). In accordance with the GRADE Working Group statement [14], these data do not support the efficacy of saw palmetto over placebo (1A recommendation).

Implications for practice and future research

In summary, there exists high-quality evidence supporting the long-term combined use of doxazosin and finasteride to reduce the risk of BPH progression. In addition, clinical trial data suggest that the combined use of tamsulosin and dutasteride provides added symptom amelioration compared with either therapy alone. As such, combination medical therapy is recommended as an initial treatment strategy in men with moderate LUTS and prostate volumes of 25 mL and greater. Further research is required to determine if a "class effect" exists by testing other combinations of alpha-1-adrenergic antagonists and 5-alpha-reductase inhibitors.

To date, the published data provide strong support for short-term safety and efficacy of tamsulosin plus tolterodine ER for men with overactive bladder and LUTS. However, long-term data are still needed before this approach can be fully recommended. Given the variety of antimuscarinic

agents available, the optimal combination and regimen remain to be determined.

Finally, since contemporary data do not support the efficacy of saw palmetto over placebo, this phytotherapy is not recommended in the management of LUTS associated with BPH. Additional randomized, placebo-controlled trials are necessary in order to determine whether other phytotherapies are useful treatments for benign prostatic hyperplasia.

References

1. Gee WF, Holtgrewe HL, Albertsen PC, et al. Subspecialization, recruitment and retirement trends of American urologists. J Urol 1998;159:509-11.
2. Roehrborn CG, Siegel RL. Safety and efficacy of doxazosin in benign prostatic hyperplasia: a pooled analysis of three double-blind, placebo-controlled studies. Urology 1996;48:406-15.
3. Roehrborn CG, Oesterling JE, Auerbach S, et al. The Hytrin Community Assessment Trial study: a one-year study of terazosin versus placebo in the treatment of men with symptomatic benign prostatic hyperplasia. HYCAT Investigator Group. Urology 1996;47:159-68.
4. Roehrborn CG. Efficacy and safety of once-daily alfuzosin in the treatment of lower urinary tract symptoms and clinical benign prostatic hyperplasia: a randomized, placebo-controlled trial. Urology 2001;58:953-9.
5. Kawabe K. Efficacy and safety of tamsulosin in the treatment of benign prostatic hyperplasia. BJU 1995;76(suppl):7.
6. McConnell JD, Bruskewitz R, Walsh P, et al. The effect of finasteride on the risk of acute urinary retention and the need for surgical treatment among men with benign prostatic hyperplasia. Finasteride Long-Term Efficacy and Safety Study Group. N Engl J Med 1998;338:557-63.
7. Jadad AR, Moore RA, Carroll D, et al. Assessing the quality of reports of randomized clinical trials: is blinding necessary? Contr Clin Trials 1996;17:1-12.
8. Lepor H, Williford WO, Barry MJ, et al. The efficacy of terazosin, finasteride or both in benign prostatic hyperplasia. Veterans Affairs Cooperative Studies Benign Prostatic Hyperplasia Study Group. N Engl J Med 1996;335:533-9.

9. Kirby RS, Roehrborn C, Boyle P, et al. Efficacy and tolerability of doxazosin and finasteride, alone or in combination, in treatment of symptomatic benign prostatic hyperplasia: the Prospective European Doxazosin and Combination Therapy (PREDICT) trial. Urology 2003;61:119-26.

10. McConnell JD, Roehrborn CG, Bautista OM, et al. The long-term effect of doxazosin, finasteride, and combination therapy on the clinical progression of benign prostatic hyperplasia. N Engl J Med 2003;349:2387-98.

11. Kaplan SA, McConnell JD, Roehrborn CG, et al. Combination therapy with doxazosin and finasteride for benign prostatic hyperplasia in patients with lower urinary tract symptoms and a baseline total prostate volume of 25 ml or greater. J Urol 220;175:217-20.

12. Siami P, Roehrborn CG, Barkin J, et al. Combination therapy with dutasteride and tamsulosin in men with moderate-to-severe benign prostatic hyperplasia and prostate enlargement: the Comb-AT Combination of Avodart and Tamsulosin. trial rationale and study design. Contemp Clin Trials 2007;28:770-9.

13. Roehrborn CG, Siami P, Barkin J, et al. The effects of dutasteride, tamsulosin and combination therapy on lower urinary tract symptoms in men with benign prostatic hyperplasia and prostatic enlargement: 2-year results from the CombAT study. J Urol 621;179:616-21.

14. Guyatt G, Vist G, Falck-Ytter Y, Kunz R, Magrini N, Schunemann H. An emerging consensus on grading recommendations? ACP J Club 2006;144:A8-A9.

15. Abrams P, Cardozo L, Fall M, et al. The standardisation of terminology in lower urinary tract function: report from the standardisation sub-committee of the International Continence Society. Urology 2003;61:37-49.

16. Abdel-Aziz KF, Lemack GE. Overactive bladder in the male patient: bladder, outlet or both? Curr Urol Rep 2002;3:445-51.

17. Chapple CR, Roehrborn CG. A shifted paradigm for the further understanding, evaluation, and treatment of lower urinary tract symptoms in men: focus on the bladder. Eur Urol 2006;49:651-8.

18. Maruyama O, Kawachi Y, Hanazawa K, et al. Naftopidil monotherapy vs naftopidil and an anticholinergic agent combined therapy for storage symptoms associated with benign prostatic hyperplasia: a prospective randomized controlled study. Int J Urol 2006;13:1280-5.

19. Abrams P, Kaplan S, de Koning Gans HJ, Millard R. Safety and tolerability of tolterodine for the treatment of overactive bladder in men with bladder outlet obstruction. J Urol 2006;175(3 pt 1):999-1004.

20. Athanasopoulos A, Gyftopoulos K, Giannitsas K, Fisfis J, Perimenis P, Barbalias G. Combination treatment with an alpha-blocker plus an anticholinergic for bladder outlet obstruction: a prospective, randomized, controlled study. J Urol 2003;169:2253-6.

21. Lee KS, Choo MS, Kim DY, et al. Combination treatment with propiverine hydrochloride plus doxazosin controlled release gastrointestinal therapeutic system formulation for overactive bladder and coexisting benign prostatic obstruction: a prospective, randomized, controlled multicenter study. J Urol 2005;174 (4 pt 1):1334-8.

22. Yang Y, Zhao XF, Li HZ, et al. Efficacy and safety of combined therapy with terazosin and tolteradine for patients with lower urinary tract symptoms associated with benign prostatic hyperplasia: a prospective study. Chinese Med J 2007;120:370-4.

23. Kaplan SA, Roehrborn CG, Rovner ES, Carlsson M, Bavendam T, Guan Z. Tolterodine and tamsulosin for treatment of men with lower urinary tract symptoms and overactive bladder: a randomized controlled trial. (Erratum appears in JAMA 2007;297(11):1195.) JAMA 2006;296:2319-28.

24. Dreikorn K, Richter R. Conservative nonhormonal treatment of patients with benign prostatic hyperplasia. In: *New Developments in Biosciences 5: prostatic hyperplasia*. Berlin: Walter de Gruyter, 1989:109-31.

25. Berges RR, Windeler J, Trampisch HJ, Senge T. Randomised, placebo-controlled, double-blind clinical trial of beta-sitosterol in patients with benign prostatic hyperplasia. Beta-sitosterol Study Group. Lancet 1995;345:1529-32.

26. Buck AC, Cox R, Rees RW, Ebeling L, John A. Treatment of outflow tract obstruction due to benign prostatic hyperplasia with the pollen extract, cernilton. A double-blind, placebo-controlled study. BJU 1990;66:398-404.

27. Champault G, Patel JC, Bonnard AM. A double-blind trial of an extract of the plant Serenoa repens in benign prostatic hyperplasia. Br J Clin Pharmacol 1984;18:461-2.

28. Fitzpatrick JM, Dreikorn K, Habib F, Mebust WK, Perrin P, Schulze HK. Medical management of benign prostatic hyperplasia other than with hormones or alpha blockers. Progr Clin Biol Res 1994;386:303-9.

29. Barnes PM, Powell-Griner E, McFann K, Nahin RL. Complementary and alternative medicine use among adults: United States, 2002. Advance Data 2004;343:1-19.

30. Delos S, Iehle C, Martin PM, Raynaud JP. Inhibition of the activity of 'basic' 5 alpha-reductase type 1 detected in DU 145 cells and expressed in insect cells. J Steroid Biochem Molec Biol 1994;48:347-52.

31. Wilt TJ, Ishani A, Stark G, MacDonald R, Lau J, Mulrow C. Saw palmetto extracts for treatment of benign prostatic hyperplasia: a systematic review. (Erratum appears in JAMA 1999;281(6):515.) JAMA 1998;280:1604-9.

32. Marks LS, Partin AW, Epstein JI, et al. Effects of a saw palmetto herbal blend in men with symptomatic benign prostatic hyperplasia. J Urol 2000;163:1451-6.

33. Debruyne F, Koch G, Boyle P, et al. Comparison of a phytotherapeutic agent Permixon with an alpha-blocker Tamsulosin in the treatment of benign prostatic hyperplasia: a 1-year randomized international study. Eur Urol 506;41:497-506.

34. Willetts KE, Clements MS, Champion S, Ehsman S, Eden JA. Serenoa repens extract for benign prostate hyperplasia: a randomized controlled trial. BJU Int 2003;92:267-70.

35. Bent S, Kane C, Shinohara K, et al. Saw palmetto for benign prostatic hyperplasia. N Engl J Med 2006;354:557-66.

11 Surgical management of benign prostatic hyperplasia

Rustom P. Manecksha and John M. Fitzpatrick

Department of Urology and Surgical Professional Unit, Mater Misericordiae University Hospital, Dublin, Ireland

Introduction

One of the most common urological issues affecting aging men is benign prostatic hyperplasia (BPH). About 80% of men will develop BPH and nearly one-third of all men will receive surgical treatment [1].

The surgical options for the treatment of moderate to severe bladder outflow obstruction (BOO) have evolved over the past decade. Standard surgical options include transurethral resection of the prostate (TURP) and open prostatectomy, i.e. adenoma enucleation through a suprapubic transvesical (Freyer) or retropubic approach (Millin). While TURP remains an effective treatment, 15–20% of patients develop a significant complication, and 10–15% require a second intervention within 10 years [2,3].

Although newer and less invasive techniques have been popularized, these should be compared with the standard surgical options, for which the rate of complication is low and long-term success in ameliorating symptoms and improving voiding function has been proven [4]. Nonetheless, for some patients, TURP and open prostatectomy is not a suitable form of treatment, because the patients are either poor surgical risks or are reluctant to undergo an invasive surgical procedure.

This chapter aims to critically appraise the alternatives to TURP and to evaluate the robustness of the evidence supporting these alternatives.

Clinical question 11.1

What are the role and long-term results of minimally invasive alternatives to TURP?

Literature search

A literature search was performed using PubMed (www.ncbi.nlm.nih.gow/pubmed/) with the following keywords: "minimally invasive," "prostatectomy," "transurethral microwave therapy," "needle ablation." Particular attention was paid to high-quality papers, i.e. systematic reviews, meta-analyses and randomized controlled trials.

Background

Transurethral resection of the prostate is the most widely performed surgery for BPH. However, it requires anesthesia and hospitalization and is associated with short- and long-term morbidity approaching 20%. It is, therefore, no surprise that the search for minimally invasive alternatives rages on. A number of techniques and procedures utilizing myriad technologies, including microwave, radiofrequency energy and lasers, have been approved by the FDA for the treatment of BPH. How do they stack up against TURP? Laser treatment (HoLEP and KTP PVP) are discussed separately. Here we present the evidence for transurethral microwave therapy (TUMT) and transurethral needle ablation (TUNA). Other emerging treatments including water-induced thermotherapy and transrectal high-intensity focused ultrasound are not discussed because of the absence of high-quality data. Until these treatments are measured against standard treatment, their use should be confined to trials and remain investigational [5].

The evidence

Transurethral microwave therapy

Transurethral microwave therapy involves the insertion of a specially designed urinary catheter into the bladder, allowing a microwave antenna to be positioned within the prostate. It then heats and destroys prostate tissue. Hoffman and colleagues conducted a systematic review of TUMT versus TURP for the treatment of BPH [6] and updated this with a further systematic review of all randomized controlled trials evaluating TUMT [7]. Six studies were identified comparing TUMT with TURP. The decrease in pooled mean urinary symptom scores favored TURP, as did the increase in pooled mean peak urinary flow. The mean length of hospitalization was 0 days for patients who had TUMT and 4 days for patients who had TURP. However, the mean length of catheterization was 13.7 days for patients who had TUMT versus 3.6 days for patients who had TURP [8]. Dysuria and urinary retention were more common in the TUMT group. There was a significantly lower incidence of retrograde ejaculation, hematuria, blood transfusions and TUR syndrome with TUMT compared with TURP [8-10]. The retreatment rate for TUMT was 19.8–29.3% and related to failure of treatment with mean follow-up of 30–60 months [5] Where retreatment after TURP was sought, it related more commonly to meatal, urethral or bladder neck strictures (9.6% for TURP versus 0.7% for TUMT) [9,11].

Transurethral needle ablation

Transurethral needle ablation involves the delivery of low-level radiofrequency energy to the prostate by placing two needles transurethrally into the prostate. The needles are deployed under direct vision using an endoscope.

Two meta-analyses of trials of TUNA provide robust evidence on its efficacy and safety [12,13]. TUNA was comparable to TURP for symptom score improvement at 3 months, but from 1 year to 4 years, the symptom score improvement favored TURP considerably. Interestingly, at 5 years, the symptom score improvement for TUNA and TURP was identical [12]. TURP outperformed TUNA for improvement in maximum flow rate (Qmax) throughout all time points: at 3 months, the improvement in Qmax for TUNA was 4.85 mL/s (57%) and for TURP 11.37 mL/s (148%). At 5 years, the improvement for TUNA was 2.6 mL/s (30%) and for TURP was 9.8 mL/s (127%) [12] TUNA fared better than TURP for adverse events – the only adverse events which were higher in patients who had TUNA were dysuria and transient urinary retention [12]. The vast majority of patients underwent TUNA as a day case and had the procedure performed with local anesthetic with or without sedation. The retreatment rate for patients who had TUNA was 10% compared with just 1% for TURP [12].

Bouza and colleagues concluded that when comparing TUNA with TURP, TUNA achieves a similar level of efficacy, especially in symptoms and quality of life scores in the short term, but in the medium and long term, TURP proved superior to TUNA in all efficacy measures. However, TUNA was significantly better in almost all safety parameters.

Comment

Transurethral microwave therapy is performed without the need for anesthesia and has a low morbidity rate, making it an attractive alternative to TURP, especially suited to patients who would be considered a high operative risk. However, the retreatment rate is higher for TUMT and the outcome measures are less favorable compared to TURP.

While TUNA does not reach the same level of efficacy as TURP, it can provide adequate short-term symptom relief and improvement in quality of life with low postoperative morbidity. Because TUNA can be performed without a spinal or general anesthetic, it may be an attractive option for selected patients, especially those with considerable anesthetic risk. The potential advantages of TUNA in symptomatic BPH must be balanced against its high rate of retreatment, which represents a substantial limitation. While it will not replace TURP as the gold standard, the available data show TUNA to be an effective and safe minimally invasive procedure for patients who are high risk for surgery or who are keen to avoid the adverse effects of TURP.

In summary, the advantages of TUMT and TUNA are that they are day-case procedures and have a lower rate of side effects and complications. The disadvantages are that they are associated with longer postoperative catheterization period and have a higher retreatment rate. The advantages of TURP are shorter postoperative catheterization period, better and more robust subjective and objective outcome and lower retreatment rate. Disadvantages are that it is an inpatient procedure with longer hospital stay and a higher side effect and complication rate. We conclude that TURP remains the preferred approach for most patients (conditional recommendation for TURP; 2B); however, in high-risk patients, the evidence supports a conditional recommendation for TUMT or TUNA (2B).

Clinical question 11.2

Have holmium laser enucleation of the prostate (HoLEP) and potassium-titanyl-phosphate (KTP) laser prostatectomy proved to be competitive compared with TURP?

Literature search

A literature search was performed using PubMed with the following keywords: "prostatectomy," "potassium-titanyl-phosphate laser," "green light laser," "KTP," "photoselective laser vaporization," "holmium laser" and "enucleation." Systematic reviews, meta-analyses and randomized controlled trials were given particular attention when formulating recommendations.

The evidence

Holmium laser enucleation of the prostate

Laser prostatectomy was pioneered by Chun [14] and Gilling [15] using a combination of holmium and Nd:YAG laser. Not long after this, techniques were developed using holmium laser exclusively. Holmium laser has a wavelength of 2140 nm and is strongly absorbed by water. The depth of thermal damage ranges from 0.5 mm to 1.0 mm, enabling excellent cutting and tissue ablation, but avoids deep coagulative tissue necrosis [16]. It is a pulsed laser which allows precise tissue vaporization at the tip of the laser fiber. It is therefore an excellent incisional tool for soft tissue [17]. Furthermore, it conducts through saline and thereby removes the risk of the TUR syndrome.

Holmium laser enucleation of the prostate involves laser dissection of the median and lateral lobes of the prostate from its capsule. Once the prostate is enucleated, the lobes are morcellated in the bladder prior to removal.

The literature on HoLEP is particularly formidable, with a significant number of randomized controlled trials (RCTs) and a meta-analysis published, providing high levels of evidence.

No less than four RCTs have been published comparing HoLEP with TURP for large prostates causing BOO. Gupta and colleagues published results of their prospective RCT of 50 patients randomized into three equal-numbered groups: TURP, transurethral vaporization of prostate (TUVP) and HoLEP [18]. All patients had BPH and prostate glands greater than 40 g (mean 58–63 g) measured with transabdominal ultrasound. Blood loss, the volume of postoperative irrigant, nursing contact time and catheter duration were all significantly less with HoLEP compared to the other two modalities. However, operative time and volume of operative irrigant were significantly greater for HoLEP. Although complication rates were no different between the three groups, bladder mucosal injury was peculiar to the HoLEP group. The outcome measures of IPSS, maximum flow rate (Qmax) and postvoid residual (PVR) volumes were comparable for the three groups, though the follow-up period was short at only 1 year.

Wilson and colleagues reported their 2-year follow-up of a RCT comparing HoLEP with TURP involving 61 patients in total [19]. Prostate volumes were measured with transrectal ultrasound and the mean volume was 77.8 ± 5.6 g (42–152) in the HoLEP group and 70.0 ± 5.0 g (46–156) in the TURP group. They reference their earlier work that found HoLEP to be superior to TURP as regards catheter time and hospital stay but took significantly longer to perform [20]. At 2 years, there was no significant difference between the two groups with respect to American Urological Association scores, quality of life scores or Qmax values. Two patients from the TURP group required reoperation. The authors concluded that HoLEP was comparable to TURP at 2 years.

Montorsi and colleagues published the first multicenter RCT comparing HoLEP and TURP [21]. One hundred patients were randomized into either HoLEP (52 patients) or TURP (48 patients) and followed for 1 year. While outcome measures and complication rates at 1 year were similar in both groups, patients who had HoLEP had shorter catheterization periods and shorter hospital stays.

Whilst the comparison of HoLEP and open prostatectomy is beyond the scope of this clinical question, we have addressed this comparison because we feel that it is at this end of the spectrum that HoLEP seems to come into its own. For patients with very large prostates, two RCTs provide robust data demonstrating superiority of HoLEP compared to open prostatectomy [22,23]. Naspro and colleagues randomized 80 men into either open prostatectomy (39 men) or HoLEP (41 men). While open prostatectomy was significantly quicker to perform and yielded a greater specimen weight, HoLEP was associated with less bleeding, less need for blood transfusion, shorter duration of catheterization (1.5 versus 4.1 days) and shorter hospital stay (2.7 versus 5.4 days). The outcome measures at 2 years were comparable between the two surgical groups. Kuntz and colleagues report a 5-year follow-up of a RCT comparing HoLEP with open prostatectomy in patients with prostates over 100 g [23]. One hundred and twenty patients were randomized to either HoLEP or open prostatectomy (60 men in each group), of which 74 men completed the 5-year follow-up. The resected weights, AUA symptom score, Qmax and PVR volumes were similar in both groups throughout the follow-up period. Complication rates were also similar in both groups. The authors were able to conclude that the outcomes for HoLEP were as durable compared with open prostatectomy.

Shah and colleagues performed a retrospective review of 354 patients who underwent HoLEP and stratified them into three groups according to prostate size (less than 60 g, 60–100 g and greater than 100 g) [24]. All outcome measures and complication rates were comparable between the three groups, demonstrating that the efficacy and safety of HoLEP were independent of prostate size. The authors showed that HoLEP efficiency (i.e. weight of tissue resected per minute) increased with the size of the prostate, with a mean of 0.36 g/min in the > 60 g group compared with a mean of 0.58 g/min in the > 100 g group (Level 4).

A RCT with 3-year follow-up reported by Ahyai and colleagues (100 patients each in the HoLEP and TURP groups) showed that the AUA symptom scores for HoLEP were better at 1 and 2 years but were similar at 3 years compared to TURP [25]. Qmax was comparable for both groups throughout the follow-up period. Although the PVR volumes were significantly better at 2 and 3 years in the HoLEP group, it is clinically irrelevant since the mean PVR volume in the TURP group was less than 30 mL.

Tan and colleagues performed a meta-analysis of HoLEP versus TURP [26]. They showed no difference between HoLEP and TURP in terms of Qmax at 6 and 12 months' follow-up. There was less blood loss, a shorter catheterization time and a shorter hospital stay in the HoLEP group. The operating time for TURP was shorter. Both operations were similar in terms of urethral stricture, stress incontinence, transfusion requirement and rate of reoperation.

Potassium-titanyl-phosphate (KTP) laser

Potassium-titanyl-phosphate laser is generated by passing Nd:YAG laser light through a KTP crystal. This has a wavelength of 532 nm, visible as a green light. High-power (80 W) KTP laser is used to remove obstructive prostatic tissue in a hemostatic fashion by photoselective vaporization of the prostate (PVP). Similar to HoLEP, KTP laser PVP is performed using saline irrigant. Barber and colleagues demonstrated the absence of TUR syndrome with PVP by using expired breath ethanol measurements [27].

The data for PVP are less robust as there are far fewer comparative studies of PVP versus TURP and follow-up periods are short. Bouchier-Hayes and colleagues published the first RCT of PVP versus TURP [28]. The mean prostate volumes were 33.2 cc for TURP and 42.4 cc for PVP. IPSS, Qmax and PVR volumes were similar in both groups. The reductions in hemoglobin, catheterization period and hospital stay were significantly shorter in the PVP group. There were fewer complications in the PVP group although three patients in the PVP group required reoperation. The authors concede, however, that the follow-up period was short and some of the data incomplete, and therefore conclusions are guarded.

Horansanli and colleagues reported a prospective RCT of PVP versus TURP involving 76 patients in total [29]. All patients had prostate volumes between 70 and 100 mL. The follow-up period was merely 6 months. While the catheterization period and hospital stay were shorter in the PVP group, the operative time was significantly longer. Furthermore, outcome measures (IPSS, Qmax and PVR volume) significantly favored the TURP group. The reoperation rate for PVP was 18% and zero for the TURP group. The authors conceded that TURP was superior to PVP for large prostates (greater than 70 g).

Sandhu and colleagues reported the use of PVP for high-risk patients on anticoagulants and antiplatelet medication [30]. The mean prostate volume was 82 cc. Warfarin was discontinued 2 days before surgery and recommenced the day after surgery. Clopidogrel and aspirin were not discontinued. No patients developed significant hematuria or clot retention. There was a significant improvement in the IPSS, Qmax and PVR volumes although 1-year follow-up was only available for 11/24 patients studied.

Comment

Given that HoLEP is associated with less blood loss, lower blood transfusion rate, shorter catheterization and

hospitalization periods, it has been proven to be competitive with TURP and is a true endoscopic alternative to open prostatectomy. There is medium-term follow-up evidence supporting the durability of HoLEP but longer term follow-up is still needed. Furthermore, due to its longer operative time and the learning curve involved, the evidence would suggest that it is unlikely to replace TURP as the standard of care; rather, its role would be defined for the larger prostates for which open prostatectomy may otherwise have been considered. Therefore, we make a conditional recommendation against HoLEP (2B).

Robust evidence is still lacking for KTP laser PVP comparing it to TURP. It is likely that KTP laser, while easier to master than HoLEP, will be limited to high-risk patients with small prostates. Due to the lack of robust evidence and long-term follow-up data, no recommendation can be made.

Clinical question 11.3

How does the Gyrus bipolar TURP compare with standard monopolar TURP?

Literature search

A literature search was performed using PubMed with the following keywords: "transurethral prostatectomy," "bipolar," "gyrus," "plasmakinetic," "transurethral resection," "saline," "monopolar." Particular emphasis was placed on high-quality papers, i.e. systematic reviews, meta-analyses and randomized controlled trials.

The evidence

In the quest to reduce complications associated with conventional monopolar transurethral resection, various bipolar devices have been developed. They include the Gyrus PlasmaKinetic system, ACMI Vista controlled tissue resection system, Olympus TURIS system, the Wolf system and the Karl Storz system. The safety, efficacy and durability of these new techniques must be compared with conventional monopolar TURP (MTURP), the benchmark against which all new techniques are evaluated.

With conventional MTURP, the active electrode is the resecting loop and the return electrode is a diathermy pad placed on the patient's thigh or buttock so the energy must travel a considerable distance through the body to complete the circuit [31]. Bipolar TURP (BTURP), however, involves the use of the active and return electrodes in close proximity to each other at the target tissue, thus limiting the distance that the energy is required to travel [31]. One of the key differences is the ability to perform BTURP using physiological saline as the irrigation fluid, thereby eliminating the risk of TUR syndrome and dilutional hyponatremia.

Of all the bipolar devices, the Gyrus system has the longest clinical experience, being first described as a vaporization technique [32]. After the initial enthusiasm for transurethral vaporization, reservations arose as a result of the lack of tissue for histology. In a prospective RCT comparing vaporization of the prostate and MTURP, Hon and colleagues reported incidental findings of prostate cancer in 8/79 (10%) men who had TURP, raising the fear that clinically significant prostate cancers may be missed with vaporization, especially important in younger men [33]. Furthermore, vaporizing prostate tissue at the apex was difficult without risk to the external urethral sphincter nearby. Tefekli and colleagues described a hybrid technique combining vaporization and resection of the prostate (Table 11.1) [34]. As medium-term results emerged, vaporization was shown to be inferior to TURP and has now been abandoned.

Starkman & Santucci reported results of a retrospective study comparing Gyrus BTURP with MTURP [35]. The catheterization period and hospital stay were shorter for BTURP and complication rates were comparable, but the retrospective nature of the study and the lack of efficacy data weaken their evidence (see Table 11.1). The first RCT comparing Gyrus BTURP with MTURP was published by Tefekli and colleagues although they employed a hybrid approach, using vaporization and resection in the bipolar group [34]. The follow-up period was 1 year. The catheterization period and hospital stay were shorter, in favor of BTURP, the short-term IPSS was equivalent to MTURP at 1 year and the Qmax was better for BTURP. However, significantly more patients reported severe irritative symptoms postoperatively and the urethral stricture rate was signi-ficantly higher for BTURP (see Table 11.1). The irritative symptoms are thought to be a complication of vaporization rather than resection. De Sio and colleagues published results of their RCT with 1-year follow-up comparing Gyrus BTURP with MTURP [36]. They showed BTURP to be comparable to MTURP in terms of operative, safety and short-term efficacy outcomes, while having a shorter catheterization period and shorter hospital stays (see Table 11.1). The largest RCT (N 240) comparing Gyrus BTURP to MTURP was published by Erturhan and colleagues [37]. They reported a faster resection time in favor of BTURP, shorter catheterization time and shorter hospital stay for BTURP (p < 0.001) and a better Qmax at 12-month follow-up for BTURP (see Table 11.1).

Comment

While efficacy outcomes seem comparable to TURP in the short to medium term, long-term data from RCTs are still not available. Therefore, the durability of Gyrus BTURP cannot yet be validated. The higher stricture rate associated with Gyrus BTURP is a worry and may offset the apparent benefit in terms of electrolyte imbalance and shorter catheterization periods. Until long-term data are available, Gyrus BTURP cannot be said to have replaced conventional MTURP as the standard of care and no recommendation can be made.

Clinical question 11.4

Is bipolar TURP in saline better than TURP?

Literature search

A literature search was performed using PubMed with the following keywords: "transurethral prostatectomy," "bipolar," "transurethral resection," "saline," "TURIS," "monopolar." Particular emphasis was placed on high-quality papers, i.e. systematic reviews, meta-analyses and randomized controlled trials.

The evidence

The transurethral resection in saline (TURIS) system utilizes the resection loop as the active electrode and the resectoscope sheath as the return electrode. It is a simpler design compared with the Gyrus system, and similarly, resection can be performed in a saline environment. A number of RCTs have been published comparing TURIS with conventional monopolar TURP, albeit fewer than with the more established Gyrus system. Ho and colleagues published the first RCT with a 1-year follow-up [38]. They showed that there was a greater decline in serum Na^+ using conventional monopolar TURP compared with TURIS (see Table 11.1). Furthermore, TUR syndrome could be avoided by resecting in saline. They also showed the technique to be comparable to TURP as regards weight of tissue resected and resection time. The efficacy parameters of IPSS and Qmax were comparable by 3 months and were sustained at 12 months (see Table 11.1). Worryingly, however, they reported a urethral stricture rate of 6.3% with TURIS. The cause of the increased incidence of urethral strictures is unclear – there are concerns about the energy exiting through the urethra/penis and the use of larger resectoscope sheaths.

Michielsen and colleagues published results of their RCT involving 238 patients randomized to either conventional monopolar TURP or TURIS [39]. Similar to Ho, they were able to show a greater decline in serum Na^+ with monopolar TURP and elimination of TUR syndrome with TURIS but did not report on the efficacy parameters (see Table 11.1).

Table 11.1 Bipolar TURP (BTURP) versus conventional monopolar TURP (MTURP). Study designs and outcome measures

Authors	Methods	Intervention	Participants	Results	Notes
Singh et al. [40]	RCT F/U 1/12, 3/12	MTURP (25.5F Wolf) v BTURP (25.6F ACMI Vista CTR)	MTURP = 30 patients BTURP = 30 patients	• Greater decline in Na^+ in MTURP group (p<0.001) • No difference in decrease in Hb • No difference in resection time or weight • Catheter time shorter in BTURP group (p=0.022) • Hospital stay shorter in BTURP group (p=0.019) • IPSS, Qmax, PVR comparable improvement • Stricture rate BTURP = 1, MTURP = 0 (NS)	• Single surgeon • No TUR syndrome in either group
Starkman et al. [35]	Retrospective F/U 18/12	MTURP v BTURP (Gyrus – hybrid vaporization & resection)	MTURP = 18 patients BTURP = 25 patients	• Low Na+ MTURP (2 patients) v BTURP (1 patient) • Resection weight MTURP = 18 g, BTURP = 15 g • Catheter time & hospital stay shorter in BTURP (NS) • Stricture rate BTURP = 1, MTURP = 1 (NS)	• Single surgeon
Tefekli et al. [34]	RCT F/U 3/12, 6/12, 12/12	MTURP(26F) v BTURP (27F Gyrus – hybrid vaporization & resection)	MTURP = 50 patients BTURP = 51 patients	• Shorter operative time with BTURP (40.3 min v 57.8 min, p<0.01) • Less intraoperative irrigant with BTURP (p<0.05) • Shorter catheter time with BTURP (2.3 days v 3.8 days, p<0.05) • IPSS comparable throughout follow-up periods • Qmax better improvement with BTURP at 12/12 (p<0.05) • More BTURP patients with severe irritative symptoms (p=0.0014) • Stricture rate BTURP > MTURP (3 v 1, p=0.002)	• 2 surgeons • Na^+ & Hb not reported • Resection weights not reported
De Sio et al. [36]	RCT F/U 3/12, 6/12, 9/12, 12/12	MTURP (26F Storz) v BTURP (Gyrus PK system)	MTURP = 35 patients BTURP = 35 patients	• Operative time, resection time, resection weight, variations in Na^+ and Hb comparable between the 2 groups • Shorter catheter time with BTURP (p<0.05) and shorter hospital stay (p<0.05) • IPSS, Qmax, PVR and QoL scores comparable between the 2 groups at 9/12 • Stricture rate BTURP = MTURP (1 each)	• No TUR syndrome in either group • 1 patient in BTURP group had massive postoperative bleeding requiring transfusion
Erturhan et al. [37]	RCT F/U 1/12, 12/12	MTURP v BTURP (Gyrus PK system)	MTURP = 120 patients BTURP = 120 patients	• Shorter resection time (for 40 mL prostates) with BTURP (36 min v 57 min, p<0.001) • Shorter catheterization time with BTURP (3 days v 4.5 days, p<0.001) • Better improvement in Qmax with BTURP (p<0.001)	
Ho et al. [38]	RCT F/U 1/12, 3/12, 6/12, 12/12	MTURP (26F) v BTURP (26F Olympus TURIS)	MTURP = 50 patients BTURP = 50 patients	• Greater decline in postoperative Na^+ with MTURP (p<0.01) • Decline in Hb comparable between both groups • 2 cases of TUR syndrome in MTURP group (p<0.05) • Resection time & resection weight comparable between both groups • IPSS and Qmax comparable between both groups • More urethral strictures with BTURP (3 v 1, NS)	• 2 surgeons
Michielsen et al. [39]	RCT F/U period not reported	MTURP (26F Olympus) v BTURP (24F Olympus TURIS)	MTURP = 120 patients BTURP = 118 patients	• Greater decline in Na^+ with MTURP (p=0.05) • Operative time was longer with BTURP (p<0.001) • Resection weight was comparable between both groups • Catheter time & hospital stay comparable • TUR syndrome – 1 case with MTURP, 0 with BTURP	• Efficacy outcome not reported

F/U, follow-up; Hb, hemoglobin; IPSS, International Prostate Symptom Score; Na+, serum sodium; NS, not significant; PVR, postvoid residual volume; Qmax, maximum flow rate; RCT, randomized controlled trial

Comment

The short-term efficacy data of TURIS is comparable to TURP with an increased safety profile in terms of electrolyte imbalance and TUR syndrome. The higher incidence of urethral strictures is a concern and there is still absence of long-term data to confirm its durability compared with TURP. Therefore, no recommendation can be made.

Conclusion and implications for further research

As life expectancy and the aging population increase, more men will seek treatment for BPH, and many of them will have significant co-morbidities. These men, regarded as a high anesthetic risk, will be denied surgical treatment with TURP. Minimally invasive techniques, such as TUMT and TUNA, as discussed earlier, provide alternatives to TURP for men in the high-risk category, as these techniques do not require anesthesia and have low morbidity and low complication rates. Furthermore, the laser alternatives may be used safely in patients on anticoagulant or antiplatelet therapy [30].

Holmium laser enucleation of the prostate and KTP laser treatment have proved competitive in comparison to TURP. The short- and medium-term data show these laser treatments to be comparable to TURP in terms of efficacy while having fewer complications. The role of TURP as the standard of care for the surgical treatment of BPH is being challenged by these treatments. In retaliation, the introduction of continuous flow resection and bipolar technology has reduced the morbidity traditionally associated with monopolar TURP. The various bipolar devices employ similar resection techniques to monopolar TURP, therefore limiting the learning curve for the adaptation of these techniques. Lasers, on the other hand, and in particular HoLEP, involve a considerable learning curve, not to mention kitting-out cost. It is our contention that TURP remains the standard of care for patients with BPH who have failed medical therapy.

Further research should be directed toward generating high levels of evidence through randomized controlled trials, with long-term follow-up. Cost–analyses should also be performed as the economic implications of new technology cannot be ignored and the widespread acceptance of new technology will be determined not solely by favorable outcomes but also by economic viability.

References

1. Rosen R, Altwein J, Boyle P, et al. Lower urinary tract symptoms and male sexual dysfunction: the multinational survey of the aging male (MSAM-7). Eur Urol 2003;44:637-49.

2. Mebust WK, Holtgrewe HL, Cockett A, et al. Transurethral prostatectomy: immediate and postoperative complications. A cooperative study of 13 participating institutions evaluating 3,885 patients. J Urol 1989;141:243.

3. Dunsmuir WD, Emberton M and the National Prostatectomy Audit Steering Group. There is significant sexual dysfunction following TURP. BJU 1996;77(suppl):39.

4. Fitzpatrick JM. Minimally invasive and endoscopic management of benign prostatic hyperplasia. In: Wein AJ (ed) *Campbell-Walsh Urology*, 9th edn. Philadelphia, PA: Saunders Elsevier, 2007.

5. De la Rosette J, Gravas S, Fitzpatrick JM. Minimally invasive treatment of male lower urinary tract symptoms. Urol Clin North Am 2008;35:505-18.

6. Hoffman RM, MacDonald R, Monga M, Wilt TJ. Transurethral microwave thermotherapy vs transurethral resection for treating benign prostatic hyperplasia: a systematic review. BJU Int 2004;94(7):1031-6.

7. Hoffman RM, Monga M, Elliot SP, et al. Microwave thermotherapy for benign prostatic hyperplasia. Cochrane Database Syst Rev 2007;4:CD004135.

8. De la Rosette J, Laguna P, Gravas S, de Wildt M. Transurethral microwave therapy: the gold standard for minimally invasive therapies for patients with benign prostatic hyperplasia? J Endourol 2003;17(4):245-51.

9. Dahlstrand C, Walden M, Geirsson G, Pettersson S. Transurethral microwave thermotherapy versus transurethral resection for symptomatic benign prostatic obstruction: a prospective randomized study with a 2-year follow-up. BJU 1995;76:614-18.

10. Ahmed M, Bell T, Lawrence WT, et al. Transurethral microwave thermotherapy (Prostatron version 2.5) compared with transurethral resection of the prostate for the treatment of benign prostatic hyperplasia: a randomized, controlled, parallel study. BJU 1997;79:181-5.

11. Floratos DL, Kiemeney LA, Rossi C, et al. Long-term follow-up of a randomized TUMT versus TURP study. J Urol 2001;165:1533-8.

12. Bouza C, Lopez T, Magro A, et al. Systematic review and meta-analysis of transurethral needle ablation in symptomatic benign prostatic hyperplasia. BMC Urol 2006;6:14.

13. Boyle P, Robertson C, Vaughan ED, et al. A metaanalysis of trials of trnasurethral needle ablation for treating symptomatic benign prostatic obstruction. BJU Int 2004;94(1):83-8.

14. [My paper]Chun SS, Razvi HA, Denstedt JD. Laser prostatectomy with the holmium:YAG laser. Tech Urol 1995;1:217.

15. Gilling PJ, Cass CB, Malcolm AR, Fraundorfer MR. Combination holmium and Nd:YAG laser ablation of the prostate initial clinical experience. J Endourol 1995;9:151.

16. Seki N, Naito S. Holmium laser for benign prostatic hyperplasia. Curr Opin Urol 2008;18:41-5.

17. Tan AHH, Gilling PJ. Holmium laser prostatectomy. BJU Int 2003;92:527-30.

18. Gupta NP, Anand A. Comparison of TURP, TUVRP and HoLEP. Curr Urol Reports 2009;10(4):276–278.

19. Wilson LC, Gilling PJ, Williams A, et al. A randomised trial comparing holmium laser enucleation versus transurethral resection in the treatment of prostates larger than 40 grams: results at 2 years. Eur Urol 2006;50:569-73.

20. Tan AHH, Gilling PJ, Kennett KM, et al. A randomized trial comparing holmium laser enucleation of the prostate with

transurethral resection of the prostate for the treatment of bladder outlet obstruction secondary to benign prostatic hyperplasia in large glands (40 to 200 grams). J Urol 2003;170:1270-4.

21. Montorsi F, Naspro R, Salonia A, et al. Holmium laser enucleation versus transurethral resection of the prostate: results from a 2-center, prospective, randomized trial in patients with obstructive benign prostatic hyperplasia. J Urol 2008;179: S87-S80.

22. Naspro R, Suardi N, Salonia A, et al. Holmium laser enucleation of the prostate versus open prostatectomy for prostates > 70 g: 24-month follow-up. Eur Urol 2006;50:563-8.

23. Kuntz RM, Lehrich K, Ahyai SA. Holmium enucleation of the prostate versus open prostatectomy for prostates greater that 100 grams: 5 year follow up results of a randomized control trial. Eur Urol 2008;53:160-8.

24. Shah HN, Sodha HS, Kharodawala SJ, et al. Influence of prostate size on the outcome of holmium laser enucleation of the prostate. BJU Int 2008;101:1536-41.

25. Ahyai SA, Lehrich K, Kuntz RM. Holmium laser enucleation versus transurethral resection of the prostate: 3-year follow-up results of a randomized clinical trial. Eur Urol 2007;52:1456-64.

26. Tan A, Liao C, Mo Z, Cao Y. Meta-analysis of holmium enucleation versus transurethral resection of the prostate for symptomatic prostatic obstruction. Br J Surg 2007;94:1201-8.

27. Barber N, Zhu G, Donohue J, et al. Use of expired breath ethanol measurements in evaluation of irrigant absorption during high-power potassium titanyl phosphate laser vaporization of prostate. Urology 2006;67(1):80-3.

28. Bouchier-Hayes DM, Anderson P, van Appledorn S, Bugeja P, Costello AJ. KTP laser versus transurethral resection: early results of a randomized trial. J Endourol 2006;20(8):580-5.

29. Horasanli K, Silay M, Altay B, et al. Photoselective potassium titanyl phosphate (KTP) laser vaporization versus transurethral resection of the prostate for prostates larger than 70 ml: a short-term prospective randomized trial. Urology 2008; 71(2):247-51.

30. Sandhu JS, Ng CK, Gonzalez RR, et al. Photoselective laser vaporization prostatectomy in men receiving anticoagulants. J Endourol 2005;19:1196-8.

31. Issa M. Technological advances in transurethral resection of the prostate: bipolar versus monopolar TURP. J Endourol 2008;22(8):1587-95.

32. Botto H, Lebret T, Barre P, et al. Electrovaporization of the prostate with the Gyrus device. J Endourol 2001;15:313-16.

33. Hon NHY, Brathwaithe D, Hussain Z, et al. A prospective, randomized trial comparing conventional transurethral prostate resection with plasmakinetic vaporization of the prostate: physiological changes, early complications and long-term follow-up. J Urol 2006;176:205-9.

34. Tefekli A, Muslumanoglu AY, Baykal M, et al. A hybrid technique using bipolar energy in transurethral prostate surgery: a prospective randomized comparison. J Urol 2005;174(4 Pt 1):1339-43.

35. Starkman JS, Santucci RA. Comparison of bipolar transurethral resection of prostate with standard transurethral prostatectomy: shorter stay, earlier catheter removal and fewer complications. BJU Int 2005;95:69-71.

36. de Sio M, Antorino R, Quarto G, et al. Gyrus bipolar versus standard monopolar transurethral resection of the prostate: a randomized prospective trial. Urology 2006;67(1):69-72.

37. Erturhan S, Erbagci A, Seckiner I, et al. Plasmakinetic resection of the prostate versus standard transurethral resection of the prostate: a prospective randomized trial with a 1-year follow-up. Prostate Cancer Prostatic Dis 2007;10:97-100.

38. Ho HS, Yip SK, Lim KB, et al. A prospective randomized study comparing monopolar and bipolar transurethral resection of prostate using transurethral resection in saline (TURiS) system. Eur Urol 2007;52(2):517-22.

39. Michielsen DPJ, Debacker T, de Boe V, et al. Bipolar transurethral resection in saline – an alternative surgical treatment for bladder outlet obstruction? J Urol 2007;178(5):2035-9.

40. Singh H, Desai MR, Shrivastav P, Vani K. Bipolar versus monopolar transurethral resection of prostate: randomized controlled study. J Endourol 2005;19(3):333-8.

12 Treatment of chronic prostatitis/chronic pelvic pain syndrome

J. Curtis Nickel

Department of Urology, Queen's University, Kingston, Ontario, Canada

Introduction

Prostatitis, by its very name, conjures up the idea of an inflamed (. . . itis) prostate (prostat . . .). For clinicians, inflammation in the urinary tract is invariably associated with infection. Therefore, it is no surprise that therapy for chronic prostatitis/chronic pelvic pain syndrome (CP/CPPS) has traditionally been directed towards a prostate-centric infectious and/or inflammatory condition of the male lower urinary tract [1]. This chapter will review the evidence available for the use of antimicrobials, anti-inflammatories and the two major classes of agents employed in treating benign prostate disease (alpha-blockers and 5-alpha-reductase inhibitors).

A quick review of the prostatitis syndromes is necessary in order to understand therapeutic approaches to CP/CPPS [2-4]. Category I acute bacterial prostatitis is an acute bacterial infection of the prostate gland associated with local pain, obstructive voiding symptoms, fever and other systemic manifestations of a serious infection. Treatment is antibiotics. Category II chronic bacterial prostatitis is a chronic infection of the prostate associated with recurrent urinary tract infections. Patients are often asymptomatic between infections. Treatment consists of long-term antibiotics, usually trimethoprim-sulfamethoxazole or preferably a fluoroquinolone (ciprofloxacin or levofloxacin). Category III CP/CPPS is characterized by chronic pelvic (and/or genitourinary) pain/discomfort that is not associated with recurrent or active infection. This chapter will discuss the treatment of this category.

Chronic prostatitis/chronic pelvic pain syndrome is a major clinical problem. The prevalence rate of physician-diagnosed prostatitis in Olmsted County was 9% [5]; population-based surveys have estimated that between 6% and 12% of men experience prostatitis-like symptoms [6,7]. The quality of life is dismal [8] and the costs to society enormous [9].The etiology of prostatitis in the majority of men whose symptoms persist longer than 3 months is believed to be noninfectious [3,4].

The literature is replete with many small, under-powered, poorly designed trials in CP/CPPS. This has changed with the general acceptance of the NIH classi-fication system and clinical definition of CP/CPPS [2], the development and validation of the NIH Chronic Prostatitis Symptom Index (CPSI) as an outcome tool [10,11] and description of a properly designed clinical trial in CP/CPPS [12,13]. Nickel described the four requirements that would constitute clinical trial data that could be used to draw evidence-based treatment recommendations in CP/CPPS [1]:
- NIH classification system for definition and characterization of patients
- randomized placebo-controlled design
- validated outcome parameters (such as the NIH-CPSI)
- peer reviewed (published in peer-reviewed literature).

Papers published or accepted for publication in the peer-reviewed journals were included in this review. Papers published in nonpeer-reviewed supplements were not included. The manuscript list was obtained through the major databases covering the last 10 years (e.g. Medline, EMBASE, Cochrane Library, Biosis, Science Citation Index). The tables of contents of the major journals of urology and other relevant journals for the previous 3 months were reviewed to take into account possible delay in indexation of papers in the databases. These approaches identified multiple references. After reviewing the titles and abstracts, articles (for the most part that met the criteria noted above) were identified for detailed review.

Clinical question 12.1

What is the role of antimicrobial therapy in CP/CPPS?

Evidence-Based Urology. Edited by Philipp Dahm, Roger R. Dmochowski.
© 2010 Blackwell Publishing.

Literature search

Search terms employed included "prostatitis," "pelvic pain," "chronic pelvic pain syndrome," "clinical trials," "antibiotics," "antimicrobials."

Evidence

Prospective nonrandomized or uncontrolled trials [14,15] have led to recommendations that antibiotics should be employed in the treatment of CP/CPPS, particularly the inflammatory subtype (Category IIIA) [16]. Two multicenter, randomized, placebo-controlled studies have assessed the efficacy of 6 weeks of levofloxacin [17] and ciprofloxacin [18] in men with CP/CPPS. In these trials the participants had chronic symptoms for a long duration (many years) and had been heavily treated (including treatment with antibiotics). In the study by Nickel and associates [17], 80 patients were randomized to levofloxacin or placebo while in the NIH-sponsored study reported by Alexander and colleagues [18], 196 men with CP/CPPS were randomized in a two-by-two factorial design to ciprofloxacin, tamsulosin, the combination of ciprofloxacin and tamsulosin or placebo. In both of these prospective controlled multicenter trials, no significant difference was reported between fluoroquinolone and placebo in terms of symptom amelioration.

Comment

Critical evaluation of the two randomized, placebo-controlled trials evaluating antimicrobials convincingly demonstrates the futility of employing antibiotics in CP/CPPS men suffering for a long duration (many years in these studies) who had been heavily pretreated (received antibiotics in the past for prostatitis) (Grade 1A). However, nonplacebo-controlled trials suggest that men with early diagnosis (4–8 weeks) who had not been previously treated with antibiotics may respond to a trial course of antimicrobial therapy [14,19] (Grade 2B).

Clinical question 12.2

What is the role of anti-inflammatory therapy in CP/CPPS?

Literature search

Search terms employed included "prostatitis," "pelvic pain," "chronic pelvic pain syndrome," "clinical trials," "anti-inflammatories," "nonsteroidal," "COX-2 inhibitors."

Evidence

The results of a North American randomized placebo-controlled trial comparing the cyclo-oxygenase-2 (COX-2) inhibitor rofecoxib to placebo [20] indicated that some men with CPPS benefited (in terms of pain and quality of life) from rofecoxib therapy compared with placebo. In this study, in which 161 patients were randomized to rofecoxib 25 mg, rofecoxib 50 mg or placebo, only patients on the high dose showed statistically clinical improvement compared to the placebo. Very few patients, however, had complete resolution of their symptoms [20].

The clinical and pathological characteristics of CP/CPPS are similar to those of interstitial cystitis and a number of small studies examining the efficacy of pentosan polysulfate, a glycosaminoglycan that has some anti-inflammatory activity used in the treatment of interstitial cystitis, suggested benefit [21]. The results of a multicenter, randomized, placebo-controlled trial that randomized 100 men to pentosan polysulfate 900 mg/day (three times the usual dose) or placebo indicated that this medication provided modest benefit for some men with CPPS [22]. Quercetin, a natural bioflavanoid with potent anti-inflammatory characteristics (for a phytotherapuetic agent), has been shown to provide a statistically and clinically significant benefit compared to placebo in a very small, single-center pilot study [23]. A very small (17 patients in total) single-center study [24] showed no obvious benefits of zafirlukast, a leukotriene antagonist, compared to placebo on the symptoms of Category IIIA CP/CPPS.

Comment

Critical evaluation of these trials would suggest that high dose anti-inflammatory therapy continued for a prolonged duration may have a modest ameliorative effect in some patients (Grade 1B). The results from the small but placebo-controlled trial with quercetin are intriguing and should be further investigated. Pentosan polysulfate might be more effective in men whose CPPS is related to a primary bladder etiology (interstitial cystitis). Anti-inflammatory therapy cannot be recommended as a monotherapy for CP/CPPS, but could be considered in a multimodal therapeutic regime.

Clinical question 12.3

What is the role of prostate-specific therapy (e.g. alpha-blockers and 5-alpha-reductase inhibitors) in the treatment of CP/CPPS?

Literature search

Search terms employed included "prostatitis," "pelvic pain," "chronic pelvic pain syndrome," "clinical trials," "alpha-blockers," "alpha-receptor antagonists," "terazosin," "alfuzosin," "doxazosin," "tamsulosin," "5-alpha-reductase" "inhibitors," "finasteride."

Evidence

There are six randomized, placebo-controlled, double-blind clinical trials evaluating alpha blockers in patients with CP/CPPS that meet the criteria outlined and one study that was presented at the 2008 American Urological Association annual meeting and should be published shortly. The first trial was a short-term study in which 58 patients with CP/CPPS were randomized to receive tamsulosin 0.4 mg once daily (OD) or placebo for 6 weeks [25]. Tamsulosin provided modest improvement in the total NIH-CPSI score (p = 0.04). There was a trend for a greater improvement in pain, voiding and quality of life (QoL) domains with tamsulosin, but the difference versus placebo did not reach significance. In the second study [26], 86 patients with CP/CPPS were randomized to receive terazosin (titration from 1–5 mg OD in 2 weeks then 5 mg OD) or placebo for 14 weeks. Terazosin significantly improved the total NIH-CPSI score compared to placebo (p < 0.01). Pain, voiding and QoL domains were all significantly improved compared with placebo (p < 0.05). The third study [27] was a long-term trial in which 37 patients were randomized to receive alfuzosin or placebo for 6 months. These two groups were compared to a positive control/standard therapy group including 29 patients who agreed to participate but not to be randomized in the trial. Standard therapy consisted of hot sitz baths and anti-inflammatory drugs (ibuprofen, ketoprofen, diclofenac). After the end of the 6-month treatment period, patients were followed for an additional 6 months. Alfuzosin administered for 6 months significantly improved total and pain NIH-CPSI scores in the alfuzosin group compared to the placebo and control groups (p < 0.01). At the end of the 6-month treatment phase, patients in both groups who had initially reported improvement in pain reported progressive deterioration in symptoms. The fourth study was another long-term trial which included 90 treatment-naive patients with CP/CPPS randomized to receive doxazosin 4 mg OD alone or a triple therapy (doxazosin 4 mg OD plus an anti-inflammatory agent – ibuprofen 400 mg per day – and a muscle relaxant – thiocolchicoside 12 mg per day) or placebo [28]. At the end of the 6-month treatment period, patients were followed for an additional 6 months. Over 6 months, total NIH-CPSI score significantly improved in the doxazosin group and triple therapy groups while it remained stable in the placebo group.

The NIH-Chronic Prostatitis Collaborative Network (NIH-CPCRN) compared tamsulosin 0.4 mg, ciprofloxacin 500 mg twice daily, ciprofloxacin plus tamsulosin 0.4 mg or placebo administered for 6 weeks in 196 patients with CP/CPPS [18]. In contrast to the randomized studies described above, no significant symptom improvement was observed with tamsulosin, alone or in combination with ciprofloxacin, compared to placebo. Patients enrolled in the NIH-CPCRN strongly differed from prior phase II studies as they had chronic symptoms (6–8 years) and were heavily pretreated, including with alpha-blockers.

These studies would suggest that benefits of alpha-blockers in CP/CPPS may not occur with short-term therapy in heavily pretreated patients with long duration of symptoms. It was hypothesized that the benefits observed in the previous studies were due to the fact that the onset of symptoms or diagnosis was more recent and the patients were relatively treatment naive, particularly in regard to alpha-blockers [29,30]. In order to test this hypothesis, the NIH-CPCRN recently reported its second phase III study in 272 newly diagnosed (< 2 years) and alpha-blocker-naive CP/CPPS patients randomized to receive alfuzosin 10 mg OD or placebo for 12 weeks [31]. The primary endpoint was defined as a 4-point decrease from baseline in the NIH-CPSI total score after the 12-week treatment period. Alfuzosin therapy in this study resulted in an identical response rate as that for placebo therapy.

A number of trials, including an RCT that did not meet the criteria for inclusion in this review [32], suggested that finasteride, a 5-alpha-reductase inhibitor used in the treatment of benign prostate hyperplasia, would be effective in CP/CPPS. A RCT that did meet the criteria set for this review compared the reduction of NIH-CPSI in 64 men with CP/CPPS randomized to finasteride or placebo [33]. Six months of finasteride resulted in a numerical but not statistically significant reduction in symptoms compared to the symptom reduction noted in the placebo group. A small, single-center, pilot study suggested that mepartricin, a drug which lowers prostatic estrogen levels, may provide some benefits [34] but a larger, well-designed multicenter trial is necessary to confirm this.

Comment

Critical evaluation of the published phase III randomized placebo-controlled trial evaluating tamsulosin demonstrates that alpha-blockers are probably not useful in heavily pretreated CP/CPPS men suffering for a long duration, but review of the four smaller phase II studies suggests that alpha-blocker-naive men who have shorter duration of symptoms may benefit from alpha-blockers, especially if they are continued for longer than 6 weeks. A subsequent large multicenter RCT assessing alpha-blocker therapy for 12 weeks in alpha-blocker-naive men failed to show any difference from placebo. The recently reported NIH trial which specifically examined this group with 12 weeks of alfuzosin did not support this hypothesis (**Grade 2B**). Finasteride shows modest benefit in some men, but the effect was not statistically significant compared to placebo. Prostate-specific therapy with alpha-blockers and/or finasteride cannot be recommended for either chronic CP/CPPS or early treatment-naive CP/CPPS. The studies were not designed or powered to determine whether these agents would be more effective in patients with a primary voiding dysfunction or those with concurrent BPH.

Discussion

High-grade evidence is available to assess the efficacy of the traditional empiric therapies used to manage CP/CPPS. Unfortunately, these traditional therapies based on an inflammation/infection prostate model do not provide the efficacy required to recommend any of them as a primary monotherapy for patients with CP/CPPS. Yet, physicians continue to use many of these therapies, in selected patients, as treatment adjuncts and in a multimodal therapeutic plan. Patients diagnosed with CP/CPPS present with multiple clinical phenotypes, likely originating from different etiologies. For example, for some men the etiology may originally be infection, for others dysfunctional voiding, while trauma and pelvic floor dysfunction could be the cause of other men's symptoms. There appears to be a progression from local inflammation and pain to peripheral sensitization with pelvic neuromuscular dysfunction and pain, to a central sensitization with further modulation from higher central nervous system cognitive mechanisms. This is the most likely explanation why various therapies that appear to be efficacious in many men in clinical practice do not seem to be that effective when subjected to prospective randomized placebo-controlled trials. The future will likely involve clinical phenotyping of patients presenting with CP/CPPS, hopefully with the development of new biomarkers and then therapy directed towards the patients' individual phenotype. These treatments may include antibiotics, anti-inflammatories, and prostate-directed therapies in some patients, while others may require various therapeutic plans that incorporate medical and minimally invasive neuromodulation, physical and cognitive behavioral therapies [35].

Implications for research

Future therapies must look beyond the traditional biomedical model of CP/CPPS and examine therapies directed towards the evolving biopsychosocial phenotyping model of CP/CPPS. Basic science studies are urgently required to examine the multiple etiologies of this condition, develop clinical phenotype models (discovery of novel biomarkers) and evaluate treatment modalities which appear to be promising (neuromodulation, physical therapy, cognitive behavioral therapy).

Implications for practice

Recommendations based on the evidence would suggest that the clinician has few options for treating patients presenting with CP/CPPS. The following is a therapeutic plan that will benefit patients while we wait for the basic and clinical science to catch up with us. The clinician should use his/her clinical evaluation to clinically phenotype CP/CPPS patients using the UPOINT phenotype classification system [36,37], a system developed for both of the urological chronic pelvic pain syndromes (interstitial cystitis and prostatitis), and then employ focused treatment based on that phenotype.

• *U*rinary phenotype – in patients with obstructive voiding (history and/or flow rate), a 12-week course of an alpha-blocker may be of benefit. In men over 45 years of age, with a large prostate (co-existing benign prostatic hyperplasia), 5-alpha-reductase inhibitor therapy could be contemplated.

• *P*sychosocial phenotype – men with CP/CPPS commonly present with evidence of clinical depression, maladaptive coping (e.g. catastrophizing) and/or evidence of abuse history. For these patients, therapy should included counseling, cognitive behavioral therapy, antidepressants, etc.

• *O*rgan (prostate)-specific phenotype – men with CP/CPPS can present with a primary symptom of deep perineal and/or ejaculatory pain as their major (or only) symptom that coincides with other organ-specific findings on clinical (pain localized to prostate on physical examination) or laboratory examination (prostate inflammation on microscopy). For these patients, anti-inflammatories (quercetin, NSAIDs), analgesics, repetitive prostate massage, surgery (only if indication) and the prostate-specific medications outlined in the urinary phenotype appear to be indicated.

• *I*nfection phenotype – in patients with a history of infection or response to antibiotics, but who have not been subjected to a long-term course of antibiotics, a 4-week course of a fluoroquinolone may be beneficial.

• *N*eurological/systemic phenotype – a significant proportion of men with CP/CPPS also present with a number of associated conditions including irritable bowel syndrome, fibromyalgia, chronic fatigue syndrome and other neurological conditions (e.g. migraines, back and/or leg pain). In these patients the following treatments should be considered: pregabalin, nortriptyline, amitriptyline, alternative or complementary neuromodulation (e.g. acupuncture).

• *T*enderness phenotype – in CP/CPPS patients with muscle spasm/trigger points related to pelvic floor, pelvis and/or abdomen during physical examination, pelvic physiotherapy, exercise, muscle relaxants, stress reduction, etc. may help.

Our understanding of CP/CPPS is evolving and our management will follow advances in clinical and basic sciences. The field, once ruled by anecdote and tradition, is now evidence based.

References

1. Nickel JC. The three A's of chronic prostatitis therapy; antibiotics, alpha-blockers, and anti-inflammatories: what is the evidence? BJU Int 2004;94:1230-3.

2. Krieger JN, Nyberg LJ, Nickel JC. NIH consensus definition and classification of prostatitis. JAMA 1999;282:236-7.

3. Nickel JC. Inflammatory conditions of the male genitourinary tract: prostatitis and related conditions, orchitis, and epididymitis. In: Walsh P (ed) *Campbell-Walsh Urology*, 9th edn. Philadelphia, PA: WB Saunders, 2006: 330-70.

4. Schaeffer AJ. Chronic prostatitis and the chronic pelvic pain syndrome. N Engl J Med 2006;355(16):1690-8.

5. Roberts RO, Lieber MM, Rhodes T, et al. Prevalence of a physician-assigned diagnosis of prostatitis: the Olmsted County study of urinary symptoms and health status among men. Urology 1998;51(40):578-84.

6. Nickel JC, Downey J, Hunter D, et al. Prevalance of prostatitis-like symptoms in a population based study employing the NIH-chronic prostatitis symptom index (NIH-CPSI). J Urol 2001;165:842-5.

7. McNaughton-Collins M, Joyce GF, Wise M, et al. Prostatitis. In: Litwin MS, Saigal CS (eds) *Urologic Diseases in America*. Washington, DC: US Government Publishing Office, 2007: 9-41.

8. McNaughton-Collins M, Pontari MA, O'Leary MP, et al. Quality of life is impaired in men with chronic prostatitis: the Chronic Prostatitis Collaborative Research Network. J Gen Intern Med 2001;16:656-62.

9. Calhoun EA, McNaughton-Collins M, Pontari MA, et al. The economic impact of chronic prostatitis. Arch Intern Med 2004;164:1231-6.

10. Litwin MS, McNaughton-Collins M, Fowler FJ, et al. The National Institutes of Health Chronic Prostatitis Symptom Index: development and validation of a new outcome measure. J Urol 1999;162(2):369-75.

11. Propert KJ, Litwin M, Wang Y, et al. Responsiveness of the NIH-CPSI. Qual Life Res 2006;15(2):299-305.

12. Nickel JC, Nyberg L, Hennennfent M. Research guidelines for chronic prostatitis: a consensus report from the first National Institutes of Health-International Prostatitis Collaborative Network (NIH-IPCN). Urology 1999;54:229-33.

13. Propert KJ, Alexander RB, Nickel JC, et al. The design of a multi-center randomized clinical trial for chronic prostatitis/chronic pelvic pain syndrome. Urology 2002;59:870-6.

14. Nickel JC, Downey J, Johnston B, et al. Predictors of patient response to antibiotic therapy for chronic prostatitis/chronic pelvic pain syndrome: a prospective multicenter clinical trial. J Urol 2001;165(5):1539-44.

15. Shoskes DA. Use of antibiotics in chronic prostatitis syndromes. Can J Urol 2001;8:24-8.

16. Bjerklund Johansen T, Gruneberg RN, Guibert J, et al. The role of antibiotics in the treatment of chronic prostatitis: a consensus statement. Eur Urol 1998;34:457-66.

17. Nickel JC, Downey J, Clark J, et al. Levofloxacin for chronic prostatitis/chronic pelvic pain syndrome in men: a randomized placebo-controlled multicenter trial. Urology 2003;62:614-17.

18. Alexander RB, Propert KJ, Schaeffer AJ, et al. Ciprofloxacin or tamsulosin in men with chronic prostatitis/chronic pelvic pain syndrome. Ann Intern Med 2004;141:581-9.

19. Nickel JC, Xiang J. Clinical significance of non-traditional uropathogens in the management of chronic prostatitis. J Urol 2008;179:1391-5.

20. Nickel JC, Pontari M, Moon T, et al. A randomized, placebo-controlled, multicenter study to evaluate the safety and efficacy of rofecoxib in the treatment of chronic nonbacterial prostatitis. J Urol 2003;169:1401-5.

21. Nickel JC, Johnston B, Downey J, et al. Pentosan polysulfate therapy for chronic nonbacterial prostatitis (chronic pelvic pain syndrome category IIIA): a prospective multicenter clinical trial. Urology 2000;56:413-17.

22. Nickel JC, Forrest JB, Tomera K, et al. Pentosan polysulfate sodium therapy for men with chronic pelvic pain syndrome: a multicenter, randomized, placebo-controlled study. J Urol 2005;173:1252-5.

23. Shoskes DA, Zeitlin SI, Shahed A, et al. Quercetin in men with category III chronic prostatitis: a preliminary prospective, double-blind, placebo control trial. Urology 1999;54(6):960-3.

24. Goldmeier D, Madden P, McKenna M, et al. Treatment of category IIIA prostatitis with zafirlukast: a randomized controlled feasiblity study. Int J STD AIDS 2005;16:196-200.

25. Nickel JC, Narayan P, McKay J, Doyle C. Treatment of chronic prostatitis/chronic pelvic pain syndrome with tamsulosin: a randomized double-blind trial. J Urol 2004;171:1594-7.

26. Cheah PY, Liong ML, Yuen KH, et al. Terazosin therapy for chronic prostatitis/chronic pelvic pain syndrome: a randomized, placebo controlled trial. J Urol 2003;169: 592-6.

27. Mehik A, Alas P, Nickel JC, et al. Alfuzosin treatment for chronic prostatitis/chronic pelvic pain syndrome: a prospective, randomized, double-blind, placebo-controlled, pilot study. Urology 2003;62:425-9.

28. Tugcu V, Tasci AI, Fazlioglu A, et al. A placebo-controlled comparison of the efficiency of triple- and monotherapy in category III B chronic pelvic pain syndrome (CPPS). Eur Urol 2007;51:1113-18.

29. Yang G, Wei Q, Li H, et al. The effect of alpha-adrenergic antagonists in chronic prostatitis/chronic pelvic pain syndrome: a meta-analysis of randomized controlled trials. J Androl 2006;27(6):847-52.

30. Mishra VC, Browne J, Emberton M. Role of alpha-blockers in type III prostatitis: a systemic review of the literature. J Urol 2007;177(1): 25-30.

31. Nickel JC, Krieger JN, McNaughton-Collins M, et al. Effect of alfuzosin on symptoms in men with chronic prostatitis/chronic pelvic pain syndrome. N Engl J Med 2008;359(25):2663-73.

32. Leskinen M, Lukkarinen O, Marttilla T. Effects of finasteride in patients with inflammatory chronic pelvic pain syndrome: a double-blind, placebo controlled, pilot study. Urology 1999;53:502-5.

33. Nickel JC, Downey J, Pontari MA, et al. Randomized placebo-controlled, multi-center study to evaluate the safety and efficacy

of finasteride in the treatment of male chronic pelvic pain syndrome: category IIIA CPPS (chronic nonbacterial prostatitis). BJU Int 2004;93:991-5.

34. De Rose AF, Gallo F, Giglio M, et al. Role of mepartricin in category III chronic nonbacterial prostatitis/chronic pelvic pain syndrome: a randomized prospective placebo-controlled trial. Urology 2004;63(1):13-16.

35. Nickel JC, Baranowski AP, Pontari M, Berger RE, Tripp DA. Management of men diagnosed with chronic prostatitis/chronic pelvic pain syndrome who have failed traditional management. Rev Urol 2007;9(2):1-10.

36. Shoskes DA, Nickel JC, Rackley RR, Pontari MA. Clinical phenotyping in chronic prostatitis/chronic pelvic pain syndrome and interstitial cystitis: a management strategy for urologic chronic pelvic pain syndromes. Prostate Cancer Prostatic Dis 2009;12:177-83.

37. Shoskes DA, Nickel JC, Dolinga R, Prots D. Clinical phenotyping of chronic prostatitis/chronic pelvic pain patients and correlation with symptom severity. Urology 2009;73:538-43.

13 Treatment of interstitial cystitis: does anything work?

Ann Oldendorf and J. Quentin Clemens
Department of Urology, University of Michigan, Ann Arbor, MI, USA

Introduction

For many clinicians, the treatment of interstitial cystitis/ painful bladder syndrome (IC/PBS) has become a lesson in learning to treat chronic pain. It is not a cancer that can be cured, nor a stone to be extracted. It is a painful triad of pelvic or bladder pain accompanied by urinary urgency and frequency. There is no perfect test to establish its diagnosis; rather, it is a diagnosis of exclusion. This is a chronic, frustrating disease which often leads patients to "doctor shop" and receive inadequate treatment for their chronic pain. Clinicians are equally frustrated due to the lack of effective treatment options for their patients.

A variety of treatments have been utilized to improve symptoms in IC/PBS patients. These include dietary modification, pelvic floor physical therapy, lifestyle interventions, oral medication, intravesical instillation therapy, neuromodulation, and surgical intervention. No single treatment has emerged as highly effective in all cases. Two frequently utilized therapies are oral pentosan polysulfate and intravesical instillations. We have reviewed the medical literature to evaluate the existing evidence to support these therapies.

Literature search

A Medline literature search was performed for the period 1980–2008 to identify all meta-analyses and systematic reviews related to the use of pentosan polysulfate for IC/PBS. These were identified by using a keyword search for "interstitial cystitis" and limiting the search to meta-analyses and systematic reviews. All abstracts identified by this process were then manually reviewed to identify publications which addressed the efficacy of pentosan polysulfate.

Clinical question 13.1

Is oral pentosan polysulfate effective in reducing IC/PBS symptoms?

The evidence

Dimitrakov and co-workers conducted a systematic review of the literature through 2007 to assess the efficacy of various pharmacological approaches to IC/PBS [1]. Included in this analysis were six randomized controlled trials and one meta-analysis which compared oral pentosan polysulfate to placebo. Treatment duration ranged from 12 to 24 weeks. The reported overall response rate varied between 15% and 67% in individual trials. Pooled analysis suggested benefit of active treatment compared with placebo, with a relative risk of 1.78 for patient-reported "global improvement" in symptoms (95% confidence interval 1.34–2.35) (Table 13.1). Improvements in pain, frequency, urgency, and Interstitial Cystitis Symptom Index scores were also reported, although many of these improvements did not reach statistical significance.

Comment

The current evidence suggests that pentosan polysulfate provides modest short-term benefit in the treatment of IC/ PBS symptoms (weak/conditional recommendation for using pentosan polysulfate: 2C). Few data exist regarding the duration of this treatment effect. It is unknown if a longer duration of therapy is beneficial in patients who do not respond to an initial 12–24-week trial.

Evidence-Based Urology. Edited by Philipp Dahm, Roger R. Dmochowski.
© 2010 Blackwell Publishing.

Table 13.1 Symptom response to pentosan polysufate therapy. Adapted from Dimitrakov et al. [1]

Outcome	Standardized mean difference (95% CI)*
Effect on patient-reported pain	
Mullholland et al. [3]	−0.15 (−0.53 to 0.22)
Parsons & Mullholland [4]	**−0.74 (−1.34 to −0.14)**
Sairanein et al. [5]	−0.48 (−1.01 to 0.04)
Sant et al. [6]	−0.11 (−0.62 to 0.40)
Effect on patient-reported urinary frequency	
Lazzeri et al. [7]	**−1.57 (−2.64 to -0.50)**
Parsons & Mullholland [4]	−0.51 (−1.06 to 0.03)
Sairanen et al. [5]	−0.27 (−0.85 to 0.31)
Sant et al. [6]	0.06 (−0.45 to 0.56)
Effect on patient-reported urinary urgency	
Parsons & Mullholland [4]	**−0.62 (−1.14 to −0.10)**
Sant et al. [6]	0.06 (−0.45 to 0.57)
Effect on Interstitial Cystitis Symptom Index [8] score	
Sairanen et al. [5]	**−0.89 (−1.49 to −0.28)**
Sant et al. [6]	−0.26 (−0.77 to 0.25)
Relative risk of overall improvement	
Holm-Bentzen et al. [9]	1.25 (0.76 to 2.04)
Mullholland et al. [3]	1.84 (0.81 to 4.17)
Parsons &Mullholland [4]	**2.67 (1.20 to 5.91)**
Parsons et al . [10]	**2.15 (1.21 to 3.82)**
Sant et al. [6]	1.91 (1.00 to 3.64)
Overall	**1.78 (1.34 to 2.35)**

* Values in bold have 95% confidence intervals which do not cross 1

Clinical question 13.2

Are intravesical therapies effective in reducing IC/PBS symptoms?

The evidence

A systematic review of intravesical treatments for IC/PBS was conducted by Dawson & Jamison [2]. Studies published through 30 May 2006 were included. Nine eligible trials were identified, with a total of 616 subjects. These included trials of six different intravesical preparations (resiniferatoxin, dimethyl sulfoxide, BCG, pentosan polysulfate, oxybutynin, and urinary pH alkalinization). Outcome measures were highly variable, and confidence intervals for effects sizes were quite wide due to small sample sizes (Table 13.2). Evidence to support any of the therapies was inconclusive.

Comment

Although intravesical instillation therapy for IC/PBS is conceptually appealing and is widely practiced, the evidence base for using this therapeutic modality is extremely limited. Very few randomized controlled trials have been performed to assess the efficacy of intravesical therapy versus placebo instillations. The available data suggest that the current agents confer no clear benefit above those obtained with placebo instillations. However, given the paucity of data, no clear recommendations can be made regarding this treatment modality.

Table 13.2 Response to intravesical instillation therapy. Adapted from Dawson & Jamison [2]

Reference	Agent	No. of subjects	Outcome	Statistical method	Effect size (95% CI)
Mayer [11]	BCG	246	Change in pain score	Weighted mean difference	−0.50 (−1.06 to 0.06)
Peters [12]	BCG	32	Improvement in pelvic pain	Relative risk	1.76 (0.78 to 4.00)
Perez-Marrero [13]	DMSO cross-over	32	Pain relieved	Odds ratio	0.22 (−1.10 to 1.55)
Mayer [11]	BCG	222	Change in bladder capacity	Weighted mean difference	−9.00 (−44.38 to 26.83)
Perez-Marrero [13]	DMSO cross-over	32	Maximum cystometric capacity	Mean difference	17.00 (−11.22 to 45.22)
Mayer [11]	BCG	246	Change in frequency	Weighted mean difference	−1.20 (−3.42 to 1.02)
Mayer [11]	BCG	246	Change in IC Symptom Index	Weighted mean difference	−0.70 (−1.70 to 0.30)
Mayer [11]	BCG	246	Change in IC Problem Index	Weighted mean difference	−0.60 (−1.56 to 0.36)
Bade [14]	Pentosan polysulfate	20	Subjective symptom improvement	Relative risk	2.00 (0.47 to 8.56)
Payne [15] Mayer [11]	Resiniferatoxin	163	Subjective symptom improvement	Relative risk	0.74 (0.43 to 1.27)
Peters [12]	BCG	295	Subjective symptom improvement	Relative Risk	1.83 (1.12 to 2.99)

BCG, bacillus Calmette–Guerin; DMSO, dimethyl sulfoxide; IC, interstitial cystitis.

Implications for research

To date, efforts to identify effective therapies for IC/PBS have been unsuccessful. Further research is needed to provide a better understanding of the pathophysiology of this enigmatic condition. Furthermore, better characterization of IC/PBS into clinically relevant subpopulations may allow more targeted intervention strategies with better clinical outcomes.

References

1. Dimitrakov J, Kroenke K, Steers WD, et al. Pharmacologic management of painful bladder syndrome/interstitial cystitis. Arch Intern Med 2007;167(22):1922-9.
2. Dawson TE, Jamison J. Intravesical treatments for painful bladder syndrome/interstitial cystitis. Cochrane Database Syst Rev 2007;4:CD006113
3. Mullholland SG, Hanno P, Parsons CL, Sant GR, Staskin DR. Pentosan polysulfate sodium for therapy of interstitial cystitis: a double-blind placebo-controlled clinical study. Urology 1990;35:552-8.
4. Parsons CL, Mulholland SG. Successful therapy of interstitial cystitis with pentosanpolysulfate. J Urol 1987;138:513-16.
5. Sairanein J, Tammela TL, Leppilahti M, et al. Cyclosporine A and pentosan polysulfate sodium for the treatment of interstitial cystitis: a randomized comparative study. J Urol 2005;174:2235-8.
6. Sant GR, Propert KJ, Hanno PM, et al. A pilot clinical trial of oral pentosan polysulfate and oral hydroxyzine in patients with interstitial cystitis. J Urol 2003;170:810-15.
7. Lazzeri M, Benefort P, Spinelli M, Zanollo A, Barbagli G, Turini D. Intravesical resiniferatoxin for the treatment of hypersensitive disorder: a randomized placebo controlled study. J Urol 2000;164:676-9.
8. O'Leary MP, Sant GR, Fowler FJ Jr, Whitmore KE, Spolarich-Kroll J. The interstitial cystitis symptom index and problem index. Urology 1997;49(5A)(suppl):58-63.
9. Holm-Bentzen M, Jacobsen F, Nerstrom B, et al. A prospective double-blind clinically controlled multicenter trials of sodium pentosanpolysulfate in the treatment of interstitial cystitis and related painful bladder disease. J Urol 1987;138:503-7.
10. Parsons CL, Benson G, Childs SJ, Hanno P, Sant GR, Webster G. A quantitatively controlled method to study prospectively interstitial cystitis and demonstrate the efficacy of pentosanpolysulfate. J Urol 1993;150:845-8.
11. Mayer R, Propert KJ, Peters KM, et al. A randomized controlled trial of intravesical bacillus Calmette–Guerin for treatment refractory interstitial cystitis. J Urol 2005;173:1186-91.
12. Peters K, Diokno A, Steinert B, et al. The efficacy of intravesical Tice strain bacillus Calmette–Guerin in the treatment of interstitial cystitis: a double-blind, prospective, placebo controlled trial. J Urol 1997;157:2090-4.
13. Perez-Marrero R, Emerson LE, Feltis JT. A controlled study of dimethyl sulfoxide in interstitial cystitis. J Urol 1988;140:36-9.
14. Bade JJ, Laseur M, Nieuwenburg A, van der Weele LT, Mensink HJ. A placebo-controlled study of intravesical pentosanpolysulfate for the treatment of interstitial cystitis. BJU 1997;79:168-71.
15. Payne CK, Mosbaugh PG, Forrest JB, et al. Intravesical resiniferatoxin for the treatment of interstitial cystitis: a randomized, double-blind, placebo-controlled trial. J Urol 2005; 173:1590-4.

14 Treatment of premature ejaculation

Chris G. McMahon
University of Sydney, Australian Centre for Sexual Health, Sydney, Australia

Introduction

Over the past 20–30 years, the premature ejaculation (PE) treatment paradigm, previously limited to behavioral psychotherapy, has expanded to include drug treatment [1,2]. Animal and human sexual psychopharmacological studies have demonstrated that serotonin and 5-HT receptors are involved in ejaculation and confirm a role for selective serotonin reuptake inhibitors (SSRIs) in the treatment of PE [3-6]. Many well-controlled evidence-based studies have demonstrated the efficacy and safety of SSRIs in delaying ejaculation, confirming their role as first-line agents for the treatment of lifelong and acquired PE [7]. More recently, there has been increased interest in the psychosocial consequences of PE, its epidemiology, its etiology and its pathophysiology from both clinicians and the pharmaceutical industry [8-13].

Clinical question 14.1

What is the definition of premature ejaculation?

The evidence

Medline, Web of Science, PsychINFO, EMBASE and the proceedings of major international and regional scientific meetings were searched for publications or abstracts using the words in the title, abstract or keywords "premature ejaculation," "rapid ejaculation," "ejaculation," "definition," "control," "distress," "sexual satisfaction," "ejaculatory latency." This search was then manually cross-referenced for all papers.

The medical literature contains several univariate and multivariate operational definitions of PE [2,14-21]. Each of these definitions characterizes men with PE using all or most of the accepted dimensions of this condition: ejaculatory latency, perceived ability to control ejaculation, and negative psychological consequences of PE including reduced sexual satisfaction, personal distress, partner distress and interpersonal or relationship distress.

The first official definition of PE was proposed in 1980 by the American Psychiatric Association (APA) in the *Diagnostic and Statistical Manual of Mental Disorders* (DSM-III) [22]. This definition was progressively revised in the DSM-III-R, DSM-IV and finally DSM-IV-TR to include "shortly after penetration" as an ejaculatory latency criterion, "before the person wishes it" as a control criterion and "causes marked distress or interpersonal difficulty" as a criterion for the negative psychological consequences of PE [14,23,24]. Although DSM-IV-TR, the most commonly quoted definition, and other definitions of PE differ substantially, they are all authority based, i.e. expert opinion without explicit critical appraisal, rather than evidence based, and have no support from controlled clinical and/or epidemiological studies [25]. The DSM definitions are primarily conceptual in nature, vague in terms of operational specificity, multi-interpretable, fail to provide any diagnostic intravaginal ejaculatory latency time (IELT) cut-off points and rely on the subjective interpretation of these concepts by the clinician [26-28]. The absence of a clear IELT cut-off point in the DSM definitions has resulted in the use of a broad range of subjective latencies for the diagnosis of PE in clinical trials ranging from 1 to 7 minutes [29-37]. The failure of DSM definitions to specify an IELT cut-off point means that a patient in the control group of one study may very well be in the PE group of a second study, making comparison of studies difficult and generalization of their data to the general PE population impossible.

This potential for errors in the diagnosis of PE was demonstrated in two recent observational studies in which PE

Evidence-Based Urology. Edited by Philipp Dahm, Roger R. Dmochowski.
© 2010 Blackwell Publishing.

was diagnosed solely by the application of the DSM-IV-TR definition [11,38]. Giuliano et al. diagnosed PE using DSM-IV-TR criteria in 201 of 1115 subjects (18%) and predictably reported that the mean and median IELT were lower in subjects diagnosed with PE compared to non-PE subjects. There was, however, substantial overlap in stopwatch IELT values between the two groups. In subjects diagnosed with PE, the IELT range extended from 0 seconds (antiportal ejaculation) to almost 28 minutes with 48% of subjects having an IELT in excess of 2 minutes and 25% of subjects exceeding 4 minutes. This study demonstrates that a subject diagnosed as having PE on the basis of DSM-IV-TR criteria has a 48% risk of not having PE if a PE diagnostic threshold IELT of 2 minutes, as suggested by community-based normative IELT trial, is used [10].

The first contemporary multivariate evidence-based definition of lifelong PE was developed in 2008 by a panel of international experts, convened by the International Society for Sexual Medicine (ISSM), who agreed that the diagnostic criteria necessary to define PE are: time from penetration to ejaculation, inability to delay ejaculation and negative personal consequences from PE. This panel defined lifelong PE as a male sexual dysfunction characterized by ". . . ejaculation which always or nearly always occurs prior to or within about one minute of vaginal penetration, the inability to delay ejaculation on all or nearly all vaginal penetrations, and the presence of negative personal consequences, such as distress, bother, frustration and/or the avoidance of sexual intimacy" [39].

This definition is supported by evidence from several controlled clinical trials.

Evidence to support inclusion of the criterion of ". . . ejaculation which always or nearly always occurs prior to or within about one minute of vaginal penetration . . ."

Operationalization of PE using the length of time between penetration and ejaculation, the IELT, forms the basis of most current clinical studies on PE [40]. IELT can be measured by a stopwatch or estimated. Several authors report that estimated and stopwatch IELT correlate reasonably well or are interchangeable in assigning PE status when estimated IELT is combined with patient-reported outcomes (PROs) [41-43].

Several studies suggest that 80–90% of men seeking treatment for lifelong PE ejaculate within 1 minute (Table 14.1) [44-46]. Waldinger et al. reported IELTs < 30 s in 77% and < 60 s in 90% of 110 men with lifelong PE, with only 10% ejaculating between 1 and 2 minutes. These data are consistent with normative community IELT data, support the notion that IELTs of less than 1 minute are statistically abnormal and confirm that an IELT cut-off of 1 minute will capture 80–90% of treatment-seeking men with lifelong PE [10]. Further qualification of this cut-off to "about

Table 14.1 Findings of key publications regarding the time-to-ejaculate in PE

Author/s	Summary of primary findings
Waldinger et al. [44]	110 men with lifelong PE whose IELT was measured by the use of a stopwatch 40% of men ejaculated within 15 seconds, 70% within 30 seconds, and 90% within 1 minute
McMahon [45]	1346 consecutive men with PE whose IELT was measured by the use of a stopwatch/wristwatch 77% of men ejaculated within 1 minute
Waldinger et al. [46]	88 men with lifelong PE who self-estimated IELT 30% of men ejaculated within 15 seconds, 67% within 30 seconds, and 92% within 1 minute after penetration Only 5% ejaculated between 1 and 2 minutes
Waldinger et al. [10]	Stopwatch IELT study in a random unselected group of 491 men in 5 countries IELT had a positive skewed distribution Application of 0.5 and 2.5 percentiles as disease standards 0.5 percentile equated to an IELT of 0.9 min and 2.5 percentile to an IELT of 1.3 min
Althof [41]	IELT estimations for PE men correlate reasonably well with stopwatch-recorded IELT
Pryor et al. [42]	IELT estimations for PE men correlate reasonably well with stopwatch-recorded IELT
Rosen et al. [43]	Self-estimated and stopwatch IELT as interchangeable Combining self-estimated IELT and PROs reliably predicts PE

1 minute" affords the clinician sufficient flexibility to also diagnose PE in the 10–20% of PE treatment-seeking men who ejaculate within 1–2 minutes of penetration without unnecessarily stigmatizing the remaining 80–90% of men who ejaculate within 1–2 minutes of penetration but have no complaints of PE.

Evidence to support inclusion of the criterion ". . . the inability to delay ejaculation on all or nearly all vaginal penetrations . . ."

The ability to prolong sexual intercourse by delaying ejaculation and the subjective feelings of ejaculatory control comprise the complex construct of ejaculatory control. Virtually all men report using at least one cognitive or behavioral technique to prolong intercourse and delay ejaculation, with varying degrees of success, and many young men reported using multiple different techniques [47]. Voluntary delay of ejaculation is most likely exerted either prior to or in the early stages of the emission phase of the reflex but progressively decreases until the point of ejaculatory inevitability [48,49].

Several authors have suggested that an inability to voluntarily defer ejaculation defines PE (Table 14.2) [50-53]. Patrick et al. reported ratings of "very poor" or "poor" for

Table 14.2 Findings of key publications regarding ejaculatory control in PE

Author/s	Summary of primary findings
Grenier & Byers [47]	Relatively weak correlation between ejaculatory latency and ejaculatory control (R = 0.31) Ejaculatory control and latency are distinct concepts
Grenier & Byers [54]	Relatively poor correlation between ejaculatory latency and ejaculatory control, sharing only 12% of their variance suggesting that these PROs are relatively independent
Waldinger et al. [44]	Little or no control over ejaculation was reported by 98% of subjects during intercourse Weak correlation between ejaculatory control and stopwatch IELT (p = 0.06)
Rowland et al. [56]	High correlation between measures of ejaculatory latency and control (R = 0.81, p < 0.001)
Patrick et al. [11]	Men diagnosed with PE had significantly lower mean ratings of control over ejaculation (p < 0.0001) 72% of men with PE reporting ratings of "very poor" or "poor" for control over ejaculation compared to 5% in a group of normal controls IELT was strongly positively correlated with control over ejaculation for subjects (R = 0.51)
Giuliano et al. [57]	Men diagnosed with PE had significantly lower mean ratings of control over ejaculation (p < 0.0001) "Good" or "very good" control over ejaculation in only 13.2% of PE subjects compared to 78.4% of non-PE subjects Perceived control over ejaculation had a significant effect on intercourse satisfaction and personal distress IELT did not have a direct effect on intercourse satisfaction and had only a small direct effect on personal distress
Patrick et al. [58]	Effect of IELT upon satisfaction and distress appears to be mediated via its direct effect upon control
Rosen et al. [43]	Control over ejaculation and subject assessed level of personal distress are more influential in determining PE status than IELT Subject reporting "very good" or "good" control over ejaculation is 90.6% less likely to have PE than a subject reporting "poor" or "very poor" control over ejaculation

control over ejaculation in 72% of men with PE compared to 5% in a group of normal controls [11]. Lower ratings for control over ejaculation were associated with shorter IELT with "poor" or "very poor" control reported by 67.7%, 10.2% and 6.7% of subjects with IELT < 1 min, > 1 min and > 2 min respectively.

However, control is a subjective measure which is difficult to translate into quantifiable terms and is the most inconsistent dimension of PE. Control has yet to be adequately operationalized to allow comparison across subjects or across studies. Grenier & Byers failed to demonstrate a strong correlation between ejaculatory latency and subjective ejaculatory control [47,54]. Several authors

report that diminished control is not exclusive to men with PE and that some men with a brief IELT report adequate ejaculatory control and vice versa, suggesting that the dimensions of ejaculatory control and latency are distinct concepts [11,47,55]. Furthermore, there is a higher variability in changes in control compared to IELT in men treated with SSRIs [7].

Contrary to this, several authors have reported a moderate correlation between the IELT and the feeling of ejaculatory control [11,43,56,57]. Rosen et al. report that control over ejaculation, personal distress and partner distress was more influential in determining PE status than IELT [43]. In addition, the effect of IELT upon satisfaction and distress appears to be mediated via its direct effect upon control [58].

However, despite conflicting data on the relationship between control and latency, the balance of evidence supports the notion that the inability to delay ejaculation appears to differentiate men with PE from men without PE [11,57,59].

Evidence to support exclusion of the criterion of sexual satisfaction

Men with PE report lower levels of sexual satisfaction compared to men with normal ejaculatory latency. Patrick et al. reported ratings of "very poor" or "poor" for sexual satisfaction in 31% of subjects with PE compared to 1% in a group of normal controls [11].

However, caution should be exercised in assigning lower levels of sexual satisfaction solely to the effect of PE and contributions from other difficult-to-quantify issues such reduced intimacy, dysfunctional relationships, poor sexual attraction, and poor communication should not be ignored. This is supported by the report of Patrick et al. that despite reduced ratings for satisfaction with shorter IELTs, a substantial proportion of men with an IELT < 1 min report "good" or very good" satisfaction ratings (43.7%).

The current data are limited but suggest that sexual satisfaction is of limited use in differentiating PE subjects from non-PE subjects and are not included in the ISSM definition of PE [11].

Evidence to support inclusion of the criterion "... the presence of negative personal consequences, such as distress, bother, frustration and/or the avoidance of sexual intimacy"

Premature ejaculation has been associated with negative psychological outcomes in men and their women partners (Table 14.3) [9,11,12,57,59-69]. Patrick et al. reported significant differences in men with and without PE in the PRO measures of personal distress (64% versus 4%) and interpersonal difficulty (31% versus 1%), suggesting that this personal distress has discriminative validity in diagnosing men with and without PE.

Table 14.3 Findings of key publications regarding the negative personal consequences of PE

Author/s	Summary of primary findings
Patrick et al. [11]	Using the validated Premature Ejaculation Profile (PEP), 64% of men in the PE group versus 4% in the non-PE group reported personal distress
Giuliano et al. [57]	On the PEP 44% of men in the PE group versus 1% of men in non-PE group reported personal distress
Rowland et al. [61]	Men in highly probable PE group reported greater distress versus men in non-PE group on PEP scale On the Self Esteem and Relationship Questionnaire (SEAR) men with highly probable PE had lower mean scores overall, for confidence and self-esteem versus non-PE men
Rowland et al. [59]	30.7% of probable PE group, 16.4% of possible PE group vs 7.7% of non-PE group found it difficult to relax and not be anxious about intercourse
Porst et al. [12]	Depression reported by 20.4% of PE group vs 12.4% of non-PE group Excessive stress in 28% of PE group vs 19% of non-PE group Anxiety in 24% of PE group vs 13% in non-PE group
McCabe. [63]	Sexually dysfunctional men, including those with PE, scored lower than sexually functional men on all measures of intimacy on the Psychological and Interpersonal Relationship Scale (PAIRS)
Symonds et al. [9]	68% reported self-esteem affected by PE. Decreased confidence in sexual encounter Anxiety reported by 36% (causing PE or because of it) Embarrassment and depression also cited due to PE
Dunn et al. [60]	Strong association of PE with anxiety and depression on the Hospital and Anxiety Scale
Hartmann et al. [66]	58% of PE group reported partner's behavior and reaction to PE was positive and 23% reported it was negative
Byers et al. 2003 [64]	Men with PE and their partners reported slightly negative impact of PE on personal functioning and sexual relationship but no negative impact on overall relationship

The personal and/or interpersonal distress, bother, frustration and annoyance that result from PE may affect men's quality of life and partner relationships, their self-esteem and self-confidence, and can act as an obstacle to single men forming new partner relationships [9,11,12,57,59-69]. McCabe reported that sexually dysfunctional men, including men with PE, scored lower on all aspects of intimacy (emotional, social, sexual, recreational and intellectual) and had lower levels of satisfaction compared to sexually functional men (p < 0.001 or p < 0.01) [63]. Rowland et al. showed that men with PE had significantly lower overall health-related quality of life, total Self-Esteem and Relationship Questionnaire (SEAR) scores and lower confidence and self-esteem compared to non-PE groups [61]. PE men rated their overall health-related quality of life lower than men without PE (p ≤ 0.001).

This definition should form the basis for the office diagnosis of lifelong PE. It is limited to heterosexual men engaging in vaginal intercourse as there are few studies available on PE research in homosexual men or during other forms of sexual expression. The panel concluded that there is insufficient published evidence to propose an evidence-based definition of acquired PE [39]. However, recent unpublished data suggest that men with acquired PE have similar IELTs and report similar levels of ejaculatory control and distress, suggesting the possibility of a single unifying definition of PE.

Comment

The evidence suggests that the multivariate evidence-based ISSM definition of lifelong PE gives the clinician a more discriminating diagnostic tool. The IELT cut-off of about 1 minute captures the 90% of men with PE who actively seek treatment and ejaculate within 1 minute but also affords the clinician sufficient flexibility to also diagnose PE in the 10% of PE treatment-seeking men who ejaculate within 1–2 minutes of penetration. If the ISSM definition is used, men who ejaculate in < 1 minute but report adequate control and no personal negative consequences related to their rapid ejaculation do not merit the diagnosis of PE. Similarly, men who have IELTs of 10 minutes but report poor control, dissatisfaction and personal negative consequences also fail to meet the criteria for PE.

Clinical question 14.2

Is psychosexual cognitive behavioral therapy effective as a treatment for premature ejaculation?

The evidence

Medline, Web of Science, PsychINFO, EMBASE and the proceedings of major international and regional scientific meetings were searched for publications or abstracts using the words in the title, abstract or keywords "premature ejaculation," "rapid ejaculation," "ejaculation," "cognitive behavioral therapy," "psychological counseling" and "sex therapy." This search was then manually cross-referenced for all papers.

The cornerstones of cognitive behavioral treatment (CBT), the Semans "stop-start" maneuver and the Masters & Johnson "squeeze technique," were first described as a treatment of PE more than 50 years ago [1,2]. Although contemporary psychotherapy research has attempted to adapt the methodology of clinical psychopharmacology randomized controlled trials (RCTs) to define empirically supported psychotherapies [70,71], the medical literature is characterized by an almost complete lack of supportive RCTs (Table 14.4). Rowland & Burek reported a trend over the past 25 years towards the publication of biological and pharmacological articles and a decline in the proportion of psychological behavior articles [72]. They suggested that researchers are missing the opportunity to investigate important biobehavioral interactions underlying ejaculatory dysfunction, and to augment the current biopharmacological paradigm by integrating cognitive behavioral and sex therapy programs into pharmacological PE treatment

The lack of psychotherapy RCT data reflects, in part, the inherent difficulties in devising a convincing psychotherapy placebo and many psychotherapy placebos are retrospectively criticized as potentially effective treatments. The problems associated with creating a suitable placebo condition in psychotherapy research are threefold [73]. First, a placebo is conceptually an inert intervention and in pharmacological trials any response to a placebo pill is regarded as being due to psychological factors. However, in psychotherapy, all change is due to psychological factors. If a change occurs in response to a psychological placebo, the "placebo" is thus not inert and the statement is self-contradictory. Furthermore, investigators who administer treatment will know that one of the treatments is a placebo, making a double-blind RCT design impossible and introducing investigator bias and treatment expectation as confounding factors. Second, it is difficult to create a psychological placebo whose credibility and expectancy generation in the subject are equivalent to that of actual therapy conditions [74]. Without such equivalence, the placebo condition fails to control for a critical aspect of the very factor for which it is being used and the central confound thus remains. Furthermore, the more credible the psychotherapy placebo becomes, the closer it becomes to qualifying as an active rather than placebo treatment. Finally, significant ethical problems exist for the use of psychological placebos which include potential harm to subjects due to the inherent deception involved, the fact that they will not be seeking effective treatment during the course of the study, and the predicted minimal improvement that they will likely experience.

Anxiety has been reported as a cause of PE by multiple authors and is entrenched in the folklore of sexual medicine as the most likely cause of PE despite scant empirical research evidence to support any causal role [50,75,76]. Several authors have suggested that anxiety activates the sympathetic nervous system and reduces the ejaculatory threshold as a result of an earlier emission phase of ejaculation [50,76]. The possibility that high levels of anxiety and excessive and controlling concerns about sexual performance and potential sexual failure might distract a man from monitoring his level of arousal and recognizing the prodromal sensations that precede ejaculatory inevitability has been suggested as a possible cause of PE by several authors [52,53,77-80].

As most men with PE are aware of their anxiety and the sources of that anxiety tend to be relatively superficial, treatment success with these behavioral approaches is anecdotally reported as relatively good in the short term but convincing short- and long-term treatment outcome data from RCTs are lacking [51,81-83]. CBT, when combined with pharmacotherapy, is an effective intervention for acquired PE related to sexual performance anxiety and a substantial proportion of men report sustained improvements in ejaculatory latency and control following cessation of pharmacotherapy [19,45,49].

However, men with lifelong PE or acquired PE due to co-morbid erectile dysfunction (ED), hyperthyroidism, chronic lower urogenital infection, prostatodynia or chronic pelvic pain syndrome (CPPS) rarely achieve symptomatic improvement with CBT alone and are best managed with either SSRIs and/or etiology-specific pharmacotherapy alone or occasionally in combination with CBT if there is a significant secondary psychogenic or relationship contribution [45,84]. In men with lifelong PE, cessation of SSRI pharmacotherapy invariably results in a return to pretreatment latency and control within 1–2 weeks. This reflects the accumulating data suggesting that ejaculatory latency

Table 14.4 Findings of key publications regarding cognitive behavioral therapy/psychotherapy

Author/s	CBT	N	Study design	Level of evidence
Semans [1]	Stop-start technique	14	CBT	Low
Masters & Johnson [2]	Squeeze technique	–	Review	Low
McCarthy [51]	CBT techniques	–	Review	Low
De Carufel & Trudel [81]	CBT techniques	36	RCT	Moderate
De Amicis et al. [82]	Long-term results of CBT	38	Observation	Moderate
Hawton et al. [83]	Long-term results of CBT	–	Observation	Moderate
McMahon et al. [19]	Systematic review	–	Review	
Perelman [49]	Combination of pharmacotherapy and CBT	–	Review	Low
McMahon [45]	Combination of pharmacotherapy and CBT	171	Drug + CBT	Moderate

time is probably a biological variable, which is genetically determined and may range from extremely rapid through average to slow ejaculation. This is supported by animal studies showing a subgroup of persistent rapidly ejaculating Wistar rats [6], an increased familial occurrence of lifelong PE [5], a moderate genetic influence on PE in the Finnish twin study [85] and the recent report that genetic polymorphism of the 5-HTT gene determines the regulation of the IELT and that men with LL genotypes have statistically shorter IELTs than men with SS and SL genotypes [86].

There is evidence to suggest that type-V phosphodiesterase inhibitor drugs (PDE5i), alone or in combination with a SSRI, may have a role in the management of acquired PE in men with co-morbid ED [87-89]. The proposed mechanism of action of PDE5is as monotherapy or in combination with a SSRI in the treatment of acquired PE in men with co-morbid ED includes a reduction in performance anxiety due to better erections, downregulation of the erectile threshold to a lower level of arousal so that increased levels of arousal are required to achieve the ejaculation threshold and reduction of the erectile refractory period [55,90,91] and reliance upon a second and more controlled ejaculation during a subsequent episode of intercourse. Treatment of acquired PE secondary to hyperthyroidism requires thyroid hormone normalization with antithyroid drugs, radio-active iodine or thyroidectomy. Although antibiotic treatment of chronic prostatitis improves lower urinary tract symptoms (LUTS), there are few published data to suggest a parallel improvement in PE and other sexual dysfunction symptoms [92-94]. El-Nashaar & Shamloul reported that antibiotic treatment of microbiologically confirmed bacterial prostatitis in men with acquired PE resulted in a 2.6-fold increase in IELT and improved ejaculatory control in 83.9% of subjects [94].

Comment

The evidence suggests that psychosexual CBT has a limited role in the contemporary management of PE with low-quality evidence and a weak/conditional recommendation (**Grade 2C**). Men with acquired PE due to sexual performance anxiety or other psychological or relationship factors can be treated with CBT alone or combined with pharmacotherapy according to patient/partner preference. Men with lifelong PE should be initially managed with pharmacotherapy and may benefit from concomitant behavioral therapy if significant contributing psychogenic or relationship factors are present. However, recurrence of lifelong PE is highly likely to occur following withdrawal of pharmacotherapy. Men with PE secondary to ED, hyperthyroidism, chronic lower urogenital infection, prostatodynia or CPPS should receive appropriate etiology-specific treatment alone or in combination with SSRIs.

Clinical question 14.3

Is pharmacotherapy an effective and safe treatment for premature ejaculation?

The evidence

Medline, Web of Science, PsychINFO, EMBASE and the proceedings of major international and regional scientific meetings were searched for publications or abstracts using the words in the title, abstract or keywords "premature ejaculation," "rapid ejaculation," "ejaculation," "treatment," "drug," "medication." This search was then manually cross-referenced for all papers.

The first publication on the pharmacological treatment of PE was the 1943 report of Schapiro that PE was a psychosomatic disturbance which could be treated with on-demand use of topical anesthetic cream to delay ejaculation [75]. The introduction of the serotonergic tricyclic clomipramine and the SSRIs paroxetine, sertraline, fluoxetine, citalopram and fluvoxamine has revolutionized the approach to and treatment of PE. These drugs block axonal reuptake of serotonin from the synaptic cleft of central and peripheral serotonergic neurons by 5-HT transporters, resulting in enhanced 5-HT neurotransmission, stimulation of postsynaptic membrane 5-HT2C autoreceptors and delayed ejaculation. Although the methodology of the initial drug treatment studies was poor, later double-blind and placebo-controlled studies confirmed the ejaculation-delaying effect of clomipramine, SSRIs and topical anesthetics (Tables 14.5-14.7). These drugs can be administered on either a chronic daily basis or "on demand," prior to planned sexual contact.

Daily treatment with SSRIs

Daily treatment with paroxetine 10–40 mg, clomipramine 12.5–50 mg, sertraline 50–200 mg, fluoxetine 20–40 mg and citalopram 20–40 mg is usually effective in delaying ejaculation (see Table 14.5) [95-100]. A meta-analysis of published data suggests that paroxetine exerts the strongest ejaculation delay, increasing IELT approximately 8.8-fold over baseline [95]. However, the use of these drugs is limited by the lack of Food and Drug Administration (FDA), European Medicines Agency (EMEA) or other regulatory agency approval as a treatment for PE and the need to prescribe "off-label." This largely reflects the failure of the pharmaceutical industry to appreciate the prevalence of PE, the unmet treatment need and the commercial opportunity of an approved drug treatment for PE [101].

Ejaculation delay usually occurs within 5–10 days of starting treatment, but the full therapeutic effect may require 2–3 weeks of treatment and is usually sustained

Table 14.5 Findings of key publications regarding daily drug treatment

Author/s	Drug	N	Study design	Level of evidence
Atmaca et al. [96]	Citalopram	26	DBRCT	Moderate
Safarinejad & Hosseini [142]	Citalopram	58	DBRCT	Moderate
Waldinger et al. [143]	Citalopram	30	DBRCT	Moderate
Goodman [100]	Clomipramine	20	DBRCT	Low
Girgis et al. [144]	Clomipramine	50	DBRCT	Low
Althof et al. [41]	Clomipramine	15	DBRCT	Low
McMahon [45]	Clomipramine, paroxetine, sertraline, fluoxetine	171	SBRCT	Moderate
McMahon & Touma [129]	Paroxetine	68	DBRCT	Moderate
Safarinejad [145]	Escitalopram	276	DBRCT	Moderate
Kara et al. [146]	Fluoxetine	17	DBRCT	Low
Haensel et al. [147]	Fluoxetine	40	DBRCT	Moderate
Yilmaz et al. [148]	Fluoxetine	40	DBRCT	Low
Waldinger et al. [138]	Fluoxetine, fluvoxamine, paroxetine, sertraline	51	DBRCT	High
Kim & Seo [149]	Fluoxetine, sertraline, clomipramine	36	DBRCT	Moderate
Waldinger [95]	Meta-analysis		DBRCT	High
Waldinger et al. [99]	Paroxetine	17	DBRCT	Moderate
Waldinger et al. [150]	Paroxetine	34	DBRCT	High
McMahon & Touma [151]	Paroxetine	94	Open	Moderate
Waldinger et al. [152]	Paroxetine, Mirtazapine	24	DBRCT	Moderate
McMahon [153]	Sertraline	37	SBRCT	Moderate
Arafa & Shamloul [154]	Sertraline	147	SBRCT, cross-over	Moderate
Mendels et al. [155]	Sertraline	52	DBRCT	Moderate
Biri et al. [156]	Sertraline	37	DBRCT	Moderate
McMahon [157]	Sertraline	46	Open	Low
Akgül et al. [158]	Sertraline, Citalopram	80	DBRCT	Moderate
Basar et al. [116]	Terazosin	90	SBRCT	Low
Cavallini [115]	Terazosin, Alfuzosin	91	DBRCT	Very Low
Safarinejad & Hosseini [118]	Tramadol	64	DBRCT	Low
Salem et al. [119]	Tramadol	60	SBRCT	Low

cross-over, cross-over study; DBRCT, double-blind randomized clinical trial; open, open label study; SBRCT, single-blind randomized clinical trial

during long-term use [45]. Although tachyphylaxis is uncommon, some patients report a reduced response after 6–12 months of treatment. Adverse effects are usually minor, start in the first week of treatment, gradually disappear within 2–3 weeks and include fatigue, yawning, mild nausea, diarrhea or perspiration. Hypoactive desire and ED are infrequently reported and appear to have a lower incidence in nondepressed PE men compared to depressed men treated with SSRIs [102].

Neurocognitive adverse effects include significant agitation and hypomania in a small number of patients and treatment with SSRIs should be avoided in men with a history of bipolar depression [103]. Systematic analysis of antidepressant RCTs demonstrates a small increase in the risk of suicidal ideation or suicide attempts in youth [104] but not adults [104,105], suggesting that SSRIs should not be prescribed as a treatment for PE to young men aged 18 years or less, and to men with a depressive disorder, particularly when associated with suicidal thoughts. Patients should be advised to avoid sudden cessation or rapid dose

reduction of SSRIs which may be associated with a SSRI withdrawal syndrome, characterized by dizziness, headache, nausea, vomiting and diarrhea and occasionally agitation, impaired concentration, vivid dreams, depersonalization, irritability and suicidal ideation [106,107]. Platelet serotonin release has an important role in hemostasis [108] and SSRIs, especially with concurrent use of aspirin and nonsteroidal anti-inflammatory drugs, are associated with an increased risk of upper gastrointestinal bleeding [109,110]. Priapism is a rare adverse effect of SSRIs and requires urgent medical treatment [111-113]. Long-term SSRIs may be associated with weight gain and an increased risk of type 2 diabetes mellitus [114].

Daily treatment with alpha-1-adrenoceptor antagonists

Ejaculation is a sympathetic spinal cord reflex which could theoretically be delayed by alpha-1- adrenergic blockers. Several authors have reported their experience with the selective alpha-1-adrenergic blockers alfuzosin and terazosin in the treatment of PE (see Table 14.5). Both drugs are approved only for the treatment of LUTS in men with obstructive benign prostatic hyperplasia (BPH). In a double-blind placebo-controlled study, Cavallini reported that both alfuzosin (6 mg/day) and terazosin (5 mg/day) were effective in delaying ejaculation in approximately 50% of cases [115]. Similarly, Basar et al. reported that terazosin was effective in 67% of men [116]. However, both studies were limited by the use of subjective study endpoints of patient impression of change and sexual satisfaction and did not evaluate objective endpoints such as IELT. Additional controlled studies are required to determine the role of alpha-1-blockers in the treatment of PE and at this stage routine use cannot be recommended.

Tramadol

Tramadol is a centrally acting synthetic opioid analgesic with an unclear mode of action which is thought to include binding of parent and M1 metabolite to μ-opioid receptors and weak inhibition of reuptake of GABA, norepinephrine and serotonin [117]. The efficacy of on-demand tramadol in the treatment of PE was recently reported in two RCTs (see Table 14.6) [118,119]. Both studies were poorly designed and although tramadol is reported to have a lower risk of dependence than traditional opioids, its use as an on-demand treatment for PE is limited by the potential risk of addiction [120]. In community practice, dependence does occur but appears minimal [121]. Adams et al. reported abuse rates of 0.7% for tramadol compared to 0.5% for nonsteroidal anti-inflammatory drugs and 1.2% for hydrocodone based upon application of a dependency

algorithm as a measure of persistence of drug use [122]. Additional flexible-dose, long-term follow-up studies are required to evaluate efficacy, safety and, in particular, the risk of opioid addiction and at this stage routine use cannot be recommended.

Topical anesthetics

The use of topical local anesthetics such as lidocaine and/or prilocaine as a cream, gel or spray is well established and is moderately effective in retarding ejaculation (see Table 14.7). They may be associated with significant penile hypoanesthesia and possible transvaginal absorption, resulting in vaginal numbness and resultant female anorgasmia unless a condom is use [123-125]. A recent study reported that a metered-dose aerosol spray containing a eutectic mixture of lidocaine and prilocaine (TEMPE®) produced a 2.4-fold increase in baseline IELT and significant improvements in ejaculatory control and both patient and partner sexual quality of life [126]. The physicochemical characteristics of this eutectic mixture and the spray delivery system have been designed to both optimize and limit tissue penetration to the mucosa of the glans penis and not the keratinized skin of the penile shaft [127].

Table 14.7 Findings of key publications regarding on-demand drug treatment

Author/s	Drug	N	Study design	Level of evidence
Haensel et al. [163]	Clomipramine	8	DBRCT	Moderate
Strassberg et al.[130]	Clomipramine	34	DBRCT	Moderate
Waldinger et al. [132]	Clomipramine, paroxetine	30	DRRCT	High
Hellstrom et al. [135]	Dapoxetine (Phase 2)	157	DBRCT	High
Hellstrom et al. [136]	Dapoxetine (Phase 2)	166	DBRCT	High
Pryor et al. [137]	Dapoxetine (Phase 3)	2614	DBRCT	High
McMahon & Touma [129]	Paroxetine	68	SBRCT	Moderate
Kim & Paick [131]	Sertraline	24	Open	Low
Fein RL [128]	Intracavernous injection therapy	16	Open	Very low
Waldinger et al. [46]	Preference study	88	OBS PREF	Very low

DBRCT, double-blind randomized clinical trial; OBS, observational study; PREF, treatment preference study; SBRCT, single-blind randomized clinical trial

Table 14.6 Findings of key publications regarding topical anesthetic treatment

Author/s	Drug	N	Study design	Level of evidence
Choi et al. [159]	SS-cream	50	DBRCT	Low
Atikeler et al. [160]	Prilocaine-lidocaine	40	Open	Low
Berkovitch et al. [123]	Prilocaine-lidocaine	11	Open	Low
Atan et al. [161]	Fluoxetine, lidocaine	43	Open	Low
Atan et al. [162]	Sildenafil, EMLA	84	SBRCT	Moderate
Busato & Galindo [125]	EMLA	42	SBRCT	Moderate
Dinsmore et al. [126]	Tempe®	42	DBRCT	High

DBRCT, double-blind randomized clinical trial; SBRCT, single-blind randomized clinical trial

Penile hypoanesthesia was reported by 12% of subjects and skin irritation or burning was not observed.

Intracavernous injection of vasoactive drugs

Intracavernous self-injection treatment of PE has been reported but is without any evidence-based support for efficacy or safety (see Table 14.6) [128]. Fein reported an open study of eight men treated with a combination of papaverine and phentolamine administered by intracavernous autoinjection where the treatment success was defined as prolongation of erection after ejaculation and not by any measure of ejaculatory latency. In the absence of well-controlled studies, treatment of PE by intracavernous autoinjection cannot be routinely recommended but may be of value in treatment-refractory informed subjects.

Comment

The evidence confirms that treatment of PE with SSRI drugs and topical anesthetics drugs is effective and safe with high-quality evidence and a strong recommendation (Grade 1A). There is little convincing evidence to support a treatment role of alpha-1-adrenoceptor antagonists, tramadol or intracavernous injection of vasoactive drugs, with very low-quality evidence and a weak/conditional recommendation (Grade 2D), and their use cannot be routinely recommended. Drug treatment fails to directly address causal psychological or relationship factors, and data are either lacking or scarce on the efficacy of combined psychosexual counseling and pharmacological treatment, and the maintenance of improved ejaculatory control after drug withdrawal.

Clinical question 14.4

Is premature ejaculation best treated by on-demand rapid-acting short-duration SSRI drugs or daily dosed SSRI drugs?

The evidence

Medline, Web of Science, PsychINFO, EMBASE and the proceedings of major international and regional scientific meetings were searched for publications or abstracts using the words in the title, abstract or keywords "premature ejaculation," "rapid ejaculation," "ejaculation," "selective serotonin reuptake inhibitor." This search was then manually cross-referenced for all papers.

Administration of clomipramine, paroxetine, sertraline and fluoxetine 4–6 hours before intercourse is modestly efficacious and well tolerated but is associated with substantially less ejaculatory delay than daily treatment (see Table 14.7) [129-132]. Following acute on-demand administration of an SSRI, increased synaptic 5-HT levels are downregulated by presynaptic 5-HT1A and 5-HT1B/1D autoreceptors to prevent overstimulation of postsynaptic 5-HT2C receptors. However, during chronic daily SSRI administration, a series of synaptic adaptive processes, which may include presynaptic 5-HT1A and 5-HT1B/1D receptor desensitization, greatly enhances synaptic 5-HT levels resulting in superior fold increases in IELT compared to on-demand administration [133]. On-demand treatment may be combined with either an initial trial of daily treatment or concomitant low-dose daily treatment [129-131].

The assertion that on-demand drug treatment of PE is preferable to daily dosing parallels the rationale for the treatment of ED but is contrary to the results of the only PE drug preference study [46]. The methodology of this trial was not ideal as it involved comparison of preference for daily paroxetine, on-demand clomipramine or topical anesthetic based only on subject information/questionnaires and not on actual use of the drug/s. Well-designed preference trials will provide additional detailed insight into the role of on-demand dosing. Whilst many men suffering from PE who infrequently engage in sexual intercourse may prefer on-demand treatment, many men in established relationships prefer the convenience of daily medication.

Dapoxetine

Dapoxetine is an investigational SSRI with a pharmacokinetic profile of a rapidly absorbed, short half-life drug with minimal plasma accumulation, suggesting a role as an on-demand treatment for PE [134-136].

In randomized, double-blind, placebo-controlled, multicenter, phase III 12-week clinical trials involving 2614 men with a mean baseline IELT ≤ 2 min, dapoxetine 30 mg or 60 mg was more effective than placebo for all study endpoints (see Table 14.7) [137]. Arithmetic mean IELT increased from 0.91 minutes at baseline to 2.78 and 3.32 minutes at study end with dapoxetine 30 and 60 mg respectively, compared to 1.75 minutes with placebo. However, as IELT in subjects with PE is distributed in a positively skewed pattern, reporting IELTs as arithmetic means may overestimate the treatment response and the geometric mean IELT is more representative of the actual treatment effect [10,45,138-140]. Pooled data from four phase III dapoxetine studies confirms this assertion and reports arithmetic and geometric mean IELTs of 1.9 and 1.2 for placebo, 3.1 and 2.0 for dapoxetine 30mg and 3.6 and 2.3 for dapoxetine 60 mg respectively. This represents a 1.6-, 2.5- and 3.0-fold increase over baseline geometric mean IELT for placebo, dapoxetine 30 and 60 mg respectively

Dapoxetine treatment is also associated with significant improvements in PROs of control, distress and sexual satisfaction. Mean patient rating of control over ejaculation as fair, good or very good increased from 2.8% at baseline to 51.8% and 58.4% at study end with dapoxetine 30 and 60 mg respectively. Treatment-related side effects were uncommon, dose dependent, included nausea, diarrhea, headache, dizziness and were responsible for study discontinuation in 4% (30 mg) and 10% (60 mg) of subjects. There was no indication of an increased risk of suicidal ideation or suicide attempts and little indication of withdrawal symptoms with abrupt dapoxetine cessation [141].

Comment

The evidence suggests that daily administration of an SSRI is more effective than on-demand administration of SSRIs including dapoxetine with moderate-quality evidence and a weak/conditional recommendation (**Grade 2B**), although this has yet to be confirmed in a well-designed head-to-head comparator trial. However, the use of SSRI drugs is off-label and limited by the lack of regulatory approval for the treatment of PE. Regulatory approval is not synonymous with superior treatment outcomes and the decision not to seek approval may be little more than a commercial decision of the manufacturer. It is likely that dapoxetine, despite its modest effect upon ejaculatory latency, has a place in the management of PE which will eventually be determined by market forces once the challenge of regulatory approval has been met.

References

1. Semans JH. Premature ejaculation: a new approach. South Med J 1956;49:353-8.
2. Masters WH, Johnson VE. *Human Sexual Inadequacy*. Boston: Little Brown, 1970.
3. Waldinger MD, Hengeveld M. Neuroseksuologie en seksuele psychofarmacologie. Tijdschr Psychiatr 2000;8:585-93.
4. Olivier B, van Oorschot R, Waldinger MD. Serotonin, serotonergic receptors, selective serotonin reuptake inhibitors and sexual behaviour. Int Clin Psychopharmacol 1998;13:S9-14.
5. Waldinger MD, Rietschel M, Nothen MM, Hengeveld MW, Olivier B. Familial occurrence of primary premature ejaculation. Psychiatr Genet 1998;8:37-40.
6. Pattij T, Olivier B, Waldinger MD. Animal models of ejaculatory behavior. Curr Pharm Des 2005;11:4069-77.
7. Waldinger MD, Zwinderman AH, Schweitzer DH, Olivier B. Relevance of methodological design for the interpretation of efficacy of drug treatment of premature ejaculation: a systematic review and meta-analysis. Int J Impot Res 2004;16:369-81.
8. Metz ME, Pryor JL, Nesvacil LJ, Abuzzahab F Sr, Koznar J. Premature ejaculation: a psychophysiological review. J Sex Marital Ther 1997;23:3-23.
9. Symonds T, Roblin D, Hart K, Althof S. How does premature ejaculation impact a man's life? J Sex Marital Ther 2003;29:361-70.
10. Waldinger MD, Quinn P, Dilleen M, Mundayat R, Schweitzer DH, Boolell M. A multinational population survey of intravaginal ejaculation latency time. J Sex Med 2005;2:492-7.
11. Patrick DL, Althof SE, Pryor JL, et al. Premature ejaculation: an observational study of men and their partners. J Sex Med 2005;2:358-67.
12. Porst H, Montorsi F, Rosen RC, Gaynor L, Grupe S, Alexander J. The Premature Ejaculation Prevalence and Attitudes (PEPA) survey: prevalence, comorbidities, and professional help-seeking. Eur Urol 2007;51:816-23.
13. Giuliano F, Patrick DL, Porst H, et al. Premature ejaculation: results from a five-country European observational study. Eur Urol 2008;53:1048-57.
14. American Psychiatric Association. *Diagnostic and Statistical Manual of Mental Disorders (DSM-IV)*, 4th edn. Washington DC: American Psychiatric Association, 1994.
15. World Health Organization. *International Classification of Diseases and Related Health Problems*, 10th edn. Geneva: World Health Organization, 1994.
16. Metz M, McCarthy B. *Coping with Premature Ejaculation: how to overcome PE, please your partner and have great sex*. Oakland, CA: New Harbinger Publications, 2003.
17. Montague DK, Jarow J, Broderick GA, et al. AUA guideline on the pharmacologic management of premature ejaculation. J Urol 2004;172:290-4.
18. Colpi G, Weidner W, Jungwirth A, et al. EAU guidelines on ejaculatory dysfunction. Eur Urol 2004;46:555-8.
19. McMahon CG, Abdo C, Incrocci I, et al. Disorders of orgasm and ejaculation in men. In Lue TF, Basson R, Rosen R, Giuliano F, Khoury S, Montorsi F (eds) *Sexual Medicine: sexual dysfunctions in men and women*. Second International Consultation on Sexual Dysfunctions. Paris: Health Publications, 2004: 409-68.
20. Waldinger MD, Zwinderman AH, Olivier B, Schweitzer DH. Proposal for a definition of lifelong premature ejaculation based on epidemiological stopwatch data. J Sex Med 2005;2:498-507.
21. Jannini EA, Lombardo F, Lenzi A. Correlation between ejaculatory and erectile dysfunction. Int J Androl 2005;28(suppl 2):40-5.
22. American Psychiatric Association. *Diagnostic and Statistical Manual of Mental Disorders (DSM-IIII)*, 3rd edn. Washington DC: American Psychiatric Association, 1980.
23. American Psychiatric Association. *Diagnostic and Statistical Manual of Mental Disorders (DSM-IIII-R)*, 3rd edn revised. Washington DC: American Psychiatric Association, 1987.
24. American Psychiatric Association. *Diagnostic and Statistical Manual of Mental Disorders (DSM-IV-R)*, 4th edn revised. Washington DC: American Psychiatric Association, 2000.
25. Centre for Evidence-Based Medicine. Oxford Centre for Evidence-based Medicine Levels of Evidence (May 2001). Available from: www.cebm.net/index.aspx?o = 1025.
26. O'Donohue W, Letourneau EJ, Geer JH. *Premature Ejaculation*. New York: Simon and Schuster, 1993.
27. Waldinger MD. The neurobiological approach to premature ejaculation. J Urol 2002;168:2359-67.
28. Althof SE, Symonds T. Patient reported outcomes used in the assessment of premature ejaculation. Urol Clin North Am 2007;34:581-9.
29. Cooper AJ, Magnus RV. A clinical trial of the beta blocker propranolol in premature ejaculation. J Psychosom Res 1984;28:331-6.

30. Spiess WF, Geer JH, O'Donohue WT. Premature ejaculation: investigation of factors in ejaculatory latency. J Abnorm Psychol 1984;93:242-5.

31. Strassberg DS, Mahoney JM, Schaugaard M, Hale VE. The role of anxiety in premature ejaculation: a psychophysiological model. Arch Sex Behav 1990;19:251-7.

32. Strassberg DS, Kelly MP, Carroll C, Kircher JC. The psychophysiological nature of premature ejaculation. Arch Sex Behav1987;16:327-36.

33. LoPiccolo J. Direct treatment of sexual dysfunction in the couple. In: Money J, Mesaph H (eds) *Handbook of Sexology: Vol 5. Selected syndromes and therapy*. New York: Elsevier, 1978: 1227-44.

34. Zeiss RA, Christensen A, Levine AG. Treatment for premature ejaculation through male-only groups. J Sex Marital Ther 1978;4:139-43.

35. Kilmann PR, Auerbach R. Treatments of premature ejaculation and psychogenic impotence: a critical review of the literature. Arch Sex Behav 1979;8:81-100.

36. Schover L, Friedman J, Weiler S, Heiman J, LoPiccolo J. Multiaxial problem-oriented system for sexual dysfunctions. Arch Gen Psychiat 1982;39:614-19.

37. Trudel G, Proulx S. Treatment of premature ejaculation by bibliotherapy: an experimental study. Sex Marital Ther 1987;2:163-7.

38. Giuliano F, Patrick DL, Porst H, et al. Premature ejaculation: results from a five-country European observational study. Eur Urol 2008;53(5):1048-57.

39. McMahon CG, Althof SE, Waldinger MD, et al. An evidence-based definition of lifelong premature ejaculation: report of the International Society for Sexual Medicine (ISSM) ad hoc committee for the definition of premature ejaculation. J Sex Med 2008;5:1590-606.

40. Waldinger MD, Hengeveld MW, Zwinderman AH. Paroxetine treatment of premature ejaculation: a double blind, randomized, placebo controlled study. Am J Psychiatr 1994;151:1377-9.

41. Althof SE, Levine SB, Corty EW, Risen CB, Stern EB, Kurit DM. A double-blind crossover trial of clomipramine for rapid ejaculation in 15 couples. J Clin Psychiatr 1995;56:402-7.

42. Pryor JL, Broderick GA, Ho KF, Jamieson C, Gagnon D. Comparison of estimated versus measured intravaginal ejaculatory latency time (IELT) in men with and without premature ejaculation (PE). J Sex Med 2005;3(54):abstract 126.

43. Rosen RC, McMahon CG, Niederberger C, Broderick GA, Jamieson C, Gagnon DD. Correlates to the clinical diagnosis of premature ejaculation: results from a large observational study of men and their partners. J Urol 2007;177:1059-64; discussion 64.

44. Waldinger M, Hengeveld M, Zwinderman A, Olivier B. An empirical operationalization of DSM-IV diagnostic criteria for premature ejaculation. Int J Psychiatr Clin Pract 1998;2:287-93.

45. McMahon CG. Long term results of treatment of premature ejaculation with selective serotonin re-uptake inhibitors. Int J Impot Res 2002;14:S19.

46. Waldinger MD, Zwinderman AH, Olivier B, Schweitzer DH. The majority of men with lifelong premature ejaculation prefer daily drug treatment: an observation study in a consecutive group of Dutch men. J Sex Med 2007;4:1028-37.

47. Grenier G, Byers ES. The relationships among ejaculatory control, ejaculatory latency, and attempts to prolong heterosexual intercourse. Arch Sex Behav 1997;26:27-47.

48. McMahon CG, Waldinger M, Rowland DL, et al. Ejaculatory disorders. In: Porst H, Buvat, J (eds) *Standard Practice in Sexual Medicine*. Oxford: Blackwell, 2006: 188-209.

49. Perelman MA. A new combination treatment for premature ejaculation: a sex therapist's perspective. J Sex Med 2006;3:1004-12.

50. Kaplan HS, Kohl RN, Pomeroy WB, Offit AK, Hogan B. Group treatment of premature ejaculation. Arch Sex Behav 1974;3:443-52.

51. McCarthy B. Cognitive-behavioural strategies and techniques in the treatment of early ejaculation. In: Leiblum SR, Rosen R. (eds) *Principles and Practices of Sex Therapy: Update for the 1990's*. New York: Guilford Press, 1988: 141-67.

52. Vandereycken W. Towards a better delineation of ejaculatory disorders. Acta Psychiatr Belg 1986;86:57-63.

53. Zilbergeld B. *Male Sexuality*. Toronto: Bantam, 1978.

54. Grenier G, Byers S. Operationalizing premature or rapid ejaculation. J Sex Res 2001;38:369-78.

55. McMahon CG, Stuckey B, Andersen ML. Efficacy of Viagra: sildenafil citrate in men with premature ejaculation. J Sex Med 2005;2:368-75.

56. Rowland DL, Strassberg DS, de Gouveia Brazao CA, Slob AK. Ejaculatory latency and control in men with premature ejaculation: an analysis across sexual activities using multiple sources of information. J Psychosom Res 2000;48:69-77.

57. Giuliano F, Patrick DL, Porst H, et al. Premature Ejaculation: Results from a Five-Country European Observational Study. Eur Urol 2008;53(5):1048-57.

58. Patrick DL, Rowland D, Rothman M. Interrelationships among measures of premature ejaculation: the central role of perceived control. J Sex Med 2007;4:780-8.

59. Rowland D, Perelman M, Althof S, et al. Self-reported premature ejaculation and aspects of sexual functioning and satisfaction. J Sex Med 2004;1:225-32.

60. Dunn KM, Croft PR, Hackett GI. Association of sexual problems with social, psychological, and physical problems in men and women: a cross sectional population survey. J Epidemiol Commun Health 1999;53:144-8.

61. Rowland DL, Patrick DL, Rothman M, Gagnon DD. The psychological burden of premature ejaculation. J Urol 2007;177:1065-70.

62. Rosen R, Althof S. Psychological consequences of PE, quality of life and impact on sexual relationships. J Sexual Medicine. 2008;5(6):1296-307.

63. McCabe MP. Intimacy and quality of life among sexually dysfunctional men and women. J Sex Marital Ther 1997;23:276-90.

64. Byers ES, Grenier G. Premature or rapid ejaculation: heterosexual couples' perceptions of men's ejaculatory behavior. Arch Sex Behav 2003;32:261-70.

65. Riley A, Riley E. Premature ejaculation: presentation and associations. An audit of patients attending a sexual problems clinic. Int J Clin Pract 2005;59:1482-7

66. Hartmann U, Schedlowski M, Kruger TH. Cognitive and partner-related factors in rapid ejaculation: differences between dysfunctional and functional men. World J Urol 2005;10:10.

67. Brock GB, Gajewski J, Carrier S, Bernard F, Lee J, Pommerville PJ. The prevalence and impact of premature ejaculation in Canada. Proceedings of Annual Meeting of the American Urological Association, Anaheim, CA, May 19–24, 2007.

68. Althof SE. Prevalence, characteristics and implications of premature ejaculation/rapid ejaculation. J Urol 2006;175:842-8.

69. Althof S. The psychology of premature ejaculation: therapies and consequences. J Sex Med 2006;3(suppl 4):324-31.

70. Chambless DL, Ollendick L. Empirically supported psychological interventions: Controversies and evidence. Ann Rev Psychol 2001:52:685-716.

71. Herbert JD, Gaudiano BA. Introduction to the special issue on the placebo concept in psychotherapy. J Clin Psychol 2005;61:787-90.

72. Rowland D, Burek M. Trends in research on premature ejaculation over the past 25 years. J Sex Med 2007;4:1454-61.

73. O'Leary KD, Borkovec TD. Conceptual, methodological, and ethical problems of placebo groups in psychotherapy research. Am Psychol 1978;33:821-30.

74. Borkovec TD, Nau SD. Credibility of analogue therapy rationales. J Behav Ther Exper Psychiatr 1972;3:257-60.

75. Schapiro B. Premature ejaculation, a review of 1130 cases. J Urol 1943;50:374- 9.

76. Williams W. Secondary premature ejaculation. Aust NZ J Psychiatr 1984;18:333-40.

77. Zilbergeld B. *The New Male Sexuality*. Toronto: Bantam, 1992.

78. Kaplan HS. *PE: how to overcome premature ejaculation*. New York: Brunner/Mazel, 1989.

79. Kockott G, Feil W, Revenstorf D, Aldenhoff J, Besinger U. Symptomatology and psychological aspects of male sexual inadequacy: results of an experimental study. Arch Sex Behav 1980;9:457-75.

80. Kaplan H. *The Evaluation of Sexual Disorders: the urologic evaluation of ejaculatory disorders*. New York: Brunner/Mazel, 1983.

81. de Carufel F, Trudel G. Effects of a new functional-sexological treatment for premature ejaculation. J Sex Marital Ther 2006;32:97-114.

82. De Amicis LA, Goldberg DC, LoPiccolo J, Friedman J, Davies L. Clinical follow-up of couples treated for sexual dysfunction. Arch Sex Behav 1985;14:467-89.

83. Hawton K, Catalan J, Martin P, Fagg J. Long-term outcome of sex therapy. Behav Res Ther 1986;24:665-75.

84. McMahon C, Abdo C, Incrocci L, et al. Disorders of orgasm and ejaculation in men. J Sex Med 2004;1(1):58-65.

85. Jern P, Santtila P, Witting K, et al. Premature and delayed ejaculation: genetic and environmental effects in a population-based sample of Finnish twins. J Sex Med 2007;4(6):1739-49.

86. Janssen PKC, Bakker SC, Réthelyi J, et al. Serotonin transporter promoter region (5-HTTLPR) polymorphism is associated with the intravaginal ejaculation latency time in Dutch men with lifelong premature ejaculation. J Sex Med 2009;6(1):276-84.

87. Chia S. Management of premature ejaculation – a comparison of treatment outcome in patients with and without erectile dysfunction. Int J Androl 2002;25:301-5.

88. Li X, Zhang SX, Cheng HM, Zhang WD. (Clinical study of sildenafil in the treatment of premature ejaculation complicated by erectile dysfunction.) Zhonghua Nan Ke Xue 2003;9:266-9.

89. Sommer F, Klotz T, Mathers MJ. Treatment of premature ejaculation: a comparative vardenafil and SSRI crossover study. J Urol 2005;173(202):abstract 741.

90. Aversa A, Mazzilli F, Rossi T, Delfino M, Isidori AM, Fabbri A. Effects of sildenafil (Viagra) administration on seminal parameters and post-ejaculatory refractory time in normal males. Hum Reprod 2000;15:131-4.

91. Mondaini N, Ponchietti R, Muir GH, et al. Sildenafil does not improve sexual function in men without erectile dysfunction but does reduce the postorgasmic refractory time. Int J Impot Res 2003;15:225-8.

92. Boneff AN. Topical treatment of chronic prostatitis and premature ejaculation. Int Urol Nephrol 1972;4:183-6.

93. Brown AJ. Ciprofloxacin as cure of premature ejaculation. J Sex Marital Ther 2000;26:351-2.

94. El-Nashaar A, Shamloul R. Antibiotic treatment can delay ejaculation in patients with premature ejaculation and chronic bacterial prostatitis. J Sex Med 2007;4:491-6.

95. Waldinger M. Towards evidenced based drug treatment research on premature ejaculation: a critical evaluation of methodology. J Impot Res 2003;15:309-13.

96. Atmaca M, Kuloglu M, Tezcan E, Semercioz A. The efficacy of citalopram in the treatment of premature ejaculation: a placebo-controlled study. Int J Impot Res 2002;14:502-5.

97. McMahon CG. Treatment of premature ejaculation with sertraline hydrochloride: a single-blind placebo controlled crossover study. J Urol 1998;159:1935-8.

98. Kara H, Aydin S, Yucel M, Agargun MY, Odabas O, Yilmaz Y. The efficacy of fluoxetine in the treatment of premature ejaculation: a double-blind placebo controlled study. J Urol 1996;156:1631-2.

99. Waldinger MD, Hengeveld MW, Zwinderman AH. Paroxetine treatment of premature ejaculation: a double-blind, randomized, placebo-controlled study. Am J Psychiatr 1994;151:1377-9.

100. Goodman RE. An assessment of clomipramine (Anafranil) in the treatment of premature ejaculation. J Int Med Res 1980;8:53-9.

101. Waldinger MD. Drug treatment of premature ejaculation: pharmacodynamic and pharmacokinetic paradigms. Drug Discovery Today: Therapeutic Strategies 2005;2:37-40.

102. Waldinger MD. Premature ejaculation: definition and drug treatment. Drugs 2007;67:547-68.

103. Marangell LB, Dennehy EB, Wisniewski SR, et al. Case-control analyses of the impact of pharmacotherapy on prospectively observed suicide attempts and completed suicides in bipolar disorder: findings from STEP-BD. J Clin Psychiatr 2008;69:916-22.

104. Khan A, Khan S, Kolts R, Brown WA. Suicide rates in clinical trials of SSRIs, other antidepressants, and placebo: analysis of FDA reports. Am J Psychiatr 2003;160:790-2.

105. Mann JJ, Emslie G, Baldessarini RJ, et al. ACNP Task Force report on SSRIs and suicidal behavior in youth. Neuropsychopharmacology 2006;31:473-92.

106. Ditto KE. SSRI discontinuation syndrome. Awareness as an approach to prevention. Postgrad Med 2003;114:79-84.

107. Black K, Shea CA, Dursun S, Kutcher S. Selective serotonin reuptake inhibitor discontinuation syndrome: proposed diagnostic criteria. J Psychiatry Neurosci 2000;25:255-61.

108. Li N, Wallen NH, Ladjevardi M, Hjemdahl P. Effects of serotonin on platelet activation in whole blood. Blood Coagul Fibrinolysis 1997;8:517-23.

109. Weinrieb RM, Auriacombe M, Lynch KG, Lewis JD. Selective serotonin re-uptake inhibitors and the risk of bleeding. Expert Opin Drug Saf 2005;4:337-44.

110. Garcia Rodriguez LA, Jick H. Risk of upper gastrointestinal bleeding and perforation associated with individual non-steroidal anti-inflammatory drugs. Lancet 1994;343:769-72.

111. Ahmad S. Paroxetine-induced priapism. Arch Intern Med 1995;155:645.

112. Rand EH. Priapism in a patient taking sertraline. J Clin Psychiatr 1998;59:538.

113. Dent LA, Brown WC, Murney JD. Citalopram-induced priapism. Pharmacotherapy 2002;22:538-41.

114. Fava M, Judge R, Hoog SL, Nilsson ME, Koke SC. Fluoxetine versus sertraline and paroxetine in major depressive disorder: changes in weight with long-term treatment. J Clin Psychiatr 2000;61:863-7.

115. Cavallini G. Alpha-1 blockade pharmacotherapy in primitive psychogenic premature ejaculation resistant to psychotherapy. Eur Urol 1995;28:126-30.

116. Basar MM, Yilmaz E, Ferhat M, Basar H, Batislam E. Terazosin in the treatment of premature ejaculation: a short-term follow-up. Int Urol Nephrol 2005;37:773-7.

117. Frink MC, Hennies HH, Englberger W, Haurand M, Wilffert B. Influence of tramadol on neurotransmitter systems of the rat brain. Arzneimittelforschung 1996;46:1029-36.

118. Safarinejad MR, Hosseini SY. Safety and efficacy of tramadol in the treatment of premature ejaculation: a double-blind, placebo-controlled, fixed-dose, randomized study. J Clin Psychopharmacol 2006;26:27-31.

119. Salem EA, Wilson SK, Bissada NK, Delk JR, Hellstrom WJ, Cleves MA. Tramadol HCL has promise in on-demand use to treat premature ejaculation. J Sex Med 2008;5(1):188-93.

120. Cossmann M, Kohnen C, Langford R, McCartney C. (Tolerance and safety of tramadol use. Results of international studies and data from drug surveillance.) Drugs 1997;53:50-62.

121. McDiarmid T, Mackler L, Schneider DM. Clinical inquiries. What is the addiction risk associated with tramadol? J Fam Pract 2005;54:72-3.

122. Adams EH, Breiner S, Cicero TJ, et al. A comparison of the abuse liability of tramadol, NSAIDs, and hydrocodone in patients with chronic pain. J Pain Symptom Manage 2006;31:465-76.

123. Berkovitch M, Keresteci AG, Koren G. Efficacy of prilocaine-lidocaine cream in the treatment of premature ejaculation. J Urol 1995;154:1360-1.

124. Xin ZC, Choi YD, Lee SH, Choi HK. Efficacy of a topical agent SS-cream in the treatment of premature ejaculation: preliminary clinical studies. Yonsei Med J 1997;38:91-5.

125. Busato W, Galindo CC. Topical anaesthetic use for treating premature ejaculation: a double-blind, randomized, placebo-controlled study. BJU Int 2004;93:1018-21.

126. Dinsmore WW, Hackett G, Goldmeier D, et al. Topical eutectic mixture for premature ejaculation (TEMPE): a novel aerosol-delivery form of lidocaine-prilocaine for treating premature ejaculation. BJU Int 2007;99(2):369-75.

127. Henry R, Morales A, Wyllie MG. TEMPE: topical eutectic-like mixture for premature ejaculation. Expert Opin Drug Deliv 2008;5:251-61.

128. Fein RL. Intracavernous medication for treatment of premature ejaculation. Urology 1990;35:301-3.

129. McMahon CG, Touma K. Treatment of premature ejaculation with paroxetine hydrochloride as needed: 2 single-blind placebo controlled crossover studies. J Urol 1999;161:1826-30.

130. Strassberg DS, de Gouveia Brazao CA, Rowland DL, Tan P, Slob AK. Clomipramine in the treatment of rapid (premature) ejaculation. J Sex Marital Ther 1999;25:89-101.

131. Kim SW, Paick JS. Short-term analysis of the effects of as needed use of sertraline at 5 PM for the treatment of premature ejaculation. Urology 1999;54:544-7.

132. Waldinger MD, Zwinderman AH, Olivier B. On-demand treatment of premature ejaculation with clomipramine and paroxetine: a randomized, double-blind fixed-dose study with stopwatch assessment. Eur Urol 2004;46:510-15.

133. Waldinger MD, Berendsen HH, Blok BF, Olivier B, Holstege G. Premature ejaculation and serotonergic antidepressants-induced delayed ejaculation: the involvement of the serotonergic system. Behav Brain Res 1998;92:111-18.

134. Dresser MJ, Lindert K, Lin D. Pharmacokinetics of single and multiple escalating doses of dapoxetine in healthy volunteers. Clin Pharmacol Ther 2004;75:113 (abstract P1).

135. Hellstrom WJ, Gittelman M, Althof S. Dapoxetine HCl for the treatment of premature ejaculation: a Phase II, randomised, double-blind, placebo controlled study. J Sex Med 2004;1:59.

136. Hellstrom WJ, Althof S, Gittelman M, et al. Dapoxetine for the treatment of men with premature ejaculation (PE):dose-finding analysis. J Urol 2005;173:238 (abstract 877).

137. Pryor JL, Althof SE, Steidle C, et al. Efficacy and tolerability of dapoxetine in treatment of premature ejaculation: an integrated analysis of two double-blind, randomised controlled trials. Lancet 2006:368:929-37.

138. Waldinger MD, Hengeveld MW, Zwinderman AH, Olivier B. Effect of SSRI antidepressants on ejaculation: a double-blind, randomized, placebo-controlled study with fluoxetine, fluvoxamine, paroxetine, and sertraline. J Clin Psychopharmacol 1998;18:274-81.

139. Waldinger MD, Zwinderman AH, Olivier B, Schweitzer DH. Geometric mean IELT and premature ejaculation: appropriate statistics to avoid overestimation of treatment efficacy. J Sex Med 2008;5:492-9.

140. McMahon CG. Clinical trial methodology in premature ejaculation: observational, interventional, and treatment preference studies—part II—study design, outcome measures, data analysis, and reporting. J Sex Med 2008;5(8):1817-33.

141. Levine L. Evaluation of withdrawal effects with dapoxetine in the treatment of premature ejaculation (PE). J Sex Med 2007;4:1:49.

142. Safarinejad MR, Hosseini SY. Safety and efficacy of citalopram in the treatment of premature ejaculation: a double-blind placebo-controlled, fixed dose, randomized study. Int J Impot Res 2006;18:164-9.

143. Waldinger MD, Zwinderman AH, Olivier B. SSRIs and ejaculation: a double-blind, randomized, fixed-dose study with paroxetine and citalopram. J Clin Psychopharmacol 2001;21:556-60.

144. Girgis SM, El-Haggar S, El-Hermouzy S. A double-blind trial of clomipramine in premature ejaculation. Andrologia 1982;14:364-8.

145. Safarinejad MR. Safety and efficacy of escitalopram in the treatment of premature ejaculation: a double-blind, placebo-controlled, fixed-dose, randomized study. J Clin Psychopharmacol 2007;27:444-50.

146. Kara H, Aydin S, Yucel M, Agargun MY, Odabas O, Yilmaz Y. The efficacy of fluoxetine in the treatment of premature

ejaculation: a double-blind placebo controlled study. J Urol 1996;156:1631-2.

147. Haensel SM, Klem TL, Hop WCL, Slob AK. Fluoxetine and premature ejaculation: a double-blind, crossover, placebo-controlled study. J Clin Psychopharmacol 1998;18:72-7.

148. Yilmaz U, Tatlisen A, Turan H, Arman F, Ekmekcioglu O. The effects of fluoxetine on several neurophysiological variables in patients with premature ejaculation. J Urol 1999;161:107-11.

149. Kim SC, Seo KK. Efficacy and safely of fluoxetine,sertraline and clomipramine in patients with premature ejaculation: a double blind, placebo controlled study. J Urol 1998;159:425-7

150. Waldinger MD, Hengeveld MW, Zwinderman AH. Ejaculation-retarding properties of paroxetine in patients with primary premature ejaculation: a double-blind, randomized, dose-response study. BJU 1997;79:592-5.

151. McMahon CG, Touma K. Treatment of premature ejaculation with paroxetine hydrochloride. Int J Impot Res 1999;11:241-5; discussion 6.

152. Waldinger MD, Zwinderman AH, Olivier B. Antidepressants and ejaculation: a double-blind, randomized, fixed-dose study with mirtazapine and paroxetine. J Clin Psychopharmacol 2003;23:467-70.

153. McMahon C. Treatment of premature ejaculation with sertraline hydrochloride: a single-blind placebo controlled crossover study. J Urol 1998;159:1935-8.

154. Arafa M, Shamloul R. Efficacy of sertraline hydrochloride in treatment of premature ejaculation: a placebo-controlled study using a validated questionnaire. Int J Impot Res 2006;18:534-8.

155. Mendels J, Camera A, Sikes C. Sertraline treatment for premature ejaculation. J Clin Psychopharmacol 1995;15:341-6.

156. Biri H, Isen K, Sinik Z, Onaran M, Kupeli B, Bozkirli I. Sertraline in the treatment of premature ejaculation: a double-blind placebo controlled study. Int Urol Nephrol 1998;30:611-15.

157. McMahon C. Treatment of premature ejaculation with sertraline hydrochloride. Int J Impot Res 1998;10:181-4.

158. Akgul T, Karakan T, Ayyildiz A, Germiyanoglu C. Comparison of sertraline and citalopram for treatment of premature ejaculation. Urol J 2008;5:41-5.

159. Choi HK, Xin ZC, Choi YD, Lee WH, Mah SY, Kim DK. Safety and efficacy study with various doses of SS-cream in patients with premature ejaculation in a double-blind, randomized, placebo controlled clinical study. Int J Impot Res 1999;11:261-4.

160. Atikeler MK, Gecit I, Senol FA. Optimum usage of prilocaine-lidocaine cream in premature ejaculation. Andrologia 2002; 34:356-9.

161. Atan A, Basar MM, Aydoganli L. Comparison of the efficacy of fluoxetine alone vs. fluoxetine plus local lidocaine ointment in the treatment of premature ejaculation. Arch Esp Urol 2000;53:856-8.

162. Atan A, Basar MM, Tuncel A, Ferhat M, Agras K, Tekdogan U. Comparison of efficacy of sildenafil-only, sildenafil plus topical EMLA cream, and topical EMLA-cream-only in treatment of premature ejaculation. Urology 2006;67:388-91.

163. Haensel SM, Rowland DL, Kallan KT. Clomipramine and sexual function in men with premature ejaculation and controls. J Urol 1996;156:1310-15.

15 Management of erectile dysfunction

Mathew D. Sorensen and Hunter Wessells

Department of Urology, University of Washington School of Medicine, Seattle, WA, USA

Introduction

Erectile dysfunction (ED) affects up to 30 million men in the United States [1]. Seven percent of men aged 18–29 years report symptoms of ED with the prevalence increasing to more than 50% of men between 40 and 70 years of age [2,3]. As the male population in the developed world ages and worsens in overall health and fitness, the risks of diabetes, obesity and cardiovascular disease will dramatically increase the incidence and prevalence of erectile dysfunction [4]. Combining these trends with men's expectations for quality of life throughout the lifespan, a significant burden will be placed on healthcare systems to diagnose and treat male sexual dysfunctions. Such expectations will increasingly come into conflict with fiscal and regulatory constraints.

Between 1994 and 2000, annual medical expenditures for ED in the United States increased substantially from $185 million to nearly $330 million [5]. The economic impact of ED has until recently excluded pharmaceutical costs, which now make up the majority of treatment-related ED costs. For example, the 2006 worldwide sales of the phosphodiesterase 5 enzyme (PDE5) inhibitors were over $3 billion: Viagra™ $1.6 billion, Cialis™ $971 million and Levitra™ $464 million. US sales represent approximately half of the global sales total (www.wikinvest.com/concept/Erectile_dysfunction_drug_market). It is certain that policy makers and third-party payers will seek evidence-based approaches to determine the feasibility and appropriateness of coverage for the treatment of ED. The stakes are not trivial: if all men in the United States sought treatment for ED, the yearly total costs, including pharmaceutical costs, could exceed $10 billion.

Release of nitric oxide from autonomic nerves and endothelial cells during sexual stimulation leads to relaxation of vascular and sinusoid smooth muscle with resultant increased inflow of blood into the cavernosal spaces [6]. Nitric oxide stimulates the formation of cyclic guanosine monophosphate (cGMP) by guanylate cyclase. cGMP, the key second messenger involved in the initiation of penile erection, is then hydrolyzed by cGMP-specific phosphodiesterase type 5 enzyme (PDE5) to terminate the erectile response.

Current pharmacological treatments target the NO-cGMP-PDE5 pathway to initiate or enhance penile erection. Treatment options for ED have expanded dramatically in the last 10 years to include psychological counseling; oral, topical, intraurethral, and intracavernosal vasoactive therapy; oral therapies with other or unknown mechanisms; hormone replacement; vacuum constriction devices; and surgery, including vascular bypass procedures and penile implants. The goal of treatment is to preserve or restore satisfactory penile erections with minimal adverse effects. Men have demonstrated a strong preference for oral treatments even if they have lower efficacy [7], suggesting that efforts to optimize treatment of ED should address patient/partner satisfaction and preference in addition to the more standard physiologic and clinical measures of improvement. Men with ED want a safe, well-tolerated, convenient treatment requiring little or no invasiveness that is reliably effective in all types of ED. Unfortunately, no single therapy is satisfactory for every patient [8].

The purpose of this chapter is to summarize and evaluate the key evidence which supports the major treatment modalities for male erectile dysfunction.

Definition and measurement of erectile dysfunction

An NIH consensus panel defined ED as the persistent "inability to achieve or maintain an erection sufficient for

Evidence-Based Urology. Edited by Philipp Dahm, Roger R. Dmochowski.
© 2010 Blackwell Publishing.

satisfactory sexual performance" [1]. The diagnosis of ED requires a detailed sexual and medical history, physical examination and laboratory tests. Comprehensive, validated scales to reproducibly quantify the presence and severity of ED have become useful adjuncts to the case history, but are not sufficient to diagnose ED correctly or treat it safely.

The International Index of Erectile Function (IIEF [9]) is an example of such a symptom-based definition; it has been fundamental to the development of objective primary endpoints for randomized clinical trials of pharmaceutical agents, and has replaced use of physiological measures of erectile function in phase II and III clinical trials. This 15-item questionnaire addresses several domains of sexual function including erectile function (EF) domain: questions 1–5 and 15, maximum score 30. Responses to the IIEF-EF domain allow categorization of ED as severe (0–10), moderate (11–16), mild to moderate (17–20), mild (21–25) or no erectile dysfunction (26–30). Trials usually also include global efficacy questions (GEQ) relating to improvement in erection and or intercourse success.

The ability to objectively measure response to ED treatments is foundational to the value of this chapter to clinicians and policy makers; while pharmaceutical trials have most successfully used these outcome measures, definitional questions limit the ability to analyze and compare results from intervention and prevention trials focused on radical prostatectomy-associated ED (10) and many studies of penile implants. Finally, the importance of partner perspective is well recognized in the clinical evaluation and treatment of ED; how these parameters are measured in clinical trials, and how the data should be interpreted, is less well defined.

Search strategy

Potentially relevant studies were identified by computerized search of Medline (1966 to February 2009), restricted to English-language human studies. Relevant text searches included: sildenafil, vardenafil, tadalafil, alprostadil, intracavernosal injection, intraurethral suppository, radical prostatectomy, penile rehabilitation or penile implant with studies restricted to randomized controlled trial, meta-analysis or controlled clinical trial article types. The reference lists of relevant articles were searched by hand to identify additional relevant articles. Studies were selected for inclusion if they focused on patients with erectile dysfunction and were randomized controlled trials, prospective or retrospective cohort studies. In the case of penile implant surgery, we included large case series of currently available devices approved by the Food and Drug Administration.

Estimates for efficacy and safety outcomes in patients treated with the various pharmacological and surgical treatments were tabulated. Levels of evidence quality were assessed for each study using the GRADE system [11] and included in the tables. Due to the widely divergent outcome measures, risks, and safety issues, we did not attempt to compare between broad categories of treatment.

Clinical question 15.1

What is the effectiveness and safety of PDE5 inhibitors in the treatment of erectile dysfunction?

The evidence

Randomized placebo-controlled trial data strongly and uniformly indicate a significant improvement in erectile function with the use of all three available oral phosphodiesterase 5 inhibitors (Table 15.1). Overall, the quality of evidence for all three agents is high. It should be noted that trials of vardenafil and tadalafil in general had higher baseline IIEF-EF domain scores compared to sildenafil; this is a known effect in studies of subsequent drugs introduced in patient populations already exposed to agents in the same drug class. Finally, results from clinical trials are not uniformly generalizable to clinical practice. Patients in clinical trials in general will have fewer and less severe co-morbid conditions, better control of diabetes, and absence of hypogonadism. Placebo run-ins, common in the PDE5 inhibitor trials, also may bias towards better responses.

Sildenafil administered on demand at either fixed doses (ranging from 25 to 100 mg) or in flexible dosing leads to statistically significant increases in the IIEF-EF domain of 6.4 to 11.7 points (all studies $p < 0.001$). This difference is of clinical significance. Sildenafil demonstrates excellent drug efficacy in patients over a wide range of ages, with different causes of ED (organic, psychogenic and mixed causes) and in all severities of ED. Patients expected to be the most refractory to treatment, such as those with diabetes, spinal cord injury, post radical prostatectomy, and with other co-morbidities, were found to have significant improvement in erectile function in clinical trials [12-14]. All studies of sildenafil included in Table 15.1 report significant improvement in erections compared to placebo as evaluated by the GEQ "Did the treatment improve your erections?". Overall, 67–87% of men receiving sildenafil reported improvement in their erections compared to 18–33% of men receiving placebo (all studies $p < 0.001$). There was a dose–response effect on both the difference in IIEF-EF score and patient-reported improvement in erections as measured by the GEQ with near normalization of erectile function for many patients [15].

Table 15.1 Efficacy and safety of oral phosphodiesterase 5 inhibitors for the treatment of erectile dysfunction

	Trial year	N	Study design	Baseline IIEF-EF domain	IIEF-EF domain (treatment vs placebo)	GEQ (treatment vs placebo)	Grade
Sildenafil							
Goldstein et al. [44]	1998	861	Multicenter, RCT, flexible dose	12	22.1 vs 12.2 (p<0.001)	74% vs 19% (p<0.001)	High
Montorsi et al. [45]	1999	514	Multicenter, RCT, fixed dose	12.5	~19–25 mg ~21–50 mg ~22.5–100 mg vs ~12.6 placebo (p<0.001)	67–86% (25–100 mg) vs 24% (p<0.0001)	High
Dinsmore et al. [15]	1999	220	Multicenter, RCT, flexible dose	10.3	21.8 vs 10.1 (p<0.0001) healthy controls 25.8	81% vs 18% (p<0.0001)	High
Tan et al. [46]	2000	254	Multicenter, RCT, flexible dose	13.3	25.1 vs 15.5 (p<0.0001)	87% vs 33% (p<0.0001)	Mod
Fink et al. [47]	2002	27 trials (6659 men)	Systematic review and meta-analysis	N/A	N/A	78% vs 25% (p<0.0001)	Low
Vardenafil							
Porst et al. [48]	2001	601	Multicenter, RCT fixed dose	14.0	20.9–5 mg 22.1–10 mg 22.8–20 mg vs 15.6 placebo	66–80% (5–20 mg) vs 30% (p<0.001)	High
Hatzichristou et al. *Eur Urol* 2004 (49)	2004	323	Multicenter, RCT, flexible dose	12.8	24.2 vs 15.6 (p<0.005)	86% vs 36% (p<0.005)	High
Hellstrom et al. [22]	2002	805	Multicenter, RCT, fixed dose	13–14	17.8–5 mg 21.2–10 mg 21.8–20 mg vs 14.8 placebo	65–85% (5–20 mg) vs 28% (p<0.0001)	Mod
Markou et al. [50]	2004	10 trials (6809 men)	Systematic review	N/A	Increase 5–7.5 points over placebo	69% vs 26% (p<0.00001)	Low
Potempa et al. [51]	2004	398	Multicenter, open-label flexible dose. No placebo	13.9	25.9	92%	Low
Tadalafil							
Padma-Natha et al. [52]	2001	179	Multicenter, RCT, fixed dose	15.0	19.3–2 mg 22.9–5 mg 23.6–10 mg 24.2–25 mg vs 14.7 placebo	51–81% (2–25 mg) vs 17% placebo (p<0.005)	High
Porst et al. [19]	2006	268	Multicenter, RCT, 5 mg or 10 mg daily dose vs placebo	13.4	22.8–5 mg 22.8–10 mg vs 15.0 placebo (p<0.001)	85% vs 28% (p<0.001)	High
Rajfer et al. [18]	2007	287	Multicenter, RCT, 2.5 or 5 mg daily dose vs placebo	13.4	19.1–2.5 mg 20.8–5 mg vs 14.6 placebo (p<0.001)	63–73% (2.5–5 mg) vs 26% placebo (p<0.001)	High
MacMahon et al. [53]	2005	140	Multicenter, RCT, 20 mg fixed dose	15.6	22.8 vs 12.7 (p<0.001)	78% vs 12.8% (p<0.001)	Mod
Carson et al. [54]	2005	195	Multicenter, RCT, 20 mg fixed dose	13.0	19.5 vs 13.5 (p<0.001)	73% vs 15% (p<0.001)	Mod

Carson et al. [55]	2004	11 trials (2102 men)	Systematic review	N/A	21.1–10 mg 23.2–20 mg vs 15.3 placebo (p<0.001)	71–84% (10–20 mg) vs 33% placebo (p<0.001)	Low
Yip et al. [56]	2006	242	Multicenter, RCT, 20 mg fixed dose	N/A	Increase 8.5 points vs 2.1 for placebo	86% vs 30%	Low
Special populations Diabetes							
Rendell et al. [57]	1999	268	Sildenafil multicenter, RCT, flexible dose	9.7	17.5 vs 10.4 (p<0.001)	74% vs 12% (p<0.001)	High
Goldstein et al. [12]	2003	452	Vardenafil multicenter, RCT, fixed dose, diabetic men	11.2	17.1–10 mg 19.0–20 mg vs 12.6 placebo	57–72% (10–20 mg) vs 13% (p<0.0001)	Mod
Vardi & Nini [13]	2009	8 trials (1759 men)	Any PDE5 inhibitor Systematic review, meta-analysis, diabetic men	N/A	Increase 6.6 points (95% CI 5.2–7.9) over placebo	3.8-fold higher in treatment group	Mod
Spinal cord injury							
DeForge et al. [14]	2006	2 trials (205 men)	Sildenafil systematic review of RCT, spinal cord injury	NA	N/A	75–76% vs 4–7% (p<0.001)	Low
Radical prostatectomy							
Montorsi et al. [73]	2004	303	Tadalafil Multicenter RCT, 20 mg fixed dose, men 12–48 months after bilateral nerve-sparing radical prostatectomy	13.0	17.1 vs 12.5 (p<0.001)	62% vs 23% (p<0.001)	High

Men administered vardenafil in a RCT had statistically and clinically significant increases in IIEF-EF score (3–8.6 points) versus placebo. They also reported significantly higher response to GEQ (65–85% improvement) compared to placebo (26–36%, all studies p < 0.005). Improvements were similarly dose responsive in patients taking 5–20 mg.

Tadalafil has been extensively studied in a variety of administration schedules. Due to the long 17.5-h half-life of this medication [16,17], efficacy has been demonstrated when taken on demand, three times per week and daily. Some men may find alternative dosing schedules attractive. Studies evaluating daily tadalafil use at various doses indicate that doses as low as 2.5 mg or 5 mg daily improve IIEF-EF scores by 6–8 points over placebo, with higher IIEF-EF scores and more patients reporting improved erections at the 5 mg dose [18]. However, no additional benefit was derived at 10 mg daily doses [19]. At fixed doses ranging from 5 to 25 mg, IIEF-EF scores were 6–10 points higher than placebo in a dose–response fashion and positive GEQ responses were 60–86% positive versus 13–33% for placebo.

Regardless of the oral PDE5 inhibitor studied, the majority of patients in flexible-dose trials concluded the trial at the highest allowed dosage. There was strong evidence across studies of improved response at higher doses, although side effects increased with increased dosages as well.

Additional comments

Mechanism of action

Sildenafil, vardenafil and tadalafil are competitive inhibitors of the PDE5. Although sildenafil and vardenafil share a closer molecular structure compared to tadalafil, each acts via inhibition of PDE5 to block cGMP hydrolysis in corporal tissues. This results in sustained increased levels of cGMP, consequent amplification of neurally mediated and endothelium-dependent NO release and smooth muscle relaxation, resulting in enhanced erectile responses.

Efficacy

Efficacy at the first attempt is an important aspect of ED therapy since this has a great effect on the patient's sexual confidence and long-term compliance with the selected ED treatment. First-time response is a marker of continued response, and these medications tend to remain effective for men even after years of medication use. With repeat challenges and counseling, a percentage of initial nonresponders may be salvaged; treatment should be continued at increased doses up to three separate attempts before conceding failure of a medication [20-22]. With improvement in erectile function, men tend to note improvements in self-esteem, confidence and relationship satisfaction which correlate with improvement in IIEF-EF scores [23].

An area of some controversy is the impact of PDE5 inhibitors on the sexual function of men without ED. One small RCT [24] administered a fixed dose of sildenafil to 47 men without significant ED. Those receiving placebo showed no improvement in erectile function, whereas those given sildenafil demonstrated a statistically significant two-point increase in IIEF-EF domain scores. However, the small sample size, lack of dose–responsiveness data, and questionable clinical significance of the increase in EF domain scores all reduce the quality of evidence.

There have been no rigorous RCTs designed to evaluate comparative efficacy of the three available PDE5 inhibitors. A recent meta-analysis attempted to pool RCT data from fixed-dose studies involving sildenafil, vardenafil and tadalafil [25]. It concluded that at maximum doses, all three drugs improve IIEF-EF scores by 7–10 points compared to placebo treatment. Scores from the pooled studies indicated that sildenafil might be slightly more efficacious than vardenafil, but the differences between drugs were slight. Other randomized cross-over studies have demonstrated similar improvements in IIEF-EF score, similar sexual attempts during treatment, and similar safety profiles, but a 52–73% patient preference for tadalafil over sildenafil or vardenafil [26,27]. Patient preference appears to be primarily due to differences in dosing schedule and reduced performance pressure. These data were of moderate and low evidence due to methodological and study design issues, with one study comparing the highest recommended dose of tadalafil to an intermediate dose of sildenafil.

Safety

Overall, oral PDE-5 inhibitors are well tolerated, with few patients in any of the studies terminating treatment due to adverse effects. The side effects of these medications tend to be dose related. In general, men may report headaches (8–14%), flushing (4–6%), dyspepsia (5–18%), rhinitis (,5%), visual effects and blue vision (3%). Sudden hearing loss is rare, as is nonarteritic anterior ischemic optic neuropathy, which may occur in patients with underlying risk factors.

Absolute contraindications to all PDE5 inhibitors include concurrent nitrate use. Caution should also be exercised in patients taking alpha-adrenergic antagonists, CYP3A4 inhibitor drugs (phenytoin, ketoconazole, rifampin, HIV protease inhibitors, erythromycin, grapefruit juice), excessive alcohol intake, and in those with low baseline blood pressure, active coronary ischemia not on nitrates, and in those with congestive heart failure.

Implications for practice: recommendations

- High-quality evidence demonstrates that PDE5 inhibitors improve erectile function in men with erectile dysfunction (strong recommendation, Grade 1A).
- PDE5 inhibitors are efficacious in men with diabetes, spinal cord injury, depression and after nerve-sparing radical prostatectomy, although their efficacy is lower than in otherwise healthy men (strong recommendation, Grade 1A).
- Treatment for ED should begin with a trial of PDE5 inhibitors with at least three attempts with drug of choice, then trial of a second PDE5 inhibitor (strong recommendation, Grade 1B).

Clinical question 15.2

What is the effectiveness and safety of alprostadil (prostaglandin E1) in the treatment of erectile dysfunction?

The evidence

Initially used off-label, intracavernosal injection (ICI) of drugs such as papaverine (a nonspecific PDE inhibitor) and phentolamine (an alpha-adrenergic antagonist) served as a comparison, albeit indirect, for the initial alprostadil studies. With the approval of alprostadil (Caverject™) by the FDA in 1996, patients were given an easily accessibly and standardized treatment for ED. After in-clinic studies showed efficacy compared to placebo controls [28], subsequent at-home testing in "responders" demonstrated success rates (GEQ, e.g.) above 90% [29]. The lack of at-home placebo controls, and selection of responders for home use studies, lowered the quality of evidence as reflected in the GRADE ratings. Nevertheless, the 90% rate of erections sufficient for sexual activity attests to the effectiveness of this second-line therapy.

The inconvenience of ICI and relatively high percentage of patients reporting pain with alprostadil (Table 15.2 [29]) led to the development of an intraurethral delivery system for alprostadil, MUSE™. Its easier application per urethra made placebo-controlled in-office and home trials more feasible. For example, the main phase III study of intraurethral alprostadil [30] consisted of an in-clinic component and a home use component. Approximately two-thirds of men respond to intraurethral alprostadil when challenged in the clinic, and of these approximately 60–70% achieve erections sufficient for sexual activity in the home setting [30,31]. Only in-clinic responders were included in an at-home RCT, thus biasing the study towards better outcomes. These selection biases may explain the lesser response to MUSE in clinical situations and comparison

Table 15.2 Efficacy and safety of alprostadil for the treatment of erectile dysfunction

	Trial year	N	Study design	Control group	Baseline IIEF-EF domain	IIEF-EF domain	GEQ (treatment vs placebo)	Pain	Grade
Intracavernosal									
Mahmoud et al. [59]	1992	52	Double blind cross-over	Papaverine	N/A	N/A	81 vs 63%		Low
Godschalk et al. [28]	1994	15	RCT	Placebo	N/A	N/A	66%#	10%	Mod
Linet et al. [29]	1996	296	Prospective	Placebo					Mod
		683	Prospective	None	N/A	N/A	94%	11%	High
Intraurethral									
Hellstrom et al.[60]	1996	68	RCT		N/A	N/A	91%	9–18.3%	Mod
Padma-Nathan et al. [30]	1997	996	RCT of in-clinic responders*	Placebo	N/A	N/A	65 vs 19%	10%	Mod
Williams et al . [31]	1998	159	RCT of in-clinic responders**	Placebo	N/A	N/A	69 vs 11%	17%	Mod
Intracavernosal vs intraurethral									
Shabsigh et al. [33]	2000	111	Randomized		N/A	N/A	85 vs 53%	34 vs 25%	Mod
Shokeir et al. [32]	1999	60	Randomized		N/A	N/A	87 vs 53%	40 vs 7%	V Low

#No placebo arm to at-home study

^In-office administration only

*Response rate in clinic was 66% of 1511 patients

**Response rate in clinic was 64% of 259 patients

trials. For example, in two studies in which subjects were randomized to ICI or MUSE, the overall intercourse success rate for MUSE was 53% [32,33].

Additional comments

Mechanism of action

Vasoactive compounds can directly initiate penile erection via intracavernosal sites of action. Alprostadil, the only FDA-approved agent for ICI or intraurethral delivery, causes cavernosal smooth muscle relaxation via cAMP-mediated mechanisms. Evidence from RCT and large prospective studies supports the proerectile effect, dose–response relationship, and at-home efficacy of intracavernosal and intraurethral PGE1 (see Table 15.2).

Safety

Priapism is a rare but serious complication of all pro-erectile pharmacological agents. The rates of priapism in the pivotal phase III trials for intracavernosal and intraurethral alprostadil were 1% and 0% respectively. Hypotension may occur with either delivery method but is very rare. Nevertheless, AUA guidelines recommend that the first dose of MUSE be administered in a clinical setting

[34]. Pain from the medication, as distinct from the route of injection, occurs via an unclear mechanism that may involve nerve sensitization. The incidence and severity of pain vary but, as shown in Table 15.2, are higher for ICI than intraurethral alprostadil. The risk of penile nodules and fibrosis is 2% with ICI.

Implications for practice: recommendations

• Second-line treatments with alprostadil are efficacious and safe (strong recommendation, **Grade 1A** evidence).
• Intraurethral delivery, although less invasive, is less efficacious than ICI (**Grade 1B**).

Clinical question 15.3

Does penile rehabilitation (PDE5 inhibitors, PGE1, etc.) improve recovery of erectile function after radical prostatectomy?

The evidence

Erectile dysfunction associated with radical prostatectomy (RP) is prevalent, severe and difficult to treat.

Even nerve-sparing techniques fail to preserve normal sexual functioning in a substantial majority of previously potent men [35]. Thus, strategies aimed at preventing post-RP ED are an important new area in urological and sexual medicine research.

Although the pathophysiology of erectile impairment after prostatectomy remains incompletely understood, neural injury, smooth muscle apoptosis, and cavernosal fibrosis are the major proposed mechanisms. A small number of trials provide evidence supporting the use of oral PDE5 inhibitors, vacuum erection devices, and alprostadil for post-RP penile rehabilitation and are shown in Table 15.3. Montorsi et al. [36] first reported the use of thrice-weekly ICI alprostadil after nerve-sparing RP using an RCT design. The small sample size, lack of objective endpoints, and lack of baseline pre-RP erectile function measures reduced the GRADE of the study but it remains a seminal publication with far-reaching impact. Two trials [37,38] involving the use of vacuum erection devices (VED) and intraurethral alprostadil respectively reported improvements in erectile function with these interventions compared to controls; however, the study design and enrollment strategies reduced the quality of evidence and therefore they received lower GRADE ratings. One small but well-executed study randomized men post RP to either observation or VED. Kohler et al. [39] showed that daily use of a VED led to preservation of erectile function compared to controls. The significant effect on erectile function, and related preservation of penile length, warrant confirmatory study. Finally, the role of PDE5 inhibitors in penile rehabilitation after RP remains controversial. One large multicenter RCT compared on-demand and nightly vardenafil with placebo in a 9-month study [40]. No differences in end-of-study erectile function were noted after a 2-month single-blind washout period. Smaller, controlled clinical studies suggest an effect of nightly sildenafil but involve single-surgeon series [41] or unexpectedly low potency rates in controls [42]. Overall, the data are intriguing. The large number of men at risk, and high cost associated with nightly drug administration, make further studies imperative.

Implications for practice: recommendations

• Oral PDE5 inhibitors, intracavernosal prostaglandins, and vacuum erection devices may be useful to treat erectile dysfunction post radical prostatectomy and are efficacious, especially if bilateral nerve sparing is performed (strong recommendation, Grade 1A).
• There are currently no high-quality data supporting the use of oral PDE5 inhibitors, intracavernosal prostaglandins or vacuum erection devices to prevent or decrease post-prostatectomy erectile dysfunction (no recommendation, inadequate evidence).

Table 15.3 Prevention trials for postradical prostatectomy-associated erectile dysfunction

	Trial year	Agent	N	Study design	Pre RRP IIEF-EF domain	End of study IIEF-EF domain (Tx vs P)	End of study GEQ (Tx vs P)	Grade
Oral PDE5-I								
Montorsi [40]	2008	Vardenafil	628	RCT	N/A	No difference	62.60%	High
59.80%								
57.10%								
Padma-Nathan et al. [42]	2008	Sildenafil	76	RCT			27% vs 4%	Mod
Bannowsky et al. [41]	2008	Sildenafil (nightly)	43	Cohort	21.0*	14.1 vs 9.3*	47% vs 28%	V. low
Intracavernosal								
Montorsi [36]	1997	Alprostadil	30	RCT	N/A	N/A	67% vs 20%	Mod
Intraurethral								
Raina [38]	2007	Alprostadil	91	Case series	21*	N/A	58% vs 37%	V. low
Vacuum device								
Kohler [39]	2007	Post NS RP	28	RCT	22.7	12.4 vs 3.0		Mod
Raina [37]	2006	Post RP	109	RCT	22.5*	16 vs 11.2*	32% vs 11%	Low

*IIEF-5 is an abbreviated five-item version of the IIEF (range 0–25)
NS, nerve sparing; P, placebo; RP, radical prostatectomy; Tx, treatment

What evidence is there to support the choice of different penile implants including malleable versus inflatable and antibiotic-coated implants?

The evidence

Surgical implantation of a mechanical device was the first and for many years only efficacious treatment for ED. Since the introduction of oral pharmacotherapy in 1998, penile implant costs have become a proportionally smaller percentage of national expenditures [5]. Early reports of the success of penile implants were in the form of case series and uncontrolled clinical studies with poorly defined endpoints [43]. The introduction of newer implant models over the last 10 years provides insight into the trial methodologies and quality of evidence supporting this treatment of ED. In general, the presence of a functioning implant is equated with efficacy; penile rigidity is not quantitatively assessed in trials, and validated self-administered symptom measures have not been used. Thus infection, mechanical failure and patient satisfaction are the primary outcomes. Given the potential risks associated with incorrect implantation, including infection, revision surgery or explantation, these studies deserve review regardless of the relative quality of evidence compared to drug trials with their more rigorous methodology.

Overall, infection occurs in less than 6% of patients, approximately 90% of patients report high satisfaction scores, and mechanical failure at 5 years is between 5–10%. A greater percentage of penile implants are inflatable rather than semi-rigid or malleable; no direct comparative studies have determined the effectiveness or satisfaction with one or the other type of device. This is unfortunate because of the significantly higher cost of inflatable devices and likely higher mechanical failure rate inferred from the study results shown in Table 15.4. All implants appear to undergo a time-dependent mechanical malfunction. Currently approved devices can be expected to provide 5–10 years of function in the majority of patients. Infection rates vary from 0.7% to 6.5%; diabetes, reoperative surgery, and surgeon experience may all contribute to increasing rates of infection.

Infectious complications of surgical procedures for ED

Infection of a penile implant is a devastating complication that requires surgical explantation and either salvage replacement with a new device or complete removal of all components. The Veterans Affairs National Surgical Quality Improvement Program provided summary data on 706 veterans undergoing surgical treatment for ED in 1998–2003 [5]. One or more complications occurring within 30 days were recorded in 42 of 706 men (5.9%), the most frequent complication being "wound events" (83% of all complications). Approximately 4% of men required a return to the operating room within 30 days; only two men (0.3%) died within 30 days of the procedure.

New modifications have added antibiotic coating to most currently approved devices; while infection rates are lower compared to historical controls, the quality of evidence to support this embellishment is relatively low (Table 15.5). No RCT data exist to support the use of antibiotic coatings on American Medical Systems (AMS) or Coloplast implants. Although the trials listed in Table 15.5

Table 15.4 Clinical studies of currently approved penile implants for the treatment of erectile dysfunction

	Trial year	N	Study design	Implant	Outcome: infection	Outcome: satisfaction*	Device survival	Grade
Inflatable								
Wilson et al. [65]	1999	971	Retrospective	Mentor Alpha 1	4.80%	N/A	93% at 5 yrs	Mod
Carson et al. [63]	2000	372	Retrospective	AMS 700 CX	3.20%	88.20%	86% at 5 yrs	Mod
Dhar et al. [62]	2006	380	Retrospective	AMS 700	N/A	N/A	81% at 10 yrs	Mod
Goldstein et al. [67]	1997	434	Retrospective	Mentor Alpha 1	2.80%	89%	85% at 3 yrs	Low
Govier et al. [66]	1998	169	Retrospective	Mentor/AMS	6.50%	N/A	N/A	Low
Montorsi et al. [64]	2000	200	Retrospective	AMS 700 CX	6%	92%	90% at 5 yrs	Low
Lux et al. [61]	2007	146	Retrospective	AMS Ambicor	0.70%	86%	91% at 4 yrs	Low
Malleable								
Kearse et al. [68]	1996	196	Prospective	Dura-II	2.60%	91%	95% at 2 yrs	Mod

*Satisfaction measures were not standardized across studies

Table 15.5 Clinical studies of antibiotic-coated penile implants

	Infection rate								
	Trial year	N	Study design	Reduction in infection risk	*De novo*	*De novo* DM	Revision w/o washout	Revision with washout	Grade
Wilson et al. [69]	2007	467	Prospective	66%	0% N 223	1.2% N 83	10.3% N 39	3.3% N 122	Low
Carson [70]	2004	4205	Retrospective cohort study	60%	–	–	–	–	Mod
Abouassaly et al. [71]	2006	53	Retrospective case series	–	N/A	–	–	1.9%	Low
Droggin et al. [72]	2005	152	Retrospective case series	100%	0% N 53	–	–	–	V. low

De novo, first time (virgin) penile implant; DM, diabetes mellitus

demonstrate lower infection rates than in earlier trials listed in Table 15.4, it is possible that selection bias may influence the findings. For example, if more *de novo* implants are performed, this will reduce the infection rate in the cohort. Similarly, high-volume implant surgeons or hospitals may explain some of the lower infection rate reported in recent clinical studies. AMS uses a combination of rifampin and minocycline in the Inhibizone? coated implants. Coloplast has created an absorptive surface modification, which allows the device to be soaked in antibiotic solution at time of implantation; no trials of the latter modification were found in our literature search. Despite a lack of high-quality evidence, current practice has shifted almost entirely to these newer, more expensive implants. Randomized controlled trials and cost-effectiveness studies would be useful additions to the literature in this area.

Implications for practice: recommendations

• Penile implants, in well-selected patients who fail other treatments, provide a satisfactory and reliable erection (strong recommendation, **Grade 1B**).
• Penile implant infection rates are lower in recent trials using antibiotic-coated devices, but the evidence supporting the use of this innovation is indirect and derivative (conditional recommendation, **Grade 2C**).

Implications for research

• A rigorous RCT comparing the various phosphodiesterase 5 inhibitors is necessary, as are studies directly comparing PDE5 inhibitors and other therapeutic options.

• Rigorous RCT methodology is still needed to determine the best approach to preserve erectile function post prostatectomy.
• Comparative satisfaction and efficacy of malleable and inflatable penile implants should be determined in a RCT.
• All future studies should assess and report baseline IIEF-EF score as well as change in IIEF-EF score for treatment versus placebo groups.

References

1. NIH Consensus Conference. Impotence. NIH Consensus Development Panel on Impote:nce. JAMA 1993;270(1):83-90.
2. Laumann EO, Paik A, Rosen RC. Sexual dysfunction in the United States: prevalence and predictors. JAMA 1999;281(6):537-44.
3. Feldman HA, Goldstein I, Hatzichristou DG, Krane RJ, McKinlay JB. Impotence and its medical and psychosocial correlates: results of the Massachusetts Male Aging Study. J Urol 1994;151(1):54-61.
4. Bacon CG, Mittleman MA, Kawachi I, Giovannucci E, Glasser DB, Rimm EB. Sexual function in men older than 50 years of age: results from the health professionals follow-up study. Ann Intern Med 2003;139(3):161-8.
5. Wessells H, Joyce GF, Wise M, Wilt TJ. Erectile dysfunction. J Urol 2007;177(5):1675-81.
6. Andersson KE, Wagner G. Physiology of penile erection. Physiol Rev 1995;75(1):191-236.
7. Jarow JP, Nana-Sinkam P, Sabbagh M, Eskew A. Outcome analysis of goal directed therapy for impotence. J Urol 1996;155(5):1609-12.
8. Lue TF. Erectile dysfunction. N Engl J Med 2000;342(24): 1802-13.

9. Rosen RC, Riley A, Wagner G, Osterloh IH, Kirkpatrick J, Mishra A. The International Index of Erectile Function (IIEF): a multidimensional scale for assessment of erectile dysfunction. Urology 1997;49(6):822-30.

10. Burnett AL, Aus G, Canby-Hagino ED, et al. Erectile function outcome reporting after clinically localized prostate cancer treatment. J Urol 2007;178(2):597-601.

11. Guyatt GH, Oxman AD, Kunz R, Vist GE, Falck-Ytter Y, Schunemann HJ. What is "quality of evidence" and why is it important to clinicians? BMJ 2008;336(7651):995-8.

12. Goldstein I, Young JM, Fischer J, Bangerter K, Segerson T, Taylor T. Vardenafil, a new phosphodiesterase type 5 inhibitor, in the treatment of erectile dysfunction in men with diabetes: a multicenter double-blind placebo-controlled fixed-dose study. Diabetes Care 2003;26(3):777-83.

13. Vardi M, Nini A. Phosphodiesterase inhibitors for erectile dysfunction in patients with diabetes mellitus. Cochrane Database Syst Rev 2007;1:CD002187.

14. Deforge D, Blackmer J, Garritty C, et al. Male erectile dysfunction following spinal cord injury: a systematic review. Spinal Cord 2006;44(8):465-73.

15. Dinsmore WW, Hodges M, Hargreaves C, Osterloh IH, Smith MD, Rosen RC. Sildenafil citrate (Viagra) in erectile dysfunction: near normalization in men with broad-spectrum erectile dysfunction compared with age-matched healthy control subjects. Urology 1999;53(4):800-5.

16. Porst H, Padma-Nathan H, Giuliano F, Anglin G, Varanese L, Rosen R. Efficacy of tadalafil for the treatment of erectile dysfunction at 24 and 36 hours after dosing: a randomized controlled trial. Urology 2003;62(1):121-5; discussion 5-6.

17. Young JM, Feldman RA, Auerbach SM, et al. Tadalafil improved erectile function at twenty-four and thirty-six hours after dosing in men with erectile dysfunction: US trial. J Androl 2005;26(3):310-18.

18. Rajfer J, Aliotta PJ, Steidle CP, Fitch WP, 3rd, Zhao Y, Yu A. Tadalafil dosed once a day in men with erectile dysfunction: a randomized, double-blind, placebo-controlled study in the US. Int J Impot Res 2007;19(1):95-103.

19. Porst H, Giuliano F, Glina S, et al. Evaluation of the efficacy and safety of once-a-day dosing of tadalafil 5mg and 10mg in the treatment of erectile dysfunction: results of a multicenter, randomized, double-blind, placebo-controlled trial. Eur Urol 2006;50(2):351-9.

20. Hatzimouratidis K, Moysidis K, Bekos A, Tsimtsiou Z, Ioannidis E, Hatzichristou D. Treatment strategy for "non-responders" to tadalafil and vardenafil: a real-life study. Eur Urol 2006;50(1):126-32; discussion 32-3.

21. Eardley I. Optimisation of PDE5 inhibitor therapy in men with erectile dysfunction: converting "non-responders" into "responders". Eur Urol 2006;50(1):31-3.

22. Hellstrom WJ, Elhilali M, Homering M, Taylor T, Gittleman M. Vardenafil in patients with erectile dysfunction: achieving treatment optimization. J Androl 2005;26(5):604-9.

23. O'Leary MP, Althof SE, Cappelleri JC, Crowley A, Sherman N, Duttagupta S. Self-esteem, confidence and relationship satisfaction of men with erectile dysfunction treated with sildenafil citrate: a multicenter, randomized, parallel group, double-blind, placebo controlled study in the United States. J Urol 2006;175 (3 pt 1):1058-62.

24. Gruenwald I, Leiba R, Vardi Y. Effect of sildenafil on middle-aged sexually active males with no erectile complaints: a randomized placebo-controlled double-blind study. Eur Urol 2009;55(4):969-76.

25. Berner MM, Kriston L, Harms A. Efficacy of PDE-5-inhibitors for erectile dysfunction. A comparative meta-analysis of fixed-dose regimen randomized controlled trials administering the International Index of Erectile Function in broad-spectrum populations. Int J Impot Res 2006;18(3):229-35.

26. Von Keitz A, Rajfer J, Segal S, et al. A multicenter, randomized, double-blind, crossover study to evaluate patient preference between tadalafil and sildenafil. Eur Urol 2004;45(4):499-507; discussion 507-9.

27. Eardley I, Mirone V, Montorsi F, et al. An open-label, multicentre, randomized, crossover study comparing sildenafil citrate and tadalafil for treating erectile dysfunction in men naive to phosphodiesterase 5 inhibitor therapy. BJU Int 2005;96(9):1323-32.

28. Godschalk MF, Chen J, Katz PG, Mulligan T. Treatment of erectile failure with prostaglandin E1: a double-blind, placebo-controlled, dose-response study. J Urol 1994;151(6): 1530-2.

29. Linet OI, Ogrinc FG. Efficacy and safety of intracavernosal alprostadil in men with erectile dysfunction. The Alprostadil Study Group. N Engl J Med 1996;334(14):873-7.

30. Padma-Nathan H, Hellstrom WJ, Kaiser FE, et al. Treatment of men with erectile dysfunction with transurethral alprostadil. Medicated Urethral System for Erection (MUSE) Study Group. N Engl J Med 1997 2;336(1):1-7.

31. Williams G, Abbou CC, Amar ET, et al. Efficacy and safety of transurethral alprostadil therapy in men with erectile dysfunction. MUSE Study Group. BJU 1998;81(6):889-94.

32. Shokeir AA, Alserafi MA, Mutabagani H. Intracavernosal versus intraurethral alprostadil: a prospective randomized study. BJU Int 1999;83(7):812-15.

33. Shabsigh R, Padma-Nathan H, Gittleman M, McMurray J, Kaufman J, Goldstein I. Intracavernous alprostadil alfadex is more efficacious, better tolerated, and preferred over intraurethral alprostadil plus optional actis: a comparative, randomized, crossover, multicenter study. Urology 2000;55(1): 109-13.

34. Montague DK, Jarow JP, Broderick GA, et al. Chapter 1: The management of erectile dysfunction: an AUA update. J Urol 2005;174(1):230-9.

35. Dalkin BL, Christopher BA. Potent men undergoing radical prostatectomy: a prospective study measuring sexual health outcomes and the impact of erectile dysfunction treatments. Urol Oncol 2008;26(3):281-5.

36. Montorsi F, Guazzoni G, Strambi LF, et al. Recovery of spontaneous erectile function after nerve-sparing radical retropubic prostatectomy with and without early intracavernous injections of alprostadil: results of a prospective, randomized trial. J Urol 1997;158(4):1408-10.

37. Raina R, Agarwal A, Ausmundson S, et al. Early use of vacuum constriction device following radical prostatectomy facilitates

early sexual activity and potentially earlier return of erectile function. Int J Impot Res 2006;18(1):77-81.

38. Raina R, Pahlajani G, Agarwal A, Zippe CD. The early use of transurethral alprostadil after radical prostatectomy potentially facilitates an earlier return of erectile function and successful sexual activity. BJU Int 2007;100(6):1317-21.

39. Kohler TS, Pedro R, Hendlin K, et al. A pilot study on the early use of the vacuum erection device after radical retropubic prostatectomy. BJU Int 2007;100(4):858-62.

40. Montorsi F, Brock G, Lee J, et al. Effect of nightly versus on-demand vardenafil on recovery of erectile function in men following bilateral nerve-sparing radical prostatectomy. Eur Urol 2008;54(4):924-31.

41. Bannowsky A, Schulze H, van der Horst C, Hautmann S, Junemann KP. Recovery of erectile function after nerve-sparing radical prostatectomy: improvement with nightly low-dose sildenafil. BJU Int 2008;101(10):1279-83.

42. Padma-Nathan H, McCullough AR, Levine LA, et al. Randomized, double-blind, placebo-controlled study of post-operative nightly sildenafil citrate for the prevention of erectile dysfunction after bilateral nerve-sparing radical prostatectomy. Int J Impot Res 2008;20(5):479-86.

43. Scott FB, Fishman IJ, Light JK. An inflatable penile prosthesis for treatment of diabetic impotence. Ann Intern Med 1980;92(2 pt 2):340-2.

44. Goldstein I, Lue TF, Padma-Nathan H, Rosen RC, Steers WD, Wicker PA. Oral sildenafil in the treatment of erectile dysfunction. Sildenafil Study Group. N Engl J Med 1998;338(20):1397-404.

45. Montorsi F, McDermott TE, Morgan R, et al. Efficacy and safety of fixed-dose oral sildenafil in the treatment of erectile dysfunction of various etiologies. Urology 1999;53(5):1011-18.

46. Tan HM, Moh CL, Mendoza JB, et al. Asian Sildenafil Efficacy and Safety Study (ASSESS-1): a double-blind, placebo-controlled, flexible-dose study of oral sildenafil in Malaysian, Singaporean, and Filipino men with erectile dysfunction. The Assess-1 Study Group. Urology 2000;56(4):635-40.

47. Fink HA, MacDonald R, Rutks IR, Nelson DB, Wilt TJ. Sildenafil for male erectile dysfunction: a systematic review and meta-analysis. Arch Intern Med 2002;162(12):1349-60.

48. Porst H, Rosen R, Padma-Nathan H, et al. The efficacy and tolerability of vardenafil, a new, oral, selective phosphodi-esterase type 5 inhibitor, in patients with erectile dysfunction: the first at-home clinical trial. Int J Impot Res 2001;13 (4):192-9.

49. Hatzichristou D, Montorsi F, Buvat J, Laferriere N, Bandel TJ, Porst H. The efficacy and safety of flexible-dose vardena-fil (Levitra) in a broad population of European men. Eur Urol 2004;45(5):634-41; discussion 41.

50. Markou S, Perimenis P, Gyftopoulos K, Athanasopoulos A, Barbalias G. Vardenafil (Levitra) for erectile dysfunction: a systematic review and meta-analysis of clinical trial reports. Int J Impot Res 2004;16(6):470-8.

51. Potempa AJ, Ulbrich E, Bernard I, Beneke M. Efficacy of varde-nafil in men with erectile dysfunction: a flexible-dose community practice study. Eur Urol 2004;46(1):73-9.

52. Padma-Nathan H, McMurray JG, Pullman WE, et al. On-demand IC351 (Cialis) enhances erectile function in patients with erectile dysfunction. Int J Impot Res 2001;13(1):2-9.

53. McMahon CG, Stuckey BG, Lording DW, et al. A 6-month study of the efficacy and safety of tadalafil in the treatment of erectile dysfunction: a randomised, double-blind, parallel-group, placebo-controlled study in Australian men. Int J Clin Pract 2005;59(2):143-9.

54. Carson C, Shabsigh R, Segal S, Murphy A, Fredlund P, Kuepfer C. Efficacy, safety, and treatment satisfaction of tadalafil versus placebo in patients with erectile dysfunction evaluated at tertiary-care academic centers. Urology 2005;65(2):353-9.

55. Carson CC, Rajfer J, Eardley I, et al. The efficacy and safety of tadalafil: an update. BJU Int 2004;93(9):1276-81.

56. Yip WC, Chiang HS, Mendoza JB, et al. Efficacy and safety of on demand tadalafil in the treatment of East and Southeast Asian men with erectile dysfunction: a randomized double-blind, parallel, placebo-controlled clinical study. Asian J Androl 2006;8(6):685-92.

57. Rendell MS, Rajfer J, Wicker PA, Smith MD. Sildenafil for treatment of erectile dysfunction in men with diabetes: a randomized controlled trial. Sildenafil Diabetes Study Group. JAMA 1999;281(5):421-6.

58. Montorsi F, Nathan HP, McCullough A, et al. Tadalafil in the treatment of erectile dysfunction following bilateral nerve sparing radical retropubic prostatectomy: a randomized, double-blind, placebo controlled trial. J Urol 2004;172(3): 1036-41.

59. Mahmoud KZ, el Dakhli MR, Fahmi IM, Abdel-Aziz AB. Comparative value of prostaglandin E1 and papaverine in treatment of erectile failure: double-blind crossover study among Egyptian patients. J Urol 1992;147(3):623-6.

60. Hellstrom WJ, Bennett AH, Gesundheit N, et al. A double-blind, placebo-controlled evaluation of the erectile response to transurethral alprostadil. Urology 1996;48(6):851-6.

61. Lux M, Reyes-Vallejo L, Morgentaler A, Levine LA. Outcomes and satisfaction rates for the redesigned 2-piece penile prosthesis. J Urol 2007;177(1):262-6.

62. Dhar NB, Angermeier KW, Montague DK. Long-term mechanical reliability of AMS 700CX/CXM inflatable penile prosthesis. J Urol 2006;176(6 pt 1):2599-601; discussion 2601.

63. Carson CC, Mulcahy JJ, Govier FE. Efficacy, safety and patient satisfaction outcomes of the AMS 700CX inflatable penile prosthesis: results of a long-term multicenter study. AMS 700CX Study Group. J Urol 2000;164(2):376-80.

64. Montorsi F, Rigatti P, Carmignani G, et al. AMS three-piece inflatable implants for erectile dysfunction: a long-term multi-institutional study in 200 consecutive patients. Eur Urol 2000; 37(1):50-5.

65. Wilson SK, Cleves MA, Delk JR 2nd. Comparison of mechanical reliability of original and enhanced Mentor Alpha I penile prosthesis. J Urol 1999;162(3 pt 1):715-18.

66. Govier FE, Gibbons RP, Correa RJ, Pritchett TR, Kramer-Levien D. Mechanical reliability, surgical complications, and patient and partner satisfaction of the modern three-piece inflatable penile prosthesis. Urology 1998;52(2):282-6.

67. Goldstein I, Newman L, Baum N, et al. Safety and efficacy outcome of Mentor Alpha-1 inflatable penile prosthesis implantation for impotence treatment. J Urol 1997;157(3):833-9.

68. Kearse WS Jr, Sago AL, Peretsman SJ, et al. Report of a multicenter clinical evaluation of the Dura-II penile prosthesis. J Urol 1996;155(5):1613-16.

69. Wilson SK, Zumbe J, Henry GD, Salem EA, Delk JR, Cleves MA. Infection reduction using antibiotic-coated inflatable penile prosthesis. Urology 2007;70(2):337-40.

70. Carson CC 3rd. Efficacy of antibiotic impregnation of inflatable penile prostheses in decreasing infection in original implants. J Urol 2004;171(4):1611-14.

71. Abouassaly R, Angermeier KW, Montague DK. Risk of infection with an antibiotic coated penile prosthesis at device replacement for mechanical failure. J Urol 2006;176(6 pt 1): 2471-3.

72. Droggin D, Shabsigh R, Anastasiadis AG. Antibiotic coating reduces penile prosthesis infection. J Sex Med 2005;2(4): 565-8.

73. Montorsi F, Nathan HP, McCullough A, et al. Tadalafil in the treatment of erectile dysfunction following bilateral nerve sparing radical retropubic prostatectomy: a randomized, double-blind, placebo controlled trial. J Urol 2004;172(3):1036-41. Erratum in: J Urol 2005;173(2):664.

16 Male infertility

Ashok Agarwal, Fnu Deepinder and Edmund S. Sabanegh Jr

Center for Reproductive Medicine, Glickman Urological and Kidney Institute, The Cleveland Clinic, Cleveland, OH, USA

The role of varicocelectomy in management of male subfertility

Background

Varicocele is present in approximately 40% of men presenting with infertility [1]. Although varicocele repair is widely used in the management of male-factor infertility, the effectiveness of varicocelectomy has been intensely debated, and there is still no consensus on the topic.

Existing literature is conflicting, and very few sufficiently large and adequately controlled prospective trials are available evaluating the efficacy of varicocelectomy in improving pregnancy outcomes. Two published meta-analyses evaluating prospective randomized trials came to the same conclusion that varicocele repairs do not improve subfertility [2,3]. A recently updated Cochrane review recommended against varicocele repair for unexplained infertility [4]. However, these meta-analyses have been criticized for methodological flaws which may have biased their results [5]. Consequently, they have not resolved the issues surrounding varicocelectomy and subfertility.

The development of assisted reproductive techniques (ART) has led to increased use of intracytoplasmic sperm injection (ICSI) for all causes of male infertility including varicoceles. However, these techniques have safety issues, deprive patients of the satisfaction of natural conception, and are less cost-effective [6].

Recent guidelines from the Best Practice Policy Committee of the American Urological Association (AUA) and the American Society for Reproductive Medicine (ASRM) have recommended varicocele repair for infertile men with a clinically palpable varicocele and at least one or more abnormal semen parameters with female partner having either normal or potentially treatable fertility [7].

Rationale for the use of varicocelectomy in management of male subfertility

The exact mechanism by which varicocelectomy improves fertility in affected men remains unknown. Oxidative stress and DNA damage to sperm, which are well-documented components of varicocele pathophysiology, have shown improvement after varicocele repair. Hurtado de Catalfo and colleagues have demonstrated elevated levels of thiobarbituric acid reactive substances which are markers of oxidative stress in both seminal and peripheral plasma of varicocele patients which returned to normal 1 month post varicocelectomy. Other markers of oxidative stress were also decreased and the total antioxidant capacity was increased 6 months after varicocelectomy in their study [8]. Confirming the increased antioxidant capacity after varicocele repair, a more recent study also found a significant decrease in the levels of 8-hydroxy-2-deoxy-guanosine (8-OHdG), another marker of oxidative stress in all post-varicocele repair patients. In this study, investigators also demonstrated a significant decline in the incidence of 4977 bp deletion in mitochondrial DNA, a marker of oxidant-mediated DNA damage after varicocele repair [9]. Shiraishi & Naito showed that elevated preoperative 4-hydroxy-2-nonenal (4-HNE) modified protein levels in the testis could predict a response to varicocele repair [10]. These landmark studies have suggested that varicocele repair decreases the levels of oxidative stress as a mechanism for improving fertility.

Literature search

We conducted new meta-analyses to assess the effect of varicocelectomy on pregnancy outcomes and semen parameters [11,12]. In these analyses, we included both randomized controlled trials and observational studies.

Although critics may object to inclusion of observational studies in a meta-analysis, we adhered to the principles of the Potsdam guidelines laid down by a group of 20 scientists for the conduct and interpretation of meta-analyses [13].

Studies were identified by performing an extensive search using BIOSIS, EMBASE, and Medline (from 1985 to the present) with the help of a professional librarian as well as by hand-searching review articles and cross-references. The following keywords were used to search the databases: "varicocelectomy," "microsurgery," "high ligation," "infertility," "semen parameters," and "pregnancy or outcome." No exclusions were made based on language. Studies were excluded if subclinical varicocele only or subclinical varicocele combined with clinical varicocele were examined or if the effect of treatment was examined only in an adolescent population.

Types of participants
Infertile males diagnosed with unilateral or bilateral varicoceles with abnormal semen parameters. The control groups were composed of infertile males with varicocele who declined to undergo surgical repair of varicocele, were randomized to no/medical treatment or randomized to receive treatment after the follow-up period.

Types of intervention
Surgical ligation (high ligation, inguinal or microsurgery).

Types of outcome measures
• *Effect of varicocelectomy on semen parameters* – change in semen parameters (count, motility and morphology) after surgery using before-and-after repeated measures studies. These studies had semen data from the same individual, before and after varicocelectomy.
• *Effect of varicocelectomy on pregnancy outcome* – proportion of couples achieving spontaneous pregnancy during follow-up of up to 24 months using observational and randomized controlled trials.

Effect of varicocelectomy on semen parameters
Blinding and scoring. All articles and reviewers were blinded during the evaluation period. Two evaluators blinded to the concluding results, authors, journal, and year of the articles evaluated each study on its methodological merits. Articles with both pre- and postoperative repeated measures of semen parameters were evaluated for methodological qual-ity by our new scoring system (Table 16.1). The questions and scores were developed to evaluate four categories of bias: selection or follow-up bias, confounding bias, information or detection bias, and other sources of bias such as misclassification. If the points for more than one category of bias totaled to below an acceptable range, the

study was automatically excluded from the final analysis. If the points for only one category totaled below the acceptable range, the study was re-examined to determine whether the overall study was likely to be biased and, if not, whether it could be included in the meta-analysis. If the follow-up time was more than 2 years after the surgery or with no follow-up within this time period or if the study did not account for time-varying confounders, then it was likely that the study would be excluded. Two reviewers scored each study independently, and the final decision on whether or not a study was to be included was determined by a discussion between the two reviewers.

Data extraction. Data were extracted by one of the investigators on a preformatted data extraction sheet. The outcomes of interest for continuous variables such as concentration, motility and morphology data were extracted, and a weighted mean was calculated. Population information (i.e. primary versus secondary infertility) and study characteristics such as the specific intervention (high ligation, microsurgery, and laparoscopy) were listed.

Data analysis. The data were then entered in the RevMan software (version 4.2.8) developed by the Cochrane Collaboration for the purpose of meta-analysis (www.cochrane.org). The semen data were segregated according to the type of surgical procedure used on these patients. Studies were included that had at least three semen analyses per patient. Since sequential semen data often demonstrate variability, a random effects model was used to adjust for the heterogeneity. A p value < 0.05 was used as a cut-off point for significance testing in all statistical tests.

Effect of varicocelectomy on pregnancy outcome To examine the effect of varicocelectomy on "spontaneous or natural" pregnancy outcome, cohorts were studied within a 2-year follow-up, after a varicocelectomy was performed on one cohort and no/medical treatment or no surgical treatment on another. Studies were retrieved in the same manner as described above for semen characteristics. They were then graded using a scoring sheet that was specifically intended to examine the research question. The development of the scoring criteria was similar to that described above with the same considerations of bias, but other questions were developed for cohort studies rather than pre/post repeated measures studies. Studies were excluded if they had men with subclinical varicoceles. Patients who had undergone ART were not included in the analysis. Studies that used embolization or sclerosis techniques for varicocele corrections were also excluded.

Extraction of data was performed without a data extraction sheet because there was only one outcome of interest.

Table 16.1 Scoring sheet used to evaluate studies

Selection/follow-up	Confounding	Information/detection bias	Other
From what, if any, underlying cohort is the study population derived? (3) From a geographical cohort (3) From a community (2) From a clinic population (1) Unable to answer	Was the time between the two follow-up periods short enough to allow for no confounding by age within subjects (under 2 years)? (3) Yes (1) No (1) Unable to answer	Was the method of follow-up the same before and after treatment? (3) Yes (2) No (1) Unable to answer	Does the study combine outcomes across groups with very heterogeneous histories/durations of infertility and across different interventions? (2)Yes (3) No (1) Unable to answer
How were subjects recruited? (3) All cases in the population were included (2) Cases were recruited consecutively over a period of time (3) Cases were randomly selected (1) Unable to answer	Do they evaluate and account for potential confounders that may vary over time, e.g. amount of follow-up time, season, smoking, alcohol consumption, original sperm count, time-varying exposures, etc.? (1) No (2) Yes, but they do not adjust (3) Yes, and they adjust for them when necessary (1) Unable to answer	Was the measurement of outcome(s) objective? Objective meaning medical records or diagnostic test, not objective/subjective meaning recall, etc. (3) Yes (2) No (1) Unable to answer	Was severity/grade of varicocele evaluated before the intervention? (3) Yes (2) No (1) Unable to answer
Did the investigators restrict against participants based on infection, previous treatment, and female factor infertility or conditions related to ART outcome and sperm parameters? (3) Yes (2) No (1) Unable to answer	Did the investigators prespecify the same procedures for analysis for before and after the intervention? (2) Yes (2) Not applicable (1) No (1) Unable to answer	Was ascertainment of outcome performed at the same location both before and after treatment? (4) Yes (2) No (1) Unable to answer	Did investigators use an established set of guidelines for semen analysis? (4) Yes (1) No (1) Unable to answer
Was there loss of follow-up or lack of participation greater than 10% of those sampled initially? (1) Yes (2) No (1) Unable to answer			
Total =	Total =	Total =	Total =

Exclusion criteria

Category	Maximum score	Minimum score	Include score	Exclude score
Selection	11	4	11–7	6–4
Confounding	8	3	8–5	4–3
Information	10	3	10–8	7–3
Other	10	3	10–8	7–3

Any study will be excluded if two or more categories score in the "exclude" range
Any studies will be re-reviewed if only one category scores in the "exclude" range

Pregnancy data were recorded for the 24-month interval after surgery and the overall odds were calculated. The data were verified by a second investigator, and analysis of the pregnancy data was performed by both random and fixed effects models.

Clinical question 16.1

What is the effect of varicocelectomy on semen parameters?

Trials included

A total of 136 studies were identified, of which only17 were included in the meta-analysis that pertained to semen parameters [14-30].

Outcomes

Of the 17 studies, only 10 examined concentration and motility of sperm before and after intervention by microsurgery. The sperm concentration was increased by 9.71×10^6/mL (95% confidence interval (CI) 7.34–12.08, p < 0.00001) in all 10 studies (Figure 16.1A). The average motility was increased by 9.92% (95% CI 4.90–14.95, p = 0.0001) in the studies that utilized microsurgery (Figure 16.1B).

The results for high ligation were similar by applying a weighted average in seven or eight studies (depending on the outcomes measured). Concentration was increased by 12.03×10^6/mL (95% CI 5.71–18.35, p = 0.0002) as calculated from reported results in eight studies (Figure 16.2A). Motility was increased by 11.72% (95% CI 4.33–19.12, p = 0.002) as averaged over reported results in seven studies (Figure 16.2B).

Morphology was only reported in seven of the 17 studies. These studies were analyzed together, but three utilized microsurgery and three used high ligation. One study had data on morphology using both of these techniques. The combined results for both the types of surgery were included in the analysis. The change in morphology was statistically significant with an estimated change of 3.16% (95% CI 0.72–5.60, p = 0.01) (Figure 16.3).

Clinical question 16.2

What is the effect of varicocelectomy on pregnancy rate?

Trials included

Out of the 101 articles retrieved, our meta-analysis was limited to five surgical studies that had data on "spontaneous" pregnancy rates [30-34].

Outcomes

The odds of "spontaneous" pregnancy after varicocelectomy compared with no/medical treatment for clinical varicocele was significantly different at 2.87 (95% CI 1.33–6.20, p = 0.007) using random effects model (Figure 16.4). A fixed effects model also yielded a significant odds ratio of 2.63 (95% CI 1.60–4.33, p = 0.00001). The test for the presence of heterogeneity between study measures was not significant (p = 0.17).

Comment

Surgical varicocelectomy in selected patients does have a beneficial effect on fertility status. In infertile men with palpable lesions and at least one abnormal semen parameter, it improves the odds of spontaneous pregnancy in their female partners. Similarly, varicocelectomy significantly improves semen parameters in infertile men with palpable varicocele and abnormal semen parameters. The couples who fail to achieve a natural pregnancy after varicocele repair may achieve better results with ART because of the increase in semen quality.

Recommendations

We support the latest best practice policy guidelines laid down by the ASRM and the AUA and recommend varicocele repair for infertile men with clinically palpable varicocele having at least one abnormal semen parameter (Grade 1B).

Efficacy of clomiphene citrate in male infertility treatment

Background

Antiestrogens are used as empiric nonspecific therapy in the management of idiopathic male infertility. The two most commonly used nonsteroidal antiestrogens are clomiphene citrate and tamoxifen. Clomiphene is a synthetic compound similar in structure to diethylstilbestrol. In spite of its mild estrogenic properties, it predominantly acts as an antiestrogen. Clomiphene citrate is usually prescribed in doses of 12.5–50 mg per day

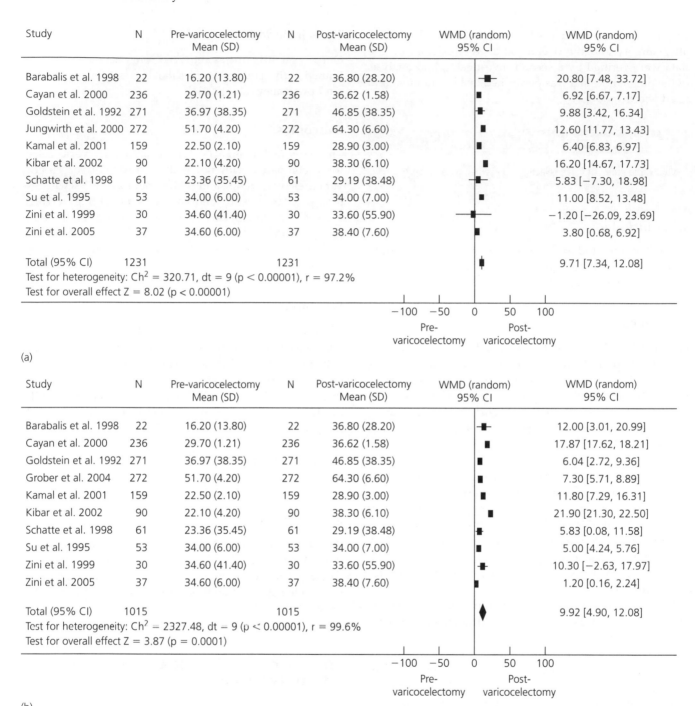

Figure 16.1 (a) Postoperative sperm concentration increased significantly following microsurgical varicocelectomy (p < 0.00001). (b) Postoperative sperm motility increased significantly following microsurgical varicocelectomy (p = 0.0001). CI, confidence interval; SD, standard deviation; WMD, weighed mean difference.

either continuously or on a 25-day cycle with a 5-day rest period each month [35,36].

Although numerous investigators have studied the effect of clomiphene on male infertility, controversy still exists regarding its efficacy. Many well-designed prospective randomized controlled trials failed to demonstrate any significant improvement with clomiphene as compared to placebo [37-43]. However, a few studies have shown a positive effect of clomiphene on pregnancy outcomes [44,45]. The Cochrane systematic review which was

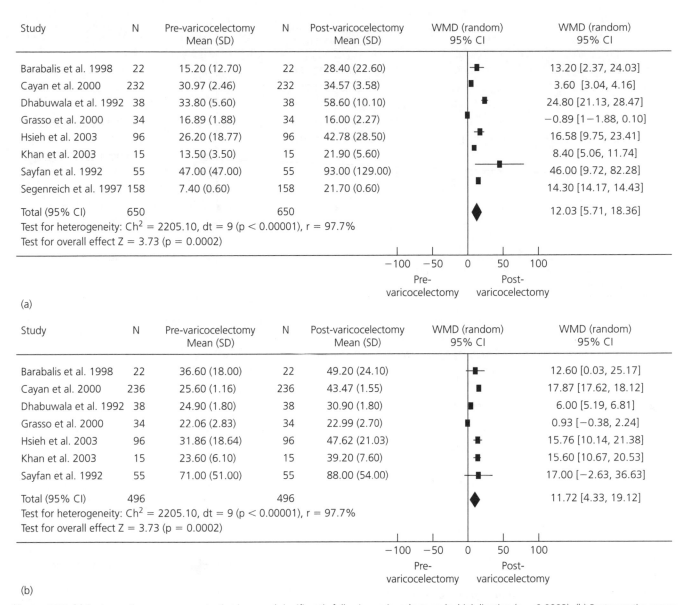

Study	N	Pre-varicocelectomy Mean (SD)	N	Post-varicocelectomy Mean (SD)	WMD (random) 95% CI	WMD (random) 95% CI
Barabalis et al. 1998	22	15.20 (12.70)	22	28.40 (22.60)		13.20 [2.37, 24.03]
Cayan et al. 2000	232	30.97 (2.46)	232	34.57 (3.58)		3.60 [3.04, 4.16]
Dhabuwala et al. 1992	38	33.80 (5.60)	38	58.60 (10.10)		24.80 [21.13, 28.47]
Grasso et al. 2000	34	16.89 (1.88)	34	16.00 (2.27)		−0.89 [1−1.88, 0.10]
Hsieh et al. 2003	96	26.20 (18.77)	96	42.78 (28.50)		16.58 [9.75, 23.41]
Khan et al. 2003	15	13.50 (3.50)	15	21.90 (5.60)		8.40 [5.06, 11.74]
Sayfan et al. 1992	55	47.00 (47.00)	55	93.00 (129.00)		46.00 [9.72, 82.28]
Segenreich et al. 1997	158	7.40 (0.60)	158	21.70 (0.60)		14.30 [14.17, 14.43]
Total (95% CI)	650		650			12.03 [5.71, 18.36]

Test for heterogeneity: $Ch^2 = 2205.10$, dt = 9 (p < 0.00001), r = 97.7%
Test for overall effect Z = 3.73 (p = 0.0002)

(a)

Study	N	Pre-varicocelectomy Mean (SD)	N	Post-varicocelectomy Mean (SD)	WMD (random) 95% CI	WMD (random) 95% CI
Barabalis et al. 1998	22	36.60 (18.00)	22	49.20 (24.10)		12.60 [0.03, 25.17]
Cayan et al. 2000	236	25.60 (1.16)	236	43.47 (1.55)		17.87 [17.62, 18.12]
Dhabuwala et al. 1992	38	24.90 (1.80)	38	30.90 (1.80)		6.00 [5.19, 6.81]
Grasso et al. 2000	34	22.06 (2.83)	34	22.99 (2.70)		0.93 [−0.38, 2.24]
Hsieh et al. 2003	96	31.86 (18.64)	96	47.62 (21.03)		15.76 [10.14, 21.38]
Khan et al. 2003	15	23.60 (6.10)	15	39.20 (7.60)		15.60 [10.67, 20.53]
Sayfan et al. 1992	55	71.00 (51.00)	55	88.00 (54.00)		17.00 [−2.63, 36.63]
Total (95% CI)	496		496			11.72 [4.33, 19.12]

Test for heterogeneity: $Ch^2 = 2205.10$, dt = 9 (p < 0.00001), r = 97.7%
Test for overall effect Z = 3.73 (p = 0.0002)

(b)

Figure 16.2 (a) Postoperative sperm concentration increased significantly following varicocelectomy by high ligation (p = 0.0002). (b) Postoperative sperm motility increased significantly following varicocelectomy by high ligation (p = 0.002). CI, confidence interval; SD, standard deviation; WMD, weighed mean difference.

updated more than a decade ago found no significant benefit with clomiphene in increasing the fertility rates of men with idiopathic oligospermia [46]. In another meta-analysis, Kamischke & Nieschlag demonstrated no significant therapeutic effect of antiestrogen therapy with clomiphene and tamoxifen on pregnancy outcomes [47].

Some investigators have found men with normal pretreatment follicle-stimulating hormone (FSH) to be more likely to respond to clomiphene treatment. They suggested utilizing pretreatment serum hormone levels to differentiate potential responders and nonresponders [38,39,45]. However, a large multicenter double-blind

randomized controlled study conducted by the World Health Organization and a multicenter prospective randomized Scottish trial found no evidence to support this hypothesis [40,43].

Rationale for the use of clomiphene citrate in male infertility

Clomiphene indirectly stimulates the secretion of gonadotropin-releasing hormone (GnRH), FSH and luteinizing hormone (LH) by binding to estrogen receptors in the hypothalamus and pituitary, thereby blocking estrogen

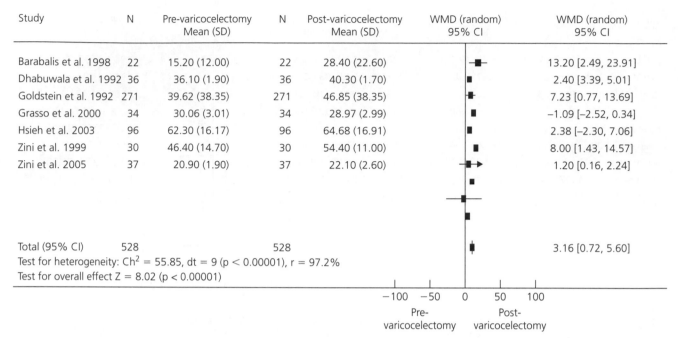

Figure 16.3 Postoperative sperm morphology increased significantly following varicocelectomy (p = 0.01).

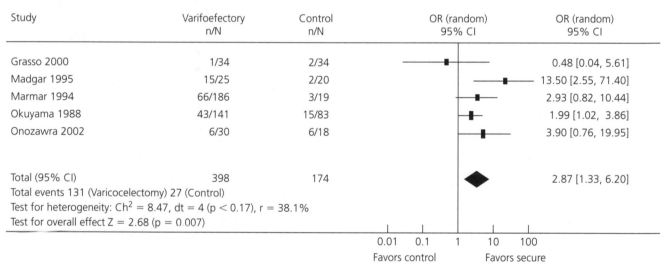

Figure 16.4 Effect of varicocelectomy on pregnancy rate using random effect model showed significant improvement (p = 0.007). CI, confidence interval; n, number of couples achieving pregnancy with male partners diagnosed with clinical varicoceles; N, total number of cases; OR, odds ratio; SD, standard deviation; WMD, weighed mean difference.

feedback inhibition. The resultant increase in intratesticular testosterone concentration is believed to boost the gametogenic function of the testis. Men treated with clomiphene consistently demonstrate an elevation in serum FSH, LH and testosterone levels. However, it is essential to maintain serum testosterone within normal limits because higher levels may negatively influence spermatogenesis [35,36]. Application of clomiphene citrate in males with non-obstructive azoospemia may result in sufficient sperm for

ICSI, either identified in the ejaculate or by successful surgical testicular sperm extraction [48].

Literature search

Studies were identified by performing an extensive Medline search (from 1975 to the present) with the help of a professional librarian as well as by hand-searching review articles and cross-references. The following keywords were used to search the databases: "clomiphene citrate," "antiestrogens," "oligospermia," "infertility," "semen parameters," and "pregnancy rate or outcome." Randomized controlled trials (RCT) of clomiphene therapy for at least 3 months or more compared to placebo or alternative treatment for subfertile males among couples where subfertility was attributed to male factor were selected.

Couples who failed to achieve pregnancy after at least 12 months of unprotected intercourse were chosen. The male partners of the couples included were diagnosed with idiopathic infertility and had oligo- and/or asthenozoospermia. Any patient with known cause for infertility, such as history of toxin or drug exposure, varicocele, undescended testis, primary germinal infertility or known endocrine disorder, was excluded. The female partners had no demonstrable cause for infertility as they had normal menstrual and ovulatory pattern and no significant mechanical abnormalities by laparoscopy or hysterosalpingography.

Pregnancy data were recorded for 6–12 months after the clomiphene empiric therapy and the overall odds were calculated. P values < 0.05 were used as a cut-off point for significance testing in all statistical tests.

Clinical question 16.3

Is clomiphene citrate effective for male infertility treatment?

Trials included

A total of 21 studies were identified, of which only seven met our inclusion criteria [38-43,45]. Five studies used placebo as a control group [39,41-43,45] whereas one each

compared antioxidant vitamin C [40] and low-dose cortisone acetate [38] to clomiphene citrate therapy.

Outcomes

The odds of "spontaneous" pregnancy after at least 3 months of clomiphene therapy compared with no or alternative empiric treatment for male subfertility did not differ significantly: 1.55 (95% CI 0.66–3.68) by fixed effect model and 1.35 (95% CI 0.75–2.42) by random effect model (Table 16.2).

However, some of the trials demonstrated significant improvement in semen parameters, especially the total motile sperm count. Unfortunately, insufficient studies and heterogeneity among these trials precluded us from conducting a meaningful meta-analysis evaluating the improved outcomes in semen parameters.

Comment

Empiric clomiphene therapy 25–50 mg/day for at least 3 months may have a beneficial effect on fertility status in subfertile men by improving semen parameters which may allow a downstaging of the required ART procedure, i.e. utilizing intrauterine insemination (IUI) instead of ICSI.

Recommendations

Empiric trial therapy with clomiphene citrate 25–50 mg/day for at least 3 months may be offered to subfertile men with oligo- and/or asthenozoospermia at the clinician's discretion before proceeding to advanced ART techniques such as ICSI (**Grade 2C**). Literature support remains inconclusive, awaiting large randomized prospective trials of empiric therapy.

Table 16.2 Effect of empiric clomiphene citrate therapy on pregnancy outcomes

Study	Clomiphene dose (mg/day)	Treatment group (n/N)	Control group	Control group (n/N)	Odds ratio (95% CI)
WHO 1992	25	7/70	Placebo	6/71	1.20 (0.39–3.75)
Sokol et al. [41]	25	1/11	Placebo	4/9	0.17 (0.02–1.21)
Micic & Dotlic [45]	50	7/56	Placebo	0/45	6.81 (1.46–31.69)
Wang et al. [42]	25 or 50	4/29	Placebo	0/7	3.89 (0.29–51.80)
Abel et al. [40]	50	15/93	Vitamin C 200 mg/day	10/86	1.45 (0.62–3.37)
Ronnberg [39]	50	1/14	Placebo	1/15	1.07 (0.06–18.10)
Paulson [38]	25	7/17	Cortisone 10 mg/day	2/15	4.55 (0.77–26.83)
Total	25–50	42/298		23/248	1.35 (0.75–2.42)

CI, confidence interval; OR, odds ratio; n, number of couples achieving pregnancy; N, total number of cases

References

1. Nagler HM, Luntz RK, Martinis FG. Varicocele. In: Lipshultz LI, Howards SS (eds) *Infertility in the Male*, 3rd edn. St Louis, MO: Mosby Year Book, 1997: 336-59.
2. Kamischke A, Nieschlag E. Varicocele treatment in the light of evidence based andrology. Hum Reprod Update 2001;7:65-9.
3. Evers JL, Collins JA. Surgery or embolisation for varicocele in subfertile men. Cochrane Database Syst Rev 2004;3:CD000479.
4. Evers JH, Collins J, Clarke J. Surgery or embolisation for varicocele in subfertile men. Cochrane Database Syst Rev 2008;16:CD000479.
5. Ficarra V, Cerruto MA, Liguori G, et al. Treatment of varicocele in subfertile men: the Cochrane Review – a contrary opinion. Eur Urol 2006;49:258-63.
6. Meng MV, Greene KL, Turek PJ. Surgery or assisted reproduction? A decision analysis of treatment costs in male infertility. J Urol 2005;174:1926-31.
7. Practice Committee of the American Society for Reproductive Medicine. Report on varicocele and infertility. Fertil Steril 2006;86:S93-S95.
8. Hurtado de Catalfo GE, Ranieri-Casilla A, Marra FA, et al. Oxidative stress biomarkers and hormonal profile in human patients undergoing varicocelectomy. Int J Androl 2007;30:519-30.
9. Chen SS, Huang WJ, Chang LS, Wei YH. Attentuation of oxidative stress after varicocelectomy in subfertile patients with varicocele. J Urol 2008;179:639-42.
10. Shiraishi K, Naito K. Generation of 4-hydroxy-2nonenal modified proteins in testes predicts improvement in spermatogenesis after varicocelectomy. Fertil Steril 2006;86:233-5.
11. Agarwal A, Deepinder F, Cocuzza M, et al. Efficacy of varicocelectomy in improving semen parameters: new meta-analytical approach. Urology 2007;70:532-8.
12. Marmar JL, Agarwal A, Prabakaran S, et al. Reassessing the value of varicocelectomy as a treatment for male subfertility with a new meta-analysis. Fertil Steril 2007;88:639-48.
13. Cook DJ, Sackett DL, Spitzer WO. Methodologic guidelines for systematic reviews of randomized control trials in health care from Potsdam Consultation on Meta-Analysis. J Clin Epidemiol 1995;48:167-71.
14. Kibar Y, Seckin B, Erduran D. The effects of subinguinal varicocelectomy on Kruger morphology and semen parameters. J Urol 2002;168:1071-4.
15. Goldstein M, Gilbert BR, Dicker AP, et al. Microsurgical inguinal varicocelectomy with delivery of the testis: an artery and lymphatic sparing technique. J Urol 1992;148:1808-11.
16. Barbalias GA, Liatsikos EN, Nikiforidis G, et al. Treatment of varicocele for male infertility: a comparative study evaluating currently used approaches. Eur Urol 1998;34:393-8.
17. Cayan S, Erdemir F, Ozbey I, et al. Can varicocelectomy significantly change the way couples use assisted reproductive technologies? J Urol 2002;167:1749-52.
18. Jungwirth A, Gogus C, Hauser G, et al. Clinical outcome of microsurgical subinguinal varicocelectomy in infertile men. Andrologia 2001;33:71-4.
19. Kamal KM, Jarvi K, Zini A. Microsurgical varicocelectomy in the era of assisted reproductive technology: influence of initial semen quality on pregnancy rates. Fertil Steril 2001;75:1013-16.
20. Schatte EC, Hirshberg SJ, Fallick ML, et al. Varicocelectomy improves sperm strict morphology and motility. J Urol 1998;160:1338-40.
21. Su LM, Goldstein M, Schlegel PN. The effect of varicocelectomy on serum testosterone levels in infertile men with varicoceles. J Urol 1995;154:1752-5.
22. Zini A, Buckspan M, Jamal M, et al. Effect of varicocelectomy on the abnormal retention of residual cytoplasm by human spermatozoa. Hum Reprod 1999;14:1791-3.
23. Zini A, Blumenfeld A, Libman J, et al. Beneficial effect of microsurgical varicocelectomy on human sperm DNA integrity. Hum Reprod 2005;20:1018-21.
24. Grober ED, Chan PT, Zini A, et al. Microsurgical treatment of persistent or recurrent varicocele. Fertil Steril 2004;82:718-22.
25. Dhabuwala CB, Hamid S, Moghissi KS. Clinical versus subclinical varicocele: improvement in fertility after varicocelectomy. Fertil Steril 1992;57:854-7.
26. Hsieh ML, Chang PL, Huang ST, et al. Loupe-assisted high inguinal varicocelectomy for sub-fertile men with varicoceles. Chang Gung Med J 2003;26:479-84.
27. Khan M, Khan S, Pervez A, et al. Evaluation of low ligation and high ligation procedures of varicocele. J Coll Physicians Surg Pak 2003;13:280-3.
28. Sayfan J, Soffer Y, Orda R. Varicocele treatment: prospective randomized trial of 3 methods. J Urol 1992;148:1447-9.
29. Segenreich E, Israilov SR, Shmueli J, et al. Correlation between semen parameters and retrograde flow into the pampiniform plexus before and after varicocelectomy. Eur Urol 1997;32:310-14.
30. Grasso M, Lania C, Castelli M, et al. Low-grade left varicocele in patients over 30 years old:the effect of spermatic vein ligation on fertility. BJU Int 2000;85:305-7.
31. Marmar JL, Kim Y. Subinguinal microsurgical varicocelectomy: a technical critique and statistical analysis of semen and pregnancy data. J Urol 1994;152:1127-32.
32. Madgar I, Weissenberg R, Lunenfeld B, et al. Controlled trial of high spermatic vein ligation for varicocele in infertile men. Fertil Steril 1995;63:120-4.
33. Onozawa M, Endo F, Suetomi T, Takeshima H, Akaza H. Clinical study of varicocele: statistical analysis of semen and pregnancy data. J Urol 1994;152:1127-32.
34. Okuyama A, Fujisue H, Matsui T, et al. Surgical repair of varicocele: effective treatment for subfertile men in a controlled study. Eur Urol 1988;14:298-300.
35. Peter LY, David HJ. The present and future state of hormonal treatment for male infertility. Hum Reprod Update 2003;9:9-23.
36. Cocuzza M, Ashok A. Nonsurgical treatment of male infertility: specific and empiric therapy. Biologics: Targ Ther 2007;3:259-69.
37. Foss GL, Tindall VR, Birkett JP. The treatment of subfertile men with clomiphene citrate. J Reprod Fertil 1973;32:167-70.
38. Paulson DF. Cortisone acetate versus clomiphene citrate in pergerminal idiopathic oligospermia. J Urol 1979;121:432-4.
39. Ronnberg L. The effect of clomiphene citrate on different sperm parameters and serum hormone levels in preselected infertile men: a controlled double-blind cross-over study. Int J Androl 1980;3:479-86.

40. Abel BJ, Carswell G, Elton R, et al. Randomized trial of clomiphene citrate treatment and vitamin C for male infertility. BJU 1982;54:780-4.

41. Sokol RZ, Steiner BS, Bustillo M, Peterson G, Swerdloff RS. A controlled comparison of the efficacy of clomiphene citrate in male infertility. Fertil Steril 1988;49,865-70.

42. Wang C, Chan CW, Wong KK, et al. Comparison of the effectiveness of placebo, clomiphene citrate, mesterolone, pentoxifylline, and testosterone rebound therapy for the treatment of idiopathic oligospermia. Fertil Steril 1983;40: 358-65.

43. World Health Organization. A double blind trial of clomiphene citrate for the treatment of idiopathic male infertility. Int J Androl 1992;15:299-307.

44. Check JH, Chase JS, Nowroozi K, et al. Empirical therapy of the male with clomiphene in couples with unexplained infertility. Int J Fertil 1989;34:120-2.

45. Micic S, Dotlic R. Evaluation of sperm parameters in clinical trial with clomiphene citrate of oligospermic men. J Urol 1985;133:221-2.

46. Vandekerckhove P, Lilford R, Vail A, Hughes E. Withdrawn: clomiphene or tamoxifen for idiopathic oligo/asthenospermia. Cochrane Database Syst Rev 2007;18:CD000151.

47. Kamischke A, Nieschlag E. Analysis of medical treatment of male infertility. Hum Reprod 1999;14(suppl 1):1-23.

48. Hussein A, Ozgok Y, Lawrence R, Neiderberger C. Clomiphene administration for cases of nonobstructive azoospermia: a multicenter study. J Androl 2005;26:787-91

17 Genitourinary trauma

Bryan B. Voelzke[1] and Jack W. McAninch[2]
[1]Department of Urology, Harborview Medical Center, Seattle, WA, USA
[2]Department of Urology, San Francisco General Hospital, San Francisco, CA, USA

Background

As a result of the acute and unpredictable nature of genitourinary trauma, there is an absence of prospective, randomized controlled trials to support evaluation and management. As such, urologists have relied on case series reports, retrospective series, trauma databases from level one trauma centers, and expert opinion. Indeed, the Society of International Urology published five consensus articles pertaining to renal, urethral, bladder, ureter, and external genitalia trauma that were authored by well-respected leaders in the field of genitourinary trauma [1-5]. Each article used a level of evidence grading system to validate evaluation and management proposals: (1) supportive evidence from randomized trials, (2) supportive evidence from prospective trials, (3) supportive evidence from retrospective studies, (4) supportive evidence from case series or case reports, (5) expert opinion. Level 3 and 4 evidence predominated in each article, with occasional mention of level 1 and 2 evidence. Despite the absence of stronger levels of evidence, we strongly encourage readers to examine the articles, as they provide a wealth of information for interested urologists.

This chapter will pose two major questions from the field of genitourinary trauma that have been answered with supported evidence. References will be made to the American Association for the Surgery of Trauma (AAST) renal grading system (Figure 17.1).

Clinical question 17.1

What is the appropriate evaluation of blunt abdominal trauma in the setting of gross or microscopic hematuria?

Literature search

We searched the PubMed database for the years 1980–2008 using the search terms "blunt trauma," "abdomen" and "hematuria."

The evidence

The kidneys are the second most common visceral organ to be injured after blunt abdominal trauma, with most renal injuries deemed low grade. In a series of 2024 blunt trauma patients, only 81 (4%) had grade 3 or higher renal injuries [6], a finding supported by other analyses [7,8]. As such, the objective is to identify when to perform radiographic imaging for evaluation of suspected renal injury after blunt abdominal trauma.

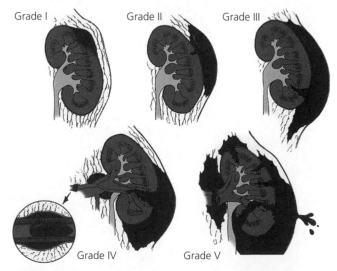

Figure 17.1 American Association for the Surgery of Trauma (AAST) organ injury severity grade for the kidney. Reproduced from Wein et al. *Campbell-Walsh Urology. Volume 2, renal and ureteral trauma*, 9th edn, 2007, p. 1274, with permission from Elsevier.

Evidence-Based Urology. Edited by Philipp Dahm, Roger R. Dmochowski.
© 2010 Blackwell Publishing.

Two large prospective studies have evaluated the appropriate setting of radiographic imaging after blunt abdominal trauma with gross/microscopic hematuria (Table 17.1) [6,8]. In both of these studies, blunt abdominal trauma patients were stratified into two groups: (1) gross hematuria or (2) microscopic hematuria and shock (systolic blood pressure < 90 mmHg). This classification system was based upon an earlier report from San Francisco General Hospital which found that radiographic imaging of blunt abdominal trauma patients with microscopic hematuria and no shock did not lead to complications from nonoperative management [9].

The largest series to prospectively evaluate the appropriate evaluation of blunt abdominal trauma in the setting of gross/microscopic hematuria included 2024 patients from San Francisco General Hospital [6]. This prospective series served as an update to the original series that first reported the algorithm for evaluation of blunt abdominal trauma referenced above. There were 78 significant renal injuries among the cohort of 422 patients with either gross hematuria or microscopic hematuria and shock. Of these, there were 25 grade 2 injuries, 30 minor lacerations (grades 3–4), and 23 vascular injuries (grade 4-5). The remaining patients (344) had renal contusions (grade 1 injury). Only 3/1588 patients with microscopic hematuria and no shock were found to have significant renal injury (grade 2 or higher). Two of these injuries (one grade 2 and one grade 3) were discovered after imaging for suspected intra-abdominal injury, while the third injury (grade 3) was discovered at the time of exploratory laparotomy for associated intra-abdominal injuries. Therefore, urologists are encouraged to perform abdominal imaging if there is suspected renal trauma even in the absence of shock or hematuria.

In the series by Hardeman and colleagues, all patients (N 506) received abdominal imaging (intravenous pyelography) after blunt abdominal trauma and any degree of hematuria regardless of the presence of shock [8]. This provides a more sensitive indicator of who would have been missed within the microhematuria and no shock cohort since everyone received abdominal imaging regardless of the presence of shock with microhematuria. After analysis, only one patient (0.27%, 1/365) with significant injury (grade 2 or more) would have been missed among the cohort with microhematuria and no shock. This patient had a minor laceration and was successfully managed by observation.

Additional reports have focused on the need for abdominal imaging in the setting of microhematuria in the *absence* of shock (Table 17.2) [6,8,10,11]. When evaluating all four studies from Tble 17.2, there were 11/2988 (0.37%) patients with renal injuries that were AAST grade 2 or greater. The AAST renal grading system had not been fully adopted at the time of three of the four studies. However, any renal injury other than a renal contusion (AAST grade 1) was assumed to be AAST grade 2 or greater.

Of these 11 patients from the above paragraph, five of the patients with renal injuries from the series by Hardeman and colleagues would have been discovered based upon their associated injures that required abdominal imaging [8]. Among the entire cohort of 2988 patients with microhematuria and absence of shock in Table 17.2, only two had renal exploration and repair. Closer review of these two patients reveals that they were diagnosed based upon clinical suspicion of their respective injuries. The ureteropelvic junction disruption from the series by Eastham was diagnosed by retrograde pyelogram that was performed based upon clinical suspicion [11]. The other repair from this group of patients with microhematuria and absence of shock after blunt abdominal injury was from the series by Miller & McAninch [6]. The patient underwent repair of an AAST renal grade 3 injury only because of an exploratory laparotomy that was performed for an associated injury. Both repairs in each respective series were successful.

Table 17.1 Radiographic assessment of blunt abdominal trauma in the setting of gross hematuria or microhematuria and shock

Authors	Methods	Intervention	Imaging at presentation	Blunt abd trauma	GH or MH/shock	Outcomes
Miller et al. [1]	Prospective	(1) GH (2) MH/shock (3) MH/no shock	Criteria based*	2024	422	– 78/422 renal injury^ (GH or MH**/shock cohort)3/1588 renal injury^ (MH/no shock cohort) 1 gr 2, 2 gr 3
Hardeman et al. [3]	Prospective	(1) GH (2) MH/shock (3) MH/no shock	All patients	506	141	– 7/141 renal injury^ (GH or MH/shock cohort) – 1/365 renal injury^ (MH/no shock cohort) minor lac w/ no contrast extravasation

*Gross hemautria, microhematuria with shock or clinical suspicion
^AAST renal grade 2 or higher
GH, gross hematuria; MH, microhematuria

Table 17.2 Radiographic assessment of blunt abdominal truama in the setting of microhematuria and no shock

Authors	Methods	Intervention	Imaging at presentation	Blunt abd trauma & hematuria	Microheme/ no shock	Outome^^
Cass et al. [5]	Prospective	(1) Microheme/no shock and no assoc injuries (2) Microheme/no shock and assoc injuries	All patients	831	(1)*160/241 (2) 334/590	(1)*1/160 (1 minor laceration) (2)5/534 (3 minor laceration, 1 deep laceration, 1 pedicle injury)
Hardeman et al. [3]	Consecutive	Microheme/no shock	All patients	506	365/506	1/365 (1 minor laceration)
Eastham et al. [6]	Retrospective, consecutive	Microheme/no shock	All patients	337**	337/337	1/337 (1 UPJ disruption)
Miller et al. [1]	Prospective	(1) Microheme/no shock and imaged (2) Microheme/no shock and not imaged	Criteria based^	2024	(1)*584/2024 (2)1004/2024	(1)*3/588 (1 gr 2, 2 gr 3) (2) 0/1004

*See under Intervention for corresponding group
**All microhematuria and no shock
^Gross hematuria, microhematuria with shock, or clinical suspicion
^^AAST grade 2 or greater, renal contusions were excluded
UPJ, ureteropelvic junction

In today's climate of an increased trend toward nonoperative management of renal injuries, one could assume that many urologists would not surgically intervene under these circumstances unless the renal injury was noted to be expanding or pulsatile intraoperatively.

All four studies from Table 17.2 utilized intravenous pyelography for the initial assessment of patients with blunt abdominal trauma and hematuria. Computed tomography was only used to further delineate suspected injuries. A compelling argument could be made that intravenous pyelography was not able to diagnose some minor renal injuries; however, if present, they were insignificant and did not require eventual surgery or result in added morbidity.

Comment

Radiographic imaging to evaluate for potential renal injury after blunt abdominal trauma should be performed for the following circumstances: (1) gross hematuria, (2) microscopic hematuria and shock (systolic blood pressure < 90 mmHg), and (3) when clinical suspicion of injury exists despite the absence of gross hematuria or microhematuria and shock (i.e. deceleration injury with renal pedicle disruption or ureteropelvic junction obstruction). Indeed, gross or microscopic hematuria may be absent in up to 50% of patients after injury to the ureteropelvic junction, further emphasizing the need to recommend abdominal imaging even

if the patient does not fulfill the criteria for abdominal imaging after blunt abdominal trauma [12]. Determination of microscopic hematuria can be performed via dipstick or microscopic analysis, as dipstick analysis has been shown to have a 97.5% specificity and sensitivity when compared with microscopic urinalysis in one large study of patients after blunt renal trauma [13].

Clinical question 17.2

What are the best predictors for nephrectomy after abdominal trauma?

Literature search

We searched the PubMed database for the years 1980–2008 using the search terms "renal trauma," "nephrectomy" and "outcome."

The evidence

The strongest predictor for nephrectomy after blunt or penetrating abdominal trauma is an increasing AAST renal grade (Table 17.3) [14-16]. As shown in all three studies from Table 17.3, as the AAST renal grade increased from grade 3 to grade 5 injuries, there was an obvious increase

Table 17.3 Predictors of nephrectomy after blunt/penetrating abdominal trauma

Authors	Methods	Number	Incidence (%)–Nephrectomy (%)				
			Gr 1*	Gr 2	Gr 3	Gr 4	Gr 5
Santucci et al. [9]	Single institution	2467	2117(86.5)–0(0)	87(3.5)–0(0)	119(4.8)–4(3.4)	99(4)–10(10.1)	28(1.1)–23(82.1)
Wright et al. [10]	NTDB	8465	4656(55)–16(0.3)	1537(18.2)–16(1)	1028(12.1)–74(7.2)	831(9.8)–268(32.3)	413(4.8)–248(60)
Shariat et al. [11]	Single institution	424	118(27.8)–0(0)	112(26.4)–0(0)	82(19.3)–4(4.9)	77(18.2)–19(24.7)	35(8.3)–32(91.4)

*AAST renal injury grade
NTDB, National Trauma Data Bank

in the nephrectomy rate. Similarly, there was an increase in renal explorations with renorrhaphy as the AAST renal grade increased.

The study design by Wright and colleagues differs from the other two studies in that the National Trauma Data Bank (NTDB) was utilized to query patients with renal injury [15]. As opposed to the other two studies, which are single institution studies, the NTDB includes over 268 trauma centers and represents a more diverse study population. The largest weakness of this database is that included trauma centers can either provide ICD-9 or Abbreviated Injury Scores (AIS) for injury identification. Software does exist to convert ICD-9 scores to AIS codes but it is unable to capture all ICD-9 injuries; therefore, only centers using AIS codes were included in the study by Wright and colleagues. While AIS and ICD-9 codes do correlate well with AAST renal grades, there are certain codes utilized by AIS and ICD-9 scores that do not have an AAST correlate (i.e. Kidney Not Further Specified, Major Contusion > 50%, and Rupture Not Further Specified). As such, there is the potential for certain renal injuries to be excluded. Additionally, the NTDB only assesses inpatient admissions; therefore, lower grade renal injuries that did not require inpatient hospitalization may have been missed. However, this last issue should not affect the assessment of predictors for nephrectomy.

Increasing AAST renal grade is the strongest predictor for nephrectomy; however, there have been other reported predictors for nephrectomy. The study by Wright and colleagues also studied extrarenal predictors of nephrectomy [15]. Spleen, liver, and/or bowel surgery were found to increase the relative risk of nephrectomy (relative risk 2.2–3.9) after blunt trauma, while bowel surgery had a lesser impact on the relative risk of nephrectomy (relative risk 1.8) after penetrating abdominal trauma. The association of nephrectomy with associated abdominal surgery is difficult to process. The nephrectomy could have been performed for either damage control or insufficient experience with renal trauma.

In the study by Shariat and colleagues, gunshot wound was also found to be associated with a higher risk of nephrectomy [16]. Stab wound and blunt injury were not associated with increased risk of nephrectomy. Penetrating renal injuries are more commonly due to gunshot over stab wounds (86% vs 14% in one study [17]). Furthermore, gunshot wounds have a higher percentage of associated injuries needing repair than stab wounds, due to concern about devascularization of peripheral tissues from the gunshot wound blast effect. Santucci and colleagues found a similar effect of gunshot wounds and increased odds of surgery with increasing AAST renal grade [14]. Surgical therapy (renorrhaphy or nephrectomy) was highest for gunshot wounds followed by stab wounds and blunt trauma.

Comment

Absolute indications for renal exploration include: (1) hemodynamic instability with shock, (2) expanding/pulsatile renal hematoma, (3) suspected renal pedicle avulsion (AAST grade 5), and (4) ureteropelvic junction disruption. Using the GRADE system, this is a strong recommendation based on moderate quality evidence (**Grade 1B**). Review of these indications for exploration aids in the understanding of how a rising AAST renal grade can predict nephrectomy.

References

1. Santucci RA, Wessells H, Bartsch G, et al. Evaluation and management of renal injuries: consensus statement of the renal trauma subcommittee. BJU Int 2004;93(7):937-54.
2. Chapple C, Barbagli G, Jordan G, et al. Consensus statement on urethral trauma. BJU Int 2004;93(9):1195-202.

3. Gomez RG, Ceballos L, Coburn M, et al. Consensus statement on bladder injuries. BJU Int 2004;94(1):27-32.

4. Brandes S, Coburn M, Armenakas N, McAninch J. Diagnosis and management of ureteric injury: an evidence-based analysis. BJU Int 2004;94(3):277-89.

5. Morey AF, Metro MJ, Carney KJ, Miller KS, McAninch JW. Consensus on genitourinary trauma: external genitalia. BJU Int 2004;94(4):507-15.

6. Miller KS, McAninch JW. Radiographic assessment of renal trauma: our 15-year experience. J Urol 1995;154(2 pt 1):352-5.

7. Eastham JA, Wilson TG, Ahlering TE. Radiographic evaluation of adult patients with blunt renal trauma. J Urol 1992;148 (2 pt 1):266-7.

8. Hardeman SW, Husmann DA, Chinn HK, Peters PC. Blunt urinary tract trauma: identifying those patients who require radiological diagnostic studies. J Urol 1987;138(1):99-101.

9. Nicolaisen GS, McAninch JW, Marshall GA, Bluth RF Jr, Carroll PR. Renal trauma: re-evaluation of the indications for radiographic assessment. J Urol 1985;133(2):183-7.

10. Cass AS, Luxenberg M, Gleich P, Smith CS. Clinical indications for radiographic evaluation of blunt renal trauma. J Urol 1986;136(2):370-1.

11. Eastham JA, Wilson TG, Ahlering TE. Radiographic assessment of blunt renal trauma. J Trauma 1991;31(11):1527-8.

12. Boone TB, Gilling PJ, Husmann DA. Ureteropelvic junction disruption following blunt abdominal trauma. J Urol 1993;150(1):33-6.

13. Chandhoke PS, McAninch JW. Detection and significance of microscopic hematuria in patients with blunt renal trauma. J Urol 1988;140(1):16-18.

14. Santucci RA, McAninch JW, Safir M, Mario LA, Service S, Segal MR. Validation of the American Association for the Surgery of Trauma organ injury severity scale for the kidney. J Trauma 2001;50(2):195-200.

15. Wright JL, Nathens AB, Rivara FP, Wessells H. Renal and extrarenal predictors of nephrectomy from the national trauma data bank. J Urol 2006;175(3 pt 1):970-5; discussion 5.

16. Shariat SF, Roehrborn CG, Karakiewicz PI, Dhami G, Stage KH. Evidence-based validation of the predictive value of the American Association for the Surgery of Trauma kidney injury scale. J Trauma 2007;62(4):933-9.

17. Kansas BT, Eddy MJ, Mydlo JH, Uzzo RG. Incidence and management of penetrating renal trauma in patients with multiorgan injury: extended experience at an inner city trauma center. J Urol 2004;172(4 pt 1):1355-60.

18 Urethral stricture disease

Bahaa S. Malaeb and Sean P. Elliott

Department of Urologic Surgery, University of Minnesota, Minneapolis, MN, USA

Background

Urethral stricture disease is one of the oldest maladies known to urology. Etiologies vary significantly and include inflammatory, infectious, traumatic, and iatrogenic as well as idiopathic. The treatment of urethral strictures has evolved over the last four decades from dilation to blind urethrotomy to direct vision internal urethrotomy and finally to the more complex procedures of urethroplasty with or without the use of grafts and flaps from various sites. The familiarity of the general urologist with endoscopic technique and the enthusiasm to apply minimally invasive procedure have led in certain situations to inappropriate methods of managing reconstructive urological conditions. We reviewed the literature and identified the areas where enough evidence is present to direct decision making.

Clinical question 18.1

What is the role of endoscopic primary realignment versus suprapubic cystostomy with delayed repair in posterior urethral disruption?

Literature search

A PubMed, Medline and Cochrane Library search was performed for all original studies published between 1990 and 2009 using the keywords/phrases: "posterior urethral disruption," "posterior urethral strictures," "posterior urethral injuries," "primary realignment of urethral stricture," "posterior urethroplasty," "endoscopic realignment." The abstracts were evaluated and the studies related to the above question were interrogated in further detail. A total of seven studies published between 1999 and 2008 was selected based on their methodology, patient numbers, and follow-up.

The evidence

The optimal management of posterior urethral distraction injuries is controversial. Early surgical intervention with primary open realignment has been associated with prolonged hospital stay, high incidence of postoperative incontinence and impotence, and large blood loss. On the other hand, delayed reconstruction with initial suprapubic cystostomy popularized by Morehouse [1] has been criticized for a high rate of stricture formation necessitating complex reconstruction done in specialized centers, which may be associated with blood loss, prolonged hospital stay and complications of long-term catheterization. Early endoscopic realignment (EER) emerged as a compromise between early open realignment and delayed treatment (DT).

When managing posterior urethral disruptions, as defined by the consensus statement on urethral trauma [2], the potential complications and outcomes of interest are urinary continence, impotence, urethral strictures and need for additional procedures.

To date, there is a paucity of prospective trials evaluating EER and no trials comparing EER to DT in a randomized fashion. Existing series are plagued by small numbers of patients, variability in degree of injury, lack of a standardized definition for outcomes measured, selection bias, lag-time bias and differential loss of follow-up. Most of these biases contribute to better perceived outcomes after EER. Selection bias results from the practice of reserving EER for the stable patient who is also the patient likely

Evidence-Based Urology. Edited by Philipp Dahm, Roger R. Dmochowski.
© 2010 Blackwell Publishing.

to have the least severe disruption. After reviewing the literature, we identified seven studies that evaluated EER and DT and the associated outcomes [3-9]. Continence after EER is reported to be 86–100% and potency is maintained in 40–88%. In the DT groups, continence and potency rates were 74–89% and 58–82% respectively. The most consistent outcome was the decreased stricture rate with EER. Almost all DT patients (83–100%) develop strictures after fibrosis and healing set in [8,9] whereas the rate of stricture formation after EER ranged between 14% and 41%. Hadjizacharia et al. [3] showed a statistically significant difference in the urethral stricture rate in EER (14.3%) compared to DT (100%) (p value < 0.0001). After EER, only 15% of those who developed strictures required urethroplasty (1–8 years of follow-up), compared to 44–47% after DT (1–22 years of follow-up) (Table 18.1). Approximating

Table 18.1 Early endoscopic realignment versus suprapubic cystostomy and delayed treatment for posterior urethral disruptions

Study	Methods	Intervention	Results	Comments
Hadjizacharia et al. [3]	1- prospective study 2- Sept 2000 to Sept 2006 3- Cross-over design 4- Single institution	• EER (14 patients, 11 partial disruption/3 complete, 7 anetrior/7 posterior) • DT (7 patients, 3 complete and posterior/4 partial and anterior)	• Statistically different results for EER vs DT respectively: 1- average SPT duration 19 vs 219 days 2- stricture rate 14.3% (2/14) vs 100% (7/7) 3- Time to spontaneous voiding 35 vs 229 days • Success rate of EER was 78%	• Mean follow-up 7 months (14 days to 1.7 years) • No difference in admission criteria among the 2 groups • Patient with DT were 4 who failed EER and 3 in which no attempt for an EER was done • Bladder neck injuries excluded
Moudouni et al. [4]	1- retrospective review 2- April 1987 to Jan 1999	• EER utilizing combined antegrade and retrograde cystourethroscopy • 29 patients (23 complete disruption, 6 partial)	• Average time to EER 3.8 days (0-8) • Operating time mean 1.15 hours (0.45 -2.25) • Continence 100% after removal of cath (4-6 weeks, assessed by patient review) • Potency preserved in 86% after EER • 41% (N 12) formed strictures after EER, mean time 6.2 months (1.5–24) • 27/29 successful EER	• 14 required additional procedures: 1- the 2 failed EER, underwent SPT and DT followed by urethroplasty 2- 10 of the 12 with strictures resolved with one VIU, 2 successfully treated with urethroplasty after 2 VIUs • Follow-up for the 14 requiring VIU or urethroplasty was 83 months (34-120) • Follow-up time 18–155 months, mean 68
Kielb et all. [5]	1- prospective study 2- May 1997 to June 1999 3- Single institution	• EER by retrograde or combined retro/antegrade cysto uretheroscopy • 10 patients (2 urethral stretch, 4 partial and 4 complete disruption) • 9 males, 1 female	• 10/10 total successful EER (8 on retrograde initial attempt, 2 combined approach) • Stretch and partial disruptions required no further interventions • 2 complete disruptions required one VIU, 1 required urethroplasty after failed VIU, and 1 lost to follow-up • Urinary continence achieved in 5/6 • Potency preserved in 2/5	• EER performed day 0-28 days • 6 of 10 available for follow-up, mean time 18 months (9-27) • Bladder neck injury in patient with residual stress incontinence

Study	Methods	Intervention	Results	Comments
Healy et al. [6]	1- retrospective review 2- May 1994 to June 2002	• EER by retrograde or combined retro/antegrade cystouretheroscopy • 10 patients with complete posterior disruption	• 8 out of 10 successful EER, 2 failed EER and underwent open primary realignment • Potency 7/8 (88%) • Continence 8/8 (100%) • 2 required dilation for urethral strictures • No urethroplasties done for EER group	• Mean follow up 41 months (12-95)
Jepson et al. [7]	1- prospective study 2- April 1991 to June 1995	• EER by retrograde or combined retro/antegrade cystouretheroscopy • No report of failed attempts • DT (7 patients, 3 complete and posterior/4 partial and anterior)	• Continence 7/8 (88%) • Impotence 3/8 (38%) • Three required 1 VIU, one required 2 VIU and one developed colovesical and vesicocutaneous fistula, necessitating colostomy and a urinary diversion at a later point	• Mean follow-up 50.4 months (35-85)
Mouraviev et al. [8]	1- comparative retrospective review 2- Sept 1980 to May 2001	• Open early realignment in 57 • DT in 39	• Stricture formation in 100% of DT group • 3.9 procedures on average required for each patient in DT group • 47% required urethroplasty in DT • Impotence and incontinence in DT were 42% and 26%	• Patients with strictures initially were started on intermittent catheterization protocol 1 month after surgery • Open realignment reduced frequency of strictures, impotence, incontinence, and average number of subsequent procedures • Follow-up 8.8 years (1-22)
Asci et al. [9]	1- comparative retrospective review 2- 1986 to 1996	• DT in 18 • Open early alignment in 20	• Stricture developed in 83.3% (15/18) of DT • 3/18 voided spontaneously • Urethroplasty in 8/18 (44.4%) • VIU in 6 (33.3%) • Dilation in 1 (5.6%) • Incontinence 11% • Impotence 17.6%	• Follow-up 37.1 months (14-78) • No SSD in rate of impotence or incontinence between open realignment and DT group • DT group had significantly higher incidence of urethral strictures

SPT, suprapubic tube; SSD, statistically significant difference the damaged ends of the urethra over a catheter allows for healing along the catheter and subsequently shorter strictures. These shorter strictures are more amenable to less invasive procedures such as internal urethrotomy (IU) or dilation, reducing the need for more complex procedures.

Comment

We suggest that clinicians consider EER in selected patient groups. Even though the risk of stricture formation is nearly half after EER compared to DT, other outcomes (potency and continence) were similar and no information is provided on cost. Methodological flaws in the observational studies make it difficult to determine the reasons for the perceived benefit of EER. Overall, the quality of the evidence supporting EER is low (Grade 2C).

Early endoscopic realignment offers a minimally invasive approach which can be performed in a retrograde, antegrade or combined fashion. It is not easy to perform and should only be attempted by urologists skilled in endoscopy and fluoroscopy. Patients likely to benefit most from EER are stable patients and those with large distraction defects.

Clinical question 18.2

Should a buccal mucosal graft (BMG) be placed ventrally or dorsally?

Literature search

A PubMed, Medline and Cochrane Library search was performed for all original studies published between 1990 and 2009 using the keywords/phrases: "buccal mucosal graft," "anterior urethroplasty," "ventral onlay urethroplasty," "dorsal onlay/inlay urethroplasty." The abstracts were evaluated and the studies related to the above question were interrogated in further detail. A total of six studies published between 2002 and 2008 was selected based on their methodology, patient number, and follow-up.

The evidence

The use of buccal mucosa for urethral reconstructive procedures has been increasing, especially for bulbar urethral strictures. Recently, debate has been extensive about the best placement of buccal mucosa. From review of the multiple studies (Table 18.2), it is noted that the initial success rate ranges from 83% to 94% for BMG in treatment of bulbar urethral strictures irrespective of the ventral/dorsal placement of the graft [10-15]. These

rates represent success defined as lack of any procedure including dilation or direct vision internal urethrotomy (VIU). If success is defined as normal voiding with a single VIU or incision of an anastomotic ring, the rate is increased to 94–100%.

The image is less clear for penile urethral strictures. Whereas in the bulbous urethra, a good vascular supply is present for the graft irrespective of placement technique, in distal bulbar and penile strictures, a dorsal placement is suggested to provide a healthier blood supply and a stronger framework to prevent ballooning of the graft [12]. Two different techniques for dorsal placement are noted. The Asopa technique is a dorsal inlay and involves performing a sagittal incision in the ventral urethra and longitudinally incising the dorsal plate to inlay the BMG followed by closure of the ventral incision [11]. The technique described by Barbagli and used in all other studies reviewed involved circumferential dissection of the urethra and rotation of the urethra 180° with dorsal onlay of the BMG [12,14]. Dorsal buccal mucosal graft urethroplasty for penile urethral strictures has a comparable success rate to bulbar strictures. In a study by Dubey et al., the reported success rate for dorsal placement of buccal graft was 87.5% for pendulous urethral strictures compared to 90% for bulbar urethral strictures [16].

Comment

A strong recommendation can be made to support both ventral and dorsal placement of BMG in bulbar urethral strictures. Low-grade evidence from retrospective case series demonstrates excellent stricture-free rates with either technique (Grade 1C). Surgical time and thus costs are similar. A comparison of other outcomes such as erectile and ejaculatory function has not been explored. The best technique to use is one with which the surgeon is most experienced. Dorsal placement for distal bulbar and penile urethral strictures offers theoretically better blood supply. The data are limited in terms of comparing dorsal and ventral placement for penile urethral.

Clinical question 18.3

What is the optimal treatment for 1–2 cm bulbar urethral strictures?

Literature search

A PubMed, Medline and Cochrane Library search was performed for all original studies published between

Table 18.2 Ventral versus dorsal placement of buccal mucosal graft (BMG) for urethral strictures

Study	Methods	Intervention	Results	Comments
Kellner et al. [10]	1- retrospective review	23 patients (18 bulbar and 5 penile strictures)	• Success achieved 20/23 (87%), no need for any urethral manipulation afterwards	• Mean follow-up 50 months (17–95)
	2- Dec 1995 to Jan 2002	Ventral placement of BMG 3- mean stricture length 4.9 cm (3-12)	• 3 patients failed by developing distal anastomotic stricture, all managed with single VIU	• 21/23 previously treated for strictures with an average of 2.8 procedures per patient
Pisapati et al. [11]	1- Prospective design	45 patients underwent BMG urethroplasty by the Asopa technique, dorsal placement	• Success rate 87% (39/45)	• Mean follow-up 42 months (12–60)
	2- Dec 2002 to Dec 2007	Stricture length 1-17 cm	• Recurrences occurred at 3-48 months, all managed with VIU and self-dilation	• 42/45 had previous procedures
Barbagli et al. [12]	1- retrospective review	50 patients with BMG urethroplasty	• 84% total success (42/50), 94% if not counting anastomotic rings	• Mean follow-up 42 months (12–76)
	2- Jan 1997 and Dec 2002	Mean stricture length 4 cm (2.5–7.5) Ventral, dorsal and lateral placement in 17, 27 and 6 consecutively	• 83% success for ventral (14/17), 85% for dorsal (23/27) and 83% for lateral (5/6)	• 47/50 had prior procedures • Dorsal placement required circumferential mobilization of corpus spongiosum and rotation of 180° • Selection of technique based on location of stricture
Elliott et al. [13]	1- retrospective review	60 patients with bulbar urethral strictures underwent ventral onlay BMG	• 90% (54/60) had initial success. Success rate of 97% (54 with initial success and 4 requiring single VIU)	• Mean follow-up 47 months (12–107)
	2- June 1993 and May 2001	Mean stricture length 5.3 cm (1.5–24)		• 49/60 had prior procedures
Kane et al. [14]	1- Retrospective review	53 patients underwent ventral onlay BMG for bulbar strictures	• 94% initial success (50/54), 3 required 1 DVIU only	• Mean follow-up 25 months (11–40)
	2- Jan 1996 to March 1998	Mean stricture length 3.6 cm (2–7.5)		
Datta et al. [15]	1- retrospective review 2- Jan 1998 to Dec 2003	43 patients managed with dorsal onlay BMG (penile and bulbar) 2- mean stricture length 4.8 cm (3–9)	• 88% (38/43) initial success, 3 treated with single VIU	• Mean follow-up 48 months (12–84) • Dorsal placement required circumferential mobilization of corpus spongiosum and rotation of 180°

1990 and 2009 using the keywords/phrases: "anterior urethroplasty," "primary anastomotic urethroplasty," "visual internal urethrotomy," "bulbar urethral stricture," "urethral strictures." The abstracts were evaluated and the studies related to the above question were interrogated in further detail. A total of six studies published between 1996 and 2007 was selected based on their methodology, patient number, and follow-up.

The evidence

In 2006, Bullock & Brandes surveyed 431 urologists nationwide to evaluate methods and patterns of evaluation and treatment of anterior urethral strictures [17]; 63% of urologists surveyed treat less than 20 urethral strictures per year. The most common treatment methods utilized were dilation (92.8% of urologists surveyed) and visual internal urethrotomy (85.6%). The survey highlighted a common

misconception among urologists that urethroplasty is only to be performed after multiple repeated failures of other less invasive methods; 74% of urologists believe that the literature supports such a reconstructive surgical ladder. Unfamiliarity with the reconstructive literature and inexperience with urethroplasty have contributed to the inappropriately common and widespread use of endoscopic methods.

We identified six studies that evaluated the utilization of primary anastomotic urethroplasty (excision with end-to-end anastomosis) (PAU) versus VIU (Table 18.3). All studies reported a superior success rate with PAU (93–99%, average follow-up 50–72 months) when compared to VIU (42–73%, average follow-up 46–98 months) [18-23]. Pansadoro & Emiliozzi reported one of the largest series evaluating outcomes of VIU [23]. Stricture length more than 1 cm and a caliber less than 15 F were associated with lower success rates (see Table 18.3). Moreover, the success rate

Table 18.3 Comparison of primary anastomosis urethroplasty (excision with end-to-end anastomosis) versus direct vision internal urethrotomy for treatment of bulbar urethral strictures

Study	Methods	Intervention	Results	Comments
Santucci et al. [18]	1- retrospective review 2- Apr 1971 – Feb 2001 3- Single surgeon	168 patients all had PAU Mean stricture length 1.7 cm (0.1–4.5)	• Success rate 95% (8/168) • 5 successfully managed by single VIU, 3 had urethroplasties • Complications: 10/168. 3 had transient thigh numbness	• Mean follow-up 72 months (6–291) • 92 underwent prior procedures: 48 had VIU and dilation, 9 had dilation, 15 had DVIU and 19 had urethroplasty
Eltahawy et al. [19]	1- retrospective review 2- Jul 1986 – May 2006 3- 3 different surgeons, same center	260 patients all had PAU Mean stricture length 1.9 cm (0.5-4.5)	• Success rate 98.8% (257/260) • 2 early recurrences and 1 late, the late recurrence managed with VIU at 4 years • Complications: neuropraxia 3.4%, UTI 5%, scrotalgia 1.5%, wound related 1.5% (all resolved within early postoperative period)	• Pelvic fracture urethral distraction strictures excluded • Mean follow-up 50.2 months (6–122) • 171 underwent prior procedures: 87 had VIU and dilation, 38 had dilation, 21 had DVIU and 25 had urethroplasty
Barbagli et al. [20]	1- retrospective review 2- 1988 – 2006 3- Single surgeon	153 patients all had PAU Stricture length was 1–2 cm in 91 patients, 2–3 cm in 58, 3–4 cm in 3, and 4–5 cm in 1	• Overall success rate was 90.8% (139/153) • 1–2 cm, 2–3 cm, and 3–5 cm strictures had 93.4%, 86.2%, and 100% success rates respectively	• Mean follow-up 68 months (12–218) • 90 patients underwent prior procedures • 1 patient had cold glans during erections, 7 had lack of glans fullness, and 11 had decreased sensation on glans

Study	Methods	Intervention	Results	Comments
Mandhani et al. [21]	1- retrospective review 2- Jan 1991 – June 2002	105 patients with VIU Mean length of stricture 0.868 cm, none over 2 cm	• Success rate 60.9% (64/105) • 28/41 underwent a second VIU, 53.5% (15/28) failed	• Mean follow-up 46.1 months (9-106) • No prior procedures. • Strictures with obliterated lumen were excluded • Daily self-dilation for a minimum of 2 years
Albers et al. [22]	1- Retrospective comaprison 2- 2 groups, 2 different hospitals 3- 1974-1989	Group 1 (357 patients) and group 2 (580 patients)	• Group 1: success rate 73.1% (261/357), 57 out of the 96 failures required only 1 additional VIU • Group 2: success rate 55.2% (320/580), 201 out of the 260 failures required only 1 additional VIU	• Follow-up 4.6 years (9 months to 16 years) and 3.2 years (4 to 72 months) in groups 1 and 2, respectively • Complications reported: bleeding (3.4% and 4%), fever, epididymitis and incontinence (0.4% and 0.5%)
Pansadoro et al. [23]	1- retrospective review 2- Jan 1975 - June 1990	224 patients underwent VIU Mean stricture length 1.6 cm (0.1-6.5)	• Overall success rate was 32% (71/224); 42% (60/142) for bulbar, 16% (6/37) for penile and 11% (5/45) for penile bulbar strictures • Bulbar strictures less than 1 cm had a 71% success rates (46/65) • 69% success rate (24/35) for strictures more than 15 F caliber versus 36% (36/107) for strictures less than 15 F • Success rate 47% (60/129) for primary (previously untreated) bulbar strictures and 0% for all recurrent bulbar strictures (0/13)	• Median follow-up 98 months (60-216) • Complications occurred in 11%: bleeding in 24, extravasation in 6, and chordee in 2 • 56% (86) of recurrences occurred within 12 months, 26% (34) in 12–24 months, 8% (12) in 24-36 months, 11% (11) in 36-60 months, and 6% (10) after 60 months

UTI, urinary tract infection

in patients who have not undergone a prior VIU is 47% compared to patients who are having a repeat VIU (success rate of 0%) [23]. According to the reviewed studies, PAU is associated with few complications, most frequently neuropraxia from positioning (less than 5%), wound complications and urinary tract infections [18-20]. The most common complication after VIU was bleeding [22-24].

Multiple studies have attempted to evaluate the cost-effectiveness of PAU compared to VIU. For bulbar urethral strictures 1–2 cm in length, Wright et al. reported that the most cost-effective approach was a single VIU before urethroplasty. The incremental cost of a second DVIU before urethroplasty was $141,962 for each additional successful outcome [24]. They also reported that urethroplasty would be the most cost-effective approach if the success of VIU is less than 35%, as is the case for longer strictures. A similar conclusion was drawn by Greenwell et al. [25]. Others reported that primary urethroplasty for a 2 cm bulbar urethroplasty was less costly than VIU. The model used included relative outcomes and reported complications of the two procedures. The cost saving per patient was $1304 [26]. The authors reported that VIU would be a preferred treatment if long-term recurrence-free rates approach 60%. Such success rate could potentially be obtained for less than 1 cm strictures not associated with significant scarring and spongiofibrosis [26].

Comment

A strong recommendation can be made for primary anastomotic urethroplasty rather than internal urethrotomy in the management of bulbar urethral strictures 1–2 cm based on clearly improved outcomes on one measure in low-quality observational data (**Grade 1C**). Multiple case series demonstrate that stricture-free rates for PAU are high despite the fact that the majority have already failed multiple procedures, including dilations, VIU or prior urethroplasty (see Table 18.3). Additionally, a cost-benefit analysis supports PAU for 1–2 cm bulbar urethral strictures. Still, studies have focused primarily on measurement of a single outcome – urethral patency. The definition of urethral patency has been inconsistent and other outcomes such as erectile function, ejaculatory function and urinary symptoms have often been ignored. While PAU should generally be favored for 1–2 cm strictures, a single internal urethrotomy may be considered in a selected patient group with short bulbar strictures, with a lumen more than 15 F, and in the absence of extensive spongiofibrosis.

References

1. Morehouse DD, Belitsky P, MacKinnon KJ. Rupture of the posterior urethra. J Urol 1972;107(2):255-8.
2. Chapple C, Barbagli G, Jordan G, et al. Consensus statement on urethral trauma. BJU Int 2004;93(9):1195-202.
3. Hadjizacharia P, Inaba K, Teixeira PG, Kokorowski P, Demetriades D, Best C. Evaluation of immediate endoscopic realignment as a treatment modality for traumatic urethral injuries. J Trauma 2008;64(6):1443-9; discussion 1449-50.
4. Moudouni SM, Patard JJ, Manunta A, Guiraud P, Lobel B, Guillé F. Early endoscopic realignment of post-traumatic posterior urethral disruption. Urology 2001;57(4):628-32.
5. Kielb SJ, Voeltz ZL, Wolf JS. Evaluation and management of traumatic posterior urethral disruption with flexible cystourethroscopy. J Trauma 2000;50:36-40.
6. Healy CE, Leonard DS, Cahill R, Mulvin D, Quinlan D. Primary endourologic realignment of complete posterior urethral disruption. Ir Med J 2007;100(6):488-9.
7. Jepson BR, Boullier JA, Moore RG, Parra RO. Traumatic posterior urethral injury and early primary endoscopic realignment: evaluation of long-term follow-up. Urology 1999;53(6):1205-10.
8. Mouraviev VB, Coburn M, Santucci RA. The treatment of posterior urethral disruption associated with pelvic fractures: comparative experience of early realignment versus delayed urethroplasty. J Urol 2005;173(3):873-6.
9. Aşci R, Sarikaya S, Büyükalpelli R, Saylik A, Yilmaz AF, Yildiz S. Voiding and sexual dysfunctions after pelvic fracture urethral injuries treated with either initial cystostomy and delayed urethroplasty or immediate primary urethral realignment. Scand J Urol Nephrol 1999;33(4):228-33.
10. Kellner DS, Fracchia JA, Armenakas NA. Ventral onlay buccal mucosal grafts for anterior urethral strictures: long-term followup. J Urol 2004;171(2 pt 1):726-9.
11. Pisapati VL, Paturi S, Bethu S, et al. Dorsal buccal mucosal graft urethroplasty for anterior urethral stricture by Asopa technique. Eur Urol 2008 Jun 9 (Epub ahead of print).
12. Barbagli G, Palminteri E, Guazzoni G, Montorsi F, Turini D, Lazzeri M. Bulbar urethroplasty using buccal mucosa grafts placed on the ventral, dorsal or lateral surface of the urethra: are results affected by the surgical technique? J Urol 2005;174(3):955-7; discussion 957-8.
13. Elliott SP, Metro MJ, McAninch JW. Long-term followup of the ventrally placed buccal mucosa onlay graft in bulbar urethral reconstruction. J Urol 2003;169(5):1754-7.
14. Kane CJ, Tarman GJ, Summerton DJ, et al. Multi-institutional experience with buccal mucosa onlay urethroplasty for bulbar urethral reconstruction. J Urol 2002;167(3):1314-17.
15. Datta B, Rao MP, Acharya RL, et al. Dorsal onlay buccal mucosal graft urethroplasty in long anterior urethral stricture. Int Braz J Urol 2007;33(2):181-6; discussion 186-7.
16. Dubey D, Kumar A, Mandhani A, Srivastava A, Kapoor R, Bhandari M. Buccal mucosal urethroplasty: a versatile technique for all urethral segments. BJU Int 2005;95(4):625-9.
17. Bullock TL, Brandes SB. Adult anterior urethral strictures: a national practice patterns survey of board certified urologists in the United States. J Urol 2007;177(2):685-90.
18. Santucci RA, Mario LA, McAninch JW. Anastomotic urethroplasty for bulbar urethral stricture: analysis of 168 patients. J Urol 2002;167(4):1715-19.
19. Eltahawy EA, Virasoro R, Schlossberg SM, McCammon KA, Jordan GH. Long-term followup for excision and primary anastomosis for anterior urethral strictures. J Urol 2007;177(5):1609-10.
20. Barbagli G, de Angelis M, Romano G, Lazzeri M. Long-term followup of bulbar end-to-end anastomosis: a retrospective analysis of 153 patients in a single center experience. J Urol 2007;178(6):2470-3.
21. Mandhani A, Chaudhury H, Kapoor R, Srivastava A, Dubey D, Kumar A. Can outcome of internal urethrotomy for short segment bulbar urethral stricture be predicted? J Urol 2005;173(5):1595-7.
22. Albers P, Fichtner J, Brühl P, Müller SC. Long-term results of internal urethrotomy. J Urol 1996;156(5):1611-14.

23. Pansadoro V, Emiliozzi P. Internal urethrotomy in the management of anterior urethral strictures: long-term followup. J Urol 1996;156(1):73-5.

24. Wright JL, Wessells H, Nathens AB, Hollingworth W. What is the most cost-effective treatment for 1 to 2-cm bulbar urethral strictures: societal approach using decision analysis. Urology 2006;67(5):889-93.

25. Greenwell TJ, Castle C, Andrich DE, MacDonald JT, Nicol DL, Mundy AR. Repeat urethrotomy and dilation for the treatment of urethral stricture are neither clinically effective nor cost-effective. J Urol 2004;172(1):275-7.

26. Rourke KF, Jordan GH. Primary urethral reconstruction: the cost minimized approach to the bulbous urethral stricture. J Urol 2005;173(4):1206-10.

19

Antimuscarinic treatments in overactive bladder

Christopher R. Chapple,[1] Dominic Muston[2] and Zoe S. Kopp[3]

[1]Sheffield Teaching Hospital NHS Trust, Royal Hallamshire Hospital, Urology Research, Sheffield, UK
[2]Health Economic Modelling Unit, Heron Evidence Development Ltd, Luton, UK
[3]Pfizer Inc, New York, NY, USA

Background

Overactive bladder (OAB) refers to the common and bothersome group of storage lower urinary tract symptoms (LUTS). The International Continence Society (ICS) defines OAB syndrome as urgency with or without urgency urinary incontinence (UUI), usually with frequency and nocturia [1]. Prevalence rates for OAB are estimated to range between 12% and 17% in the United States and Europe. Both men and women are equally affected by OAB, and the incidence rate increases with age [2-4]. This condition has a serious impact on both individuals and society [5,6]. OAB can be managed with bladder and behavioral training, biofeedback, electrical stimulation, pharmacological treatments or a combination of therapies [7]. Antimuscarinic agents are the first-line pharmacotherapy for OAB treatment [8]. This systematic review of the tolerability, safety, and efficacy of licensed antimuscarinic treatments in OAB, which is based on a recent article published in *European Urology*, provides an up-to-date summary of the efficacy, tolerability, and safety of licensed antimuscarinic treatments in OAB, and describes the effects of treatment on health-related quality of life (HRQL).

Overactive bladder (symptomatic diagnosis) is often assumed to be caused by detrusor overactivity (DO), even if this does not always seem to be the case [9-12]. DO/OAB can occur as a result of sensitization of afferent nerve terminals in the bladder or outlet region, changes of the bladder smooth muscle secondary to denervation, or consequent upon damage to the central nervous system (CNS) inhibitory pathways, as can be seen in various neurological disorders, such as multiple sclerosis, cerebrovascular disease, Parkinson's disease, brain tumors, and spinal cord injury.

Normal bladder contraction in humans is mediated mainly through stimulation of muscarinic receptors in the detrusor muscle. The neurotransmitter acetylcholine (ACh) acts on two classes of receptors: the nicotinic and the muscarinic. While the former play a role in the signal transduction between neurons or between neurons and skeletal muscle (e.g. in the distal urethra), the signal transduction between parasympathetic nerves and smooth muscle of the detrusor involves muscarinic receptors [13]. Importantly, the endogenous muscarinic receptor agonist ACh is not necessarily derived only from parasympathetic nerves in the urinary bladder, but can also be formed and released non-neuronally by the urothelium [14-16]. Five subtypes of muscarinic receptors have been cloned in humans and other mammalian species, which are designated M_{1-5} [17]. Based upon structural criteria and shared preferred signal transduction pathways, the subtypes can be grouped into M_1, M_3 and M_5 on the one hand and M_2 and M_4 on the other. However, most muscarinic receptors in the urinary bladder are located on smooth muscle and urothelial cells.

While the detrusor expresses far more M_2 than M_3 receptors, it appears that detrusor contraction under physiological conditions is largely if not exclusively mediated by the M_3 receptor [18-23]. Previous reviews have demonstrated mode-rate efficacy for muscarinic receptor antagonists relative to placebo in controlled clinical studies [24-28].

Literature search

This chapter is based on a recently published systematic review and meta-analysis by our group [25]. For this review, we undertook a comprehensive search of all major literature databases and the abstract books from several major conferences: American Urological Association, ICS, European Association of Urology, International Urogynaecological

Evidence-Based Urology. Edited by Philipp Dahm, Roger R. Dmochowski.
© 2010 Blackwell Publishing.

Association, International Consultation of Incontinence and Societe Internationale d'Urologie. As with the 2005 review, there were no restrictions on the inclusion of publications by language; publications in languages other than English were translated into English.

The literature database search updated a previous 2005 review which was carried out on 31 August 2004 for publications published since 1966 in the Medline, EMBASE, Cochrane Controlled Trials Register, and Cumulative Index to Nursing and Allied Health Literature databases [24]. The literature database search for this review was carried out on 18 October 2007 and included all publications published in 2004 or later in the same databases. Conference proceedings had previously been searched to the end of 2004. For the review update, we added evidence from further proceedings of each conference up to October 2007. There were seven drugs included in the review (darifenacin, fesoterodine, oxybutynin, propiverine, solifenacin, tolterodine, and trospium), each of which could be delivered through various European-licensed formulations, doses and frequencies.

Clinical question 19.1

What is the efficacy of antimuscarinic therapy?

The evidence

Findings of this analysis are summarized in Table 19.1. A greater proportion of patients treated with antimuscarinics than with placebo returned to continence. The pooled relative risk (RR) varied between 1.3 and 3.5 across treatments. There were no statistically significant differences between treatments in meta-analyses of active-controlled trials for this outcome. Active treatments were more effective than placebo in terms of the mean change in the number of incontinence episodes per day. Pooled differences in mean change ranged from 0.4 to 1.1 incontinence episodes per day. Active treatments were more effective than placebo in terms of the mean change in the number of micturitions per day. Pooled differences in mean changes ranged from 0.5 to 1.3 episodes per day. Fesoterodine, propiverine, solifenacin, and tolterodine were statistically significantly more effective than placebo in terms of the mean change in the number of urgency episodes per day, where reported. Pooled differences in mean changes varied between 0.64 and 1.56 episodes per day. Active treatments were all statistically significantly more effective than placebo in terms of the mean change in the volume voided per micturition (mL) where reported for each licensed drug other than trospium chloride,

for which this outcome was not reported. Differences in pooled mean changes were 13 to 40 mL.

Clinical question 19.2

What is the tolerability of antimuscarinic therapy?

The evidence

Findings of this analysis are summarized in Table 19.2. Withdrawals due to any cause were frequent in both the intervention and the control placebo arms of the studies examined. Only oxybutynin immediate release (IR) 15 mg/day and oxybutynin IR 7.5–10 mg/day were associated with statistically significantly higher risk of withdrawal from the trial due to any cause than placebo (RR 1.33, 95% confidence interval (CI) 1.01–1.76, $p = 0.04$; and RR 1.72, 95% CI 1.18–2.49, $p < 0.01$, respectively). Otherwise, no statistically significant differences in proportions of patients who withdrew from trials for any causes were found between placebo and any active treatments.

When different forms of active treatment were compared, the following statistically significant differences between active treatments were found: oxybutynin IR 7.5–10 mg/day was associated with a significantly greater risk of withdrawal due to any cause than oxybutynin extended release (ER) 5 mg/day (RR 2.22, 95% CI 1.08–4.57, $p = 0.03$); oxybutynin IR 7.5–10 mg/day carried a greater risk of withdrawal than tolterodine ER 4 mg/day (RR 2.22, 95% CI 1.45–3.45, $p < 0.01$) and tolterodine IR 4 mg/day (RR 1.41, 95% CI 1.02–1.92, $p = 0.04$); oxybutynin IR 15 mg/day carried a greater risk of withdrawal than tolterodine IR 4 mg/day (RR 2.44, 95% CI 1.64–3.57, $p < 0.01$) and oxybutynin ER 15 mg/day (RR 1.83, 95% CI 1.02–3.30, $p = 0.04$).

Tolterodine ER 4 mg/day was the only formulation found to be associated with a statistically significantly lower risk than placebo of withdrawal due to an adverse event (RR 0.71, 95% CI 0.53–0.95, $p = 0.02$). Four formulations were found to be associated with a statistically signi-ficantly higher risk of withdrawal due to adverse events than placebo: oxybutynin IR 7.5–10 mg/day (RR 1.91, 95% CI 1.18–3.10, $p = 0.01$), oxybutynin IR 15 mg/day (RR 1.89, 95% CI 1.23–2.90, $p < 0.01$), propiverine ER 20 mg/day (RR 2.39, 95% CI 1.20–4.78, $p = 0.01$) and solifenacin 10 mg/day (RR 1.53, 95% CI 1.02–2.30, $p = 0.04$). Additionally, tolterodine ER 4 mg/day was associated with lower risk of this outcome than oxybutynin tds 3.9 mg/day (RR 0.15, 95% CI 0.03–0.66, $p = 0.01$) and oxybutynin IR 15 mg/day (RR 0.32,

Table 19.1 Efficacy of antimuscarinics compared to placebo: results from meta–analyses*

	Fesoterodine 4 mg/day vs placebo	Fesoterodine 8 mg/day vs placebo	Oxybutynin IR 7.5–10 mg/day vs placebo	Oxybutynin IR 15 mg/day vs placebo	Oxybutynin tds 3.9–4.0 mg/day vs placebo	Propiverine IR 45 mg/day vs placebo	Propiverine IR 30 mg/day vs placebo
Mean change in incontinence episodes/day	−0.81 −1.27 to −0.35 p<0.01 410 (1)	−1.08 −1.52 to −0.64 p<0.01 434 (1)	–	−0.74 −1.23 to −0.26 p<0.01 312 (2)	−0.58 −1.05 to −0.11 p=0.02 612 (2)	–	–
Mean change in micturitions/day	−0.81 −1.27 to −0.35 p<0.01 544 (1)	−0.93 −1.37 to −0.49 p<0.01 555 (1)	–	−0.92 −1.43 to −0.4 p<0.01 431 (3)	−0.54 0.09 to −0.1 p=0.02 608 (2)	0 −1.33 to 1.33 98 (1)	–
Mean change in urgency episodes/day	−0.81 −1.35 to −0.27 p<0.01 544 (1)	−1.29 −1.83 to −0.75 p<0.01 555 (1)	–	–	–	–	–
Mean change in volume voided per micturition (mL)	18.35 9.01 to 27.69 p<0.01 543 (1)	24.25 14.99 to 33.51 p<0.01 553 (1)	–	39.52 30.19 to 48.85 p<0.01 382 (2)	23 10.3 to 35.7 p<0.01 355 (1)	27.9 −8.18 to 63.98 p=0.13 98 (1)	–
Patients returned to continence at endpoint	–	–	3.53 1.94 to 6.41 p<0.01 110 (1)	–	1.75 1.26 to 2.43 p<0.01 355 (1)	1.8 0.96 to 3.38 p=0.07 76 (1)	1.33 1.09–1.63 p<0.01 597 (1)
Patients with improvement in disease	1.49 1.09 to 2.03 p=0.01 544 (1)	1.51 1.11 to 2.05 p=0.01 555 (1)	4.11 1 to 16.89 p=0.05 44 (1)	–	–	–	–

Row 1: effect size (RR for dichotomous outcomes, unstandardized (weighted) mean difference for continuous outcomes). Row 2: 95% CI
Row 3: P–value vs a null hypothesis of no difference in effect (RR 1, mean difference 0). Row 4: number of patients (studies) which contributed to
meta–analysis. CI, confidence interval; ER, extended release; IR, immediate release; RR, risk ratio
*Only data suitable for meta–analysis are presented in this table

Propiverine ER 20 mg/day vs placebo	Propiverine ER 30 mg/day vs placebo	Solifenacin 5 mg/day vs placebo	Solifenacin 10 mg/day vs placebo	Tolterodine ER 4 mg/day vs placebo	Tolterodine IR 2 mg/day vs placebo	Tolterodine IR 4 mg/day vs placebo	Trospium chloride 40 mg/day vs placebo
−0.53	–	−0.77	−0.81	−0.4	−0.21	−0.5	–
−0.92 to −.14		−1.02 to −0.52	−1.06 to −0.56	−0.42 to −0.38	−0.56 to 0.14	−0.67 to −0.32	
p=0.01		p<0.01	p<0.01	p<0.01	p=0.23	p<0.01	
578 (1)		1157 (2)	1170 (2)	3095 (5)	605 (3)	2614 (7)	
−0.93	–	−0.99	−1.3	−0.77	−0.67	−0.71	–
−1.28 to −0.58		−1.23 to −0.75	−1.56 to −1.04	−0.96 to −0.58	−1.07 to −0.27	−0.93 to −0.5	
P<0.01		p<0.01	p<0.01	p<0.01	p<0.01	p<0.01	
779 (1)		1803 (2)	1789 (2)	3223 (5)	637 (3)	3121 (7)	
−1.02	–	−1.25	−1.56	−1.05	–	−0.64	–
−1.44 to −0.6		−1.57 to −0.93	−1.88 to −1.23	−1.37 to −0.73		−1.16 to −.12	
p<0.01		p<0.01	p<0.01	p<0.01		p=0.02	
779 (1)		1786 (2)	1771 (2)	1416 (2)		994 (1)	
24.95	–	24.71	31.87	16.92	13.07	17.21	–
19.89 to 30.01		20.58 to 28.85	27.58 to 36.16	13.17 to 20.66	6.63 to 19.51	13.95 to 20.47	
p<0.01		p<0.01	p<0.01	p<0.01	p<0.01	p<0.01	
776 (1)		1799 (2)	1785 (2)	3091 (5)	637 (3)	3120 (7)	
1.51	1.42	1.51	1.61	1.72	–	–	2
1.26 to 1.81	1.16 to 1.73	1.26 to 1.82	1.34 to 1.93	1.24 to 2.39			1.4 to 2.86
p<0.01	p<0.01	p<0.01	p<0.01	p<0.01			p<0.01
578 (1)	593 (1)	557 (1)	553 (1)	357 (1)			821 (2)
–	–	–		1.34	–	–	
				0.98 to 1.83			
				p=0.07			
				562 (1)			

Table 19.2 Tolerability of antimuscarinics compared to placebo control: results from meta-analyses*

	Darifenacin 7.5 mg/day vs placebo	Darifenacin 7.5 mg/day titrated vs placebo	Darifenacin 15 mg/day vs placebo	Fesoterodine 4 mg/day vs placebo	Fesoterodine 8 mg/day vs placebo	Oxybutynin IR 5 mg/day vs placebo	Oxybutynin IR 7.5–10 mg/day vs placebo	Oxybutynin IR 15 mg/day vs placebo	Propiverine IR 30 mg/day vs placebo
Total withdrawals	0.74 0.43 to 1.27 p=0.27 938 (2)	1.25 0.62 to 2.51 p=0.54 398 (1)	0.98 0.70 to 1.36 p=0.88 1416 (4)	1.3 0.85 to 2 p=0.23 557 (1)	1.08 0.69 to 1.68 p=0.73 573 (1)	1.6 0.59 to 4.33 p=0.36 60 (1)	1.33 1.01 to 1.76 p=0.04 1054 (5)	1.72 1.18 to 2.49 p<0.01 751 (5)	1.21 0.61 to 2.4 p=0.59 597 (1)
Withdrawals due to adverse events	0.67 0.11 to 3.95 p=0.66 217 (1)	2.16 0.75 to 6.25 p=0.16 398 (1)	1.83 0.95 to 3.55 p=0.07 657 (2)	1.4 0.69 to 2.82 p=0.35 926 (2)	1.33 0.65 to 2.71 p=0.44 929 (2)	1.5 0.27 to 8.34 p=0.64 60 (1)	1.91 1.18 to 3.1 p=0.01 488 (1)	1.89 1.23 to 2.9 p<0.01 743 (4)	7.67 1.02 to 57.66 p=0.05 597 (1)

	Propiverine IR 45 mg/day vs placebo	Propiverine ER 20 mg/day vs placebo	Propiverine ER 30 mg/day vs placebo	Solifenacin 5 mg/day vs placebo	Solifenacin 10 mg/day vs placebo	Tolterodine ER 4 mg/day vs placebo	Tolterodine 2 mg/day vs placebo	Tolterodine IR 4 mg/day vs placebo	Trospium chloride 40 mg/day vs placebo
Total withdrawals	1.31 0.68 to 2.52 p=0.41 293 (1)	1.07 0.69 to 1.68 p=0.76 805 (1)	1.08 0.54 to 2.17 p=0.83 593 (1)	0.83 0.64 to 1.07 p=0.15 2710 (4)	0.81 0.63 to 1.05 p=0.1 2689 (4)	0.87 0.68 to 1.1 p=0.24 2113 (5)	1.32 0.66 to 2.65 p=0.44 398 (2)	0.98 0.76 to 1.26 p=0.87 2261 (6)	1 0.73 to 1.37 832 (2)
Withdrawals due to adverse events	–	2.39 1.20 to 4.78 p=0.01 805 (1)	5.68 0.74 to 43.71 p=0.1 593 (1)	1.16 0.79 to 1.72 p=0.44 3575 (5)	1.53 1.02 to 2.3 p=0.04 2689 (4)	0.71 0.53 to .95 p=0.02 3777 (5)	0.9 0.44 to 1.83 p=0.77 851 (5)	0.88 0.66 to 1.17 p=0.39 3973 (11)	1.27 0.86 to 1.88 p=0.23 1490 (3)
Withdrawals due to deaths	–	–	–	0.34 0.01 to 8.20 p=0.5 600 (1)	1.55 0.29 to 8.21 p=0.61 1678 (2)	1 0.06 to 15.98 p=0.31 1015 (1)	0.21 0.01 to 4.29 p=0.31 251 (1)	1 0.22 to 4.49 1324 (2)	–

Row 1: effect size (risk ratio for dichotomous outcomes, unstandardized (weighted) mean difference for continuous outcomes). Row 2: 95% CI. Row 3: P-value vs a null hypothesis of no difference in effect (RR 1, mean difference 0). Row 4: number of patients (studies) which contributed to meta-analysis
ER, extended release; IR, immediate release
*Only data suitable for meta-analysis are presented in this table

95% CI 0.17– 0.57, p < 0.01); tolterodine IR 4 mg/day was associated with a lower risk than oxybutynin IR 15 mg/day (RR 0.47, 95% CI 0.33–0.69, p < 0.01); and oxybutynin ER 5 mg/day was associated with a lower risk than oxybutynin ER 15 mg/day (RR 0.27, 95% CI 0.08–0.92, p = 0.04). There were no other statistically significant differences between active treatments.

Withdrawal due to death was infrequently reported, possibly due to the low incidence of mortality relative to other outcomes in OAB patients in trials of this length. No statistically significant differences were reported between treatments (active and placebo) in any of the analyses conducted.

Clinical question 19.3

What is the safety of antimuscarinic therapy?

The evidence

Safety information on antimuscarinics is summarized in Table 19.3. Every treatment in the review, with two exceptions, was statistically significantly associated with a greater risk of adverse events than placebo. The two exceptions were tolterodine IR 2 mg/day (RR 1.00, 95% CI 0.89–1.12, p = 0.97) and oxybutynin tds 3.9 mg/day (RR 1.59, 95% CI 0.96–2.63, p = 0.07). Where statistically significant, the pooled RR for any adverse event in comparison with placebo varied between 1.13 and 2.00. No treatment was shown to be significantly associated with serious adverse events.

When comparing adverse events rates of different forms of active treatment, there were favorable results for tolterodine formulations relative to other active treatments: the risk of adverse events was statistically significantly lower with tolterodine IR 2 mg/day than oxybutynin ER 5 mg/day (RR 0.59, 95% CI 0.43–0.82, p < 0.01) and lower with tolterodine IR 4 mg/day than oxybutynin IR 7.5–10 mg/day (RR 0.83, 95% CI 0.75–0.91, p < 0.01) and oxybutynin IR 15 mg/day (RR 0.86, 95% CI 0.79–0.95, p < 0.01). One trial provided data suggestive of a higher risk of adverse events with fesoterodine 8 mg/day than fesoterodine 4 mg/day (RR 1.17, 95% CI 1.00–1.37, p = 0.04) and tolterodine ER 4 mg/day (RR 1.18, 95% CI 1.01–1.37, p = 0.04). The remaining statistically significant result favored trospium 40 mg/day over oxybutynin IR 7.5–10 mg/day (RR 0.85, 95% CI 0.73–0.98, p = 0.02).

Serious adverse events were uncommon. No treatment in the review was statistically significantly associated with a greater risk of serious adverse events than placebo or other active treatment. Dry mouth of any severity (mild, moderate or severe) was found to be highly statistically significantly more common in all interventions than placebo (p ≤ 0.01). Where significant, the pooled RR varied between 2.15 and 5.90. It was apparent that the RR generally increased with drug dose for darifenacin, fesoterodine, solifenacin, and tolterodine, although this trend was not apparent for oxybutynin and propiverine. Some adverse events were reported at statistically significantly higher levels in active treatments than in placebo: blurred vision (oxybutynin IR 15 and 20 mg/day; propiverine 20, 30, and 45 mg/day; solifenacin 10 mg/day; and tolterodine ER 4 mg/day); constipation (darifenacin 7.5 mg/day, with and without titration, and 15 mg/day; propiverine ER 20 mg/day and IR 3 and 4.5 mg/day; solifenacin 5 and 10 mg/day; tolterodine 4 mg/day; and trospium 40 mg/day); erythema (oxybutynin tds 3.9 mg/day); fatigue (tolterodine ER 4 mg/day); pruritus (oxybutynin tds 3.9 mg/day); increased sweating (solifenacin 5 mg/day); and urinary retention (oxybutynin IR 7.5 to 10 mg/day).

Implications for clinical practice

Findings presented in this chapter are based on an up-to-date systematic review on the efficacy, safety, and tolerability of antimuscarinic treatments for OAB. Conclusions derived from this review must be interpreted with some caution, taking into account the different inclusion and exclusion criteria, investigative sites, geographical locations, and study durations for individual trials. This being said, the existing body of evidence to date suggests that antimuscarinics as a class are efficacious in terms of improving patient-relevant outcomes. Antimuscarinics are also safe and well tolerated. Overall, the potential for patient benefit clearly outweighs the potential risks, but there are still a number of unknowns, for instance, potentially important CNS adverse events, such as memory impairment, have traditionally not been evaluated in antimuscarinic trials. Antimuscarinics are therefore strongly recommended as a first-line treatment option for patients with overactive bladder (Grade 1A). Newer agents (darifenacin, solifenacin and fesoterodine) may offer the potential for greater improvement in patient-perceived outcomes by allowing more dose flexibility compared to oxybutynin.

Conflict of interest

CRC is a scientific consultant and researcher with Allergan, Astellas, Novartis, and Pfizer; ZSK is a Senior Director at Pfizer Inc; DM is an employee of Heron Evidence Development Ltd, which was contracted by Pfizer Inc for this work.

Table 19.3 Adverse events of antimuscarinics compared with placebo: results from meta-analyses*

	Darifenacin 7.5 mg/day vs placebo	Darifenacin 7.5 mg/day titrated vs placebo	Darifenacin 15 mg/day vs placebo	Fesoterodine 4 mg/day vs placebo	Fesoterodine 8 mg/day vs placebo	Oxybutynin IR 5 mg/day vs placebo	Oxybutynin 7.5–10 mg/day vs placebo	Oxybutynin IR 15 mg/day vs placebo	Oxybutynin IR 20 mg/day vs placebo	Oxybutynin tds 3.9–4.0 mg/day vs placebo
Any adverse event	1.26 1.10 to 1.44 p<0.01 938 (2)	2.0 1.38 to 2.91 p<0.01 395 (1)	1.32 1.18 to 1.48 p<0.01 1262 (3)	1.31 1.08 to 1.59 p=0.01 555 (1)	1.54 1.29 to 1.84 p<0.01 570 (1)	–	1.72 1.38 to 2.14 p<0.01 289 (1)	1.29 1.19 to 1.40 p<0.01 748 (4)	–	1.59 0.96 to 2.63 p=0.07 355 (1)
Any serious adverse event	2.62 0.91 to 7.56 p=0.08 938 (2)	0.59 0.16 to 2.17 p=0.43 395 (1)	0.60 0.19 to 1.84 p=0.37 1262 (3)	–	–	–	15.00 0.86 to 261.2 p=0.06 488 (1)	0.74 0.29 to 1.91 p=0.53 568 (2)	–	–
Dry mouth (any severity)	2.57 1.79 to 3.68 p<0.01 938 (2)	2.15 1.16 to 3.99 p=0.01 395 (1)	4.40 3.34 to 5.79 p<0.01 1611 (5)	3.01 2.17 to 4.20 p<0.01 1010 (3)	3.95 2.87 to 5.44 p<0.01 1016 (3)	1.08 0.90 to 1.29 p=0.41 57 (1)	2.96 2.46 to 3.55 p<0.01 923 (4)	4.42 3.53 to 5.53 p<0.01 1006 (7)	2.9 1.73 to 4.87 p<0.01 62 (1)	1.41 0.73 to 2.73 p=0.31 612 (2)

	Propiverine IR 30 mg/day vs placebo	Propiverine IR 45 mg/day vs placebo	Propiverine ER 20 mg/day vs placebo	Propiverine ER 30 mg/day vs placebo	Solifenacin 5 mg/day vs placebo	Solifenacin 10 mg/day vs placebo	Tolterodine ER 4 mg/day vs placebo	Tolterodine 4 mg/day vs placebo	Tolterodine IR 2 mg/day vs placebo	Tolterodine IR 4 mg/day vs placebo	Trospium chloride 40 mg/day vs placebo
Any adverse event	1.90 1.40 to 2.56 p<0.01 597 (1)	1.42 1.17 to 1.74 p<0.01 457 (3)	1.58 1.02 to 2.43 p=0.04 62 (1)	1.69 1.24 to 2.29 p<0.01 593 (1)	1.23 1.10 to 1.37 p<0.01 1230 (3)	1.32 1.06 to 1.66 p=0.02 488 (2)	1.19 1.06 to 1.32 p<0.01 2634 (4)	1.13 1.05 to 1.21 p<0.01 2119 (10)	1.00 0.89 to 1.12 p=0.97 851 (5)	–	1.30 1.15 to 1.45 p<0.01 1409 (4)
Any serious adverse event	15.89 0.96 to 264.24 p=0.05 597 (1)	–	–	–	–	–	0.88 0.58 to 1.33 p=0.53 3199 (4)	0.82 0.50 to 1.36 p=0.45 2335 (6)	2.06 0.60 to 7.03 p=0.25 398 (2)	–	2.24 0.49 to 10.25 p=0.3 517 (2)
Dry mouth (any severity)	3.54 2.03 to 6.18 p<0.01 597 (1)	3.13 1.27 to 7.71 p=0.01 164 (2)	4.10 2.76 to 6.07 p<0.01 867 (2)	3.38 1.93 to 5.9 p<0.01 593 (1)	3.32 2.55 to 4.32 p<0.01 3691 (6)	5.90 4.59 to 7.59 p<0.01 2951 (5)	3.00 2.47 to 3.64 p<0.01 4129 (6)	3.44 2.92 to 4.04 p<0.01 4071 (11)	2.41 1.67 to 3.49 p<0.01 838 (5)	–	3.17 2.37 to 4.24 p<0.01 1389 (3)

Row 1: effect size (risk ratio for dichotomous outcomes, unstandardized (weighted) mean difference for continuous outcomes). Row 2: 95% CI. Row 3: P-value vs a null hypothesis of no difference in effect (RR 1, mean difference 0). Row 4: number of patients (studies) which contributed to meta-analysis
ER, extended release; IR, immediate release
*Only data suitable for meta-analysis are presented in this table

References

1. Abrams P, Cardozo L, Fall M, et al. The standardisation of terminology of lower urinary tract function: report from the Standardisation Sub-co:mmittee of the International Continence Society. Neurourol Urodyn 2002:21:167-78.

2. Irwin DE, M ilsom I, Hunskaar S, et al. Population-based survey of urinary incontinence, overactive bladder, and other lower urinary tract symptoms in five countries: results of the EPIC study. Eur Urol 2006:50:1306-14; discussion 14-15.

3. Milsom I, Abrams P, Cardozo L, Roberts RG, Thuroff J, Wein AJ. How widespread are the symptoms of an overactive bladder and how are they managed? A population-based prevalence study. BJU Int 2001:87:760-6.

4. Stewart WF, van Rooyen JB, Cundiff GW, et al. Prevalence and burden of overactive bladder in the United States. World J Urol 2003:20:327-36.

5. Coyne KS, Payne C, Bhattacharyya SK, et al. The impact of urinary urgency and frequency on health-related quality of life in overactive bladder: results from a national community survey. Value Health 2004:7:455-63.

6. Tubaro A. Defining overactive bladder: epidemiology and burden of disease. Urology 2004: 64:2-6.

7. Wein AJ, Rackley RR. Overactive bladder: a better understanding of pathophysiology, diagnosis and management. J Urol 2006:175:S5-10.

8. Andersson KE. Antimuscarinics for treatment of overactive bladder. Lancet Neurol 2004:3:46-53.

9. Aschkenzai S, Botros S, Miller J, Gamble T, Sand P, Goldberg R. Overactive bladder symptoms are not related to detrusor overactivity. Neurourol Urodyn 2007:26:abstract 35.

10. Digesu GA, Khullar V, Cardozo L, Salvatore S. Overactive bladder symptoms: do we need urodynamics? Neurourol Urodyn 2003:22:105-8.

11. Hashim H, Abrams P. Do symptoms of overactive bladder predict urodynamics detrusor overactivity? Neurourol Urodyn 2004:23:484-6.

12. Hyman MJ, Groutz A, Blaivas JG. Detrusor instability in men: correlation of lower urinary tract symptoms with urodynamic findings. J Urol 2001:166:550-2; discussion 553.

13. Abrams P, Andersson KE. Muscarinic receptor antagonists for overactive bladder. BJU Int 2007:100:987-1006.

14. Bschleipfer T, Schukowski K, Weidner W. Expression and distribution of cholinergic receptors in the human urothelium. Life Sci 2007:80:2303-7.

15. Mansfield KJ, Liu L, Mitchelson FJ, Moore KH, Millard RJ, Burcher E. Muscarinic receptor subtypes in human bladder detrusor and mucosa, studied by radioligand binding and quantitative competitive RT-PCR: changes in ageing. Br J Pharmacol 2005:144:1089-99.

16. Zarghooni S, Wunsch J, Bodenbenner M, et al. Expression of muscarinic and nicotinic acetylcholine receptors in the mouse urothelium. Life Sci 2007:80:2308-13.

17. Caufield MP, Birdsall N. Classification of muscarinic acetylcholine receptors. Pharmacol Rev 1998:50:279-90.

18. Chess-Williams R, Chapple CR, Yamanishi T, Yasuda K, Sellers DJ. The minor population of M3-receptors mediate contraction of human detrusor muscle in vitro. J Auton Pharmacol 2001:21: 243-8.

19. Fetscher C, Fleichman M, Schmidt M, Krege S, Michel MC. M(3) muscarinic receptors mediate contraction of human urinary bladder. Br J Pharmacol 2002:136:641-3.

20. Hedge S, Choppin A, Bonhaus D. Functional role of M2 and M3 muscarinic receptors in the urinary bladder of rats in vitro and in vivo. Br J Pharmacol 1997:120:1409-17.

21. Kories C, Czyborra C, Fetscher C, Schneider T, Krege S, Michel MC. Gender comparison of muscarinic receptor expression and function in rat and human urinary bladder: differential regulation of M2 and M3 receptors? Naunyn Schmiedebergs Arch Pharmacol 2003:367:524-31.

22. Schneider T, Fetscher C, Krege S, Michel MC. Signal transduction underlying carbachol-induced contraction of human urinary bladder. J Pharmacol Exp Ther 2004:309:1148-53.

23. Schneider T, Hein P, Michel MC. Signal transduction underlying carbachol-induced contraction of rat urinary bladder. I. Phospholipases and Ca2 + sources. J Pharmacol Exp Ther 2004:308:47-53.

24. Chapple C, Khullar V, Gabriel Z, Dooley JA. The effects of antimuscarinic treatments in overactive bladder: a systematic review and meta-analysis. Eur Urol 2005:48:5-26.

25. Chapple CR, Khullar V, Gabriel Z, Muston D, Bitoun CE, Weinstein D. The effects of antimuscarinic treatments in overactive bladder: an update of a systematic review and meta-analysis. Eur Urol 2008:54:543-62.

26. Herbison P, Hay-Smith J, Ellis G, Moore K. Effectiveness of anticholinergic drugs compared with placebo in the treatment of overactive bladder: systematic review. BMJ 2003:326: 841-4.

27. Novara G, Galfano A, Secco S, et al. A systematic review and meta-analysis of randomized controlled trials with antimuscarinic drugs for overactive bladder. Eur Urol 2008:54:740-63.

28. Shamliyan TA, Kane RL, Wyman J, Wilt TJ. Systematic review: randomized, controlled trials of nonsurgical treatments for urinary incontinence in women. Ann Intern Med 2008:148: 459-73.

20 Medical management of urinary incontinence in women

Ryan Hutchinson, Roger R. Dmochowski and Harriette Scarpero

Department of Urologic Surgery, Vanderbilt Medical Center, Nashville, TN, USA

Background

Urinary incontinence (UI) is an important health concern that has a substantial effect on an individual's perception of well-being, body image, and quality of life (QoL). It is estimated that 13 million people in the United States, of which 11 million are women, suffer from UI [1]. The actual prevalence of urinary incontinence in women is not known. Most women who experience urinary incontinence never seek or receive treatment [2,3]. A limitation of existing national databases is that they capture only the minority of incontinent women who are treated for incontinence [4]. Despite underestimation, UI is a prevalent condition in the female population in the United States. It affects 15–50%, and prevalence increases with age. In younger age groups under 25 years, the prevalence is low, less than 5%. Prevalence rises steadily until the postmenopausal years when it is greater than 30%. Stress urinary incontinence (SUI) is the most common type of urinary incontinence and is present in approximately 50% of incontinent women whereas pure urge incontinence exists in approximately 22% of women [4].

Urinary incontinence may be managed in a variety of medical and surgical ways. Medical management of female urinary incontinence is a broad term that encompasses several modalities including behavioral therapy, pelvic floor muscle therapy (PFMT), with or without the assistance of electrical stimulation or biofeedback, and pharmacological therapy. Antimuscarinic agents are the standard treatment for urge incontinence, but there is no Food and Drug Administration-approved drug for stress urinary incontinence.

The Agency for Healthcare Research Quality (AHRQ) clinical practice guideline on UI in adults recommends behavioral modification as first-line intervention for UI [5]. Behavioral modification includes a variety of activities such as education, lifestyle changes, keeping micturition charts and diaries, development of timed voiding and bladder training regimens, and physiotherapy with or without biofeedback. The AHRQ recommendations are based on available high-level evidence supporting the effectiveness of these interventions. However, less outcomes evidence is available about use of these interventions in clinical practice.

Pelvic floor muscle therapy for UI is the best studied nonsurgical treatment. It is useful for both stress and urge incontinence because it improves the strength of pelvic floor musculature and thus urethral support, whereas contraction of striated paraurethral musculature simultaneously causes reflex inhibition of detrusor contractions. A variety of PFMT protocols exist, which hampers comparison between studies.

Clinical question 20.1

Is there a role for education, behavioral and lifestyle modification alone for female urinary incontinence (stress and urge)?

Literature search

Evidence for the following clinical recommendations was obtained using three separate methods to ensure completeness and timeliness. First, Medline searches were conducted including all forms of published, English-language studies using the keywords: "education," "behavioral modification," "lifestyle modification," "female urinary incontinence." The references of these studies were in turn examined for further relevant studies that may have been missed in the search. Next, texts considered authoritative in the field were reviewed with specific attention to the studies used to form those resources' clinical recommendations.

Evidence-Based Urology. Edited by Philipp Dahm, Roger R. Dmochowski.
© 2010 Blackwell Publishing.

This also included searches at meta-analyses clearing houses. Finally, active practitioners and researchers within the field were queried about recent evidence on the topic and what studies they used to inform their own clinical decision making. The sum of information found through all the above means was reviewed and the following clinical recommendations are made based on this evidence.

The evidence

Lifestyle interventions for the treatment of UI are of significant interest to patients, yet there is limited high-level evidence to guide practice recommendations. Weight reduction is the behavioral and lifestyle change that has received the most attention as a treatment option for urinary incontinence. Hunskaar has published a well-researched review of the epidemiological literature of urinary incontinence with respect to overweight and obesity as risk factors [6]. The association of overweight and obesity with urinary incontinence is well established but epidemiological evidence is only fair (Level 2 and 3). Many of the studies are composed of samples of patients planning bariatric surgery; thus, they are biased populations and contain a large number of very obese patients who are not found in population-based studies. However, credible evidence from longitudinal studies that link high Body Mass Index (BMI) to the later development of new urinary incontinence is present. The connection between obesity and incontinence is greater for stress and mixed incontinence than for urge incontinence and overactive bladder (OAB) [6].

Three randomized controlled trials (RCTs) of weight reduction as treatment for urinary incontinence have been published. The first large-scale RCT to examine weight loss was the Program to Reduce Incontinence by Diet and Exercise (PRIDE) study. This was carried out at two US sites and enrolled 338 overweight or obese women reporting > 10 episodes of incontinence weekly [7]. Participating women were randomized 2:1 to an intensive 6-month lifestyle and behavior change weight intervention program (N 226) or to a structured education group (control group, N 112). Stratification was also performed according to clinical center. Participants were aware of their treatment of course, but staff members who collected the outcome data were blinded. All women received an instructional guide of standard behavioral therapy for incontinence and were trained to complete a 7-day voiding diary. The primary outcome measure was the percentage change in the number of incontinence episodes reported in the 7-day diary at 6 months after randomization. Results showed that the characteristics of the participants in the two groups were similar at baseline and rates of urge incontinence were greater than stress incontinence. At 6 months,

the weight loss group had a mean loss of 8.0% of bodyweight from baseline and a 47.4% mean decrease in the total number of incontinence episodes per week compared to a 1.6% weight loss (p < 0.001) and 28.1% mean decrease in incontinence episodes in the control group (p = 0.01). The main reduction in incontinence episodes from baseline was within episodes of stress incontinence, although the frequency of episodes of urge incontinence was greater in the weight loss group but not by a statistically significant extent. Women in the weight loss group also perceived a greater decrease in the frequency of urinary incontinence episodes and a lower volume of urine loss and reported higher satisfaction with change (p < 0.001). However, the increased awareness of bladder habits resulting from voiding diary compliance could contribute to improvement in both groups.

Fluid restriction is typically supported for the treatment of urge incontinence but there are few published randomized trials to support its use. Hashim & Abrams reported a small randomized, two-group, prospective, cross-over trial in adults with symptoms of OAB [8]. Twenty-four adult men and women with significant OAB symptoms on frequency/volume charts and having urgency and/or urge incontinence were assigned to either an increased or a decreased fluid intake regimen. The primary endpoint was the change in the frequency of urgency and/or urge incontinence events during a 24-hour period. A key finding was that adults find it easier to increase or decrease fluid intake by 25% of baseline rather than 50% (a target in earlier trials that led to poor compliance with study design) [9]. Additionally, there was a significant reduction in frequency, urgency, and nocturia when patients decreased their fluid input by 25%, but no statistically significant improvement in quality of life. With regard to whether caffeine intake contributes to OAB symptomatology, Swithinbank et al. conducted a 4-week prospective, randomized cross-over study in 30 women with urodynamically confirmed detrusor overactivity to determine the effect of caffeine restriction as well as fluid volume manipulation on urinary symptoms [10]. Interestingly, no significant difference between the baseline week and caffeine-free week was found for any outcome measures. Fluid restriction from baseline did achieve a statistically significant decrease in voiding frequency and urgency episodes, supporting the Hashim & Abrams study results.

Pelvic floor muscle therapy is a commonly prescribed conservative treatment for urinary incontinence, but a recent meta-analysis reveals the limitations of the existing evidence. In 2008, Shamliyan et al. published a large-scale review synthesizing evidence on the effectiveness of nonsurgical clinical interventions for the treatment of urinary incontinence in women [11]. Ninety-six RCTs and three systematic reviews were examined and of those,

31 addressed PFMT. Four RCTs supported PFMT over "regular care" for improvement in UI with moderate level of evidence, defined as the confidence that the estimate of effect would likely change with future research. Within these studies, pooled relative risk for continence after PFMT and PFMT with biofeedback was significant and consistent. However, pooled absolute risk differences of resolved or improved UI were inconsistent across the studies. Analysis between studies is hampered by the difference in behavioral training/PFMT protocol between studies.

Moderate-level evidence also exists to support PFMT and bladder training compared to regular care, although improvement effect was inconsistent across the studies. The authors compared results of individual studies to analyze the effectiveness of PFMT by population and treatment characteristics, and factors that portend a favorable prognosis/outcome were: PFMT in groups with skilled physical therapists, individualized behavioral intervention with PFMT, and community-based interventions including education, bladder training and PFMT [11].

The Cochrane Incontinence Group Specialized Trials Register searched randomized or quasi-randomized trials in women with stress, urge or mixed incontinence in which one arm of the trial included PFMT (defined simply as a program of repeated voluntary pelvic floor muscle contractions taught and supervised by a healthcare professional) and another arm was a no-treatment, placebo, sham or other inactive control [12]. Thirteen trials involving 714 women (375 PFMT, 339 controls) met the inclusion criteria, but only six trials (403 women) contributed data to the analysis. The reviewers identified limitations in the studies including moderate to high risk of bias in most as well as considerable variation in interventions used, study populations, and outcome measures. Results suggest that women who did PFMT were more likely to report they were cured or improved as compared to women who did not participate. Women who underwent PFMT also experienced about one fewer incontinent episodes per day. Conclusions drawn include support for the widespread recommendation that PFMT be included in first-line conservative management of stress, urge or mixed UI in women, yet tempered by recognition of statistical heterogeneity from variations in incontinence type, training, and outcome measurement between studies.

Biofeedback uses visual cues and verbal coaching to teach patients how to control the physiological responses of the bladder and pelvic floor muscles that control continence. Biofeedback-assisted PFMT has been shown to be as effective as pharmacotherapy for urge incontinence, and superior to immediate-release oxybutynin in one randomized trial [13]. There is low Level 1 evidence that biofeedback-assisted PFMT is no more effective than PFMT alone for women with stress and mixed incontinence. Nonetheless, in clinical practice, physicians may find biofeedback a useful adjunct to PFMT, particularly in women who have difficulty isolating pelvic floor muscles. Large-scale RCTs are needed to study the best use of biofeedback in PFMT. Data in support of electrical stimulation for UI are insufficient, and electrical stimulation with PFMT seems not to offer benefit. Further investigation of these modalities is necessary.

The literature on predictors of response to behavioral therapy is sparse and inconsistent. In an attempt to identify predictors of outcome of a multicomponent behavioral training program for urinary incontinence (stress and urge), a secondary analysis of data from three prospective, randomized clinical trials was performed [14]. In multivariable regression analyses, all the factors relied upon for diagnostic evaluation, such as age, race, type of incontinence, obstetric history, medications, pelvic exam, BMI, urodynamic parameters or distress level with the condition, were not associated with outcomes. Overall, previous treatment and indicators of severity, number of incontinence episodes at baseline, and lack of need for incontinence pads showed an association with outcomes of behavioral therapy. Behavioral treatment resulted in a mean 80.7% reduction of incontinence episodes compared to a mean 68.8% reduction with drug treatment and mean 39.4% reduction in the placebo control. Behavioral treatment also produced the greatest patient-perceived improvement. The investigators conclude that behavioral therapy is applicable to patients in any age group, and since most motivated patients do receive benefit from behavioral treatment without any risk, no incontinent woman should be discouraged from exploring this therapeutic option.

Recommendations

Behavioral therapies of education, diet modification, fluid restriction and weight loss are low risk to all populations, easy to access and inexpensive relative to other forms of therapy (pharmacological and surgical). There is little reason not to offer these modalities as options in the care of urinary incontinence, especially in light of the excellent risk/benefit ratios associated with these interventions and the presence of randomized, prospective evidence supporting them (Grade 1B recommendation). However, as these modalities are often not curative and are dependent on patient motivation, counseling should include a discussion of reasonable expectations as well as options in the event of treatment failure. Women should be made aware of efficacy in relation to other therapies, any risks associated with behavioral therapy, and limitations in available evidence.

Clinical question 20.2

Is there any evidence to support pharmacological treatment of stress incontinence?

Literature search

Evidence for this question was obtained in a similar manner to the previous section, starting with a Medline search using the keywords: "stress incontinence," "medical management," "anticholinergics," "estrogen," "alpha-adrenergic," "imipramine," "duloxetine" and "SNRI." The references of these papers were also evaluated for studies missed by the search. Authoritative texts and meta-analyses clearing houses were then consulted for the identification of further studies. Finally, practicing researchers and clinicians in the field were asked about studies they used to inform their own decision making.

The evidence

Estrogens

While rarely used as primary therapy for SUI, estrogens have been advocated for UI. The rationale behind their use is based on the presence of estrogen receptors in the bladder base and urethra. Estrogens may affect continence by increasing urethral resistance, raising the sensory threshold of the bladder, increasing alpha-adrenoreceptor sensitivity in the urethral smooth muscle or promoting beta-3-adreno-receptor mediated relaxation of the detrusor muscle [15,16]. Hormone replacement therapy (HRT) is also thought to increase the number of epithelial cells lining the bladder and urethra, improve the thickness and quality of the subepithelial vascular plexus and thus improve the coaptation of urethral walls and urethral resistance [17]. Recent data from several large studies have finally elucidated the effect of conjugated estrogens on the condition of SUI.

According to the Cochrane Database of Systemic Reviews, 28 trials including 2926 women report using estrogens for urinary incontinence in a variety of combinations, dosages, routes of administration and durations of therapy [18]. The consensus of these trials was that the rate of subjective improvement and cure of both stress and urge incontinence was statistically higher in women receiving estrogens compared to women receiving placebo. However, a subsequent meta-analysis of 87 articles on the use of estrogens for SUI revealed that estrogens were not effective treatment for SUI [19].

The Heart and Estrogen/Progestin Replacement Study (HERS) was designed as a RCT to evaluate daily oral conjugated estrogen plus medroxyprogesterone acetate therapy for the prevention of coronary heart disease events in postmenopausal women with known coronary disease [20]. As a separate evaluation in this population, 1525 (55%) of the 2763 women who had at least weekly urinary incontinence at the initiation of the study were evaluated for change in the severity of incontinence. Women were randomly assigned to HRT or placebo and followed for 4.1 years. Incontinence improved in 26% of the placebo group compared to 21% in the HRT group. Conversely, 27% of the placebo group and 39% of the HRT group realized a worsening of symptoms which was a statistically significant difference. Furthermore, the incidence of incontinence episodes per week increased in the HRT group by an average of 0.7 and decreased by 0.1 in the placebo group, also a difference that was statistically significant.

Additionally, a recent report from the Women's Health Initiative (WHI), a multicenter double-blind placebo-controlled randomized trial of HRT in 27,347 women, states that occurrence of both stress and urge incontinence increased in postmenopausal women placed on either conjugated equine estrogens (CEE) plus medroxyprogesterone acetate (MPA) or CEE alone compared to placebo [21]. Relative risks of developing SUI (excluding mixed incontinence) were 1.87 and 2.15, respectively. The authors concluded that HRT increased the risk of UI among continent women and worsened the characteristics of UI among asymptomatic women after 1 year. HRT also worsened pre-existing UI at 1 year. A reasonable conclusion from the more recent clinical trials is that conjugated estrogens with or without medroxyprogesterone are not indicated for the treatment of SUI.

Imipramine

The tricyclic antidepressant imipramine is indicated for nocturnal enuresis and is often used off-label for SUI, mixed urinary incontinence (MUI), and urgency urinary incontinence (UUI). Despite its long use for urinary incontinence, the exact mechanism most responsible for action on the lower urinary tract is not clear because it has so many pharmacological actions [22,23]. In theory, imipramine is used for the treatment of SUI due to its alpha-stimulating effect at the urethra, which can increase the urethral closure pressure and functional urethral length. Available data on the use of imipramine are largely anecdotal. No randomized placebo-controlled trials of imipramine for SUI have been published. In small uncontrolled studies, cure rates of 35–70% have been reported [24,25]. Side effects are numerous and related to its anticholinergic properties: dry mouth, weakness, fatigue, sedation or mania, parkinsonian effects, orthostatic hypotension, sweating, arrhythmia, and sexual dysfunction, which may preclude use of the drug [26]. Imipramine is toxic in high doses and overdose can produce lethal cardiac dysrhythmia or conduction blocks [27]. Although studies demonstrating myriad actions by imipramine on the lower urinary tract exist, there are few clinical data showing a significant positive effect for SUI.

Alpha-adrenergic agonists

Increased outlet resistance theoretically should be possible with the use of alpha-adrenergic agonists to stimulate the large number of alpha-1 receptors at the proximal urethra and sphincter. Contraction of the alpha-1 receptors in the proximal urethra leads to an increase in the maximum urethral pressure and maximum urethral closure pressure. However, currently available agents are nonselective and produce significant adverse side effects including blood pressure elevation, anxiety, insomnia, headache, tremor, weakness, palpitations, cardiac arrhythmias, and respiratory difficulties. These drugs must be used with caution in women with hypertension, cardiovascular disease or hyperthyroidism. Side effects have been so prevalent and dangerous that in 2000, the FDA issued a public health advisory concerning phenylpropanolamine (PPA). The FDA requested that all drug companies discontinue marketing products containing PPA and PPA has now been removed from the market.

Ephedrine and its stereoisomer pseudoephedrine are sympathomimetic agents that increase the release of norepinephrine from sympathetic neurons and stimulate alpha- and beta-adrenergic receptors. Few studies exist to support the use of ephedrine. In a small study of 38 patients with sphincteric incontinence, 27 achieved a "good to excellent" result with ephedrine sulfate [28]. Continence was improved mostly in the patients who experienced mild SUI. Weil et al. showed no improvement in objective measurements of urinary function in a 1998 RCT of the alpha-1 agonist midodrine [29]. With these agents, tachyphylaxis may develop after prolonged use, perhaps due to depletion of norepinephrine stores.

Serotonin and norepinephrine reuptake inhibitors

Duloxetine is not available in the United States but is approved for the treatment of SUI elsewhere. Its mechanism of action is inhibition of serotonin (5-HT) and norepinephrine reuptake in Onuf's nucleus where the pudendal motor neurons are located in the spinal cord. Resultant higher levels of 5-HT and norepinephrine increase activity on a greater number of postsynaptic receptors, a greater activation of pudendal nerve motor neurons, and increased urethral sphincter tone. Duloxetine has shown little or no inhibition of dopamine reuptake or affinity for histaminergic, dopaminergic, adrenergic or cholinergic receptors; therefore, potentially it may produce few side effects. It has been shown to be beneficial, with relative risk of decreased incontinent episode frequency 1.24 vs placebo in a meta-analysis using data from a number of large trials

[30]. The largest of these studies included 3327 women and compared duloxetine to placebo with endpoints of subjective cure of SUI and results of pad tests. Duloxetine was significantly better than placebo in improving quality of life and perception of improvement. Incontinence frequency decreased by approximately 50%, but subjective cure had a much lower success rate, at 3% over placebo.

Recommendations

Randomized trial evidence refutes the claim that oral conjugated estrogens improve stress incontinence; in light of the side effects profile of these medications and absence of efficacy, we recommend against their use (Grade 2B recommendation) in patients in whom they are not otherwise indicated. There exists no high-level evidence to support the off-label use of imipramine or alpha-agonists for stress incontinence, though there are anecdotal reports of their efficacy. Again, in light of the side effects of these medications, especially in the age range of typical SUI patients, we conditionally recommend against their use as agents used to treat SUI in isolation (Grade 2C recommendation). Duloxetine has been shown in prospective, randomized studies to both decrease frequency of incontinent episodes and increase quality of life in patients with SUI. These effects are typically small and the chance for cure remote. As this medication is not approved by the FDA for this indication due to concerns about suicidal events and liver toxicity, the off-label use of duloxetine for SUI is recommended only in selected patients who are not surgical candidates or who do not desire surgery and after extensive counseling, including depression screening, and the formation of a care plan to cover adverse effects (Grade 2B). Where this medication is approved for SUI, our recommendations remain the same, with emphasis that it be used with counseling for patients on realistic expectations.

Clinical question 20.3

What are the efficacy and side effects profiles of the anticholinergic class of drugs in premenopausal versus postmenopausal adult women?

Literature search

Evidence for this question was obtained in a similar manner to that of the previous sections, starting with a Medline search using the keywords: "anticholinergic," "detrusor overactivity," "side effects," "urge incontinence," "oxybutynin," "tolterodine," "trospium," "darifenacin" and "solifenacin." The references of these papers were used to broaden the search. Texts and meta-analysis clearing houses aided in the identification of further studies. Finally, practicing researchers and clinicians in the field were asked about studies they used to inform their own decision making.

The evidence

Anticholinergics are the standard of care for OAB and UUI treatment. The efficacy and side effects of this class of drugs have been well studied in multiple randomized placebo-controlled studies and in subsequent meta-analyses. Studies on individual anticholinergics consistently show statistically significant improvement versus placebo, both in subjective measures such as perception of cure and objective measures such as maximum cystometric capacity [31].

Across all age groups, a 2003 meta-analysis found the relative risk of cure or improvement on OAB to be 1.41, the difference in number of leakage events per day was –0.58, the maximum cystometric capacity improved 54.34 and the bladder volume at first contraction increased 52.25 [32]. With respect to which anticholinergic is best in the general population, a 2007 Cochrane review concluded that there were no statistically significant differences for patient-perceived improvement but fewer withdrawals due to adverse events with tolterodine versus oxybutynin [33]. The same review found the rates of cure/improvement to be 44% for oxybutynin and 47% for tolterodine across all age groups.

A later 2008 review and meta-analysis concluded that extended-release anticholinergic formulations should be preferred to immediate-release formulations. More clinical studies are needed to indicate which of the drugs should be used as first, second or third line [34]. Of note, many studies show a marked effect of placebo. This has been postulated to be a result of increased awareness and the therapeutic effect of keeping a bladder diary. Study effects of anticholinergics often seem small in comparison to what is seen clinically; it is worth noting that often medications are given in the clinic in combination with behavioral training, which has also been shown to be effective [13].

When looking specifically at older women aged 55–92, drug treatment with oxybutynin resulted in a 29.1% greater reduction in accidents than did placebo (68.5% reduction vs 39.4%) in a 1998 trial of 197 women. This same group of women had a smaller improvement in their perceptions of efficacy, with a 21.1% improvement over placebo in the percentage of patients who were "completely satisfied" (49.1% vs 28.0%) [13]. Another study of oxybutynin in 57 elderly women showed 31% more patients describing improvement versus placebo (86% vs 55%) [35]. When comparing efficacy in pre- versus postmenopausal women, younger women tend to have better results, both objectively and subjectively.

Side effects of anticholinergic medications include dry mouth, inability to void, constipation, blurred vision and confusion; dry mouth is the most common. Across all age groups studied, the relative risk of having dry mouth was 2.56 with anticholinergics versus placebo; when trials of exclusively elderly patients were removed from this meta-analysis, the relative risk rose to 2.88 [32]. In the elderly, dry mouth was also the most common side effect but the difference in risk between placebo and treatment was smaller than in the general population, as addressed below. In one trial, 96.9% of elderly women taking oxybutynin experienced dry mouth compared to 54.8% of those taking placebo [35]. In older patients, rates of reported dry mouth are high even in the placebo groups; this is thought to be due to the polypharmacy and physiological changes that often accompany advanced age. This higher baseline makes the relative increase in rates of dry mouth (and indeed, all side effects) greater for a younger population. Practically, dry mouth is very common in all age groups treated with anticholinergics.

Urinary retention or inability to void was similarly increased in the older age groups in both the drug and placebo arms, 21.5% to 3.2%, respectively. Interestingly, blurred vision and confusion were seen at similar percentages in the drug and placebo arms, 15.4% to 9.7%. This result has the important caveats of small sample sizes and participant criteria that excluded those with dementia and so is not generalizable for all elderly patients, but it does suggest a more benign side effects profile in cognitively intact elderly patients with incontinence.

Other studies examining cognitive function and sleep while using anticholinergics have suggested that differential binding to the muscarinic receptor M1 subtype may be a determining factor for these drugs. A RCT in young, healthy volunteers showed that sleep architecture and random eye movement sleep were not affected by trospium or tolterodine and none of the drugs studied had significant differences in subjective or cognitive assays [36]. A 2008 meta-analysis of five RCTs also supports the use of M3 selective drugs, concluding that there is compelling evidence of cognitive impairment with oxybutynin whereas darifenacin stands out by demonstrating no impairment of memory or other cognitive functions [37]. Of note, this trial made conclusions only on oxybutynin and darifenacin, citing incomplete evidence to allow judgment on tolterodine, solifenacin and trospium [37].

Recommendations

The anticholinergics are well-studied and effective drugs in the treatment of urge incontinence, with multiple trials with Grade 1A evidence showing their efficacy in both increasing cure and decreasing incontinent episodes over placebo [32]. There is no strong evidence that one agent is more effective than another. Choice of individual agent should be tailored to the individual patient and may be best made based on side effects profile, dosing regimen and patient means. Cognitive effects of anticholinergics in both young and old patients need further study. It is unclear whether previous trials have been designed to adequately capture the effect of these drugs on the brain. These drugs should be used with caution and close monitoring in elderly and cognitively impaired patients until they are better studied in this patient population.

References

1. Nygaard I, Thom DH, Calhoun EA. Urinary incontinence in women. In: Litwin MS, Saigal CS (eds) *Urologic Diseases in America*. NIH Publication No. 07-5512 [157-191].Washington, DC: US Government Printing Office, 2007.

2. Kinchen KS, Burgio K, Diokno AC, et al. Factors associated with women's decisions to seek treatment for urinary incontinence. J Women's Health 2003;12:687-98.

3. Hunskaar S, Lose G, Sykes D, et al. The prevalence of urinary incontinence in women in four European countries. BJU Int 2004;93:324-30.

4. Thom DH, Nygaard IE, Calhoun EA. Urologic Diseases in America Project: urinary incontinence in women – national trends in hospitalization, office visits, treatment and economic impact. J Urol 2005;173:1295-301.

5. Fantl JA, Newman DK, Colling J, et al. *Urinary Incontinence in Adults: acute and chronic management. Clinical Practice Guideline No. 2, 1996 Update*. AHCPR Publication No. 96-0682. Rockville, MD: US Department of Health and Human Services, Public Health Service, Agency for Health Care Policy and Research, 1996.

6. Hunskaar S. A systematic review of overweight and obesity as risk factors and targets for clinical intervention for urinary incontinence in women. Neurourol Urodyn 2008;27(8):749-57.

7. Subak LL, Wing R, West DS, et al. Weight loss to treat urinary incontinence in overweight and obese women. N Engl J Med 2009;360:481-90.

8. Hashim H, Abrams P. How should patients with an overactive bladder manipulate their fluid intake? BJU Int 2008;102: 62-6.

9. Dowd TT, Campbell JM, Jones JA. Fluid intake and urinary incontinence in older community-dwelling women. J Commun Health Nurs 1996;13:179-86.

10. Swithinbank L, Hashim H, Abrams P. The effect of fluid intake on urinary symptoms in women. J Urol 2005;174:187-9

11. Shamliyan TA, Kane RL, Wyman J, et al. Systematic Review: randomized, controlled trials of nonsurgical treatments for urinary incontinence in women. Ann Intern Med 2008;148: 459-73.

12. Hay-Smith EJ, Dumoulin C. Pelvic floor muscle training vs no treatment, or inactive control treatments for urinary incontinence in women. Cochrane Database Syst Rev 2006;1:CD005654.

13. Burgio KL, Locher JL, Goode PS, et al. Behavioral versus drug treatment for urge incontinence in older women: a randomized controlled trial. JAMA 1998;280(23):1995-2000.

14. Burgio KL, Goode PS, Locher JL, et al. Predictors of outcome in the behavioral treatment of urinary incontinence in women. Obstet Gynecol 2003;102:940-7.

15. Kinn AC, Lindskog M. Oestrogens and phenylpropanolamine in combination for stress incontinence. Urology 1988;32:273-80.

16. Matsubara S, Okada H, Shirakawa GA, et al. Oestrogen levels influence beta-3-adrenoreceptor mediated relaxation of the female rat detrusor muscle. Urology 2002;59:621-5.

17. Smith PJB. The effect of oestrogens on bladder function in the female. In: Campbell S (ed) *The Management of the Menopause and Postmenopausal Years*. Carnforth: MTP, 1976: 291-8.

18. Moeher B, Hextall A, Jackson S. Oestrogens for urinary incontinence in women. Cochrane review. In: Cochrane Library, Issue 3. Oxford: Update Software.

19. Hextall A. Oestrogens and lower urinary tract functions. Maturitas 2002;36:83-7.

20. Grady D, Brown JS, Vittinghoff E, et al. Postmenopausal hormones and incontinence: the heart and estrogen/progestin replacement study. Obstet Gynecol 2001;97:116-20.

21. Hendrix SL, Cochrane BB, Nygaard IE, et al. Effects of estrogen with and without progestin in urinary incontinence. JAMA 2005;293:935-48.

22. Khanna OP, Heber D, Gonick P. Cholinergic and adrenergic neuroreceptors in urinary tract of female dogs: evaluation of function with pharmaco-dynamics. Urology 1975;5:616-23.

23. Hunsballe JM, Djurhuus JC. Clinical options for imipramine in the management of urinary incontinence. Urol Res 2001;29: 118-25.

24. Gilja I, Radej M, Kovacic M, et al. Conservative treatment of female stress incontinence with imipramine. J Urol 1984;132:909-11.

25. Lin HH, Sheu BC, Lo MC, et al. Comparison of treatment outcomes for imipramine for female genuine stress incontinence. Br J Obstet Gynaecol 1999;106:1089-92.

26. Frazer A. Pharmacology of antidepressants. J Clin Psychopharmacol 1997;17:2S-18S.

27. Viktrup L, Bump RC. Pharmacological agents used for the treatment of stress urinary incontinence in women. Curr Med Res Opin 2003;19:485-90.

28. Diokno A, Taub M. Ephedrine in treatment of urinary incontinence. Urology 1975;5:624-7.

29. Weil EH, Eerdmans PH, Dijkman GA, et al. Randomized double-blind placebo-controlled multicenter evaluation of efficacy and dose finding of midodrine hydrochloride in women with mild to moderate stress urinary incontinence: a phase II study. Int Urogynecol J Pelvic Floor Dysfunct 1998;9(3):145-50.

30. Latthe PM, Foon R, Khan K. Nonsurgical treatment of stress urinary incontinence (SUI): grading of evidence in systematic reviews. Br J Obstet Gynaecol 2008;115(4):435-44.

31. Dmochowski RR, Miklos JR, Norton PA, et al. Duloxetine versus placebo for the treatment of North American women with stress urinary incontinence. J Urol 2003;170(4):1259-63.

32. Herbison P, Hay-Smith J, Ellis G, et al. Effectiveness of anticholinergic drugs compared with placebo in the treatment of overactive bladder: systematic review. BMJ 2003;326(7394): 841-4.

33. Sand P, Zinner N, Newman D, et al. Oxybutynin transdermal system improves the quality of life in adults with overactive bladder: a multicentre, community-based, randomized study. BJU Int 2007;99(4):836-44.

34. Novara G, Galfano A, Secco S, et al. A systematic review and meta-analysis of randomized controlled trials with antimuscarinic drugs for overactive bladder. Eur Urol 2008;54(4): 740-63.

35. Szonyi G, Collas DM, Ding YY, et al. Oxybutynin with bladder retraining for detrusor instability in elderly people: a randomized controlled trial. Age Ageing 1995;24(4):287-91.

36. Diefenbach K, Donath F, Maurer A, et al. Randomised, double-blind study of the effects of oxybutynin, tolterodine, trospium chloride and placebo on sleep in healthy young volunteers. Clin Drug Invest 2003;23(6):395-404.

37. Kay GG, Ebinger U. Preserving cognitive function for patients with overactive bladder: evidence for a differential effect with darifenacin. Int J Clin Pract 2008;62(11):1792-800.

21 Surgical treatment of female urinary incontinence

Alexander Gomelsky[1] and Roger R. Dmochowski[2]

[1]Department of Clinical Urology, Louisiana State University Health Sciences Center, Shreveport, LA, USA
[2]Department of Urologic Surgery, Vanderbilt Medical Center, Nashville, TN, USA

Background

Stress urinary incontinence (SUI) is defined by the International Continence Society as the involuntary loss of urine through an intact urethra in response to a sudden increase in intra-abdominal pressure, in the absence of a detrusor contraction or an overdistended bladder [1]. While the pathophysiological mechanism responsible for SUI is complex and incompletely understood, it is accepted that continence depends on the interaction of urethral and bladder neck support, intrinsic urethral properties, urethral sphincter mechanism, and pelvic floor musculature. At rest, a "mucosal" seal composed of submucosal connective tissue and luminal secretions from the periurethral glands compresses mucosal urethral folds to create a watertight closure. During stress maneuvers, a reflex contraction of the levator ani musculature and urogenital diaphragm elevates suburethral supporting tissue and compresses the proximal urethra ("hammock hypothesis") [2]. Additionally, the urethropelvic ligaments augment the muscular closure of the pelvic floor by enveloping the proximal urethra and bladder neck medially and inserting laterally onto the arcus tendineus fascia pelvis. Furthermore, striated muscles in the urethrovaginal sphincter and compressor urethrae compress the urethra during stress maneuvers. The net effect of these changes is equal transmission of abdominal pressure to the bladder and urethra, leading to increased outlet resistance and continence. Conversely, in women with loss of anatomic support, the proximal urethra descends during stress maneuvers and rotates out of the pelvis.

A novel continence mechanism proposed by Petros & Ulmsten suggested that the mid-urethra, rather than the bladder neck, may be the linchpin for urinary continence [3]. Their "integral theory" proposed that contraction of the pubococcygeus pulls the anterior vaginal wall forward and closes off the urethra during an increase in intra-abdominal pressure. This response is contingent on an intact attachment between the anterior vaginal wall and the pubourethral ligaments, which act as a fulcrum at the mid-urethra. Laxity in the pubourethral ligaments contributes to incontinence during increases in intra-abdominal pressure.

The purpose of anti-incontinence surgery is to prevent involuntary urine loss during periods of increased intra-abdominal pressure. Procedures can be broadly divided into several classes, based on the mechanism they address. Buttress operations, such as anterior colporrhaphy, support the urethrovesical junction by plicating the pubocervical fascia. Bladder neck suspensions (retropubic (RBNS) and transvaginal needle suspensions (TNS)) provide support by suspending and elevating lateral periurethral tissues. Slings placed at the bladder neck (pubovaginal sling: PVS) not only replace and augment normal lateral urethral support structures, but also buttress the bladder neck to prevent descent and funneling during stress maneuvers. Mid-urethral slings (MUS; retropubic (RP) and transobturator (TO)) support the mid-urethra in a tension-free fashion to prevent SUI. Finally, urethral bulking procedures augment the "mucosal seal" mechanism to aid in apposition of the urethra in a watertight fashion.

The purpose of this chapter is to review the available evidence regarding the efficacy of surgical treatment options for female SUI. The specific procedures and materials compared in this chapter are summarized in Table 21.1. Due to length constraints, neither a comparison of perioperative morbidity and treatment side effects, nor an assessment of the cost-effectiveness of a particular procedure has been included. Grading of the quality of evidence and strengths of recommendations in this chapter are based on the guidelines proposed by the international

Evidence-Based Urology. Edited by Philipp Dahm, Roger R. Dmochowski.
© 2010 Blackwell Publishing.

Table 21.1 Procedures for female SUI included in this chapter

Procedure		
Buttress procedures	Anterior colporrhaphy (AR)	
Retropubic suspensions (RBNS)	Burch colposuspension	
	Marshall–Marchetti–Krantz (MMK)	
	Laparoscopic colposuspension (lap RBNS)	
Transvaginal needle suspensions (TNS)	Raz, Stamey, Gittes, Pereyra	
Pubovaginal (bladder neck) slings (PVS)	Autologous	Rectus fascia (ARF)
		Fascia fata (AFL)
	Allograft	Cadaveric fascia lata (CFL)
	Xenograft	Porcine dermis (PD)
	Synthetic	
Mid-urethral slings (MUS)		
Retropubic (RP)	Tension-free vaginal tape (TVT)	Gynecare, Ethicon
	SPARC	AMS
	Intravaginal slingplasty (IVS)	Tyco Healthcare
Transobturator (TO)	TVT-obturator (TVT-O)	Gynecare, Ethicon
	Monarc	AMS
Bulking agents	Autologous fat cells	
	Bovine collagen (Contigen)	Bard
	Carbon-coated zirconium beads (Durasphere)	Coloplast
	Silicone (Macroplastique)	Uroplasty Inc.
	Calcium hydroxyapatite (Coaptite)	Bioform Medical
	Porcine dermal collagen (Permacol)	Tissue Science Laboratories

Grading of Recommendations, Assessment, Development, and Evaluation Working Group (Grade) [4].

Literature search

Potentially relevant studies were identified by a computerized search of the Medline electronic database (PubMed, 1966–2008). Relevant text and keywords were: incontinence OR stress urinary incontinence OR female incontinence, AND randomized controlled trial OR controlled trial OR meta-analysis. The search was limited to the English-language literature. Several recently updated Cochrane reviews represented a starting point for the evidence-based evaluation of the treatment of female SUI. In their assessment, relevant studies were identified from a register of controlled trials gathered from Medline, CINAHL, the Cochrane Central Register of Controlled Trials, and hand-searching of journals and conference proceedings. Details regarding review methods, including identification of primary studies, quality assessments, and data extraction, are described in each Cochrane review. The findings in the Cochrane reviews were augmented by additional meta-analyses and randomized controlled trials

(RCTs) located by a hand-search of the Medline database by the authors.

Despite RCTs and meta-analyses of RCTs representing the highest level of evidence, interpretation of these types of trials poses some challenges. First, lack of blinding procedures is common in the surgical literature and may not be practical in many trials. Second, randomization procedures may be inappropriate or simply not described. Third, outcome measures, such as nonvalidated questionnaires, may not be appropriate. Fourth, short-term follow-up periods may not be representative of durable, long-term cure rates. Fifth, significant heterogeneity may exist between trials, contributing to wide confidence intervals (CI) (95% CI). Additionally, dropout or failure-to-follow-up rates may be substantial in some trials. Furthermore, many trials are small and underpowered to detect a significant difference between two treatment arms.

Stress urinary incontinence literature presents additional unique challenges during interpretation. First, patient populations may be different between trials. Women may present with SUI only or with mixed (urge and stress) incontinence. Some women may have also undergone previous anti-incontinence surgery or have pelvic organ prolapse (POP) eligible for concomitant repair. Second, the type of SUI may be different, as well. Women may have the symptoms of SUI based on clinical evaluation alone or urodynamic stress incontinence. Additionally, some women may have "occult" SUI, which is diagnosed only after concomitant POP has been reduced. Third, extensive procedural variations may exist even for established surgeries, making a meta-analysis difficult. Fourth, the generalizability of the results of a particular operation may be brought into question, as the results of many trials represent the experience of a single surgeon or single institution. Additionally, the follow-up period may be variable. For the purpose of this chapter, follow-up periods are defined as short term (< 12 months), medium term (12–60 months), and long term (> 60 months).

Perhaps the most difficult issue in evaluating SUI literature is a consistent definition of success or cure. Measures may be subjectively based on a woman's report or a validated questionnaire or objectively based on a voiding diary, pad tests, cough stress testing or urodynamics. At present, there is no consensus on which measures are vital to a trial's validity, but it is widely accepted that both subjective and objective outcomes should be reported. In some trials, definitions of success may include improved patients as well, while in some studies, cure of SUI may be at the expense of worsened postoperative urge incontinence or an increased incidence of obstructive symptoms and urinary retention. Unfortunately, issues germane to outcomes of anti-incontinence procedures, such as a review of perioperative complications, will not be addressed in this chapter due to space constraints.

Clinical question 21.1

What is the efficacy of anterior vaginal repair in the surgical treatment of female SUI?

The evidence

Buttressing procedures such as an anterior vaginal repair (AR) involve the plication of the pubocervical fascia in the midline. A Cochrane review (updated 28 February 2007) summarized the outcomes of 10 trials encompassing 1012 women, of whom 385 underwent AR [5]. All but one of the trials excluded women who had previously undergone anti-incontinence surgery, and one trial comparing 16 women after AR versus pelvic floor muscle training did not provide enough data for statistical analysis.

In eight trials comparing AR to RBNS, 353 of 627 women were randomized to RBNS. For statistical analysis, women undergoing a Marshall–Marchetti–Krantz procedure (MMK) in one study were combined with the remainder of women who underwent a Burch. Subjective failure rates were

lower for women undergoing RBNS at all follow-up periods: short term (10% vs 19%; relative risk (RR) 0.51, 95% CI 0.34–0.76), medium term (16% vs 36%; RR 0.43, 95% CI 0.32–0.57), and long term (28% vs 53%; RR 0.49, 95% CI 0.32–0.75). Likewise, objective cure rates were lower for women undergoing RBNS at all follow-up periods: short term (10% vs 25%; RR 0.41, 95% CI 0.27–0.63), medium term (19% vs 44%; RR 0.40, 95% CI 0.30–0.53), and long term (26% vs 54%; RR 0.48, 95% CI 0.31–0.73).

In six trials comparing AR with Burch in women with concomitant POP, women undergoing Burch had lower subjective failure rates than women undergoing AR, both in medium-term (RR 2.49, 95% CI 1.83–3.39) and long-term (RR 3.39, 95% CI 1.4–8.22) follow-up. More women who underwent AR (25 of 107, 23%) required repeat anti-incontinence surgery when compared with women undergoing Burch (4 of 164, 2%) (RR 8.87, 95% CI 3.28–23.94). In three trials, women undergoing AR (64 of 181, 35%) and TNS (50 of 156, 32%) had similar subjective incontinence rates after 1 year (RR for failure 1.16, 95% CI 0.86–1.56); however, these trials may have been underpowered to detect a statistical difference. There were no trials comparing AR with sham procedure, laparoscopic RBNS, PVS or MUS.

Clinical question 21.2

What is the efficacy of TNS in the surgical treatment of female SUI?

The evidence

In addition to the four principal TNS procedures (see Box 21.1), some surgeons have modified these operations by varying the site of initial approach (abdominal vs vaginal) and incorporating spacers or sheaths. A Cochrane database (updated 11 May 2008) included 10 trials encompassing 864 women, 375 of whom underwent one of six different TNS procedures [6]. In addition to the principal TNS, trials also included a Raz four-corner repair and a "modified" Raz procedure, where needle sutures were placed under direct vision [7]. A comparison of TNS with AR is included in Clinical Question 21.

There were no studies comparing TNS with a sham procedure or conservative intervention. In seven trials, TNS was compared with RBNS (five Burch, one obturator shelf repair, and one MMK) [6,8]. Of 570 women, 278 underwent RBNS. Fewer women did not achieve subjective cure after RBNS (10.8%) than after TNS (15.3%) in short-term follow-up (RR 0.66, 95% CI 0.42–1.03). A similar relationship was seen in medium-term (13.7% vs 22.7%; RR 0.56, 95% CI 0.39–0.81) and long-term (18.2% vs 56.7%; RR 0.32, 95% CI 0.15–0.71) follow-up. Likewise, fewer women did not achieve objective cure after RBNS than after TNS in short-term (8.7% vs 14.4%; RR 0.56, 95% CI 0.32–0.97), medium-term (12.9% vs 21%; RR 0.59, 95% CI 0.40–0.88), and long-term follow-up (18.2% vs 56.7%; RR 0.32, 95% CI 0.15–0.71) from a single trial. In three trials including only women who had not previously undergone an anti-incontinence surgery, fewer women failed after RBNS (23 of 190, 12%) than after TNS (57 of 218, 26%) in medium-term follow-up (RR 2.37, 95% CI 1.54–3.66). Four small trials that included some women who had previously undergone anti-incontinence surgery also revealed that more women failed after TNS (34 of 95, 36%) than after RBNS (24 of 107, 22%) (RR 1.61, 95% CI 1.04–2.49). A single comparison between TNS and PVS was underpowered to detect a statistical difference. One small trial compared a standard Raz suspension with a modified Raz procedure ("transvaginal Burch") [7]. While outcomes were similar, the trial was underpowered to detect a statistical difference.

Clinical question 21.3

What is the efficacy of RBNS in the surgical treatment of female SUI?

The evidence

Retropubic bladder neck suspensions have been evaluated extensively in a Cochrane database (updated 25 May 2005), encompassing 39 trials and 3301 women [8]. Dropout rates ranging from 1.3% to 28.4% have been reported in 19 of these trials. In two small trials, women undergoing RBNS had higher subjective (RR 0.24, 95% CI 0.08–0.71) and objective (RR 0.26, 95% CI 0.13–0.53) cure rates than women undergoing pelvic floor muscle training. A comparison of RBNS and AR is provided in Clinical Question 21.1, while a comparison of RBNS and TNS is in Clinical Question 21.2.

In the Cochrane review, RBNS was compared to sling procedures in 12 trials encompassing 945 women, of whom 454 underwent RBNS [8]. Seven trials compared RBNS to tension-free vaginal tape (TVT), while five trials included PVS constructed from different materials. In three of these trials with short-term follow-up (TVT, polytetrafluoroethylene (PTFE), and rectus fascia), there was no significant difference in subjective failure between RBNS and slings (RR 0.87, 95% CI 0.62–1.22). Likewise, in three different trials with medium-term follow-up (TVT (2) and lyophilized dura mater), there was no significant difference in subjective failure rates between RBNS and slings (RR 0.96, 95% CI 0.71–1.31). Objective failure rates between RBNS and slings were not significantly different in short-term (RR 1.19, 95% CI 0.79–1.78) and medium-term (RR 1.28, 95% CI 0.78–2.08) follow-up periods.

At present, two trials have reported long-term outcomes comparing Burch and slings [9,10]. In a small trial of 28 women, objective cure rates were 84.6% and 100%, for Burch and PTFE sling, respectively (p = 0.17) [9]. In a large, high-quality trial, Ward & Hilton reported no significant difference in objective cure of SUI between women undergoing TVT (58 of 72, 81%) and Burch (44 of 49, 90%) at 5-year follow-up [10]. In a recently published landmark RCT, investigators of the Urinary Incontinence Treatment Network evaluated 655 women who underwent either Burch or autologous rectus fascia (ARF) PVS [11]. At 24 months of follow-up, 520 women (79%) completed the outcome assessment. Overall success rates were significantly higher for women in the sling group (47% vs 38%), as were SUI-specific success rates (66% vs 49%). Results of a recent trial comparing TO-MUS and Burch revealed similar subjective and objective cure rates at 1 and 2 years of follow-up [12].

Ten trials compared RBNS with laparoscopic (lap) RBNS [8,13]. Within the 18-month follow-up period, subjective cure rates were 58–96% in the RBNS group and 62–100% in the lap RBNS group. There was a nonsignificant 5% lower relative subjective cure rate for lap RBNS (RR 0.95, 95% CI 0.90–1.00). The 18-month objective cure rate (as measured by pad testing) statistically favored women undergoing RBNS (RR 0.91, 95% CI 0.6–0.96). The analysis for objective cure rate in medium-term follow-up revealed no significant differences between lap RBNS and RBNS (RR 1.01, 95% CI 0.88–1.16). A recent meta-analysis by Tan et al. encompassing 16 studies and 1807 women revealed similar cure rates between these procedures at 2 years of follow-up [14].

A single trial compared surgery (including Burch) with periurethral injections [15]. In short-term follow-up, there was a 19.1% difference in terms of success rates favoring surgery; however, it was not possible to extract data pertaining to RBNS specifically. In two trials, women undergoing Burch (3 of 54, 5.5%) were less likely to fail subjectively than women undergoing MMK (8 of 51, 15.7%) in short-term (RR 0.35, 95% CI 0.10–1.26) and medium-term (9 of 94 (9.6%) vs 23 of 91 (25.3%); RR 0.38, 95% CI 0.18–0.76) follow-up. Objective failure rates at medium-term follow-up also statistically favored Burch procedure (14.9% vs 34.1%; RR 0.44, 95% CI 0.25–0.77). There were insufficient data to draw conclusions regarding the efficacy of Burch compared to a paravaginal repair in one small trial.

Lap RBNS has been evaluated in a Cochrane database (updated 31 October 2007) [13]. This procedure has the theoretical advantage of smaller incisions that may result in less postoperative discomfort and shorter convalescence. As with any new technology, laparoscopic procedures are associated with a learning curve and the loss of tactile feedback enjoyed with traditional open surgery. Most of the 22 eligible RCTs had less than 50 women in each arm and 11 studies reported dropout rates and lost-to-follow-up rates.

There were no studies comparing lap RBNS to no treatment, conservative management, sham surgery, AR, TNS, PVS or periurethral injection. A comparison of RBNS versus lap RBNS is presented above.

The Cochrane database isolated eight trials comparing lap RBNS with MUS [13]. Overall, there was no statistically significant difference in the reported subjective cure rates between lap RBNS and MUS within 18 months (RR 0.91, 95% CI 0.80–1.02). Objective cure rates (according to diary, pad testing or urodynamics) assessed in all but one study were higher for women after MUS when compared with lap RBNS using sutures (RR 0.92, 95% CI 0.85–0.99) and mesh (RR 0.66, 95% CI 0.51–0.86). The use of more sutures was associated with greater cure rates. Of note, a trial by Valpas et al. comparing lap RBNS and TVT reported a significant difference in favor of TVT in both objective (cough stress test) and subjective (King's Health Questionnaire) outcome measures [16]. This trial presented 1-year data and there was a lack of appropriate blinding procedures; however, randomization technique was appropriate and subjective and objective outcome criteria were used. The inclusion of data from two recent trials, one comparing lap RBNS with the suprapubic arch (SPARC) sling procedure and another comparing lap RBNS with TVT, did not change the conclusions of the analysis [17,18].

Clinical question 21.4

What is the efficacy of PVS in the surgical treatment of female SUI?

The evidence

Traditional PVS placed at the bladder neck have been evaluated in a Cochrane database (updated 25 May 2005) [19]. Thirteen trials including 760 women were identified, of whom 627 underwent PVS. Most trials were small and had short-term follow-up periods. There were no trials comparing PVS with AR or lap RBNS. In the single small trial comparing porcine dermis PVS with TNS, there were no differences in cure rates at 3 and 24 months [20]. Six trials comparing PVS with RBNS are reviewed in Clinical Question 21.3.

Five trials compared one type of PVS against an autologous PVS constructed from rectus fascia or fascia lata [19]. Failure rates were similar both in short-term and long-term follow-up. In their recent meta-analysis, Novara et al. identified five RCTs comparing PVS to TVT [21]. Two of these trials were from the same group at various follow-up periods. TVT and PVS showed similar continence rates, by any definition of continence (odds ratio (OR) 0.82, 95% CI OR 0.42–1.59; p = 0.55), and similar results were obtained when only autologous slings were considered (OR 1.03, 95% CI OR 0.42–2.55; p = 0.94). Further sensitivity analyses limited to RCTs with > 12 months of follow-up did not significantly change the conclusions.

Two additional trials comparing PVS with MUS have since been identified. In a trial randomizing 100 women to TVT and ARF PVS, 61 women completed 12-month follow-up [22]. There was no significant difference in objective cure rate between the two procedures. In the second trial, 139 women were randomized to cadaveric fascia lata (CFL) PVS or intravaginal slingplasty (IVS), a multifilament polypropylene MUS [23]. In short-term follow-up, the overall success rates of the two procedures were not statistically different. One additional trial randomized 81 women to receive a "full-length" autologous PVS and 84 women to undergo autologous "sling-on-a-string" [24]. At short-term and long-term follow-up, both techniques offered similar improvements in SUI.

Clinical Question 21.5

What is the efficacy of MUS in the surgical treatment of female SUI?

The evidence

To date, one multicenter prospective RCT has compared MUS to no treatment. Campeau et al. randomized women over 70 years of age to undergo immediate TVT or to wait 6 months to undergo the same surgery (control group) [25]. Although continence was not an endpoint, quality of life indices were significantly higher in the immediate surgery group. There are no comparisons of MUS with AR or TNS. The comparison of RBNS and lap RBNS with MUS is reviewed in Clinical Question 21.3. The comparison of PVS and MUS is reviewed in Clinical Question 21.4.

Although the results of the Cochrane database evaluating MUS outcomes are not yet mature, Novara et al. recently published a systematic review of RCTs after MUS surgery [21]. Most of the procedures have been compared with TVT, the original RP MUS. Three RCTs compared TVT to IVS. The IVS is a multifilament, polypropylene RP MUS possessing smaller pore size and greater rigidity than the TVT. Mainly due to the findings of a large, well-designed trial by Meschia et al. [26], women undergoing TVT had greater success rates by any definition of incontinence (OR 0.51, 95% CI OR 0.31–0.83; p = 0.007) and by a negative cough stress test (OR 0.47, 95% CI OR 0.28–0.82; p = 0.007). The subjective cure rates were similar (OR 0.63, 95% CI OR 0.37–1.09; p = 0.10). Further sensitivity analyses limited to RCTs with follow-up exceeding 12 months reconfirmed these results.

Four RCTs compared TVT to SPARC, a monofilament polypropylene RP MUS with characteristics similar to the TVT [21]. With regard to continence rates, TVT was better than SPARC in terms of subjective cure rate (OR 0.56, 95% CI OR 0.35–0.92; p = 0.02) and objective cure rates by multiple definitions (OR 0.53, 95% CI OR 0.34–0.82; p = 0.005). However, the comparison data were significantly influenced by the findings from a single study. [27] Lord et al. enrolled almost half of the analyzed patients and the women were evaluated at only 2 months of follow-up. If this RCT is excluded from analysis, only a nonstatistically significant trend in favor of TVT was identified considering objective cure rates (OR 0.41, 95% CI OR 0.14–1.14; p = 0.09).

Although the TO MUS is a relatively novel procedure, a number of RCTs have compared it with the RP MUS. A systematic review by Sung et al. revealed six RCTs and 11 cohort studies comparing the two types of procedures [28]. The authors found insufficient evidence in objective outcomes to support one approach over another. Likewise, there was no difference in subjective failure between the two approaches after pooling data from RCTs (pooled OR 0.85, 95% CI 0.38–1.92). A recent systematic review and meta-analysis by Latthe et al. reported that subjective cure for the inside-out TO technique (TVT-O; five RCTs) and outside-in TO technique (Monarc; six RCTs) at 2–12 months was not better than the TVT (OR 0.85, 95% CI 0.60–1.21) [29].

Novara et al. assessed 14 RCTs comparing various RP and TO MUS, with half of the trials comparing TVT and TVT-O [21]. Most of these studies suffered from inaccurate randomization and blinding procedures, were underpowered for most of their endpoints, had short-term follow-up, and some were published only in abstract form. Results reveal that women randomized to RP or TO MUS yielded similar postoperative objective (OR 0.81, 95% CI OR 0.53–1.24; p = 0.34), subjective (OR 0.98, 95% CI OR 0.65–1.48; p = 0.92), and overall (OR 0.91, 95% CI OR 0.41–2.00; p = 0.81) continence rates. If only studies available as full-text publications or with follow-up of at least 12 months were evaluated, the results were similar.

Since the aforementioned meta-analysis, seven additional RCTs totaling 1166 women have been published comparing RP and TO MUS [30-36]. Three of these trials are full-text versions of abstracts initially included in the Novara meta-analysis [34-36]. In six of the trials there was no significant difference in subjective or objective cure rates between RP and TO MUS. In the Araco et al. trial, women with intrinsic sphincter deficiency were significantly more likely to achieve cure after TVT than the TVT-O [30]. Three RCTs compared the TVT-O to the Monarc, revealing no significant difference in success rates at 4–12 months of follow-up [37-39].

Clinical question 21.6

What is the efficacy of urethral bulking therapy in the surgical treatment of female SUI?

The evidence

A Cochrane database (updated 21 May 2007) addressing the efficacy of periurethral bulking therapy included 12 trials and 1318 women [40]. Five of these trials were in abstract form and the available data were not suitable for meta-analysis. One study compared paraurethral injection of autologous fat with placebo injection of saline in 68 women [41]. At 3 months, six of 27 (22%) women reported cure or improvement compared to six of 29 (21%) women after saline injection (RR 0.98, 95% CI 0.75–1.29). There was a similar reduction in 1-hour pad weight for both groups.

Two trials compared bulking therapy with surgical therapy. In one trial, subjective complete satisfaction was not significantly different in women undergoing bulking therapy and surgery with Burch, PVS or TNS [15]. More women were cured in the surgery group objectively based on the pad weight test. In another trial, nine of 22 women (41%) were not satisfied after Macroplastique injections compared to four of 21 (19%) after PVS (NS; RR 2.15, 95% CI 0.78–5.92) [42]. When cure was defined as subjective incontinence occurring once or less per week, there was no statistically significant difference between the two therapies.

Eight trials compared one bulking agent to another. Lightner et al. reported that 76 of 115 women (66%) undergoing injection of Durasphere reported cure or improvement in their SUI compared to 79 of 120 (66%) women having injection of bovine collagen (NS; RR 0.99, 95% CI 0.70–1.42) [43]. Andersen reported a trend toward better outcomes after 1 year of treatment with Durasphere with regard to cure (40% vs 14.3%; RR 0.70, 95% CI 0.49–1.01) and improvement of symptoms (80% vs 61.9%; RR 0.53, 95% CI 0.20–1.36); however, the results were not statistically significant [44]. There was no significant difference in objective urine loss between the two groups in the first study, and there were no data on quantification of symptoms in the second study.

A meta-analysis of two trials revealed that 65 of 145 women (44.8%) reported being dry/cured following injection of Macroplastique, compared to 46 of 134 women (34.3%) injected with bovine collagen at 12 months of follow-up [40]. Analysis suggested a nonstatistically significant trend towards better outcomes after Macroplastique injections (RR 0.85, 95% CI 0.71–1.03). Also not statistically significant, 36 of 111 women (32.4%) had no improvement following Macroplastique, compared to 48 out of 108 women (44.4%) injected with collagen (RR 0.73, 95% CI 0.52–1.03). Urinary loss as measured by pad test decreased in both groups following treatment, but there were no significant differences found between the two groups at 1, 6 or 12 months of follow-up.

Calcium hydroxyapatite (Coaptite) was compared to bovine collagen in a large multicenter RCT [45]. At 12 months of follow-up, 83 of 131 women (63.4%) receiving Coaptite reported improvement of one Stamey grade or more, compared with 57 of 100 (57%) receiving bovine collagen injections (NS; p = 0.34). In another study, porcine dermal implant (Permacol) was compared with Macroplastique [46]. There was no significant difference in improvement using a validated questionnaire or an objective pad test. In addition, although not statistically significant, women who underwent transurethral injection may have a greater rate of improvement than those treated with a periurethral injection technique.

Comments and conclusions

Although there is a multitude of publications evaluating surgical options for female SUI, RCTs are relatively uncommon. Additionally, the quality of the RCTs may be questionable due to inadequate randomization or blinding, underpowering, and short follow-up periods. Despite these observations, several conclusions may be drawn from the RCT literature. The evidence supporting the use of AR for primary SUI in women is limited and, typically, of low quality. In medium-term follow-up, more women were subjectively continent after Burch procedure than after AR (83% vs 63%). TNS and AR appeared to have similar efficacy; however, these outcomes were based on three small trials and these studies may be underpowered to detect a significant difference. AR has not been compared to the procedures more commonly used today, such as PVS or MUS. Limited evidence indicates that TNS is less effective than RBNS, in women with both primary and secondary SUI.

Current evidence suggests that RBNS, especially the Burch colposuspension, is an effective treatment for SUI. Within the first year of treatment, the overall continence rate approaches 90%, and may be near 70% 5 years after treatment. The literature review revealed significantly better subjective and objective cure and improvement rates after RBNS compared to conservative management, AR, and TNS. Despite laparoscopy being a relatively novel technique, eight of the 10 trials comparing lap RBNS and RBNS were of good quality. Subjective outcomes between RBNS and lap RBNS are similar; however, objective cure rates may be lower in the laparoscopic group.

Although the number of RCTs involving bladder neck PVS is limited, most of the short- and medium-term

outcomes suggest that this therapy is as effective as RBNS and MUS. However, a recent, large, high-quality trial from the UITN has demonstrated significantly better success rates for the ARF PVS compared to the Burch. MUS appear to have similar efficacy in short- and medium-term follow-up when compared to the Burch. When compared with women undergoing lap RBNS, women undergoing MUS appear to have similar or better subjective cure rates and higher objective cure rates. Overall, both procedures were associated with good cure rates; however, owing to their novelty, there are few long-term results. The TVT is associated with better results than the IVS, and there is some evidence that the TVT may be associated with better results than the SPARC. However, the latter conclusion is based on a study with 2-month follow-up. At this time, the RP and TO approaches are associated with similar short- and medium-term outcomes, although women with more intact intrinsic urethral function may have better outcomes after RP MUS than TO MUS. At this time, the inside-out and outside-in TO approaches appear to yield similar results.

The trials of bulking therapy were typically small and generally of moderate quality. No clear conclusions can be drawn from trials comparing alternative agents. A single small trial suggested that periurethral injection technique may carry more risks than transurethral technique. Surgery provided greater symptomatic improvement; however, it may be associated with higher risks (not a focus of this chapter).

Implications for practice and recommendations

• There is no evidence to support the use of AR over RBNS, PVS or MUS in women with primary SUI (no recommendation can be made).
• There is no evidence to support the use of TNS over RBNS, PVS or MUS in women with primary SUI (no recommendation can be made).
• Open RBNS, specifically the Burch, is a successful procedure and should be considered for the treatment of SUI in women (Grade 1B: strong recommendation in support of the procedure, based on moderate-quality evidence and favorable risk/benefit profile).
• Laparoscopic RBNS (performed with more sutures) is as effective as RBNS in the short and medium term. Surgeon preference and experience should guide the choice of the approach (Grade 1B: strong recommendation in support of the procedure, based on moderate-quality evidence and favorable risk/benefit profile).
• Bladder neck autologous PVS may be more effective than RBNS for SUI in the medium term. No one type

of PVS is statistically better than another and there are numerous variations in surgical technique and materials. Porcine dermis PVS may be as effective as TVT in the medium term (**Grade 1B**: strong recommendation in support of the procedure, based on moderate-quality evidence and favorable risk/benefit profile).

• Although long-term data are lacking, MUS appear to be as effective as RBNS and may be associated with better objective results than lap RBNS. MUS appear to be as effective as PVS. RP MUS were associated with similar outcomes as TO MUS (**Grade 1C**: recommendation in support of the procedure, based on low-quality evidence and favorable risk/benefit profile).

• There are few data to support periurethral injection over other surgical approaches to SUI. This procedure may be acceptable as a first-line therapy in women who are not able to undergo a surgical intervention (no recommendation can be made).

Implications for research

As technology advances exponentially, well-designed RCTs are not just welcome in the comparison of surgical options for female SUI, they are vital to the future of our field. Blinding and randomization procedures should be standardized. Trials should be powered to detect a significant difference where one exists. Dropout rates and lost-to-follow-up rates should be minimized, and statistical analyses should report the status of these patients. Patients should undergo long-term follow-up to demonstrate the durability of a surgical procedure. To allow comparisons between trials, results should be represented by both subjective and objective standardized, validated, and simple outcome measures. Additionally, quality of life, psychological, and economic outcomes should be incorporated. More specifically, trials of surgical intervention for SUI should include information on perioperative morbidity, length of hospital stay, short- and long-term urinary retention rates, worsened or *de novo* urinary storage symptoms, and the need for additional surgery or intervention. Finally, multi-institutional efforts should be applauded and encouraged.

References

1. Abrams P, Cardozo L, Fall M, et al. Standardization of terminology of lower urinary tract function: report from the standardization sub-committee of the International Continence Society. Neurourol Urodyn 2002;21:167-78.
2. DeLancey JOL. Structural support of the urethra as it relates to stress urinary incontinence: the hammock hypothesis. Am J Obstet Gynecol 1994;170:1713-23.
3. Petros PE, Ulmsten U. An integral theory of female urinary incontinence. Acta Obstet Gynecol Scand 1990;69(suppl):7-31.
4. Guyatt GH, Oxman AD, Vist GE, et al. GRADE: what is "quality of evidence" and why is it important to clinicians? BMJ 2008;336:995-8.
5. Glazener CMA, Cooper K. Anterior vaginal repair for urinary incontinence in women. Cochrane Database Syst Rev 2001;1:CD001755.
6. Glazener CMA, Cooper K. Bladder neck needle suspension for urinary incontinence in women. Cochrane Database Syst Rev 2004;2:CD003636.
7. Gilja I, Puskar D, Mazuran B, et al. Comparative analysis of bladder neck suspension using Raz, Burch and transvaginal Burch procedures. A 3-year randomized prospective study. Eur Urol 1998;33:298-302.
8. Lapitan MC, Cody DJ, Grant AM. Open retropubic colposuspension for urinary incontinence in women. Cochrane Database Syst Rev 2005;3:CD002912.
9. Culligan PJ, Goldberg RP, Sand PK. A randomized controlled trial comparing a modified Burch procedure and a suburethral sling: long-term follow-up. Int Urogynecol J Pelvic Floor Dysfunct 2003;14:229-33.
10. Ward KL, Hilton P. Tension-free vaginal tape versus colposuspension for primary urodynamic stress incontinence: 5-year follow-up. Br J Obstet Gynaecol 2008;115:226-33.
11. Albo ME, Richter HE, Brubaker L, et al. Burch colposuspension versus fascial sling to reduce urinary stress incontinence. N Engl J Med 2007;356:2143-55.
12. Sivaslioglu AA, Caliskan E, Dolen I, et al. A randomized comparison of transobturator tape and Burch colposuspension in the treatment of female stress urinary incontinence. Int Urogynecol J Pelvic Floor Dysfunct 2007;18:1015-19.
13. Dean NM, Ellis G, Wilson PD, et al. Laparoscopic colposuspension for urinary incontinence in women. Cochrane Database Syst Rev 2006;3:CD002239.
14. Tan E, Tekkis PP, Cornish J, et al. Laparoscopic versus open colposuspension for urodynamic stress incontinence. Neurourol Urodyn 2007;26:158-69.
15. Corcos J, Collet JP, Shapiro S, et al. Multicenter randomized clinical trial comparing surgery and collagen injections for treatment of female stress urinary incontinence. Urology 2005;65:898-904.
16. Valpas A, Kivela A, Penttinen J, et al. Tension-free vaginal tape and laparoscopic mesh colposuspension for stress urinary incontinence. Obstet Gynecol 2004;104:42-9.
17. Foote AJ, Maughan V, Carne C. Laparoscopic colposuspension versus vaginal suburethral slingplasty: a randomised prospective trial. Aust NZ J Obstet Gynaecol 2006;46:517-20.
18. Jelovsek JE, Barber MD, Karram MM, et al. Randomised trial of laparoscopic Burch colposuspension versus tension-free vaginal tape: long-term follow up. Br J Obstet Gynaecol 2008;115:219-25.
19. Bezerra CA, Bruschini H, Cody DJ. Traditional suburethral sling operations for urinary incontinence in women. Cochrane Database Syst Rev 2005;3:CD001754.
20. Hilton P. A clinical and urodynamic study comparing the Stamey bladder neck suspension and suburethral sling procedures in the treatment of genuine stress incontinence. Br J Obstet Gynaecol 1989;96:213-20.

21. Novara G, Ficarra V, Boscolo-Berto R, et al. Tension-free midurethral slings in the treatment of female stress urinary incontinence: a systematic review and meta-analysis of randomized controlled trials of effectiveness. Eur Urol 2007;52:663-79.

22. Sharifiaghdas F, Mortazavi N. Tension-free vaginal tape and autologous rectus fascia pubovaginal sling for the treatment of urinary stress incontinence: a medium-term follow-up. Med Princ Pract 2008;17:209-14.

23. Basok EK, Yildirim A, Atsu N, et al. Cadaveric fascia lata versus intravaginal slingplasty for the pubovaginal sling: surgical outcome, overall success and patient satisfaction rates. Urol Int 2008;80:46-51.

24. Guerrero K, Watkins A, Emery S, et al. A randomised controlled trial comparing two autologous fascial sling techniques for the treatment of stress urinary incontinence in women: short, medium, and long-term follow-up. Int Urogynecol J Pelvic Floor Dysfunct 2007;18:1263-70.

25. Campeau L, Tu LM, Lemieux MC, et al. A multicenter, prospective, randomized clinical trial comparing tension-free vaginal tape surgery and no treatment for the management of stress urinary incontinence in elderly women. Neurourol Urodyn 2007;26:990-4.

26. Meschia M, Pifarotti P, Bernasconi F, et al. Tension-free vaginal tape (TVT) and intravaginal slingplasty (IVS) for stress urinary incontinence: a multicenter randomized trial. Am J Obstet Gynecol 2006;195:1338-42.

27. Lord HE, Taylor JD, Finn JC, et al. A randomized controlled equivalence trial of short-term complications and efficacy of tension-free vaginal tape and suprapubic urethral support sling for treating stress incontinence. BJU Int 2006;98:367-76.

28. Sung VW, Schleinitz MD, Rardin CR, et al. Comparison of retropubic versus transobturator approach to midurethral slings: a systematic review and meta-analysis. Am J Obstet Gynecol 2007;197:3-11.

29. Latthe PM, Foon R, Toozs-Hobson P. Transobturator and retropubic tape procedures in stress urinary incontinence: a systematic review and meta-analysis of effectiveness and complications. Br J Obstet Gynaecol 2007;114:522-31.

30. Araco F, Gravante G, Sorge R, et al. TVT-O vs TVT: a randomized trial in patients with different degrees of urinary stress incontinence. Int Urogynecol J Pelvic Floor Dysfunct 2008;19:917-26.

31. Wang AC, Lin YH, Tseng LH, et al. Prospective randomized comparison of transobturator suburethral sling (Monarc) vs suprapubic arc (Sparc) sling procedures for female urodynamic stress incontinence. Int Urogynecol J Pelvic Floor Dysfunct 2006;17:439-43.

32. Barber MD, Kleeman S, Karram MM, et al. Transobturator tape compared with tension-free vaginal tape for the treatment of stress urinary incontinence: a randomized controlled trial. Obstet Gynecol 2008;111:611-21.

33. Barry C, Lim YN, Muller R, et al. A multi-centre, randomised clinical control trial comparing the retropubic (RP) approach versus the transobturator approach (TO) for tension-free, suburethral sling treatment of urodynamic stress incontinence: the TORP study. Int Urogynecol J Pelvic Floor Dysfunct 2008;19:171-8.

34. Porena M, Constantini E, Frea B, et al. Tension-free vaginal tape versus transobturator tape as surgery for stress urinary incontinence: results of a multicentre randomised trial. Eur Urol 2007;52:1481-90.

35. Rinne K, Laurikainen E, Kivelä A, et al. A randomized trial comparing TVT with TVT-O: 12-month results. Int Urogynecol J Pelvic Floor Dysfunct 2008;19:1049-54.

36. Zhu L, Lang J, Hai N, et al. Comparing vaginal tape and transobturator tape for the treatment of mild and moderate stress incontinence. Int J Gynaecol Obstet 2007;99:14-17.

37. Debodinance P. Trans-obturator urethral sling for surgical correction of female stress urinary incontinence: outside-in (Monarc) versus inside-out (TVT-O). Are both ways safe? J Gynecol Obstet Biol Reprod 2006;35:571-7.

38. But I, Faganelj M. Complications and short-term results of two different transobturator techniques for surgical treatment of women with urinary incontinence: a randomized study. Int Urogynecol J Pelvic Floor Dysfunct 2008;19:857-61.

39. Liapis A, Bakas P, Creatsas G. Monarc vs TVT-O for the treatment of primary stress incontinence: a randomized study. Int Urogynecol J Pelvic Floor Dysfunct 2008;19:185-90.

40. Keegan PE, Atiemo K, Cody J, et al. Periurethral injection therapy for urinary incontinence in women. Cochrane Database Syst Rev 2007;3:CD003881.

41. Lee PE, Kung RC, Drutz HP. Periurethral autologous fat injection as treatment for female stress urinary incontinence: a randomized double-blind controlled trial. J Urol 2001;165:153-8.

42. Maher CF, O'Reilly BA, Dwyer PL, et al. Pubovaginal sling versus transurethral Macroplastique for stress urinary incontinence and intrinsic sphincter deficiency: a prospective randomised controlled trial. Br J Obstet Gynaecol 2005;112:797-801.

43. Lightner D, Calvosa C, Andersen R, et al. A new injectable bulking agent for treatment of stress urinary incontinence: results of a multicenter, randomized, controlled, double-blind study of Durasphere. Urology 2001;58:12-15.

44. Andersen RCM. Long-term follow-up comparison of Durasphere and Contigen in the treatment of stress urinary incontinence. J Lower Gen Tract Dis 2002;6:239-43.

45. Mayer RD, Dmochowski RR, Appell RA, et al. Multicenter prospective randomized 52-week trial of calcium hydroxyapatite versus bovine collagen for treatment of stress urinary incontinence. Urology 2007;69:876-80.

46. Bano F, Barrington JW, Dyer R. Comparison between porcine dermal implant (Permacol) and silicone injection (Macroplastique) for urodynamic stress incontinence. Int Urogyn J Pelvic Floor Dysfunct 2005;16:147-50.

22 Medical management of stone disease

Timothy Y. Tseng and Glenn M. Preminger

Comprehensive Kidney Stone Center, Division of Urologic Surgery, Duke University Medical Center, Durham, NC, USA

Background

The management of renal and ureteral calculi has most often been thought to be limited to surgical removal techniques. While there have been significant advances in the minimally invasive management of symptomatic calculi, equally impressive progress has been made in medical management of stone disease. The following chapter will highlight the medical management of ureteral calculi in the acute setting and the prevention of stone recurrences with medical management strategies in the long term.

Ureteral muscle spasm is thought to be one factor contributing to the impaction of ureteral stones. The physiology of ureteral smooth muscle is well studied. Numerous investigations have demonstrated that both alpha-adrenergic receptors and calcium channel antagonist binding sites exist in ureteral smooth muscle [1]. Inhibition of alpha-adrenergic receptors results in a decrease in basal tone, ureteral contractions, and ureteral peristalsis [2]. Inhibition of the voltage-dependent smooth muscle calcium channel results in a blunted rise in intracellular calcium ion concentrations during activation, leading to decreased electrical and contractile activity [3]. Because of their relatively low side effect profile, these drugs have been explored as a means to treat the ureteral spasm component of stone impaction.

Two recent meta-analyses have demonstrated statistically significant increases in spontaneous ureteral stone passage with the use of alpha-blockers and calcium channel blockers [4,5]. Many of the primary studies have also utilized corticosteroids concurrently in an effort to decrease ureteral edema and to enhance ureteral stone expulsion. In the first half of this chapter, the recent evidence supporting such medical expulsive therapy (MET) is reviewed.

Medical management strategies for the prevention of recurrent stone disease have been investigated for several decades. Several medications including thiazide diuretics, allopurinol, potassium citrate, acetohydroxamic acid, phosphate, and magnesium have been evaluated in randomized controlled trials (RCTs). Thiazide diuretics stimulate resorption of calcium with concomitant excretion of sodium in the distal nephron, thereby reducing urinary calcium concentration. As an inhibitor of xanthine oxidase, allopurinol decreases the conversion of xanthine and hypoxanthine to uric acid, which results in a decrease in urinary uric acid concentration. Alkali therapy with potassium citrate increases urinary pH which improves urinary saturation of calcium oxalate and uric acid. Additionally, alkali therapy results in an increase in urinary citrate, which is a known inhibitor of calcium stone formation. Acetohydroxamic acid is an urease inhibitor and is thought to inhibit stone formation due to chronic urea-splitting organisms [6]. A lack of proven efficacy of phosphate and magnesium treatments has led to a lack of use of these two medications in the current era and they are not reviewed [7]. The current evidence supporting preventive medical therapy for recurrent stone disease is reviewed in the second half of the chapter.

Clinical question 22.1

What is the effect of alpha-adrenergic antagonist therapy on expulsion of ureteral stones?

Literature search

A search of the PubMed electronic database using the terms "drug therapy" and "nephrolithiasis or urinary calculi" limited to the "clinical trial, randomized controlled trial, or comparative study" publication types found 13 unique randomized trials dealing with the use of an alpha-blocker for MET of ureteral stones. Similar searches of CINAHL and the Cochrane Central Register of Controlled Trials did not identify any additional published randomized studies. A search of the American Urological Association (AUA) online meeting abstracts from 2002 to 2008 and the European Association of Urology (EAU) online meeting abstracts from 2004 to 2008 identified an additional three unique unpublished RCTs. One additional unpublished RCT was identified from a meta-analysis by Hollingsworth et al. [4,8].

The evidence

Of the 17 randomized trials that used an alpha-adrenergic antagonist for MET of stones, 13 studies utilized tamsulosin, three studies used terazosin and doxazosin, and one study used alfuzosin (Table 22.1). All trials examined patients with distal ureteral stones that ranged in size up to 18 mm who had not been previously treated with shock-wave lithotripsy. Follow-up was performed between 7 days and 6 weeks. In all but one trial, the alpha-blocker was used as the initial treatment. The exception was one trial that studied the use of the alpha-blocker after previously failed MET.

There were 10 RCTs that compared the use of tamsulosin to no additional treatment for initial MET for distal ureteral stones. An additional two randomized trials compared the use of tamsulosin to historical antispasmodics. Spontaneous stone passage rates for tamsulosin as initial therapy in individual trials ranged from a low of 53% to a high of 100%, with the overall stone passage rate being 85%. Spontaneous stone passage rates for controls in these studies ranged from a low of 20% to a high of 73%, with the overall stone passage rate being 54%. The relative risk (RR) of stone passage for initial treatment with tamsulosin ranged from 1.18 to 2.67 with an overall relative risk of 1.51 (95% confidence interval (CI) 1.38–1.65) (all relative risk calculations were performed using RevMan 5.0 available at www.cc-ims.net/RevMan/). All but two trials demonstrated a statistically significant improvement in stone expulsion rates with tamsulosin. Mean/median time to stone passage ranged from 2.7 to 8.2 days versus 4.6 to 14.2 days for controls. Among those trials that examined analgesic usage, the majority demonstrated a statistically significant decrease in analgesic consumption with tamsulosin. Among the three trials that examined the number of pain/colic episodes, each showed a trend toward a decreased number of pain episodes with tamsulosin, but in only one trial was this difference statistically significant.

Porpiglia et al. studied the use of tamsulosin for 10 days after one previous failed 10-day cycle of tamsulosin as MET [9]. This trial demonstrated a RR of stone passage of 1.65 (95% CI 1.18–2.29), suggesting a statistically significant benefit to a secondary cycle of tamsulosin. There was,

however, no statistical benefit in terms of the number of colic episodes and diclofenac usage with a second cycle of tamsulosin. Furthermore, the first failed cycle of tamsulosin was generally shorter than the follow-up in most studies, suggesting that a longer initial cycle of tamsulosin would have been beneficial. Erturhan et al. further studied the addition of tolterodine to tamsulosin for MET and found no statistical benefit over tamsulosin alone with regard to stone passage rate, time to stone passage, analgesic usage, and hospitalization rate, suggesting that anticholinergic usage is not beneficial [10].

Three RCTs studied the use of doxazosin as initial MET for distal ureteral stones. Spontaneous stone passage rates with doxazosin ranged from 76% to 93%, with the overall stone passage rate being 82%. Spontaneous stone passage rates for controls in these studies ranged from 52% to 61%, with an overall stone passage rate of 56%. The RR for stone passage with doxazosin ranged from 1.42 to 1.52, with an overall RR of 1.49 (95% CI 1.21–1.83). Liatsikos et al. distinguished the use of doxazosin with stones ≤ 5 mm and those 6–10 mm in size [11]. There was no statistical difference in either group when compared to controls. However, a combined analysis did demonstrate a statistically significant benefit with doxazosin. Time to stone passage was decreased with the use of doxazosin in all three studies. Yilmaz et al. also demonstrated a decreased number of pain episodes and diminished analgesic usage with doxazosin [12].

Three RCTs studied the use of terazosin as initial MET. Spontaneous stone passage rates were 78–79% with terazosin and 44–54% for controls. The RR for stone passage with terazosin ranged from 1.42 to 1.78, with only the unpublished trial by Tekin et al. demonstrating a statistically significant benefit [13]. When combined, the RR for stone passage across all three trials was 1.56 (95% CI 1.25–1.95). Mean time to stone passage ranged from 5.8 to 6.3 days for terazosin compared to 10.1 to 10.5 days for controls. The number of pain episodes also appeared to be improved with terazosin.

The RCT by Pedro et al. examined the use of alfuzosin as initial MET and found no statistical benefit in terms of spontaneous stone passage or opioid usage [14]. However, there was a statistically significant decrease in time to stone passage with alfuzosin.

Comment

The quality of the evidence for initial MET for distal ureteral stones using alpha-adrenergic antagonists is relatively high. The evidence strongly suggests that such agents are well tolerated and can significantly improve spontaneous stone passage rates, time to stone passage, and analgesic usage. The evidence is less compelling regarding decreasing the number of pain/colic episodes. The majority of

Table 22.1 Effect of alpha-adrenergic antagonists on ureteral stone passage

Authors	Methods*	Intervention	Participants	Outcomes	Results	Notes
Cervenakov et al. [33]	• RCT • Distal ureteral stones 1–10 mm • FU: 7-day inpatient monitoring	NSAIDs and benzodiazepines ± tamsulosin	• Tamsulosin – 51 pts • Control – 53 pts	• Spontaneous stone passage	• RR stone passage 1.28 (95% CI 1.00–1.65)	• All inpatient • 2 control pts excluded due to pyelonephritis
Dellabella et al. [34]	• Randomized trial • Distal ureteral stones 3.8–13 mm, colic lasting ≦1 day • FU: 28 days	NSAIDs and glucocorticoid ± tamsulosin or FGTMB	• Tamsulosin – 30 pts • FGTMB – 30 pts	• Spontaneous stone passage • Time to stone passage • Diclofenac usage	• RR stone passage tamsulosin vs FGTMB 1.42 (95% CI 1.12–1.80) • Mean time to expulsion 66 h (tamsulosin), 111 h (FGTMB), p=0.020 • Mean diclofenac injections 0.1 (tamsulosin), 2.8 (FGTMB), p<0.001	• Single blind
Porpiglia et al. [35]	• RCT • Distal ureteral stones 3–10 mm • FU: 4 weeks	NSAIDs and glucocorticoid ± nifedipine or tamsulosin	• Tamsulosin – 28 pts • Nifedipine – 30 pts • Control – 28 pts	• Spontaneous stone passage • Time to stone passage • Diclofenac usage	• RR stone passage vs control 2.00 (95% CI 1.27–3.15) (tamsulosin), 1.87 (95% CI 1.17–2.97) (nifedipine) • Mean time to expulsion 7.9 days (tamsulosin), 9.3 days (nifedipine), 12 days (control) • Mean diclofenac usage 26 mg (tamsulosin), 19.5 mg (nifedipine), 105 mg (control)	• 1 pt each in nifedipine and tamsulosin groups discontinued treatment due to side effects
Kupeli et al. [36]	• RCT • Distal ureteral stones <5 mm • FU: 15 days	NSAIDs ± tamsulosin	• Tamsulosin – 15 pts • Control – 15 pts	• Spontaneous stone passage	• RR stone passage 2.67 (95% CI 0.87–8.15)	• Small sample sizes • Differences in stone passage rates not statistically significant
Resim et al. [37]	• RCT • Distal ureteral stones 5–13 mm • FU: 6 weeks	NSAIDs ± tamsulosin	• Tamsulosin – 30 pts • Control – 30 pts	• Spontaneous stone passage • No. of colic episodes • Severity of colic episodes using visual analog scale	• RR stone passage 1.18 (95% CI 0.91–1.53) • Mean no. colic episodes 2.0 (tamsulosin), 2.6 (control), p=0.038 • Severity of colic episodes by visual analog scale 5.7 (tamsulosin), 8.3 (control), p<0.001	• Differences in stone passage rates not statistically significant
Autorino et al. [38]	• RCT • Distal ureteral stones 3–10 mm • FU: 14 days	NSAIDs ± tamsulosin	• Tamsulosin – 32 pts • Control – 32 pts	• Spontaneous stone passage • Time to stone passage • Need for additional analgesics • Need for hospitalization	• RR stone passage 1.47 (95% CI 1.08–2.02) • Mean time to stone passage 4.8 days (tamsulosin), 7.4 days (control), p=0.005 • Need for additional analgesics 9% (tamsulosin), 31% (control), p=0.003 • Need for hospitalization 9% (tamsulosin), 21% (control), p=0.01	

(Continued on p. 198)

Table 22.1 (Continued)

Authors	Methods*	Intervention	Participants	Outcomes	Results	Notes
Yilmaz et al. [12]	• RCT • Distal ureteral stones ≤10 mm • FU: 1 month	NSAIDs ± tamsulosin, terazosin or doxazosin	• Tamsulosin – 29 pts • Terazosin – 28 pts • Doxazosin – 29 pts • Control – 28 pts	• Spontaneous stone passage • Time to stone passage • No. pain episodes • Analgesic use	• RR stone passage vs control 1.48 (95% CI 1.00–2.19) (tamsulosin), 1.47 (95% CI 0.99–2.18) (terazosin), 1.42 (95% CI 0.95–2.12) (doxazosin), 1.45 (95% CI 1.01–2.09) (combined) • Mean time to stone passage 6.3 days (tamsulosin), 5.8 days (terazosin), 5.9 days (doxazosin), 10.5 days (control) • No. pain episodes 1.7 (tamsulosin), 1.6 (terazosin), 1.7 (doxazosin), 2.4 (control) • Mean analgesic usage 129 mg (tamsulosin), 118 mg (terazosin), 119 mg (doxazosin), 182 mg (control)	• Differences in stone passage rates not statistically significant for individual alpha-blockers
Dellabella et al. [39]	• Randomized trial • Distal ureteral stones 4–18 mm, colic lasting ≤1 day • FU: 28 days	NSAIDs ± tamsulosin, nifedipine or phloroglucinol	• Tamsulosin – 70 pts • Nifedipine – 70 pts • Phloroglucinol – 70 pts	• Spontaneous stone passage • Time to stone passage • Diclofenac usage • Need for hospitalization • No. workdays lost	• RR stone passage vs phloroglucinol 1.51 (95% CI 1.26–1.81) (tamsulosin), 1.20 (95% CI 0.97–1.49) (nifedipine) • Median time to stone passage 72 h (tamsulosin), 120 h (nifedipine), 120 h (phloroglucinol), p<0.001 • Median no. PRN diclofenac vials used 0 (tamsulosin), 1 (nifedipine), 2 (phloroglucinol), p<0.001 • Need for urgent hospitalization 0% (tamsulosin), 4% (nifedipine), 16% (phloroglucinol), p=0.001 • Need for delayed hospitalization 1.4% (tamsulosin), 16% (nifedipine), 19% (phloroglucinol), p=0.004 • Median workdays lost 2 (tamsulosin), 3 (nifedipine), 5 (phloroglucinol), p<0.001	
De Sio et al. [40]	• RCT • Distal ureteral stones ≤10 mm • FU: 2 weeks	NSAIDs ± tamsulosin	• Tamsulosin – 50 pts • Control – 46 pts	• Spontaneous stone passage • Time to stone passage • Analgesic usage • Need for hospitalization • Adverse reactions	• RR stone passage 1.53 (95% CI 1.18–1.99) • Mean time to stone passage 4.4 days (tamsulosin), 7.5 days (control), p=0.005 • Analgesic use 10% (tamsulosin), 37% (control), p=0.003 • Need for hospitalization 10% (tamsulosin), 28% (control), p=0.01 • Adverse reactions 6% (tamsulosin), 4% (control), p=0.05	• Analgesic use not defined • No adverse reactions resulted in discontinuation of treatment regimen

Study	Design	Groups	Outcomes	Results	Comments
Erturhan et al. [10]	• RCT • Distal ureteral stones 4–10 mm • FU: 3 weeks	NSAIDs ± tamsulosin ± tolterodine	• Tamsulosin – 30 pts • Tamsulosin and tolterodine – 30 pts • Tolterodine – 30 pts • Control – 30 pts	• Spontaneous stone passage • Time to stone passage • Analgesic use • Need for hospitalization	• RR stone passage tamsulosin vs control 1.83 (95% CI 1.12–2.99) • RR stone passage tamsulosin + tolterodine vs control 1.75 (95% CI 1.06–2.88) • Mean time to stone passage 6.4 days (tamsulosin), 7.5 days (tamsulosin + tolterodine), 11.4 days (tolterodine), 12.2 days (control) • Mean daily analgesic use 40 mg (tamsulosin), 55 mg (tamsulosin + tolterodine), 120 mg (tolterodine), 155 mg (control) • Hospitalization 3% (tamsulosin), 0% (tamsulosin + tolterodine), 7% (tolterodine), 7% (control)	• Addition of tolterodine does not confer an advantage over tamsulosin alone • 4 pts did not complete the study due to severe colic, obstruction, and fever
Liatsikos et al. [11]	• RCT • Distal ureteral stones ≤5 mm and 6–10 mm, colic <1 day • FU: 4 weeks	± Doxazosin	• Doxazosin ≤5 mm – 20 pts • Doxazosin 6–10 mm – 22 pts • Control ≤5 mm – 15 pts • Control 6–10 mm – 16 pts	• Spontaneous stone passage • Time to stone passage	• RR stone passage, stones ≤5 mm, 1.42 (95% CI 0.90–2.23) • RR stone passage, stones 6–10 mm, 1.66 (95% CI 0.90–3.06) • RR stone passage, overall, 1.52 (95% CI 1.05–2.22) • Mean time to stone passage 7.6 days (doxazosin ≤5 mm), 7.1 days (doxazosin 6–10 mm), 8.8 days (control ≤5 mm), 12.1 days (control 6–10 mm)	• Small sample sizes • Unblinded • Randomization based on date of presentation with increased allocation to intervention arms • Relative risk of stone passage not statistically significant in original subset analysis
Pedro et al. [11]	• RCT • Distal ureteral stones <8 mm • FU: 4 weeks	± Alfuzosin	• Alfuzosin – 34 pts • Placebo – 35 pts	• Spontaneous stone passage • Time to stone passage • Need for opioid analgesics	• RR stone passage 0.95 (95% CI 0.73–1.25) • Mean time to stone passage 5.2 days (alfuzosin), 8.5 days (placebo), p=0.003 • Morphine equivalents consumed 7.6 (alfuzosin), 8.4 (placebo), p=0.83	• Differences in stone passage rates and opioid usage not statistically significant • 7 pts did not complete study
Wang et al. [41]	• RCT • Distal ureteral stones <10 mm • FU: 2 weeks	NSAIDs ± tamsulosin or terazosin	• Tamsulosin – 32 pts • Terazosin – 32 pts • Control – 31 pts	• Spontaneous stone passage • Time to stone passage • No. colic episodes	• RR stone passage vs control 1.48 (95% CI 1.03–2.12) (tamsulosin), 1.42 (95% CI 0.99–2.06) (terazosin), 1.45 (95% CI 1.03–2.05) (combined) • Mean time to stone passage 6.3 days (tamsulosin), 6.3 days (terazosin), 10.1 days (control), p<0.001 • No. colic episodes 1.97 (tamsulosin), 1.84 (terazosin), 2.16 (control), p>0.05	• Differences in stone passage rates not statistically significant for terazosin

(Continued on p. 200)

Table 22.1 (Continued)

Authors	Methods*	Intervention	Participants	Outcomes	Results	Notes
Tekin et al. [13]	• RCT • Distal ureteral stones 5–15 mm • FU: 4 weeks	± Terazosin	• Terazosin – 36 pts • Control – 39 pts	• Spontaneous stone passage	• RR stone passage 1.78 (95% CI 1.20–2.66)	• Unpublished meeting abstract
Taghavi et al. [8]	• RCT • Distal ureteral stones <10 mm • FU: not stated	± Tamsulosin or nifedipine	• Tamsulosin – 20 pts • Nifedipine – 20 pts • Control – 24 pts	• Spontaneous stone passage • Time to stone passage	• RR stone passage vs control 1.96 (95% CI 1.24–3.11) (tamsulosin), 1.64 (95% CI 0.99–2.71) (nifedipine) • Mean time to stone passage 8.2 days (tamsulosin), 10 days (nifedipine), 14.2 days (control)	• Unpublished meeting abstract
Ayubov et al. [42]	• RCT • Distal ureteral stones, size unspecified • FU: 4 weeks	NSAIDs ± doxazosin	• Doxazosin – 30 pts • Control – 31 pts	• Spontaneous stone passage • Time to stone passage • Diclofenac usage	• RR stone passage 1.52 (95% CI 1.13–2.05) • Mean time to stone passage 5.4 days (doxazosin), 8.4 days (control), p<0.001 • Mean diclofenac usage 80 mg (doxazosin), 375 mg (control), p<0.001	• Unpublished meeting abstract
Porpiglia et al. [9]	• RCT • Distal ureteral stones >5 mm • Failed one 10-day cycle tamsulosin MET • FU: 10 days	NSAIDS and glucocorticoid ± tamsulosin	• Tamsulosin – 46 pts • Control – 45 pts	• Spontaneous stone passage • No. colic episodes • Diclofenac usage	• RR stone passage 1.65 (95% CI 1.18–2.29) • Mean no. colic episodes 1.4 (tamsulosin), 1.0 (control), p>0.05 • Mean diclofenac usage 123 mg (tamsulosin), 127 mg (control), p>0.05	• Unpublished meeting abstract • First cycle of tamsulosin shorter than that used in other trials • No statistical benefit to second cycle tamsulosin in colic episodes and diclofenac usage • Earlier report from earlier subset of pts showed no statistical difference in stone passage rates

*Actual ranges for stone size are given where available

FGTMB, fluoroglucine trimetossibenzene; FU, follow up; MET, medical expulsive therapy; NSAIDS, nonsteroidal anti-inflammatory drugs; pts, patients; RCT, randomized controlled trial; RR, relative risk.

studies utilized tamsulosin. The evidence for the use of other alpha-blockers in this setting is of moderate quality and will require further study.

In summary, a strong recommendation can be made for the use of tamsulosin as MET for distal ureteral stones based upon high-quality evidence (Grade 1A). A strong recommendation can be made for the use of other alpha-adrenergic antagonists as MET based upon moderate-quality evidence (Grade 1B).

Clinical question 22.2

What is the effect of calcium channel antagonist therapy on expulsion of ureteral stones?

Literature search

The same PubMed search used above found five unique RCTs dealing with the use of a calcium channel antagonist for MET of ureteral stones. Searches of CINAHL and the Cochrane Central Register of Controlled Trials did not identify any additional published randomized studies. A search of AUA and EAU online meeting abstracts identified an additional two unique unpublished RCTs. One additional unpublished RCT was identified from a meta-analysis by Hollingsworth et al. [4,15].

The evidence

All eight RCTs using calcium channel antagonists as initial MET used nifedipine. Three trials utilized nifedipine in conjunction with other medications including glucocorticoids, antibiotics, and acetaminophen (Table 22.2). Three studies were performed with a tamsulosin arm as well. Most trials examined patients with distal ureteral stones that ranged in size up to 18 mm. One study did not specify the size of the stones and one did not specify location in the ureter. None of the studies included patients who had undergone previous shock-wave lithotripsy or prior MET. Follow-up, which was stated for all but two studies, was performed between 28 and 45 days.

Spontaneous stone passage rates for nifedipine ranged from 75% to 91%, with the overall stone passage rate being 81%. Spontaneous stone passage rates for controls in these studies ranged from 35% to 64%, with the overall stone passage rate being 58%. The RR for stone passage with nifedipine versus controls ranged from 1.20 to 2.24, with an overall RR of 1.52 (95% CI 1.35–1.71). Mean time to stone passage was generally shorter for nifedipine arms (5.0–12.2 days) compared to controls (5.0–20.0 days). Porpiglia et al. found a statistically decreased analgesic requirement with nifedipine [16]. Additionally, Cooper et al.

found a statistically significant decrease in the number of workdays lost with nifedipine [17].

Although relatively well tolerated, nifedipine usage was associated with adverse reactions resulting in discontinuation of treatment in a small number of patients. Nifedipine usage was also associated with an up to 21% incidence of minor side effects including headache, palpitations, asthenia, and stomach ache [16]. In each of the three studies that compared nifedipine to tamsulosin, tamsulosin was superior in spontaneous stone passage rates and time to stone passage.

Comment

The evidence for MET for distal ureteral stones using calcium channel antagonists is of moderate quality. The evidence suggests that nifedipine can improve spontaneous stone passage rates and time to stone passage. However, it does appear to be associated with an increased risk of minor side effects as well as a small risk of adverse reactions leading to discontinuation of therapy. Furthermore, in all studies in which nifedipine and tamsulosin were compared, nifedipine was the inferior treatment option. In light of the superior efficacy of alpha-adrenergic antagonists and their relatively more benign side effect profile, the recommendation to use a calcium channel antagonist as MET for ureteral stones is weak. However, in the setting of a patient who cannot tolerate alpha-adrenergic antagonists, a strong recommendation to use calcium channel antagonists can be made based upon moderate-quality evidence (Grade 1B).

Clinical question 22.3

What is the effect of corticosteroid therapy on expulsion of ureteral stones?

Literature search

The PubMed literature search used above yielded one RCT that specifically studied the use of a corticosteroid in MET for distal ureteral stones. Searches of CINAHL and the Cochrane Central Register of Controlled Trials did not identify any additional published randomized studies. A search of EAU online meeting abstracts identified two additional unpublished trials. A search of AUA online meeting abstracts did not yield any additional studies.

The evidence

Of the three trials studying corticosteroid treatment for MET of distal ureteral stones, two used deflazacort and one used methylprednisolone (Table 22.3). These trials

Table 22.2 Effect of calcium channel antagonists on ureteral stone passage

Authors	Methods*	Intervention	Participants	Outcomes	Results	Notes
Borghi et al. [43]	• RCT • RCT • Ureteral stones ≤15 mm • RCT • FU: 45 days	• ± Nifedipine and methylprednisolone	• Intervention – 43 pts • Placebo – 43 pts	• Spontaneous stone passage • Time to stone passage	• RR stone passage 1.42 (95% CI 1.04–1.93) (intention to treat) • Mean time to stone passage 11.2 days (intervention), 16.4 days (placebo), p=0.036 • Diclofenac usage in both groups was similar • Decrease in systolic blood pressure (−20 mmHg), decrease in diastolic blood pressure (−8 mmHg), and increase in heart rate (+8 bpm) with nifedipine statistically significant	• 4 pts in intervention arm did not complete study due to adverse reactions • 2 pts with adverse reactions, 2 pts with bacteriuria, and 2 pts lost to follow-up in placebo arm did not complete the study • Multiple drugs given in intervention arm
Cooper et al. [17]	• RCT • RCT • Private practice urology patients • Ureteral stones 2–6 mm • FU: 6 weeks	• NSAIDs ± nifedipine, prednisone, trimethoprim-sulfamethoxazole, and acetaminophen	• Intervention – 35 pts • Control – 35 pts	• Spontaneous stone passage • Time to stone passage • Workdays lost	• RR stone passage 1.63 (95% CI 1.18–2.26) • Mean time to stone passage 12.6 days (intervention), 11.2 days (control) • Mean workdays lost 1.8 days (intervention), 5.0 days (control), p=0.024	• No IRB approval • 6 patients did not complete study • Analysis was not intention to treat • Multiple drugs given in intervention arm • Time to stone passage shorter in control group
Porpiglia et al. [16]	• RCT • Distal ureteral stones ≤10 mm • FU: 4 weeks	• ± Glucocorticoid and nifedipine	• Intervention – 48 pts • Control – 48 pts	• Spontaneous stone passage • Time to stone passage • Diclofenac usage	• RR stone passage 2.24 (95% CI 1.49–3.36) • Mean time to stone passage 7 days (intervention), 20 days (control), p<0.05 • Mean diclofenac usage 15 mg (intervention), 105 mg (control), p<0.05	• 2 pts in intervention arm discontinued therapy due to adverse reactions • 10 pts in intervention arm had minor side effects • Multiple drugs given in intervention arm
Porpiglia et al. [35]	• RCT • Distal ureteral stones 3–10 mm • FU: 4 weeks	• NSAIDs and glucocorticoid ± nifedipine or tamsulosin	• Tamsulosin – 28 pts • Nifedipine – 30 pts • Control – 28 pts	• Spontaneous stone passage • Time to stone passage • Diclofenac usage	• RR stone passage vs control 2.00 (95% CI 1.27–3.15) (tamsulosin), 1.87 (95% CI 1.17–2.97) (nifedipine) • Mean time to expulsion 7.9 days (tamsulosin), 9.3 days (nifedipine), 12 days (control) • Mean diclofenac usage 26 mg (tamsulosin), 19.5 mg (nifedipine), 105 mg (control)	• 1 pt each in nifedipine and tamsulosin groups discontinued treatment due to side effects • Tamsulosin superior to nifedipine in time to stone passage

Study	Design	Intervention	Outcomes	Results	Comments
Dellabella et al. [39]	• Randomized trial • Distal ureteral stones 4–18 mm, colic lasting ≤1 day • FU: 28 days	NSAIDs ± tamsulosin, nifedipine or phloroglucinol • Tamsulosin – 70 pts • Nifedipine – 70 pts • Phloroglucinol – 70 pts	• Spontaneous stone passage • Time to stone passage • No. PRN diclofenac vials used • Need for hospitalization • No. workdays lost	• RR stone passage vs phloroglucinol 1.51 (95% CI 1.26–1.81) (tamsulosin), 1.20 (95% CI 0.97–1.49) (nifedipine) • Median time to stone passage 72 h (tamsulosin), 120 h (nifedipine), 120 h (phloroglucinol), p<0.001 • Median no. PRN diclofenac vials used 0 (tamsulosin), 1 (nifedipine), 2 (phloroglucinol), p<0.001 • Need for urgent hospitalization 0% (tamsulosin), 4% (nifedipine), 16% (phloroglucinol), p=0.001 • Need for delayed hospitalization 1.4% (tamsulosin), 16% (nifedipine), 19% (phloroglucinol), p=0.004 • Median workdays lost 2 (tamsulosin), 3 (nifedipine), 5 (phloroglucinol), p<0.001	• No control group • Difference in stone passage rate with nifedipine not statistically significant • Tamsulosin superior to nifedipine in all outcomes
Skrekas et al. [44]	• RCT • Distal ureteral stones 3–9 mm • FU: 30 days	NSAIDs ± nifedipine • Nifedipine – 46 pts • Control – 46 pts	• Spontaneous stone passage • Time to stone passage	• RR stone passage 1.46 (95% CI 1.10–1.95) • Mean time to stone passage 6 days (nifedipine), 18 days (control)	• Unpublished meeting abstract
Staerman et al. [15]	• RCT • Distal ureteral stones, size unspecified • FU: not stated	NSAIDs, phloroglucinol ± nifedipine • Nifedipine – 23 pts • Control – 25 pts	• Spontaneous stone passage • Time to stone passage • Time to "pain relief"	• RR stone passage 1.43 (95% CI 1.04–1.96) • Mean time to stone passage 5.1 days (nifedipine), 12.9 days (control), p=0.001 • Mean time to "pain relief" 1.4 days (nifedipine), 3.8 days (control)	• Unpublished abstract • Difference in stone passage rate not statistically significant per authors' report
Taghavi et al. [8]	• RCT • Distal ureteral stones <10 mm • FU: not stated	± Tamsulosin or nifedipine • Tamsulosin – 20 pts • Nifedipine – 20 pts • Control – 24 pts	• Spontaneous stone passage • Time to stone passage	• RR stone passage vs control 1.96 (95% CI 1.24–3.11) (tamsulosin), 1.64 (95% CI 0.99–2.71) (nifedipine) • Mean time to stone passage 8.2 days (tamsulosin), 10 days (nifedipine), 14.2 days (control)	• Unpublished meeting abstract

*Actual ranges for stone size are given where available

Table 22.3 Effect of corticosteroids on ureteral stone passage

Authors	Methods*	Intervention	Participants	Outcomes	Results	Notes
Dellabella et al. [18]	• RCT • Distal ureteral stones ≥4 mm, colic lasting ≤1 day • FU: 28 days	Tamsulosin 28 days ± deflazacort 10 days	• Deflazacort – 30 pts • Control – 30 pts	• Spontaneous stone passage • Time to stone passage • Need for hospitalization • Analgesic usage • Workdays lost • Side effect prevalence	• RR stone passage 1.07 (95% CI 0.94–1.23) • Median time to stone passage 72 h (deflazacort), 120 h (control), p=0.036 • Need for urgent hospitalization 0% for both arms • Need for delayed hospitalization 3.3% (deflazacort), 10% (control), p=0.612 • Analgesic usage, 0 vials in each arm, p=0.625 • Workdays lost, 2 days in each arm, p=0.994 • Side effect prevalence 6.7% dyspepsia (deflazacort), 0% (control), p=0.492	• Need for delayed hospitalization for tamsulosin alone significantly greater than in Dellabella et al. [39] • No significant differences except for time to stone passage
Salehi et al. [45]	• RCT • Distal ureteral stones 2–9 mm • FU: 21 days	NSAIDs and hydrochlorothiazide (HCTZ) ± methylprednisolone	• Methylprednisolone – 40 pts • Control – 45 pts	• Spontaneous stone passage	• RR stone passage 1.80 (95% CI 1.25–2.58)	• Unpublished meeting abstract
Porpiglia et al. [46]	• Allocation method unspecified • Distal ureteral stones, size unspecified • Initial presentation at emergency department • FU: 10 days	± Tamsulosin ± deflazacort	• Tamsulosin – 33 pts • Deflazacort – 24 pts • Tamsulosin + deflazacort – 33 pts • Control – 24 pts	• Spontaneous stone passage • Analgesic usage	• RR stone passage deflazacort vs control 1.13 (95% CI 0.52–2.42) • RR stone passage tamsulosin vs control 1.64 (95% CI 0.86–3.12) • RR stone passage tamsulosin + deflazacort vs control 2.55 (95% CI 1.42–4.56) • RR stone passage tamsulosin + deflazacort vs tamsulosin 1.56 (95% CI 1.10–2.19) • Median diclofenac usage 43 mg (tamsulosin), 50 mg (deflazacort), 27.3 mg (tamsulosin + deflazacort), 81 mg (control)	• Unpublished meeting abstract • 3 pts in tamsulosin alone arm did not complete the study • Short follow-up • Deflazacort improves stone passage rate only in conjunction with tamsulosin

* Actual ranges for stone size are given where available

examined patients with distal ureteral stones that were 2–9 mm in size, ≥ 4 mm in size or size unspecified. Follow-up ranged from 10 to 28 days. Two of the studies examined the use of a corticosteroid in conjunction with tamsulosin. The spontaneous stone passage rate with corticosteroid treatment alone ranged from 38% to 80% versus 33% to 44% with controls. When tamsulosin was given in addition to a corticosteroid, the stone passage rates ranged from 85% to 97% compared to 55% to 90% without the corticosteroid. The RR of stone passage with a corticosteroid alone versus controls ranged from 1.13 to 1.80 with an overall RR of 1.60 (95% CI 1.15–2.22). The RR of stone passage for a corticosteroid with tamsulosin versus tamsulosin alone ranged from 1.07 to 1.71 with an overall RR of 1.27 (95% CI 1.07–1.50). In these limited studies, need for hospitalization, analgesic usage, and workdays lost were not significantly different between treatment arms. Dellabella et al. found that two out of 30 patients (7%) receiving deflazacort developed dyspepsia as a side effect [18].

Comment

The evidence for MET for distal ureteral stones using corticosteroids is of low quality. Efficacy rates among studies varied widely and statistically significant differences between intervention and control arms were seen primarily in conjunction with an alpha-adrenergic antagonist. Although corticosteroids have been used in multiple studies as adjuncts to alpha-adrenergic antagonists and calcium channel antagonists for MET, no recommendation to use corticosteroids in this setting can be made and this issue will require further study.

Clinical question 22.4

What is the effect of medical therapy on expulsion of renal and ureteral stones after shock-wave lithotripsy (SWL)?

Literature search

A PubMed literature search combining the terms "shock-wave lithotripsy" and "alpha-adrenergic antagonist or calcium channel blocker or medical expulsive therapy" identified six RCTs that studied the use of a calcium channel antagonist or an alpha-adrenergic antagonist as adjunctive MET after SWL. Searches of CINAHL and the Cochrane Central Register of Controlled Trials did not identify any additional published randomized studies. A search of EAU online meeting abstracts identified two additional unpublished trials. One of these

abstracts did not provide any quantitative outcomes data and was excluded from this review. A search of AUA online meeting abstracts identified one additional unpublished trial.

The evidence

Of the eight RCTs using MET as an adjunct to SWL, four studies utilized tamsulosin, two utilized doxazosin, and one utilized nifedipine (Table 22.4). Most trials examined MET in conjunction with primary SWL. One trial by Resim et al. included only patients who had developed steinstrasse after SWL [19]. Stone location varied from the renal collecting system to the distal ureter and stone size varied from 4 mm to 30 mm. Follow-up was performed between 15 days and 12 weeks.

The primary measure of success in these studies was variously defined as stone-free status, residual fragments < 3 mm in size or asymptomatic residual fragments < 3 mm in size. It should be noted, however, that "success" in these trials did not equal "stone free." Using these definitions, successful stone clearance rates for adjunctive MET ranged from 65% to 100%, with an overall stone clearance rate of 81%. Successful stone clearance rates for controls ranged from 33% to 81%, with an overall stone clearance rate of 63%. The RR for successful stone clearance with adjunctive MET ranged from 1.05 to 2.13 with an overall RR of 1.28 (95% CI 1.15–1.41). In three trials, the increased rate of stone clearance was not statistically significant. Mean/median time to successful stone clearance was generally shorter in intervention arms (7–13 days) compared to controls (10–14 days) in the four studies that reported such information. In no study was this difference reported as being statistically significant. Among the five trials that examined analgesic usage, all but one demonstrated a statistically significant decrease in analgesic consumption with adjunctive MET. Four trials recorded the number of patients with colic episodes or the number of colic episodes per patient. A statistically significant decrease in the prevalence of colic was found in only two trials. Among all trials, only two patients – one intervention patient and one control patient – discontinued treatment due to an adverse reaction. In their trial examining tamsulosin, Resim et al. found that the proportion of patients without any adverse reactions was similar between their intervention (60%) and control (57%) arms [19].

Comment

Using the definitions of successful stone clearance above, the evidence for the use of MET as an adjunct to SWL is of moderate quality. Although time to stone clearance may not be significantly enhanced, the evidence suggests that adjunctive MET may improve stone clearance rates

Table 22.4 Effect of medical expulsive therapy on stone passage after shock-wave lithotripsy

Authors	Methods*	Intervention	Participants	Outcomes	Results	Notes
Porpiglia et al. [47]	• RCT • Solitary ureteral stones in any location • Mean size 11.6 mm (intervention), 10.1 mm (control) • FU: 45 days	SWL and NSAIDs ± nifedipine and glucocorticoid	• Nifedipine – 40 pts • Control – 40 pts	• Success defined as residual fragments <3 mm in size • Percent of pts with colic episodes • Diclofenac usage	• RR success 1.50 (95% CI 1.05–2.15) • Percent of pts with colic episodes 37.5% (nifedipine), 42.5% (control) • Mean diclofenac usage 38 mg (nifedipine), 86 mg (control), p=0.020	• 4 pts in nifedipine group experienced side effects including asthenia and headache but did not discontinue therapy
Kupeli et al. [36]	• RCT • Solitary distal ureteral stones 6–15 mm • FU: 15 days	SWL and NSAIDs ± tamsulosin	• Tamsulosin – 24 pts • Control – 24 pts	• Stone-free status	• RR stone-free 2.13 (95% CI 1.14–3.96)	
Gravina et al. [48]	• RCT • Solitary renal stones 4–20 mm • FU: 12 weeks	SWL, glucocorticoid, and NSAIDs ± tamsulosin	• Tamsulosin – 65 pts • Control – 65 pts	• Success defined as asymptomatic residual fragments <3 mm in size • Percent of pts with colic episodes • Diclofenac usage	• RR success 1.31 (95% CI 1.03–1.66) • Percent of pts with colic episodes 26.1% (tamsulosin), 76.9% (control), p<0.001 • Mean diclofenac usage 375 mg (tamsulosin), 675 mg (control), p<0.001	• Differences in stone-free status not statistically significant at 4 and 8 weeks FU • Differences in stone-free status not statistically significant in subset of pts with stones ≤10 mm in size
Resim et al. [19]	• RCT • SWL-induced distal ureteral steinstrasse from stones originally 10–30 mm in diameter • Pts without severe pain or hydronephrosis • FU: 6 weeks	NSAIDs ± tamsulosin	• Tamsulosin – 32 pts • Control – 35 pts	• Resolution of steinstrasse • Time to resolution of steinstrasse • No. colic episodes • Pain scores • Side effect profile	• RR resolution of steinstrasse 1.05 (95% CI 0.77–1.43) • Median time to resolution of steinstrasse 9 days (tamsulosin), 10 days (control), p>0.05 • Median no. colic episodes 0 (tamsulosin), 1 (control), p<0.01 • Median visual analog pain score 4 (tamsulosin), 6 (control), p<0.001 • Percent of pts without side effects 60% (tamsulosin), 57% (control)	• Sample population limited to nonobese pts not taking psychiatric medications or antihistamines • Differences in steinstrasse resolution not statistically significant • Differences in colic episodes may not be clinically significant
Bhagat et al. [49]	• RCT, placebo controlled, double blind • Renal stones 6–24 mm or ureteral stones 6–15 mm • FU: 1 month	SWL, narcotics, and NSAIDs ± tamsulosin	• Tamsulosin – 30 pts • Placebo – 30 pts	• Success defined as asymptomatic residual stone fragments <3 mm • No. analgesic doses given	• RR success 1.22 (95% CI 0.98–1.52) • Mean no. analgesic doses 1 (tamsulosin), 2 (placebo), p=0.3	• 1 pt in each group discontinued therapy • Differences not statistically significant with intention-to-treat analysis • Time to clearance in the 18 pts who developed steinstrasse was longer with tamsulosin

Study	Design/Population	Intervention	Groups	Outcomes	Results	Comments
Gravas et al. [50]	• RCT • Distal ureteral stones 6–13 mm • FU: 4 weeks	SWL and NSAIDs ± tamsulosin	• Tamsulosin – 31 pts • Control – 31 pts	• Success defined as asymptomatic residual stone fragments <3 mm • Time to success • Diclofenac usage	• RR success 1.11 (95% CI 0.75–1.65) • Median time to success 13.0 days (tamsulosin), 13.2 days (control), $p>0.05$ • Mean diclofenac usage 57 mg (tamsulosin), 119 mg (control), $p=0.02$	• Randomization based on hospital record number • Study enrolled fewer pts than required by their preset sample size calculation • Unblinded • Differences not statistically significant
Mukhtarov et al. [51]	• RCT • Distal ureteral stones 6–15 mm • FU: 28 days	SWL and NSAIDs ± doxazosin	• Doxazosin – 24 • Control – 21	• Stone-free status • Time to stone-free status • Analgesic usage	• RR stone-free 1.23 (95% CI 0.99–1.53) • Mean time to stone-free status 8.0 days (doxazosin), 13.5 days (control), $p>0.05$ • Mean diclofenac usage 75 mg (doxazosin), 270 mg (control), $p<0.001$	• Unpublished meeting abstract • Differences in stone-free rate and mean time to stone-free status not statistically significant
Shaaban et al. [52]	• RCT • Renal and upper ureteral stones 5–20 mm • FU: 12 weeks	SWL and NSAIDs ± doxazosin	• Doxazosin – 52 pts • Control – 53 pts	• Success defined as asymptomatic residual stone fragments <3 mm • Time to success • Percent of pts with colic episodes	• RR success 1.22 (95% CI 1.03–1.45) • Mean time to stone passage 7 days (doxazosin), 14 days (control) • Percent of pts with colic episodes 26% (doxazosin), 75% (control)	• Unpublished meeting abstract • 15% of pts in the intervention arm experienced minor side effects but did not discontinue treatment

*Actual ranges for stone size are given where available

after SWL and decrease patients' analgesic requirements. As opposed to the definitions of successful stone clearance involving residual fragments < 3 mm in size, a more clinically appropriate definition of success would be true stone-free status. Only two of the eight trials on MET after SWL utilized this definition of success. Nevertheless, as these medications are relatively well tolerated, the recommendation to use MET as an adjunct to SWL can be considered strong based upon moderate-quality evidence (Grade 1B). Further study will be required to more accurately and definitively determine the benefits of MET in this setting.

Clinical question 22.5

What is the effect of thiazide and nonthiazide diuretic therapy on recurrence of urinary calculi?

Literature search

A PubMed literature search combining the terms "nephrolithiasis, urolithiasis, urinary calculi, or kidney calculi" with the terms "random" or the "randomized controlled trial" publication type identified seven RCTs that studied the effect of a thiazide diuretic or the nonthiazide diuretic indapamide on the recurrence of urinary calculi. Indapamide is included in the thiazide diuretic group because of its similar mechanism of action. A search of the Cochrane Central Register of Controlled Trials identified one additional published randomized controlled trial [20]. Searches of CINAHL, EAU and AUA online meeting abstracts did not identify any additional published or unpublished randomized studies. Two additional trials that were presented at the Fifth International Symposium on Urolithiasis and Related Clinical Research in 1984 were identified from a review of reference lists from retrieved articles [21,22].

The evidence

Of the nine trials studying thiazide and nonthiazide diuretic treatment for medical prophylaxis of stone disease, three studies used hydrochlorothiazide, three used bendroflumethiazide, and one study each used trichloromethiazide, chlorthalidone, and indapamide (Table 22.5). Only five studies limited their study populations to calcium stone formers and only two studies limited their study population to those patients with documented hypercalciuria. Two studies limited the study population to patients who were stone free at the start of the study [20,23]. The remainder utilized radiographic imaging to document pre-existing stones. Primary outcomes involved "stone events" that were variously defined to include spontaneous passage of stones, radiographic evidence of new stones, and/or growth of pre-existing stones. Many of the studies were of poor quality. Most suffered from small sample sizes, many had exceedingly high attrition rates, and several were reported prior to completion of enrollment or used incomplete datasets. Additionally, randomization methodology was sparsely reported and, in at least one study, resulted in the intervention arm having a significantly more favorable baseline stone formation rate. The majority of studies, however, were placebo controlled.

The stone event rate ranged from 0.05 to 0.24 stones/patient/year for thiazide and indapamide therapy versus 0.11 to 0.58 stones/patient/year for controls. In only three of the eight studies where such data were provided were the differences in stone event rates reported as being statistically significant. Remission rates for thiazide and indapamide therapy, where calculable, ranged from 70% to 100%, with an overall remission rate of 82%. Remission rates for controls ranged from 52% to 83%, with an overall remission rate of 64%. The RR of remission with treatment ranged from 0.95 to 17.31 with an overall RR of 2.49 (95% CI 1.53–4.05). In the study by Ettinger et al., up to 21% of chlorthalidone patients discontinued therapy due to side effects that included fatigue, impotence, and lightheadedness [24].

Comment

The evidence for the use of thiazides and nonthiazide diuretics as medical prophylaxis for recurrent stone disease in the general stone-forming population is of low quality. Many of the studies involving these drugs suffer from serious methodological deficiencies. Nevertheless, six of the nine RCTs utilizing such therapy demonstrated an advantage with treatment in either the rate of stone events/patient/year or the stone remission rate. In five of these studies, the differences were statistically significant. Because of the poor quality of the available studies and the variability in the efficacy rates among the different trials, a recommendation to use thiazides and nonthiazide diuretics for stone prophylaxis is a weak one (Grade 2C). With the current understanding of the mechanism of action of thiazides and the nonthiazide diuretic indapamide on urinary calcium excretion, a greater benefit from treatment might be expected in appropriately selected hypercalciuric patients. Further studies should focus on this patient population. Although the rate of minor adverse reactions leading to discontinuation of therapy was moderately high in some trials, given the significant morbidity associated with recurrent stone disease, a trial of a thiazide derivative or indapamide may be warranted in hypercalciuric recurrent stone formers.

Table 22.5 Effect of thiazide and nonthiazide diuretic therapy on urinary calculi formation

Authors	Methods	Intervention	Participants	Outcomes	Results	Notes
Brocks et al. [53]	• RCT, placebo controlled, double blind • Any pt with radiographic history of ≥2 upper urinary tract stones • FU: planned 4 years, actual mean FU 1.6 years	Bendroflumethiazide (BFMZ)	• BMFZ – 33 pts • Placebo – 29 pts	• Newly formed stones/pt/yr • Remission rate	• Stones/pt/yr 0.09 (BFMZ), 0.11 (placebo) • Remission rate 84.8% (BFMZ), 82.8% (placebo) • RR remission 1.17 (95% CI 0.30–4.52)	• Randomization resulted in intervention group having significantly fewer stones/pt/yr prior to treatment • Study reported prior to completion of the study period • Not selected for pts with hypercalciuria • Differences in remission rate not statistically significant
Scholz et al. [54]	• RCT, placebo controlled • Pts with "metabolically active calcium stone formation" • FU: 12 months	Hydrochloro-thiazide (HCTZ)	• HCTZ – 25 pts • Control – 26 pts	• Spontaneous passage of newly formed stones • Remission rate	• Stones/pt/yr 0.24 (HCTZ), 0.23 (placebo) • Remission rate 76.0% (HCTZ), 76.9% (placebo) • RR remission 0.95 (95% CI 0.26–3.47)	• Method of assessing outcome not stated • Not selected for pts with hypercalciuria • 2 pts in intervention group and 1 pt in placebo group discontinued therapy due to side effects • Differences in remission rate not statistically significant
Laerum et al. [55]	• RCT, placebo controlled, double blind • Any pt with history of ≥2 urinary tract stones with most recent one radiographically documented • FU: 3 years	HCTZ	• HCTZ – 25 pts • Placebo – 25 pts	• Spontaneously passed and newly formed radiographically identified stones/pt/yr • Remission rate	• Passed and newly formed stones/pt/yr 0.21 (HCTZ), 0.32 (placebo) • Remission rate 78.3% (HCTZ), 52.0% (placebo), p=0.05 • RR remission 3.32 (95% CI 0.94–11.76)	• 2 pts in intervention group lost to follow-up • Not selected for pts with hypercalciuria • Differences in remission rates not statistically significant
Robertson et al. [22]	• RCT • Recurrent idiopathic calcium stone formers • FU: planned 3–5 years, actual not stated	± BFMZ, potassium, and dietary and fluid intake advice	• BFMZ – 13 pts • Control – 9 pts	• Stone "episodes" per pt per yr	• Stone episodes/pt/yr 0.22 (BFMZ), 0.58 (placebo)	• Study report published using data from less than 30% of total study enrollment • Stone "episodes" not defined • Control group did not receive dietary and fluid intake advice • Not selected for pts with hypercalciuria
Wilson et al. [21]	• RCT, open-label • Recurrent idiopathic calcium stone formers • FU: planned ≥1 year, actual mean FU 2.8 years	± HCTZ	• HCTZ – 23 pts • Control – 21 pts	• Stones/pt/yr • Remission rate	• Stones/pt/yr 0.15 (HCTZ), 0.32 (control), p<0.05 • Remission rate 69.6% (HCTZ), 61.9% (control) • RR remission 1.41 (95% CI 0.40–4.91)	• Unpublished meeting abstract • Not selected for pts with hypercalciuria • Differences in remission rates not statistically significant

(Continued on p. 210)

Table 22.5 (Continued)

Authors	Methods	Intervention	Participants	Outcomes	Results	Notes
Mortensen et al. [20]	• RCT, placebo controlled, double blind • Stone-free pts with radiographic history of ≥1 stone • FU: 2 years	BFMZ and potassium	• BFMZ – 12 pts • Placebo – 10 pts	• Remission rate	• Remission rate 100% (BFMZ), 60% (placebo) • RR remission 17.3 (95% CI 0.80–373.45)	• Study enrolled less than 50% of planned enrollment • 15% of pts lost to follow-up • Not selected for pts with hypercalciuria • Differences in remission rates not statistically significant
Ettinger et al. [24]	• RCT, placebo controlled, double blind • Pts with active recurrent stone disease • FU: 3 years	Low-dose chlorthalidone, high-dose chlorthalidone or placebo	• Low-dose chlorthalidone – 19 pts • High-dose chlorthalidone – 23 pts • Placebo – 31 pts	• Stone events (defined as growth of previous calculi, appearance of new calculi or passage of calculi) per pt per yr • Remission rate	• Stone events/pt/yr 0.07 (low-dose chlorthalidone), 0.05 (high-dose chlorthalidone), 0.22 (placebo) • Remission rate 84.2% (low-dose chlorthalidone), 87.0% (high-dose chlorthalidone), 85.7% (chlorthalidone overall), 54.8% (placebo) • RR remission 4.94 (95% CI 1.62–15.10)	• Randomization based on hospital record number • 38% of intervention pts did not complete the study (18% lost interest, 21% developed side effects including fatigue, impotence, and light-headedness • 16% of placebo pts did not complete the study • Not selected for pts with hypercalciuria
Ohkawa et al. [56]	• RCT • Calcium stone formers with idiopathic hypercalciuria • FU: actual mean FU 2 years	Trichlor-methiazide (TMZ)	• TMZ – 82 pts • Control – 93 pts	• Spontaneously passed and newly formed radiographically identified stones/pt/yr • Remission rate defined as total relapse-free pt-yrs per total pt-yrs	• Passed and newly formed stones/pt/yr 0.13 (TMZ), 0.31 (placebo), p<0.05 • Remission rate 91.7% (TMZ), 85.9% (placebo), p>0.05 • RR remission cannot be calculated from these data	• 17% of pts did not complete the study • 2 pts in intervention group discontinued therapy because of side effects • Differences in relapse-free rates not statistically significant
Borghi et al. [23]	• RCT • Stone-free recurrent calcium stone formers with idiopathic hypercalciuria • FU: 3 years	± Indapamide ± allopurinol	• Indapamide – 25 pts • Indapamide + allopurinol – 25 pts • Control	• Spontaneous passage and newly formed radiographically identified stones/pt/yr • Remission rate	• Passed and newly formed stones/pt/yr 0.06 (indapamide), 0.04 (indapamide + allopurinol), 0.28 (control), p<0.01 • Remission rate 84.2% (indapamide), 87.5% (indapamide + allopurinol), 57.2% (control) • RR remission vs control 4.13 (95% CI 1.09–15.59) (indapamide), 5.76 (95% CI 1.36–24.36) (indapamide + allopurinol)	• 44% of control pts, 24% of indapamide pts, and 4% of indapamide + allopurinol pts did not complete the study

Clinical question 22.6

What is the effect of allopurinol therapy on recurrence of urinary calculi?

Literature search

The PubMed literature search used above yielded three RCTs that studied the use of allopurinol for prevention of recurrent stone disease. Searches of CINAHL and the Cochrane Central Register of Controlled Trials did not identify any additional published randomized studies. A search of EAU and AUA online meeting abstracts did not yield any additional unpublished studies. Two additional trials that were presented at the Fifth International Symposium on Urolithiasis and Related Clinical Research in 1984 were identified from a review of reference lists from retrieved articles [21,25].

The evidence

Five RCTs utilizing allopurinol for medical prophylaxis of stone disease were identified (Table 22.6). Only one of these trials selected for hyperuricosuric patients [26]. One trial assessed the effect of allopurinol in conjunction with indapamide [23]. Stone events were variously defined to include spontaneous passage of stones, radiographic evidence of new stones, and/or growth of pre-existing stones. Most studies suffered from small sample sizes. The stone event rate in trials comparing allopurinol to no treatment ranged from 0.12 to 0.96 stone events/patient/year versus 0.26 to 0.66 stone events/patient/year for controls. The remission rates, where calculable, for allopurinol treatment ranged from 53% to 69%, with an overall remission rate of 63%. The remission rates for controls ranged from 42% to 62%, with an overall remission rate of 50%. The RR of remission with allopurinol treatment ranged from 0.69 to 3.08, with an overall RR of 1.68 (95% CI 0.40–4.91). In two trials, the stone event rate was higher in the allopurinol arm compared to the control arm. Only in the study by Ettinger et al. that selected for hyperuricosuric patients was the benefit from allopurinol treatment statistically significant [26]. There did not appear to be a significant benefit to the addition of allopurinol to a regimen of indapamide in hypercalciuric patients [23]. Up to 15% of patients taking allopurinol had adverse reactions, including gastrointestinal discomfort, rash, and fatigue, leading to discontinuation of therapy.

Comment

The evidence for the use of allopurinol for the purposes of stone prevention in a nonhyperuricosuric patient population is of low quality and a recommendation for its use in this setting is weak (Grade 2C). A statistically significant benefit to allopurinol therapy was found only in the trial by Ettinger et al. that limited the study population to hyperuricosuric patients [26]. Further research is necessary to more definitively determine the merits of allopurinol therapy for stone prophylaxis. Although minor adverse reactions may occur with a low frequency, a trial of allopurinol treatment in hyperuricosuric stone formers may be warranted.

Clinical question 22.7

What is the effect of alkali citrate therapy on recurrence of urinary calculi?

Literature search

The PubMed literature search used above yielded three RCTs that studied the use of alkali therapy for prevention of recurrent stone disease. Searches of CINAHL, the Cochrane Central Register of Controlled Trials, and EAU and AUA online meeting abstracts did not identify any additional published or unpublished randomized studies.

The evidence

Of the three placebo-controlled RCTs utilizing alkali citrate therapy for medical prophylaxis of stone disease, one trial used potassium citrate, one used sodium-potassium citrate (Na-K-Cit), and one used potassium-magnesium citrate (K-Mg-Cit) (Table 22.7). All three studies suffered from a high rate of patient noncompliance. In the only trial that selected for hypocitraturic patients, Barcelo et al. measured radiographically identified new stone formation events and found that potassium citrate therapy resulted in a stone event rate of 0.1 stones/patient/year compared to 1.1 stones/patient/year for placebo [27]. Hofbauer et al. did not define their stone event outcome and found no difference in stone formation rates between Na-K-Cit and placebo (0.9 and 0.7 stones/patient/year, respectively). The remission rates for alkali citrate therapy ranged from 31% to 88%, with an overall remission rate of 60%. The remission rates for placebo patients ranged from 20% to 36%, with an overall remission rate of 29%. The RR of remission with alkali citrate therapy ranged from 1.21 to 12.44, with an overall RR of 4.83 (95% CI 2.13–10.92). Minor adverse reactions, primarily gastrointestinal, occurred in up to 42% of patients. Significant gastrointestinal adverse reactions resulting in discontinuation of therapy occurred in up to 16% of patients.

Table 22.6 Effect of allopurinol therapy on urinary calculi formation

Authors	Methods	Intervention	Participants	Outcomes	Results	Notes
Robertson et al. [22]	• RCT • Recurrent idiopathic calcium stone formers • FU: planned 3–5 years, actual not stated	± Allopurinol and dietary and fluid intake advice	• Allopurinol – 12 pts • Control – 9 pts	• Stone "episodes" per pt per yr	• Stone episodes/pt/yr 0.54 (allopurinol), 0.58 (placebo)	• Study report published using data from less than 30% of total study enrollment • Stone "episodes" not defined • Control group did not receive dietary and fluid intake advice • Not selected for pts with hyperuricosuria
Wilson et al. [21]	• RCT, open-label • Recurrent idiopathic calcium stone formers • FU: planned ≥1 year, actual mean FU 2.8 years	± Allopurinol	• Allopurinol – 17 pts • Control – 21 pts	• Stones/pt/yr • Remission rate	• Stones/pt/yr 0.48 (allopurinol), 0.32 (control), p<0.05 • Remission rate 52.9% (allopurinol), 61.9% (control) • RR remission 0.69 (95% CI 0.19–2.53)	• Unpublished meeting abstract • Not selected for pts with hyperuricosuria • Differences in stones/pt/yr statistically favor control • Differences in remission rates not statistically significant
Miano et al. [25]	• RCT, placebo controlled, double blind • Recurrent stone formers, ≥2 stones/year for 3 years • FU: 3 years	Allopurinol	• Allopurinol – 8 pts • Placebo – 7 pts	• Stones/pt/yr	• Stones/pt/yr 0.96 (allopurinol), 0.66 (placebo)	• Allopurinol arm had significantly greater stone event rate at baseline • Not selected for pts with hyperuricosuria
Ettinger et al. [26]	• RCT, placebo controlled, double blind • Hyperuricosuric, normocalciuric pts with ≥2 calcium oxalate stones in the prior 5 years with 1 stone in the prior 2 years • FU: 2 years	Allopurinol	• Allopurinol – 29 pts • Placebo – 31 pts	• Stone events (defined as growth of previous calculi, appearance of new calculi or passage of calculi) per pt per yr • Remission rate	• Stone events/pt/yr 0.12 (allopurinol), 0.26 (placebo), p<0.05 • Remission rate 69.0% (allopurinol), 41.9% (placebo) • RR remission 3.08 (95% CI 1.06–8.90)	• 15% of enrolled intervention pts discontinued therapy within the first 6 months due to gastrointestinal discomfort, rash or fatigue and were not included in the results • 10% of intervention pts did not complete the study • 6% of placebo pts did not complete the study
Borghi et al. [23]	• RCT • Stone-free recurrent calcium stone formers with idiopathic hypercalciuria • FU: 3 years	± Indapamide ± allopurinol	• Indapamide – 25 pts • Indapamide + allopurinol – 25 pts • Control	• Spontaneous passage and newly formed radiographically identified stones/pt/yr • Remission rate	• Passed and newly formed stones/pt/yr 0.06 (indapamide), 0.04 (indapamide + allopurinol), 0.28 (control), p<0.01 • Remission rate 84.2% (indapamide), 87.5% (indapamide + allopurinol), 57.2% (control) • RR remission vs control 4.13 (95% CI 1.09–15.59) (indapamide), 5.76 (95% CI 1.36–24.36) (indapamide + allopurinol) • RR remission indapamide + allopurinol vs indapamide 1.40 (95% CI 0.28–7.00)	• 44% of control pts, 24% of indapamide pts, and 4% of indapamide + allopurinol pts did not complete the study • Not selected for hyperuricosuria • Differences in remission rates not statistically significant between indapamide + allopurinol and indapamide alone arms

Table 22.7 Effect of alkali therapy on urinary calculi formation

Authors	Methods	Intervention	Participants	Outcomes	Results	Notes
Barcelo et al. [27]	• RCT, placebo controlled • Idiopathic hypocitraturic active calcium stone formers with ≥2 stones in previous 2 years • FU: 3 years	Potassium citrate	• Potassium citrate – 18 pts • Placebo – 20 pts	• Newly formed radiographically identified stones/pt/yr • Growth of stones ≥100% increase in stone size • Remission rate	• Stones/pt/yr 0.1 (potassium citrate), 1.1 (placebo), p<0.001 • Growth of stones 16.7% (potassium citrate), 20.0% (placebo) • Remission rate 72.2% (potassium citrate), 20% (placebo) • RR remission 10.40 (95% CI 2.31–46.83)	• 28% of pts excluded due to noncompliance • 17% of potassium citrate pts reported minor GI adverse reactions • 4% of potassium citrate and 2% of placebo pts discontinued therapy due to GI intolerance
Hofbauer et al. [57]	• RCT, placebo controlled • Recurrent idiopathic calcium stone formers ≥1 stone/yr in previous 3 years • FU: 3 years	Sodium-potassium citrate (Na-K-Cit)	• Na-K-Cit – 22 pts • Placebo – 16 pts	• Stones/pt/yr • Remission rate	• Stones/pt/yr 0.9 (Na-K-Cit), 0.7 (placebo), p=0.65 • Remission rate 31% (Na-K-Cit), 27% (placebo) • RR remission 1.21 (95% CI 0.29–3.47)	• Stone events not defined • 16% of pts excluded due to noncompliance • 16% of Na-K-Cit pts discontinued therapy due to GI intolerance • Differences in remission rates not statistically significant • Not selected for pts with hypocitraturia
Ettinger et al. [58]	• RCT, placebo controlled • Recurrent idiopathic calcium stone formers • FU: 37 months	Potassium-magnesium citrate (K-Mg-Cit)	• K-Mg-Cit – 16 pts • Placebo – 25 pts	• Remission rate	• Remission rate 87.9% (K-Mg-Cit), 36.4% (placebo) • RR remission 12.44 (95% CI 2.29–67.56)	• 16% of K-Mg-Cit pts discontinued therapy due to GI intolerance • 42% of K-Mg-Cit pts and 40% of placebo pts reported minor GI adverse reactions • Not selected for pts with hypocitraturia

Comment

The quality of the evidence for alkali therapy for the prevention of recurrent calcium stone disease is relatively high. Remission rates favor alkali therapy in all three trials and are statistically significant in two of these trials. The evidence suggests that potassium citrate is effective in hypocitraturic patients and that potassium-magnesium citrate may be useful in an unselected population of calcium stone formers. Sodium-potassium citrate, however, did not show a statistically significant benefit in either stone event rate or remission rate and may be less useful than potassium citrate and potassium-magnesium citrate. Although gastrointestinal side effects limit the tolerability of alkali citrate therapy, a recommendation to use such therapy in recurrent calcium stone-forming patients is strong and is based upon moderate-quality evidence (**Grade 1B**).

Clinical question 22.8

What is the effect of acetohydroxamic acid (AHA) therapy on the course of struvite stone disease?

Literature search

The PubMed literature search used above yielded three RCTs that studied the use of acetohydroxamic acid for prevention of recurrent stone disease. Searches of CINAHL, the Cochrane Central Register of Controlled Trials, and EAU and AUA online meeting abstracts did not identify any additional published or unpublished randomized studies.

The evidence

All patients in each of the three placebo-controlled RCTs that used AHA for the treatment and/or prevention of struvite stone disease had chronic urinary tract infections due to urea-splitting organisms (Table 22.8). The primary outcome in each trial was the variably defined growth of stones and

ranged from 0% to 42% for AHA groups versus 37% to 60% for placebo groups. In two of these trials, these differences were statistically significant [28,29]. In these two trials, the RR of stone growth with AHA treatment were 0.04 and 0.23, with an overall RR of 0.18 (95% CI 0.08–0.44). The third trial, which was limited to patients with spinal cord injuries in a Veterans' Affairs hospital setting, suffered from an extremely high dropout rate of 49% [30]. However, this study illustrates the relatively high rate of toxicity associated with AHA with up to 20% of patients discontinuing therapy due to severe or recurrent gastrointestinal, neurological or hematological adverse reactions.

Table 22.8 Effect of acetohydroxamic acid (AHA) therapy on urinary calculi formation

Authors	Methods	Intervention	Participants	Outcomes	Results	Notes
Williams et al. [29]	• RCT, placebo controlled • Stone analysis-confirmed struvite stone formers or staghorn calculi pts with persistent urea-splitting organism UTI • FU: mean 15.8 months (AHA), 19.6 months (placebo)	Suppressive antibiotics ± AHA	• AHA – 20 pts • Placebo – 19 pts	• Doubling of 2-dimensional stone area or formation of new stones • Number of surgical interventions for obstruction or infection • Adverse reactions	• Doubling of stone area 0% (AHA), 37% (placebo), p=0.008 • RR doubling of stone area 0.04 (95% CI 0.00–0.77) • Number of surgical interventions 0% (AHA), 11% (placebo), p NS • Adverse reactions 45% (AHA), 5% (placebo), p=0.008	• Adverse reactions included tremulousness, deep venous thrombosis, and intolerable headache
Griffith et al. [30]	• RCT, placebo controlled, double blind • Spinal cord injury patients with chronic urea-splitting organism UTI • FU: planned 2 years, actual not stated	AHA	• AHA – 121 pts • Control – 89 pts	• Freedom from stone growth • Doubling of stone area or increase in stone size to ≥100 mm2	• Freedom from stone growth at 1 year 67% (AHA), 40% (placebo), p=0.017 • Freedom from stone growth at 2 years 58% (AHA), 40% (placebo), p NS • Doubling of stone area at 1 year 17% (AHA), 33% (placebo) • Doubling of stone area at 2 years 4% (AHA), 31% (placebo)	• 49% of pts did not complete the study • 20% of AHA pts did not complete the study due to severe or recurrent adverse reactions including gastrointestinal, neurological, and hematological side effects • 1-year analysis includes only 85 pts, 2-year analysis includes only 59 pts
Griffith et al. [28]	• RCT, placebo controlled, double blind • Struvite stone formers with urea-splitting organism UTI • FU: mean 18 months	AHA	• AHA – 45 pts • Placebo – 49 pts	• Stone area growth ≥25%	• Stone area growth 17% (AHA), 46% (placebo), p<0.005 • RR stone area growth 0.23 (95% CI 0.09–0.63)	• 4% of AHA pts discontinued treatment due to toxic reactions including hemolytic anemia and phlebitis

Comment

Although there are only a limited number of studies on the use of AHA, the evidence is of moderate quality. There appears to be a significant benefit to AHA therapy in the setting of struvite stone disease with chronic urinary tract infections due to urea-splitting organisms. These benefits are partially offset by the risk of significant adverse reactions. Given the considerable potential morbidity of recurrent stone disease of an infectious etiology, however, a recommendation to treat recurrent struvite stone patients with AHA is a strong one and is based upon moderate-quality evidence (Grade 1B).

Implications for practice

In the setting of acute distal ureteral calculi up to 10 mm in diameter in patients with normal renal function, no hydronephrosis, and no evidence of infection, the evidence suggests that MET can improve spontaneous stone passage rates and time to stone passage. In 2007, Bensalah et al. demonstrated that MET with tamsulosin was associated with a $1132 cost advantage per patient over observation in the United States [31]. Most patients should therefore be given a trial of an alpha-adrenergic antagonist for up to 4–6 weeks. Those patients who cannot tolerate an alpha-adrenergic antagonist may be placed on a calcium channel blocker as an alternative. Patients who do not pass their stones spontaneously or who develop intractable pain, hydronephrosis, and/or infection will subsequently require an intervention such as ureteroscopic stone removal or SWL. For those patients undergoing SWL, the evidence suggests that MET can improve stone clearance rates and therefore such patients should also be given a trial of an alpha-adrenergic antagonist or a calcium channel blocker.

In the long-term setting, the evidence suggests that empiric medical therapy may decrease rates of stone formation and improve stone-free rates in a general stone-forming population. Although the evidence is less extensive, directed medical therapy may provide a significant benefit in appropriately metabolically selected patients even when the therapy does not show a significant benefit in an unselected population. In particular, a thiazide derivative may be useful in hypercalciuric patients, allopurinol may be useful in hyperuricosuric patients, and AHA may be useful in struvite stone patients with chronic urinary tract infections due to urea-splitting organisms. For patients with recurrent stone formation in the setting of hypocitraturia or gouty diathesis, alkali citrate therapy would be appropriate.

In an international cost-effectiveness assessment of medical therapy, Lotan et al. found that, except in the United Kingdom where medication costs were the lowest, conservative management strategies were more cost-effective than drug therapy [32]. Nevertheless, medical management strategies resulted in significantly lower rates of stone formation. Because of the cost advantage of conservative management, patients should be fully informed regarding the potential benefits, risks, and costs of medical management prior to initiation of therapy.

Implications for research

The evidence for MET using alpha-adrenergic antagonists and calcium channel antagonists for distal ureteral stones and after SWL is of moderate to high quality. Based on these results, it would be logical to extend their use to the postureteroscopy and postpercutaneous lithotripsy settings. The evidence supporting improved stone clearance rates after SWL further suggests a basis for the use of MET for proximal and mid-ureteral stones. Future research focusing on spontaneous stone passage of proximal and mid-ureteral stones as well as stone clearance after ureteroscopy and percutaneous nephrolithotomy will be necessary to determine the efficacy of MET in these settings. Further studies on the efficacy and safety of MET using corticosteroids in patients with ureteral calculi are also needed.

In contrast to the investigations on MET, studies of prophylactic medical therapy are generally of lower quality and no new RCTs have been published since 1997. This limitation is mainly due to the concern of withholding apparently effective therapy in stone-forming patients. Many of the studies that have been reported did not show a significant benefit for prophylactic medical therapy. The majority of these trials were performed in unselected patient populations. Future research should address these issues with well-designed RCTs in appropriately metabolically selected patients.

References

1. Weiss RM. Physiology and pharmacology of the renal pelvis and ureter. In: Wein AJ (ed) *Campbell-Walsh Urology*, vol 3, 9th edn. Philadelphia: Saunders, 2007: 1905-20.
2. Morita T, Wada I, Saeki H, Tsuchida S, Weiss RM. Ureteral urine transport: changes in bolus volume, peristaltic frequency, intraluminal pressure and volume of flow resulting from autonomic drugs. J Urol 1987;137:132.
3. Andersson KE, Forman A. Effects of calcium channel blockers on urinary tract smooth muscle. Acta Pharmacol Toxicol (Copenh) 1986;58(suppl 2):193.

4. Hollingsworth JM, Rogers MA,Kaufman SR, et al. Medical therapy to facilitate urinary stone passage: a meta-analysis. Lancet 2006;368:1171.

5. Parsons JK, Hergan LA, Sakamoto K, Lakin C. Efficacy of alpha-blockers for the treatment of ureteral stones. J Urol 2007;177:983.

6. Pietrow PK, Preminger GM. Evaluation and medical management of urinary lithiasis. In: Wein AJ (ed) *Campbell-Walsh Urology*, vol 2, 9th edn. Philadelphia: Saunders, 2007: 1393-30.

7. Pearle MS, Roehrborn CG, Pak CY. Meta-analysis of randomized trials for medical prevention of calcium oxalate nephrolithiasis. J Endourol 1999;13:679.

8. Taghavi R, Darabi MR, Tavakoli K, Keshvari M. Survey of the effect of tamsulosin and nifedipine on facilitating juxtavesical ureteral stone passage. Paper presented at the Endourology Society Annual Meeting. Amsterdam, 2005.

9. Porpiglia F, Vaccino D, Billia M, et al. Second cycle of medical expulsive therapy with tamsulosin in patients non responders to a first cycle for distal ureteral stones: results of a prospective randomised trial. Paper presented at the 23rd Annual European Association of Urology Congress. Milan, 2008.

10. Erturhan S, Erbagci A, Yagci F, et al. Comparative evaluation of efficacy of use of tamsulosin and/or tolterodine for medical treatment of distal ureteral stones. Urology 2007;69:633.

11. Liatsikos EN, Katsakiori PF, Assimakopoulos K, et al. Doxazosin for the management of distal-ureteral stones. J Endourol 2007;21:538.

12. Yilmaz E, Batislam E, Basar MM, et al. The comparison and efficacy of 3 different alpha1-adrenergic blockers for distal ureteral stones. J Urol 2005;173:2010.

13. Tekin A, Alkan E, Beysel M, et al. Alpha-1 receptor blocking therapy for lower ureteral stones: a randomized prospective trial. Paper presented at the 2004 Annual Meeting of the American Urological Association, San Francisco, 2004.

14. Pedro RN, Hinck B, Hendlin K, et al. Alfuzosin stone expulsion therapy for distal ureteral calculi: a double-blind, placebo controlled study. J Urol 2008;179:2244.

15. Staerman F, Bryckaert P, Colin J, et al. Nifedipine in the medical treatment of symptomatic distal ureteral calculi. Avail-able online at: www.urobel.uroweb.ru/meeting/pass/brussels/?page = 110.

16. Porpiglia F, Destefanis P, Fiori C, Fontana D. Effectiveness of nifedipine and deflazacort in the management of distal ureter stones. Urology 2000;56:579.

17. Cooper JT, Stack GM, Cooper TP. Intensive medical management of ureteral calculi. Urology 2000;56:575.

18. Dellabella M, Milanese G, Muzzonigro G. Medical-expulsive therapy for distal ureterolithiasis: randomized prospective study on role of corticosteroids used in combination with tamsulosin-simplified treatment regimen and health-related quality of life. Urology 2005;66:712.

19. Resim S, Ekerbicer HC, Ciftci A. Role of tamsulosin in treatment of patients with steinstrasse developing after extracorporeal shock wave lithotripsy. Urology 2005;66:945.

20. Mortensen JT, Schultz A, Ostergaard AH. Thiazides in the prophylactic treatment of recurrent idiopathic kidney stones. Int Urol Nephrol 1986;18:265.

21. Wilson DR, Strauss AL, Manuel MA. Comparison of medical treatments for the prevention of recurrent calcium nephrolithiasis. Urol Res 1984;12:39.

22. Robertson WG, Peacock M, Selby PL, et al. A multicentre trial to evaluate three treatments for recurrent idiopathic calcium stone disease – a preliminary report. In: Schwille PO (ed) *Urolithiasis and Related Clinical Research*. New York: Plenum Press, 1985: 545-8.

23. Borghi L, Meschi T, Guerra A, Novarini A. Randomized prospective study of a nonthiazide diuretic, indapamide, in preventing calcium stone recurrences. J Cardiovasc Pharmacol 1993;22(suppl 6): S78.

24. Ettinger B, Citron JT, Livermore B, Dolman LI. Chlorthalidone reduces calcium oxalate calculous recurrence but magnesium hydroxide does not. J Urol 1988;139:679.

25. Miano L, Petta S, Paradiso-Galatioto G, Goldoni S, Tubaro A. A placebo controlled double-blind study of allopurinol in severe recurrent idiopathic renal lithiasis. Preliminary results. In: Schwille PO (ed) *Urolithiasis and Related Clinical Research*. New York: Plenum Press, 1985: 521-4.

26. Ettinger B, Tang A, Citron JT, Livermore B, Williams T. Randomized trial of allopurinol in the prevention of calcium oxalate calculi. N Engl J Med 1986;315:1386.

27. Barcelo P, Wuhl O, Servitge E, Rousaud A, Pak CY. Randomized double-blind study of potassium citrate in idiopathic hypocitraturic calcium nephrolithiasis. J Urol 1993;150:1761.

28. Griffith DP, Gleeson MJ, Lee H, Longuet R, Deman E, Earle N. Randomized, double-blind trial of Lithostat (acetohydroxamic acid) in the palliative treatment of infection-induced urinary calculi. Eur Urol 1991;20:243.

29. Williams JJ, Rodman JS, Peterson CM. A randomized double-blind study of acetohydroxamic acid in struvite nephrolithiasis. N Engl J Med 1984;311:760.

30. Griffith DP, Khonsari F, Skurnick JH, James KE. A randomized trial of acetohydroxamic acid for the treatment and prevention of infection-induced urinary stones in spinal cord injury patients. J Urol 1988;140:318.

31. Bensalah K, Pearle M, Lotan Y. Cost-effectiveness of medical expulsive therapy using alpha-blockers for the treatment of distal ureteral stones. Eur Urol 2008;53 411.

32. Lotan Y, Cadeddu JA, Pearle MS. International comparison of cost effectiveness of medical management strategies for nephrolithiasis. Urol Res 2005;33:223.

33. Cervenakov I, Fillo J, Mardiak J, Kopecny M, Smirala J, Lepies P. Speedy elimination of ureterolithiasis in lower part of ureters with the alpha 1-blocker Tamsulosin. Int Urol Nephrol 2002;34:25.

34. Dellabella M, Milanese G, Muzzonigro G. Efficacy of tamsulosin in the medical management of juxtavesical ureteral stones. J Urol 2003;170:2202.

35. Porpiglia F, Ghignone G, Fiori C, Fontana D, Scarpa RM. Nifedipine versus tamsulosin for the management of lower ureteral stones. J Urol 2004;172:568.

36. Kupeli B, Irkilata L, Gurocak S, et al. Does tamsulosin enhance lower ureteral stone clearance with or without shock wave lithotripsy? Urology 2004;64:1111.

37. Resim S, Ekerbicer H, Ciftci A. Effect of tamsulosin on the number and intensity of ureteral colic in patients with lower ureteral calculus. Int J Urol 2005;12:615.

38. Autorino R, de Sio M, Damiano R, et al. The use of tamsulosin in the medical treatment of ureteral calculi: where do we stand? Urol Res 2005;33:460.

39. Dellabella M, Milanese G, Muzzonigro G. Randomized trial of the efficacy of tamsulosin, nifedipine and phloroglucinol in medical expulsive therapy for distal ureteral calculi. J Urol 2005;174:167.

40. De Sio M, Autorino R, di Lorenzo G, et al. Medical expulsive treatment of distal-ureteral stones using tamsulosin: a single-center experience. J Endourol 2006;20:12.

41. Wang CJ, Huang SW, Chang CH. Efficacy of an alpha1 blocker in expulsive therapy of lower ureteral stones. J Endourol 2008;22:41.

42. Ayubov B, Arustamov D, Mukhtarov S. Efficacy of doxazosin in the management of ureteral stones. Paper presented at the 22nd Annual European Association of Urology Congress. Berlin, 2007.

43. Borghi L, Meschi T, Amato F, et al. Nifedipine and methyl-prednisolone in facilitating ureteral stone passage: a randomized, double-blind, placebo-controlled study. J Urol 1994;152:1095.

44. Skrekas T, Liapis D, Kalantzis A, et al. Increasing the success rate of medical therapy for expulsion of distal ureteral stones using adjunctive treatment with calcium channel blocker. Paper presented at the 18th Annual European Association of Urology Congress, Madrid, 2003.

45. Salehi M, Fouladi Mehr M, Shiery H, Mokhtari G, Dejabad V. Does methylprednisolone acetate increase the success rate of medical therapy for passing distal ureteral stones? Paper presented at the 20th Annual European Association of Urology Congress, Istanbul, 2005.

46. Porpiglia F, Vaccino D, Billia M, et al. What is the role of corticosteroid therapy in the management of distal ureteral stones in emergency? Paper presented at the 21st Annual European Association of Urology Congress, Paris, 2006.

47. Porpiglia F, Destefanis P, Fiori C, Scarpa RM, Fontana D. Role of adjunctive medical therapy with nifedipine and deflazacort after extracorporeal shock wave lithotripsy of ureteral stones. Urology 2002;59:835.

48. Gravina GL, Costa AM, Ronchi P, et al. Tamsulosin treatment increases clinical success rate of single extracorporeal shock wave lithotripsy of renal stones. Urology 2005;66:24.

49. Bhagat SK, Chacko NK, Kekre NS, et al. Is there a role for tamsulosin in shock wave lithotripsy for renal and ureteral calculi? J Urol 2007;177:2185.

50. Gravas S, Tzortzis V, Karatzas A, Oeconomou A, Melekos MD. The use of tamsulozin as adjunctive treatment after ESWL in patients with distal ureteral stone: do we really need it? Results from a randomised study. Urol Res 2007;35:231.

51. Mukhtarov S, Turdiev A, Fozilov A, Arustamov D, Ayubov B. Using doxazosin for distal ureteral stone clearance with or without shock wave lithotripsy. Paper presented at the 22nd Annual European Association of Urology Congress, Berlin, 2007.

52. Shaaban AM, Barsoum NM, Sagheer GA, Anwar AZ. Is there a role for alpha blockers after SWL for renal and upper ureteral stones? Paper presented at the Annual Meeting of the American Urological Association, Orlando, 2008.

53. Brocks P, Dahl C, Wolf H, Transbol I. Do thiazides prevent recurrent idiopathic renal calcium stones? Lancet 1981;2:124.

54. Scholz D, Schwille PO, Sigel A. Double-blind study with thiazide in recurrent calcium lithiasis. J Urol 1982;128:903.

55. Laerum E, Larsen S. Thiazide prophylaxis of urolithiasis. A double-blind study in general practice. Acta Med Scand 1984;215:383.

56. Ohkawa M, Tokunaga S, Nakashima T, Orito M, Hisazumi H. Thiazide treatment for calcium urolithiasis in patients with idiopathic hypercalciuria. BJU 1992;69:571.

57. Hofbauer J, Hobarth K, Szabo N, Marberger M. Alkali citrate prophylaxis in idiopathic recurrent calcium oxalate urolithiasis – a prospective randomized study. BJU 1994;73:362.

58. Ettinger B, Pak CY, Citron JT, Thomas C, Adams-Huet B, Vangessel A. Potassium-magnesium citrate is an effective prophylaxis against recurrent calcium oxalate nephrolithiasis. J Urol 1997;158:2069.

23 Surgical management of renal stone disease

Adam C. Mues,[1] Bodo E. Knudsen[1] and Benjamin K. Canales[2]

[1]Department of Urology, Ohio State University Medical Center, Columbus, OH, USA
[2]Department of Urology, University of Florida, Gainesville, FL, USA

Clinical question 23.1

What is the most effective treatment therapy for small and medium-sized lower pole (LP) kidney stones?

Literature search

Relevant studies were retrieved from electronic databases including Cochrane Central Register of Controlled Trials, Medline 1996–current, and EMBASE 1980–current. Reference lists were also made from urology and nephrology textbooks, review articles and relevant studies as well as electronic communications seeking information about unpublished or incomplete studies to investigators known to be involved in previous studies. Search terms included all forms and abbreviations of "percutaneous nephrolithotomy (PCNL)," "shock-wave lithotripsy (SWL)," "ureteroscopy (URS)," "lithotripsy," "lower pole," and "nephrolithiasis."

The evidence

The gravity-dependent nature of the renal lower pole and its anatomy, including infundibular length, width, and infundibulopelvic angle, is thought to reduce spontaneous passage of stone fragments following lithotripsy. Two prospective randomized multicenter clinical trials have evaluated SWL, URS, and PCNL treatment modalities for small and medium-sized kidney stones in the lower pole (Table 23.1). When comparing SWL to PCNL for stones < 3 cm in the Lower Pole I study [1], KUB stone-free rate (SFR) is considerably higher for PCNL (95%) than SWL (37%, $p < 0.001$). These effects were also seen with

stones < 1 cm, with SFR for PCNL 100% and SWL at 63%. In fact, this is the only size range where SWL demonstrated SFR > 50%. Quality of life assessments and complications rates are similar for both modalities.

When considering URS for treatment of symptomatic LP stones < 1 cm (Lower Pole II study [2]), no statistically significant difference in computed tomography SFR was seen when compared to SWL. This remains true for ureteroscopy patients who had residual stone fragments manually extracted or left in place to spontaneously pass. In addition, there was no difference in the need for secondary procedures between URS and SWL cohorts. Operative time, hospital stay, and quality of life measures significantly favored patients treated with SWL.

Comment

These multicenter studies demonstrate the lack of standardization in SWL treatment. Variability occurs in the number of shocks and power settings used. Similarly, ureteral stent placement during the procedures was at surgeon discretion and not standardized. The imaging modality used for follow-up must be carefully considered, as patients in the Lower Pole II study underwent noncontrast CT scan [2] while patients in the Lower Pole I study had traditional abdominal imaging [1]. The increased sensitivity of CT compared to other imaging techniques lowers the stone free rates, 20–30% compared to less sensitive ultrasound or abdominal imaging and makes extrapolation to previous studies more difficult. Due to methodological inconsistencies, the quality of evidence is rated a Level B.

In summary, no recommendation can be given regarding small lower pole stone clearance since PCNL, SWL or URS are all reasonable options that lead to acceptable SFR. PCNL provides the highest SFR at the expense of being more invasive and associated with higher postoperative morbidity. Quality of life measures favor the less invasive approach with SWL. Ureteroscopy and laser lithotripsy with or without manual extraction of stone fragments offer

Evidence-Based Urology. Edited by Philipp Dahm, Roger R. Dmochowski.
© 2010 Blackwell Publishing.

Table 23.1 Surgical outcomes for lower pole kidney stones

Authors	Methods	Intervention	Participants	Outcomes	Results	Notes
Albala et al. [1]	RCT, multicenter FU: 3 months annually for 3 years	SWL (settings and number of shocks variable) PCNL (lithotriptors variable)	Symptomatic LP calculi ≤3.0 cm SWL: N 68 PCNL: N 60	SFR LP anatomy Complication rates Quality of life (SF-36)	• Overall SFR: • SWL -37% • PCNL -95% • (p<0.001) • SFR not influenced by LP anatomy • QOL changes were not statistically significant • No significant differences in complication rate (p=0.087) or QOL changes (p=0.7)	• Failures were treatments other than assigned treatment • Stenting at surgeon discretion • Tomography follow-up imaging
Pearle et al. [2]	RCT, multicenter FU: 2–6 weeks 3 months	SWL (settings and number of shocks variable) URS (scopes, stent, access sheaths variable)	Symptomatic LP stone <1cm SWL: N 32 URS: N 35	SFR QOL (RAND 36 Health Survey) Secondary procedures	• SFR not statistically significantly different (p 0.92) • QOL – SWL favored over URS (difference statistically significant in all categories) • Secondary treatments not significantly different	• URS – 60% pts stones manually removed • Stent placement variable • Noncontrast CT follow-up imaging

a less invasive alternative to PCNL with SFR similar to SWL. Developments in ureteroscope technology are ongoing and may lead to further improvements in SFR.

Clinical question 23.2

What is the effect of adjuvant therapies following surgery for kidney stones?

Literature search

Relevant studies were retrieved from electronic databases including Cochrane Central Register of Controlled Trials, Medline 1996–current, and EMBASE 1980–current. Reference lists were also made from urology and nephrology textbooks, review articles and relevant studies as well as electronic communications seeking information about unpublished or incomplete studies to investigators known to be involved in previous studies. Search terms included all forms and abbreviations of "percussion, diuresis, and inversion (PDI)," "PCNL," SWL," "URS," "lithotripsy," "nephrolithiasis," "medical," "therapy," "niruri."

The evidence

Evidence that ureteral stone clearance may be enhanced with medication has been increasing for several years,

and indeed multiple RCTs comparing SFR of SWL with or without tamsulosin in the setting of ureteral stones have now been performed [3-8]. Evidence for adjuvant therapy following kidney stone surgery has also demonstrated a benefit in SFR following SWL using adjuvant alpha-blocker therapy, dietary supplements (*P. niruru*) or mechanical assistance.

Gravina et al. [9] reported the first and most convincing evidence for adjunctive tamsulosin following SWL for kidney stones. Their group studied 130 patients who were randomized to standard therapy alone (control) or in combination with tamsulosin for a total of 12 weeks or until another intervention occurred. They report higher KUB SFR and less pain and analgesic use in the tamsulosin group compared to controls. Subjects with larger diameter renal stones (> 10 mm) benefited most from therapy (81% vs 55%, p = 0.009) compared to stones ≤ 10 mm (75% vs 68%, p > 0.05). Incidence of repeat SWL or ureteroscopy (31% total) was less in the tamsulosin group but not statistically significant (p > 0.05). In this trial, subjects were not randomized to placebo pills, which may have affected self-reporting. Most recently, Naja et al. [10] reported a very similar study design to that of Gravina. Following randomization to SWL only or SWL with tamsulosin, patients had SWL done every 3 weeks for up to 12 weeks or until radiographic success. Success rates after the first, second and third SWL sessions increased more in the tamsulosin arm (53%, 78%, 94%) than in controls (31%, 52%, 75%; p = 0.016, p = 0.004, p = 0.005 respectively), but overall success at study end was similar across groups. In addition to earlier clearance of fragments, subjects on tamsulosin required fewer SWL sessions, had less pain, and developed fewer episodes of steinstrasse than controls.

In 2007, Bhagat et al. [7] reported higher KUB SFR after randomizing patients with both ureteral and renal stones to tamsulosin (96.6%) or placebo (79.3%) after SWL, although analgesic administration between the groups was similar. Subgroup analysis revealed that patients with stones > 10 mm had significantly higher SFR (93.3% vs 58.3%, p = 0.03) compared to stones ≤ 10 mm (100% vs 94.1%, p = 0.35). Methods for analgesic dosing in the study were unclear, and location of stone clearance was not evaluated.

Micali et al. [11] hypothesized that the plant *Phyllanthus niruri* would improve SFR after SWL in patients with calcium oxalate stones. *P. niruri* belongs to the Euphorbiaceae family and has been shown to reduce urinary calcium by inhibiting calcium oxalate crystal adhesion and growth. Patients in the study were randomized to receive either the *P. niruri* extract Uriston® or no medical therapy. Overall SFR was improved after a 6-month follow-up in the *P. niruri* group but did not reach statistical significance (p = 0.48). When divided into location, patients taking Uriston who had stones in the lower pole had SFR of 93.7% compared to 70.8% (p = 0.001) in patients receiving no oral therapy. Similarly, patients in the Uriston arm achieved significantly higher SFR when the stones were ≤ 10 mm (p = 0.02). No significant difference was seen in retreatment rates between groups.

In 1990, Brownlee et al. [12] first introduced the concept that residual stone debris in dependent portions of the kidney could be manipulated by changing body position. Pace et al. [13] first demonstrated Level 1 evidence by using percussion, diuresis, and inversion (PDI) therapy as adjunctive treatment for patients with residual lower pole stone fragments < 4 mm who were more than 3 months post SWL. Patients were randomized to receive therapy or observation and were followed for 4 weeks. Patients in the treatment arm underwent percussion and inversion therapy once per week. All patients were followed with an imaging study (x-ray and tomography or CT) read by a radiologist blinded to the treatment groups in order to determine stone-free status. SFR for the treatment group and observation group were 40% and 3% respectively (p < 0.001). Patients undergoing observation who had residual stones at 4 weeks were offered cross-over into the treatment arm, and these patients also experienced improvement in SFR. Chiong et al. [14] corroborated their findings by demonstrating significantly higher SFR in patients undergoing PDI with small, post-SWL residual lower pole stones.

Comment

Six prospective randomized trials have demonstrated that adjunctive therapy after SWL improves SFR. Uriston (*P. niruri*) is a safe, well-tolerated medication that may augment KUB SFR, especially in patients with stones < 1 cm and for those located in the lower pole. However, this study was only positive in subset analysis and was flawed as it included patients with multiple SWL sessions. Tamsulosin appears to safely increase stone fragment clearance rate and time while having a positive impact on pain. Several trials suggest it may increase SFR for stones > 10 mm in size, and its dosage and side effect profile are well known to urologists. PDI adjunctive therapy has been shown in two randomized prospective trials to increase SFR in patients with small residual lower pole stones after SWL. Despite the evidence, this therapy has not become routine practice due to the intensity and time required for this intervention. We give these adjuncts (except Uriston) a strong recommendation based on moderate-quality evidence (Grade 1B).

Clinical question 23.3

What is the benefit of SWL for small asymptomatic renal calyceal stones?

Literature search

Relevant studies were retrieved from electronic databases including Cochrane Central Register of Controlled Trials, Medline 1996–current, and EMBASE 1980–current. Reference lists were also made from urology and nephrology textbooks, review articles and relevant studies as well as electronic communications seeking information about unpublished or incomplete studies to investigators known to be involved in previous studies. Search terms included all forms and abbreviations of "SWL," "lithotripsy," "nephrolithiasis," "calyceal," and "kidney stone."

The evidence

In a prospective RCT by Keeley et al. [15] (Table 23.3), patients with a stone burden of ≤ 1.5 cm and who were asymptomatic received either prophylactic SWL or observation. Patients were treated with repeated SWL if residual fragments ≤ 5 mm were present on KUB or until three treatment sessions were completed. A median follow-up of 2.2 years demonstrated no statistically significant differences in SFR for the SWL group (28%) compared to the observation cohort (16%, p = 0.06).

Table 23.2 Adjuvant therapies following kidney stone surgery

Authors	Methods	Intervention	Participants	Outcomes	Results	Notes
Micali et al. [11]	RCT, single center FU: 1, 2, 3, 6 months (KUB/U/S)	Uriston (*P. niruri*) + SWL SWL alone	Any size calcium oxalate renal calculi Uriston: N 78 No Uriston: N 72	KUB SFR and KUB fragments ≤3 mm Retreatment rate	• No KUB SFR (94% vs 83%, p=0.48) or small fragment (89% vs 76%, p=0.08) differences • LP KUB SFR higher in Uriston (94%) compared to no Uriston (71%, p<0.001) • KUB SFR higher with stones <10 mm (97% vs 85%, p=0.02) • No difference in retreatment rate (40% vs 43%, p=0.2)	• Stents placed for stones >2.0 cm • Variable SWL sessions (1-3) • Dornier S lithotripter • 3,000 shocks/ session • Uriston group had faster stone clearance rates at 1 month (54% vs 19%, p=0.02) and 2 month FU (69% vs 35%, p=0.03)
Pace et al. [13]	RCT, single center, single blinded FU: 3 months	Mechanical PDI + SWL SWL alone	Residual lower pole fragments <4 mm, 3 or more months after SWL PDI: N 35 SWL: N 34	KUB SFR Adverse effects of intervention Prognostic factors affecting outcome	• KUB SFR: PDI 40% compared to SWL alone 3% • (p<0.001) • No adverse effects in either group • Independent predictors of outcome: stone area, location, and infundibular width	• Observation group offered crossover if persistent stones after 1 month • Blinded radiologist-determined SFR • Intervention effect at randomization and crossover was identical
Chiong et al. [14]	RCT, single blind FU: 1, 3 months	Mechanical PDI + SWL SWL alone	Radiopaque lower pole calculi ≤ 2 cm that fragmented during SWL to ≤4 mm PDI: N 59 SWL: N 49	KUB SFR Adverse effects of intervention Prognostic factors affecting outcome	• KUB SFR: PDI 63% compared to SWL alone 35% (p=0.006) • One patient found PDI painful until resolution of a SWL hematoma	• Blinded radiologist-determined SFR • 16% PDI received 5 or more sessions • Variable SWL sessions (1-4)
Bhagat et al. [7]	RCT- single center, double blinded FU: 1 month	Tamsulosin + SWL SWL + placebo	Renal and ureteral stones 6–24 mm Tam: N 29 SWL: N 29	KUB SFR Adverse events Median dose analgesics	• KUB SFR: Tam 97% compared to placebo 79% (p=0.04) • Stones >10 mm had higher clearance rates	• No differences noted in mean analgesic dose • Unable to separate renal from ureteral stones in results
Gravina et al. [9]	RCT -single center, no blinding FU: 3 months	Tamsulosin + SWL SWL alone	Renal stones 4–20 mm Tam: N 65 SWL: N 65	KUB, renal ultrasound, intravenous pyelography SFR Adverse events Analgesic use	• KUB SFR: Tam 79% compared to SWL alone 60% (p=0.0037) • Stones >10 mm had higher clearance rates	• Decreased episodes of pain and diclofenac use • Significant improvement in first (p=0.015, Tam) and last follow-up visits
Naja et al. [10]	RCT – single center, no blinding FU: ≤ 3 months	Tamsulosin + SWL SWL alone	Single, radiopaque renal stone 6–15 mm Tam: N 51 SWL: N 65	KUB SFR Rapidity of clearance	• KUB SFR at 3 months: Tam 94% vs SWL alone 85% (p=0.14) • Higher success rate at 3 weeks in Tam arm	• Power calculation performed • Up to 4 SWL performed • No blinding

The SWL group did have an overall decrease in stone burden, defined as an improvement on KUB compared with patients under observation (p = 0.026). The requirement for additional procedures, quality of life measures, and renal function tests were not significantly different between the groups, but 49 additional procedures were required in 20 patients in the observation group. Of these procedures, 10 would be considered invasive (ureteroscopy

Table 23.3 Outcome of SWL for small, asymptomatic calyceal stones

Authors	Methods	Intervention	Participants	Outcomes	Results	Notes
Keeley et al. [15]	RCT, multicenter FU: 3, 26 months	SWL: retreatment until fragments ≤5 mm (no more than three sessions) Observation group	Asymptomatic patients, combined renal stone burden of ≤1.5 cm SWL: N 113 Observation: N 115	SFR (stone free) Need for additional treatment/ procedures	• Similar KUB SFR (p=0.29) with improved stone burden in SWL pts (p=0.026) • Large residual fragments • improved with SWL (p=0.001) • No significant differences in need for additional treatment	• Two centers with different lithotriptors • 88% pts completed 1 year FU • Invasive intervention: 10 pts in observation group no patients in SWL group • No difference in symptoms, QOL or renal function tests

or stenting). In contrast, only nine additional procedures in three patients were required in the SWL group, none of which was invasive.

Comment

The evidence from this RCT suggests that treatment with SWL for small asymptomatic calyceal stones provides marginal benefit over observation when considering SFR, symptoms, renal function, and the need for subsequent procedures. Although not statistically significant, patients being observed may require both an increased number of secondary procedures as well as a greater number of subsequent invasive procedures. Patients undergoing SWL demonstrated a decrease in stone burden on KUB following the procedure. However, the clinical significance of this finding is unknown as SFR were similar in both groups. Overall, no recommendation can be made with level of evidence Grade B.

Clinical question 23.4

What is the effect of shock-wave delivery on SWL kidney stone outcomes?

Literature search

Relevant studies were retrieved from electronic databases including Cochrane Central Register of Controlled Trials, Medline 1996–current, and EMBASE 1980–current. Reference lists were also made from urology and nephrology textbooks, review articles and relevant studies. Search terms

included all forms and abbreviations of "SWL," "lithotripsy, " "nephrolithiasis," "rate," and "kidney stone."

The evidence

Four RCTs have been performed examining the effect of shock-wave rate on the outcome of SWL (Table 23.4). Three of these studies demonstrated higher success rates when the rate of shock-wave delivery was slowed to either 60 or 90 shocks/min compared to the typical 120 shocks/min. The fourth study showed no differences between the 60 and 120 shock groups. A recent meta-analysis of all four of these RCTs demonstrated that patients who were treated at 60 shocks/min experienced a 10.2% (95% confidence interval (CI) 3.7–16.8) increase in the likelihood of a successful treatment outcome (p = 0.002) over those who had 120 shocks/min.

Comment

Based on these four studies, it appears that slowing the rate of SWL leads to ,10% higher success rates for renal stones, and subset analysis demonstrated a trend of higher success rates in patients with larger stones (≥ 8 mm). Unfortunately, the standard definition of "success" among these studies varied from 99% to 61%, and no comment can be made on SFR as only two studies included this as an outcome. Additionally, there was significant disparity between study methodologies, as all four studies had different inclusion criteria, used different lithotripters, had varying anesthetic protocols, and used an assortment of imaging modalities for follow-up. Therefore, only a conditional recommendation can be made based on low-quality evidence (Grade 2C).

Table 23.4 Outcomes for SWL at varying delivery rates

Authors	Methods	Intervention	Participants	Outcomes	Results	Notes
Madbouly et al. [16]	RCT, single center FU: 3 month KUB (100%)	SWL at 60 shocks per minute SWL at 120 shocks per minute	Single <30 mm radiopaque renal or ureteral stone 60 shocks/min: N 76 pts 120 shocks/min: N 80 pts	Success: <2 mm fragments or stone free	• Success rate 99% vs 90% (p=0.034)	• Ureteral stones 40% • Electromagnetic lithotripter and general/regional anesthesia • Mean stone length 13 mm
Pace et al. [13]	RCT, single center FU: 2 weeks and 3 month KUB (95%), CT (3%) or IVP (2%)	SWL at 60 shocks per minute SWL at 120 shocks per minute	Single ≤5 mm radiopaque kidney stone 60 shocks/min: N 110 pts 120 shocks/min: N 108 pts	Success (<5 mm residual) Stone-free rate Complications Retreatment	• Success rate 75% vs 61% (p=0.027) • Stone-free rate 60% vs 44% (p=0.065) • Complications 11% vs 19% (p=0.079) • Retreatment rate 18% vs 32% (p=0.018)	• Electrohydraulic lithotripter and sedation • Mean stone size 80 mm²
Yilmaz et al. [17]	RCT, single center FU: 10 days with KUB and RUS (100%)	SWL at 60 shocks per minute SWL at 90 shocks per minute SWL at 120 shocks per minute	Single <20 mm radiopaque kidney stone 60 shocks/min: N 56 pts 90 shocks/min: N 57 pts 120 shocks/min: N 57 pts	Success: <3 mm residual Sedation requirement Stone location and mineral composition	• Higher success rates with 60 (89%, p=0.015) and 90 (88%, p=0.032) compared to 120 (73%) • More sedation used with 120 (41%) vs 90 (16%, p=0.018) and 60 (14%, p<0.01) • No differences for location nor composition	• Electrohydraulic lithotripter and local +/-sedation • Mean stone size 13 mm
Davenport et al. [18]	RCT, multicenter FU: 3 months with KUB (100%)	SWL at 60 shocks per minute SWL at 120 shocks per minute	Single uncomplicated radiopaque kidney stone 60 shocks/min: N 49 pts 120 shocks/min: N 51 pts	Success <4 mm residual	• Success rate 61% vs 59% (p=0.87) • Stone-free rate 60% vs 44% (p=0.065) • Complications 11% vs 19% (p=0.079) • Retreatment rate 18% vs 32% (p=0.018)	• Electromagnetic lithotripter and sedation • 49% retreatment rate • Mean stone size 60 mm²

References

1. Albala DM, Assimos DG, Clayman RV, et al. Lower Pole I: a prospective randomized trial of extracorporeal shock wave lithotripsy and percutaneous nephrostolithotomy for lower pole nephrolithiasis-initial results. J Urol 2001;166:2072-80.
2. Pearle MS, Lingeman JE, Leveillee R, et al. Prospective, randomized trial comparing shock wave lithotripsy and ureteroscopy for lower pole caliceal calculi 1 cm or less. J Urol 2005;173:2005-9.
3. Kupeli B, Irkilata L, Gurocak S, et al. Does tamsulosin enhance lower ureteral stone clearance with or without shock wave lithotripsy? Urology 2004;64:1111-15.
4. Gravas S, Tzortzis V, Karatzas A, Oeconomou A, Melekos MD. The use of tamsulozin as adjunctive treatment after ESWL in patients with distal ureteral stone: do we really need it? Results from a randomised study. Urol Res 2007;35:231-5.
5. Kobayashi M, Naya Y, Kino M, et al. Low dose tamsulosin for stone expulsion after extracorporeal shock wave lithotripsy: efficacy in Japanese male patients with ureteral stone. Int J Urol 2008;15:495-8.
6. Resim S, Ekerbicer HC, Ciftci A. Role of tamsulosin in treatment of patients with steinstrasse developing after extracorporeal shock wave lithotripsy. Urology 2005;66:945-8.
7. Bhagat SK, Chacko NK, Kekre NS, Gopalakrishnan G, Antonisamy B, Devasia A. Is there a role for tamsulosin in shock wave lithotripsy for renal and ureteral calculi? J Urol 2007;177:2185-8.
8. Porpiglia F, Destefanis P, Fiori C, Scarpa RM, Fontana D. Role of adjunctive medical therapy with nifedipine and deflazacort

after extracorporeal shock wave lithotripsy of ureteral stones. Urology 2002;59:835-8.

9. Gravina GL, Costa AM, Ronchi P, et al.Tamsulosin treatment increases clinical success rate of single extracorporeal shock wave lithotripsy of renal stones. Urology 2005;66:24-8.

10. Naja V, Agarwal MM, Mandal AK, et al. Tamsulosin facilitates earlier clearance of stone fragments and reduces pain after shockwave lithotripsy for renal calculi: results from an open-label randomized study. Urology 2008;72:1006-11.

11. Micali S, Sighinolfi MC, Celia A, et al. Can Phyllanthus niruri affect the efficacy of extracorporeal shock wave lithotripsy for renal stones? A randomized, prospective, long-term study. J Urol 2006;176:1020-2.

12. Brownlee N, Foster M, Griffith DP, Carlton CE Jr. Controlled inversion therapy: an adjunct to the elimination of gravity-dependent fragments following extracorporeal shock wave lithotripsy. J Urol 1990;143:1096-8.

13. Pace KT, Tariq N, Dyer SJ, et al. Mechanical percussion, inversion and diuresis for residual lower pole fragments after shock wave lithotripsy: a prospective, single blind, randomized controlled trial. J Urol 2001;166:2065-71.

14. Chiong E, Hwee ST, Kay LM, Liang S, Kamaraj R, Esuvaranathan K. Randomized controlled study of mechanical percussion, diuresis, and inversion therapy to assist passage of lower pole renal calculi after shock wave lithotripsy. Urology 2005;65:1070-4.

15. Keeley FX Jr, Tilling K, Elves A, et al. Preliminary results of a randomized controlled trial of prophylactic shock wave lithotripsy for small asymptomatic renal calyceal stones. BJU Int 2001;87:1-8.

16. Madbouly K, El-Tiraifi AM, Seida M, El-Faqih SR, Atassi R, Talic RF. Slow versus fast shock wave lithotripsy rate for urolithiasis: a prospective randomized study. J Urol 2005;173:127-30.

17. Yilmaz E, Batislam E, Basar M, Tuglu D, Mert C, Basar H. Optimal frequency in extracorporeal shock wave lithotripsy: prospective randomized study. Urology 2005;66:1160-4.

18. Davenport K, Minervini A, Keoghane S, Parkin J, Keeley FX, Timoney AG. Does rate matter? The results of a randomized controlled trial of 60 versus 120 shocks per minute for shock wave lithotripsy of renal calculi. J Urol 2006;176:2055-8; discussion 2058.

24 Surgical management of ureteral stone disease

Jay D. Raman[1] and Margaret S. Pearle[2]
[1]Division of Urology, Penn State Milton S. Hershey Medical Center, Hershey, PA, USA
[2]Department of Urology, University of Texas Southwestern Medical Center, Dallas, TX, USA

Background

Nephrolithiasis occurs with an estimated overall prevalence of 5.2% and there is evidence that stone disease is on the rise [1]. However, many stones in the kidney go undetected because they cause no symptoms or obstruction. Conversely, ureteral stones rarely remain silent, and they have greater potential for causing pain and obstruction. As such, ureteral stones that fail to pass spontaneously require surgical intervention. Although the introduction of medical expulsive therapy (MET, the use of pharmacological agents to promote spontaneous stone passage) has changed the natural history of ureteral stone disease [2], not all ureteral stones respond to MET. Indications for surgical intervention to remove ureteral calculi include stones that are unlikely or fail to pass spontaneously with or without MET, stones that cause unremitting pain regardless of the likelihood of spontaneous passage, stones associated with persistent, high-grade obstruction, stones in patients with an anatomically or functionally solitary kidney or in those with renal insufficiency or stones in patients for whom their occupation or circumstances mandate prompt resolution (i.e. pilots, frequent travelers, etc.).

Once the decision has been made to intervene surgically for a patient with a ureteral stone, treatment options include shock-wave lithotripsy, ureteroscopy, percutaneous antegrade ureteroscopy and open or laparoscopic ureterolithotomy. Although special cirumstances may dictate the application of percutaneous antegrade ureteroscopy or ureterolithotomy (large, impacted stones, stones in patients with urinary diversions or stones that fail less invasive approaches), the two most widely practiced treatment modalities for ureteral stones are shock-wave lithotripsy (SWL) and ureteroscopy (URS). Both are associated with high success rates and low morbidity. However, the optimal treatment for ureteral stones remains controversial because of passionate advocates on both sides of the controversy. Proponents of SWL cite the noninvasiveness, high patient satisfaction and ease of treatment, while URS advocates favor the short operative times, high success rates and short time interval to become stone free. This chapter weighs the evidence in favor of SWL or URS for the treatment of ureteral stones, and also explores some of the nuances of each treatment that have evidence-based support.

Clinical question 24.1

What is the optimal surgical management for proximal, middle, and distal ureteral calculi (SWL versus URS)?

The optimal treatment modality for ureteral calculi depends on the size, location and composition of the stone, as well as the availability of equipment and expertise of the practitioner. For example, cystine stones respond poorly to SWL; consequently, URS is the preferred treatment for cystine ureteral calculi [3]. Likewise, proximal ureteral stones in a male patient may be difficult to access with a semi-rigid ureteroscope; therefore, practitioners without access to a flexible ureteroscope might not choose URS for the treatment of a proximal ureteral calculus in a male patient. Extenuating circumstances aside, however, the optimal treatment modality for noncystine, nonuric acid stones in patients with normal ureteral anatomy who are otherwise appropriate candidates for either treatment modality will be considered. Of note, however, stone size and location are important variables that affect treatment outcomes for both URS and SWL.

Evidence-Based Urology. Edited by Philipp Dahm, Roger R. Dmochowski.
© 2010 Blackwell Publishing.

Literature search

A search of the Medline database was performed using the terms "ureteral calculi," "shock-wave lithotripsy," "ureteroscopy" and "randomized, controlled trials (RCTs)." The search was limited to the English-language literature published between 1948 and 2008 and focused primarily on RCTs comparing SWL and URS.

The evidence

Despite extensive literature reporting outcomes of single-institution series of SWL or URS for the treatment of patients with ureteral calculi, as well as retrospective series comparing the two treatment modalities, only five RCTs have directly compared SWL and URS. While three RCTs focused exclusively on patients with distal ureteral calculi, only a single trial each addressed patients with proximal ureteral calculi and middle/distal ureteral stones (Table 24.1).

Lee and colleagues randomized 42 patients with large (> 15 mm) proximal ureteral calculi to undergo SWL (N 22) or URS (N 20) [4]. Single-procedure stone-free rates for both SWL and URS were poor, at 32% and 35%, respectively, Complication rates were higher in the URS group (70%) than in the SWL group (9%). Among the URS complications were five ureteral perforations and one

ureteral stricture, perhaps as a result of using a semi-rigid ureteroscope. Hospital stay (1.8 versus 4.7 days), visual analog pain scores (1.86 versus 4.35) and patient satisfaction scores (4.12 versus 3.86) all favored SWL over URS, although only length of stay reached statistical significance. Of note, the degree of hydronephrosis correlated negatively with SWL success ($p = 0.005$). The authors concluded that in the absence of hydronephrosis, both SWL and URS were reasonable therapies for large proximal ureteral stones. However, with the use of current small, flexible ureteroscopes, it is likely that the outcomes would be substantially different, since ureteral perforation, inaccessible stone and retrograde stone migration accounted for the majority of URS failures. Such factors are now routinely overcome with the use of a flexible ureteroscope.

Hendrikx and associates randomized patients with extended-middle and distal ureteral calculi to SWL (N 69) or URS (N 87) [5]. Overall, URS was associated with higher stone-free and lower retreatment rates than SWL (91% and 9%, respectively, for URS versus 51% and 45%, respectively, for SWL). This held true when outcomes were stratified by stone location: stone-free rates for URS and SWL were 81% versus 51%, respectively, for extended-middle ureteral calculi and 96% versus 50%, respectively, for distal ureteral calculi. On the other hand, complication rates and hospital length of stay favored SWL (4.3% and 2.2 days for SWL

Table 24.1 Randomized controlled trials of URS versus SWL for ureteral calculi

Author	Location (size)	F/U	Lithotripter	Patients	Stone-free rates	p-value
Hendrikx [5]	Extended-mid and distal (5–11 mm)	12 wks	Dornier HM4	69 SWL	51% (35/69) Ext-mid 51% (20/39) Distal 50% (15/30)	–
				87 URS	91% (79/87) Ext-mid 81% (26/32) Distal 96% (50/52)	
Peschel [6]	Distal (40 >5 mm; 40 <5 mm)	43 days	Dornier MFL 5000	40 SWL	85% (17/20) <5 mm 95% (19/20) >5 mm	–
				40 URS	100% (20/20) <5 mm 100% (20/20) >5 mm	
Pearle [8]	Distal (<15 mm)	3 mos	Dornier HM3	32 SWL	100% (32/32)	NS
				32 URS	100% (32/32)	
Zeng [7]	Distal (6–21 mm)	28 days	HB-ESWL-V	210 SWL	78% (164/210) RTx 12%	<0.05
				180 URS	93% (168/180) RTx 2%	
Lee [4]	Proximal (≥15 mm)	N/A	Siemans AG Lithostar 2	22 SWL	32% (14/22) single Tx	–
				20 URS	35% (7/20) single Tx	

NS, not significant; RTx, retreatment rates; Tx, treatment

versus 25.2% and 4.4 days for URS). Although stone-free and retreatment rates strongly favored URS, the lower complication rate and shorter length of stay make SWL a reasonable alternative, particularly for smaller stones.

A total of three RCTs compared SWL and URS for the management of distal ureteral calculi. Peschel and colleagues randomized 80 patients with distal ureteral stones that failed to pass to SWL (N 40) or URS (N 40) [6]. Although stone-free rates were high in both groups (90% for SWL versus 100% for URS), the authors recommended URS over SWL for distal ureteral calculi because the time to become stone free was shorter in the URS group (1.8 days) compared with the SWL group (10 days).

Zeng and co-workers also favored URS for the treatment of distal ureteral calculi based on their RCT comparing 180 patients treated by URS to 210 patients treated with SWL [7]. The stone-free rate was higher for URS than SWL (93% versus 78%, respectively, $p < 0.05$), and the retreatment rate was fivefold higher for SWL than URS (11.9% versus 2.2%, retrospectively, $p < 0.05$).

In contrast, Pearle and colleagues, in a multicenter study, randomized 64 patients with distal ureteral calculi to URS or SWL using an HM3 lithotripter (N 32 for each group) [8]. Stone-free rates were 100% in both groups, but secondary outcomes, including operating time ($p < 0.05$), outpatient procedure rate and patient satisfaction, favored SWL. As such, although SWL was more costly than URS at their institution, the authors recommended HM3 SWL over ureteroscopy since it was equally efficacious, more efficient, and less morbid.

Using these five RCTs, Nabi and colleagues performed a meta-analysis using stone-free rate, retreatment rate, need for auxiliary procedures, efficiency quotient, length of stay, complications, and patient satisfaction as endpoints [9]. Their analysis revealed lower stone-free rates in the SWL arm compared to the URS arm (RR 0.84, 95% confidence interval (CI) 0.70–0.98, $p = 0.03$). In addition, the retreatment rate was lower but not significantly so in the URS group (RR 2.28, 95% CI 0.53–14.71, $p = 0.23$), complication rate was lower in the SWL group (RR 0.45, 95% CI 0.21–0.92, $p = 0.03$), and hospital length of stay was shorter for SWL treatment (RR –2.10, 95% CI –2.55 to –1.64, $p < 0.00001$). The authors concluded that URS is associated with a higher stone-free rate, but at a cost of a higher complication rate and a longer length of stay. It should be noted, however, that combining the treatment arms of these studies may be problematic because of the heterogeneity of patient groups (i.e. stone location differs in the studies, one study included only patients with > 15 mm stones, lithotripters were different in each study). Consequently, conclusions should be interpreted with caution.

Perhaps a more applicable analysis comparing SWL and URS for the treatment of ureteral calculi can be gleaned from the 2007 American Urological Association (AUA)/

European Association of Urology (EAU) Clinical Guidelines for the Management of Ureteral Calculi [10,11]. These guidelines were derived from analysis of 348 articles published between 1996 and 2006, of which 244 contained extractable data suitable for inclusion in the meta-analysis. Despite the lack of a large number of RCTs, this analysis is less susceptible to the inherent biases associated with smaller series and provides the best available evidence to guide surgical treatment decisions for ureteral calculi.

Overall, median stone-free rates for SWL and URS were 82% versus 81%, respectively, for proximal ureteral calculi, 73% versus 86%, respectively, for middle ureteral calculi and 74% versus 94% for distal ureteral calculi (Table 24.2). The more distal the stone, the greater the gap in outcomes between the two treatment modalities, in favor of URS. When stratified by stone size (≤ 10 mm and > 10 mm), stone-free rates were consistently higher for smaller than larger stones: 90% and 68%, 84% and 76%, and 86% and 74%, respectively, for proximal, middle and distal ureteral calculi. URS stone-free rates showed less stringent size dependence: 80% and 79% for proximal ureteral stones, 91% and 78% for middle ureteral stones, and 97% and 93% for distal ureteral stones ≤ 10 and > 10 mm, respectively. Notably, sample size for middle ureteral stones, particularly when stratified by stone size, was small, only 1607 overall for SWL and 1024 for URS. The number of patients treated with SWL for ≤ 10 mm stones was only 44 and those with > 10 mm stones was only 15. Likewise, only 80 and 73 patients comprised the ≤ 10 and > 10 mm URS groups, respectively. Consequently, the stratified data for middle ureteral calculi may not be as reliable as the overall outcome data.

Table 24.2 Stone-free rates for SWL and URS of ureteral calculi from the 2007 Ureteral Stones Clinical Guidelines [7,8]

Stone location/size	Stone-free rate (primary Tx) Median (95% CI)	
	SWL	URS
Distal ureter	74% (73–75)	94% (93–95)
<10 mm	86% (81–90)	97% (96–98)
>10 mm	74% (57–87)	93% (88–96)
Middle ureter	73% (66–79)	86% (81–89)
<10 mm	84% (65–95)	91% (81–96)
>10 mm	76% (36–97)	78% (61–90)
Proximal ureter	82% (79–85)	81% (77–85)
<10 mm	90% (85–93)	80% (73–85)
>10 mm	68% (55–79)	79% (71–87)

Tx, treatment

Taking into account the total number of procedures per patient associated with treatment of the target stone, including the primary procedure (and retreatments), secondary procedures to remove stones and auxiliary, nonstone removal procedures, the number is not remarkably different between SWL and URS (1.62 versus 1.45 for proximal ureteral stones, 1.52 versus 1.2 for middle ureteral stones and 1.37 versus 1.4 for distal ureteral stones, respectively). However, the number of primary procedures (the intended treatment modality) was fewer for URS compared to SWL at all ureteral locations, indicating higher retreatment rates for SWL.

Complication rates were low with both treatment modalities and largely involved infection and obstruction with SWL and infection and ureteral injury/stricture with URS.

Comment

Data derived from individual RCTs and from the 2007 AUA/EUA Ureteral Stone Clinical Guidelines Panel provide **Grade 1B** evidence that both SWL and URS are reasonable first-line treatment options for ureteral stones not amenable to medical therapy. Success rates are sufficiently high and morbidity rates acceptably low to recommend either treatment modality in most cases. However, URS is associated with higher stone-free rates overall in each ureteral location and for most size stratifications. Furthermore, the number of primary procedures required to achieve a stone-free state is lower for URS than SWL, although the total number of procedures is comparable between the two treatments, likely because stent removal constitutes an additional procedure required for most URS patients. Consequently, a conditional recommendation for URS can be made based on moderate-quality (**Grade 2B**), evidence, particularly for middle and distal ureteral calculi and for large proximal ureteral calculi.

Clinical question 24.2

Is postprocedure stenting mandatory after ureteroscopy?

Placement of a ureteral stent following ureteroscopy for the treatment of renal/ureteral calculi is common practice for most urologists [12]. There are some clear indications for stent placement following URS, including ureteral injury, dilation of stricture, presence of an anatomically or functionally solitary renal unit, renal insufficiency or treatment of a large stone burden [13]. However, need for ureteral stent placement after routine, uncomplicated ureteroscopy is controversial. Because ureteral stents are associated with lower urinary tract symptoms and flank pain, require an office procedure for removal and may be complicated by stent migration, breakage, encrustation,

obstruction, and urinary tract infection/sepsis, identification of patients who can be safely left unstented is desirable.

Literature search

A search of the Medline database was performed using the terms "ureteral calculi," "ureteroscopy," "ureteral stent" and "randomized, controlled trials." The search was limited to the English-language literature published between 1948 and 2008.

The evidence

Over the last 8 years, 10 RCTs have compared clinical outcomes and quality of life measures with or without ureteral stent placement after uncomplicated ureteroscopy (Table 24.3) [14-22]. Uniformly, no differences in complication rates or stone-free rates have been identified between the stented and unstented groups in these individual trials. However, stent placement was associated with significant lower urinary tract symptoms that affected quality of life in the immediate postoperative period.

Two recent meta-analyses identified RCTs comparing stented and unstented ureteroscopy and both concluded that routine stent placement does not improve outcomes after URS [23,24.] Nabi and colleagues identified nine RCTs, comprising 831 patients, comparing stented with unstented URS [23]. Among these trials, none reported differences in stone-free rates between the two groups. However, with regard to the most important parameter, the need for unplanned emergency room visits or need for hospitalization, pooled analysis revealed a reduced rate among stented patients (0.53, 95% CI 0.17–1.60, p = 0.26) although the difference was not statistically significant. On the other hand, lower urinary tract symptoms, including frequency, urgency and dysuria, were more commonly associated with ureteral stents.

Makarov and co-workers performed a meta-analysis of 10 RCTs specifically comparing complication rates after URS in stented and unstented patients [24]. Although these authors found that stented patients had a 4% lower risk of experiencing complications than the unstented group (95% CI –10.1 to –1.8, p = 0.175), the difference did not reach statistical significance.

Finally, Hollenbeck and colleagues recently performed a multivariable logistic regression analysis of 219 ureteroscopic cases performed for stones at their institution for which no stent was left in place in order to identify factors predictive of postoperative morbidity [25]. When taking into account patient, operative and stone characteristics, they found that bilateral stentless procedures, history of recent/recurrent infections and history of stones were independently associated with postoperative complications in patients undergoing stentless URS.

Table 24.3 Randomized, prospective trials comparing stent versus no stent after ureteroscopy

Author	No. patients	Stone location (size)	URS intervention	F/U	Outcomes	Comments
Borboroglu [14]	113 53 stent 60 no stent	Distal (mean 6.6 mm)	6.0–9.5 Fr ureteroscope (~50% 9.5 Fr) Ho:YAG or EHL 6 Fr stent × 3–10 days	48 h, 1 wk, 4 wks	Stented with more OP, FP, BP, USx, and NU	4 nonstent readmitted and 2 required stent 6 unstented withdrawn due to intraop ureteral trauma
Denstedt [47]	58 29 stent 29 no stent	Variable (mean 9 mm)	6.9–7.5 Fr Ho:YAG or EHL Stent × 1 week	1, 6 and 12 wks	SFR 100% in both At 1 wk, stented with more FP, BP, USx	No difference in USx or pain at any other timepoints 1 patient in each group readmitted
Netto [22]	295 133 stent 162 no stent	Variable (2–50 mm)	7.5 Fr Ultrasonic lithotripter Stent × 2–3 days	3 mos	No difference in SFR, OP, complications Stented with longer OR	Cost higher for stent cases
Chen [15]	60 30 stent 30 no stent	Variable (mean 6.2 mm)	6.0 Fr ureteroscope EHL 7 Fr stent × 3 days	3 and 7 days	No difference in SFR, OP, AU 83% stented vs 13% nonstented with USx or BP	–
Cheung [16]	58 29 stent 29 no stent	Variable (mean 9.7 mm)	6.5–7.0 Fr ureteroscope Ho:YAG 6 Fr stent × 2 wks	1 and 3 days	No difference in SFR, OR Stented with more OP, USx, H	No difference in % of unplanned medical visits (17% nonstent vs 21% stent)
Srivastava [21]	48 26 stent 22 no stent	Distal (mean 7.6 mm)	8.5 Fr ureteroscope SL 6 Fr stent × 3 wks	3 wks	No difference in SFR, OR, AU Stented with more FP, USx	–
Damiano [17]	104 52 stent 52 no stent	Variable (mean 10.5 mm)	8.9 Fr ureteroscope SL 4.8 or 6 Fr stent × 2 wks	3, 7, and 15 days	No difference in SFR, OR, USx, H Nonstent with less pain on day 3, but not 7 or 10	22.8% (11/52) nonstented required readmission with 6 ureteral stents placed
Jeong [20]	45 23 stent 22 no stent	Variable (mean 5.3 mm stent, 7.1 mm no stent)	8.5 Fr ureteroscope EHL 7 Fr stent × 7 days	7 and 28 days	No difference in OR, HOSP, FP, USx Presence of H only difference between groups	–
Grossi [18]	56 28 stent 28 no stent	Variable (mean 9.2 mm)	8.5 Fr ureteroscope Ballistic lithotripsy 6 Fr stent for 3–10 days	3 and 7 days	No difference in SFR, OP, complications	1 nonstent required stenting POD#1
Ibrahim [19]	220 110 stent 110 no stent	Distal (mean 13 mm)	7.5–10.5 Fr ureteroscope Ho:YAG or SL 6 Fr stent × 2 weeks	48 h and 1 wk	No difference in SFR, HOSP, H, complications Stented group with more USx	–

AU, analgesic use; BP, bladder/suprapubic pain; EHL, electrohydraulic lithotripsy; FP, flank pain; H, hematuria; HOSP, hospital stay; Ho: YAG, holmium-YAG laser; OP, overall pain; OR, operative time; POD, post-operative day; SFR, stone-free rate; SL, Swiss Lithoclast; USx, urinary symptoms

Comment

Grade 1B evidence by way of a meta-analysis of 10 RCTs suggests that routine stent placement following uncomplicated ureteroscopy does not provide an advantage with regard to postoperative complications and/or need for emergency room visits or hospitalization, nor does it improve stone-free rates. However, it does lead to significant postoperative lower urinary tract symptoms including frequency, urgency, and dysuria. As such, a strong recommendation (Grade 1B) against routine stenting after uncomplicated ureteroscopy can be made. However, while these data are convincing, lack of uniformity among trials with regard to inclusion/exclusion criteria still prevents establishment of a clear definition of uncomplicatd URS.

Clinical question 24.3

Is there an advantage to placement of a ureteral stent in conjunction with SWL of ureteral calculi?

Placement of a ureteral stent in conjunction with SWL was historically thought to facilitate stone fragmentation and prevent post-SWL steinstrasse or obstruction. Stone impaction and the lack of an adequate stone–fluid interface was thought to account for the poorer fragmentation and need for greater numbers of shock waves when treating ureteral stones. Consequently, push-back of the stone into the kidney or placement of a ureteral stent to bypass the stone, thereby creating a better stone–fluid interface, was advocated. However, a number of RCTs have demonstrated no advantage to stent placement for the treatment of ureteral stones.

Literature search

A search of the Medline database was performed using the terms "ureteral calculi," "shock-wave lithotripsy," "*in situ* shock-wave lithotripsy," "stent bypass," "push-back," "push-bang," "ureteral stent" and "randomized, controlled trials." The search was limited to the English-language literature published between 1948 and 2008.

The evidence

Although many clinical series have demonstrated good stone-free rates with *in situ* SWL, RCTs directly comparing stent bypass/push-back with *in situ* SWL are limited primarily to patients with proximal ureteral calculi. Among seven randomized trials comparing stent bypass/manipulation with *in situ* SWL for patients with proximal ureteral calculi, none showed a significant or substantial

difference in stone-free rates between groups (Table 24.4) [26-32]. However, one trial found that stented patients were less likely to return to the hospital or require an emergency room visit than *in situ* treated (unstented) patiets. Chandhoke and colleagues randomized 97 patients undergoing SWL for 10–20 mm renal or < 20 mm proximal ureteral calculi to no stent, 4.7 F stent or 7 Fr stent [31]. Although outcomes were not stratified by stone location (renal or ureteral) and ureteral calculi comprised only 33–40% of stones in each group, the authors found no difference in stone-free rates (85%, 80% and 77%, respectively) or retreatment rates between the three groups. However, patients in the unstented group required rehospitalization more frequently than patients in the stented groups (22% versus 7% and 7%, respectively), Likewise, the need for an emergency room visit was significantly lower in the 4.7 Fr stent group than in the unstented group (5% versus 19%, respectively). Stented patients did, however, experience more lower urinary tract symptoms (uregency, frequency, nocturia) than the unstented patients. Of note, the mean stone size in the three groups was quite large (13.3 mm, 11.3 mm and 12.7 mm, respectively) which could account for the more frequent need for medical attention postoperatively in the unstented patients.

In the most recent RCT comparing stent bypass with *in situ* SWL, El-Assmy and co-workers randomized 186 patients with solitary < 2 cm ureteral calculi and moderate to severe hydronephrosis to undergo 6 Fr stent placement or no stent at the time of SWL [32]. Although the study included patients with ureteral stones in any location, 73% of patients in each group had proximal ureteral calculi. No signficant differences between groups were found with regard to stone-free rates (85% versus 91%, respectively, p = 0.25), number of SWL sessions (1.6 versus 1.8, respectively, p = 0.43), flank pain (35% versus 61%, p = 0.75) or postoperative urinary tract infections (32% versus 6.5%, respectively, p < 0.0001). However, patients with ureteral stents experienced more frequent side effects attributable to the stent, including dysuria, suprapubic pain, hematuria, pyuria, and urinary tract infection.

The 1997 Ureteral Stone Clinical Guidelines Panel reviewed the available literature for outcomes on SWL of proximal ureteral stones and found no significant difference in stone-free rates among patients treated with *in situ*, stent bypass or push-back: 82%, 82% and 88%, respectively [33]. Likewise, stone-free rates for *in situ* and stent bypass SWL for distal ureteral calculi were comparable (86% for each group). Patient numbers for push-back SWL for distal ureteral calculi were too small to be meaningful.

No RCTs have directly compared stent bypass with *in situ* SWL for patients with middle and distal ureteral caluli. Visualization of middle ureteral calculi is often hindered by the underlying pelvic bone, thereby necessitating use of intravenous contrast or placement of a ureteral stent

Table 24.4 Randomized, clinical trials comparing stent manipulation (bypass or push-back) with no stent (*in situ*) for SWL treatment of proximal ureteral calculi

Author	Lithotripter	*In situ*				Stent bypass or push-back			
		No. pts	Stone free	Auxiliary procedure	Retreatment	No. pts	Stone free	Auxiliary procedure	Retreatment
Hendrikx[#] [26]	Lithostar	23	91%	–	–	24	83%	–	–
Danuser [27]	Dornier HM3	48	96%	2%	2%	48[+]	94%	0%	0%
Albala [28]	Lithostar	19	74%	11%	0%	18	89%	11%	0%
	Dornier HM3	10	80%	10%	0%	15	67%	13%	20%
Chang [29]	Lithostar	26	77%	8.5%	33.3%	51[^]	61%	2.8%	35%
Kumar [30]	Lithostar Plus	35	80%	–	0%	35	88.5%	–	0%
Chandhoke[a] [31]	Dornier HM3	31	84%	–	–	60[*]	78.5%	–	–
El-Assmy [32]	Dornier MFL 5000	93	91%	8%	21.5%	93	85%	15%	20%

[#]Series included 8 patients in the *in situ* group and 6 patients in the manipulated group with middle ureteral stones; only 9 of 24 patients in the push-back group underwent successful push-back of the stone into the kidney and the remaining stones were treated *in situ*. Of the 9 stones treated with push-back, 100% were stone free. Of the 15 failing push-back and treated *in situ*, 73% were stone free

[+]All patients except 4 had stone pushed back into kidney. Of the remaining 4, 3 were treated with stent bypass and 1 was treated with catheter just distal to stone

[^]Includes 27 patietns treated with stent bypass and 24 patients treated with placement of a catheter below the stone with continuous manipulation

[a]Series includes patients with renal calculi. Patients with ureteral calculi comprised 33–40% of patients in the 3 groups

[*]Includes 30 patients each with 4.7 Fr stent and 7 Fr stent. All patients in this group underwent SWL with stent bypass

or catheter to facilitate targeting of the stone. Nonetheless, retrospective, single-institution series have reported satisfactory success rates with *in situ* SWL in patients with middle and distal ureteral calculi [34,35]. Indeed, in a large series of over 18,000 patients treated with SWL for ureteral calculi, Mobley and colleagues found no difference in stone-free, retreatment and auxiliary procedure rates between *in situ* and stent bypass SWL [35]. Stone-free rates in this series for *in situ* versus stent bypass treatment of patients with ≤ 20 mm ureteral calculi were 86% versus 82% for proximal, 83% versus 84% for middle and 84% versus 78% for distal ureteral stones.

Comment

Grade 1B evidence suggests that ureteral stent placement in conjunction with SWL of most proximal ureteral calculi does not affect stone fragmentation or clearance, but is associated with more symptoms. Although one RCT did find that unstented patients were more likely to require rehospitalization or an emergency room visit, this series was not limited to patients with ureteral calculi. Consequently, a strong recommendation can be made against placement of a ureteral stent prior to SWL of proximal ureteral calculi based on moderate-quality (**Grade 1B**) evidence.

Although there are no RCTs comparing SWL outcomes of patients with middle and distal ureteral calculi treated with or without stents, results of large observational clinical series have demonstrated good outcomes in patients with stones in these locations treated with *in situ* SWL, thereby suggesting that *in situ* SWL is as efficacious as stent bypass SWL. Based on low-quality (**Grade 1C**) evidence, *in situ* SWL for middle and distal ureteral receives a conditional recommendation.

Clinical question 24.4

Does medical expulsive therapy improve stone-free rates following SWL?

Alpha-adrenergic receptor antagonists inhibit basal tone in the ureter and decrease peristaltic activity. Of the known alpha-receptors, the alpha-1a and alpha-1d subtypes mediate pronounced detrusor contraction and have been shown to promote spasm of the lower ureter and intramural tunnel. Consequently, these receptors represent ideal targets for pharmacotherapy as they are concentrated in the anatomical location of the ureter that presents the greatest impediment to stone passage. In addition, smooth muscle cells of the ureter respond to changes in intracellular calcium levels by contracting. As such, calcium channel blockade has also been proposed as a means of decreasing ureteral contraction and facilitating stone passage while minimizing the pain of ureteral colic. Selective alpha-1-antagonists, such as tamsulosin, and calciuim channel blockers, such as nifedipine, have been shown in clinical trials to facilitate spontaneous stone passage [2].

Literature search

A search of the Medline database was performed using the terms "ureteral calculi," "shock-wave lithotripsy," "medical expulsive therapy," "alpha-blocker," "calcium channel blocker," "tamsulosin," "nifedipine" and "randomized, controlled trials." The search was limited to the English-language literature published between 1948 and 2008.

The evidence

Based on the success of alpha-adrenergic receptor antagonists and calcium channel blockers in promoting spontaneous stone passage, medical expulsive therapy has been used as an adjunct to SWL to promote clearance of fragments from the ureter. To date, five published RCTs have evaluated tamsulosin (N 4), nifedepine (N 2) or both (N 1) in conjunction with SWL of ureteral calculi (Table 24.5) [36-40]. Among the five trials comprising 392 patients, rates of stone clearance ranged from 28% to 79% in the control arms compared with 64% to 97% in the adjuvant MET groups. In all but one of these studies [37], a statistically significant improvement in stone clearance rates was observed with the initiation of adjuvant MET. In this particular study, although stone-free rates were not improved by tamsulosin, patients in the treatment arm required less supplemental diclofenac for pain than the control patients.

One study selectively compared ketoprofene and nifedipine to ketoprophene alone in conjunction with SWL for proximal/middle ureteral calculi and ketoprofene and tamsulosin with ketoprofene alone for patients with distal ureteral calculi [38]. Both MET regimens were associated with higher stone-free rates than their respective control arms (86% versus 51% for the nifedipine and control arms,

Table 24.5 Prospective trials of adjunctive tamsulosin or nifedipine for SWL of ureteral calculi

Author/ study design	No. pts	Location, size (mm)	Therapy regimen	Additional therapy	Follow-up	Stone clearance rates	Comments
Tamsulosin							
Kupeli [38] R/C	78	Distal ureter (1–15 mm)	TAM 0.4 mg daily × 15 days (N 39) CON (N 39)	Diclofenac	15 days	TAM 64.1% CON 28.2%	Best stone clearance for stones >5 mm
Gravas [37] R/C	61	Distal ureter (6–13 mm)	TAM 0.4 mg daily × 30 days (N 30) CON (N 31)	Diclofenac	1–4 wks	TAM 66.7% CON 58.1%	No difference in stone clearance rates, but TAM group required less diclofenac
Bhagat [36] R/C/DB	60	Renal (6–24 mm) All ureter (6–15 mm)	TAM 0.4 mg daily × 30 days (N 30) Placebo (N 30)	Proxyvon	1 month	TAM 96.6% CON 79.3%	Includes renal stones (67%) in each arm Best clearance rates for stone >10 mm
Nifedipine							
Porpiglia [40] R/C	80	All ureter (mean 10.5 mm)	NIF 30 mg daily × 10 days (N 40) CON (N 40)	Deflazacort	45 days	NIF 75% CON 50%	NIF group required less deflazacort (37.5 mg vs 86.25 mg)
Tamsulosin and nifedipine							
Micali [39] C	113	Upper/mid ureter Distal ureter (6–14 mm)	NIF 30 mg daily × 14 days (N 35) CON (N 29) TAM 0.4 mg daily × 14 days (N 28) CON (N 21)	Ketoprofene	1 and 2 mos	NIF 85.7% CON 51.7% TAM 82.1% CON 57.1%	SWL/endoscopy retreatment rate NIF 14.3% TAM 17.8% CON 46%

C, controlled; CON, control; DB, double-blind; NIF, nifedipine; PC, placebo controlled; R, randomized; TAM, tamsulosin p = 0.005) and (82% versus 58% for the tamsulosin and control arms, p = 0.05).

In a related trial, Resim and colleagues randomized patients with steinstrasse occurring after SWL for renal calculi to either tamsulosin and tanoxicam or tanoxicam alone [41]. Although the rate of resolution of steinstrasse was slightly higher in the tamsulosin group compared with the control group (75% versus 66%), the difference was not statistically significant. However, tamsulosin was associated with fewer episodes of renal colic and lower visual analog pain scores than the control group.

Comment

The balance of data from randomized trials supports a strong recommendation in support of adjuvant MET, both nifedipine and tamsulosin, in facilitating clearance of fragments after SWL of ureteral calculi and perhaps in reducing pain medication requirements (Grade 1B). However, it should be recognized that the individual RCTs vary in the drug regimens used (both dose and duration), the study population (patients with only distal ureteral stones or all ureteral stones) and the use of other potentially active drugs in both the control and treatment arms (nonsteroidal anti-inflammatory agents or corticosteroids), thereby making comparison between trials somewhat problematic. Indeed, variation in the stone-free rates in the control arms of these trials may in part be accounted for by the use of no treatment in some trials and potentially active agents in other trials (i.e. corticosteroids). Finally, data on retreatment rates and interval to stone passage were only sporadically reported and therefore no meaningful conclusions can be derived regarding these endpoints. These limitations notwithstanding, the use of adjuvant MET in conjunction with SWL is strongly recommended based on moderate-quality (Grade 1B) evidence.

Clinical question 24.5

Does slowing the rate of shock-wave (SW) delivery improve stone-free rates for SWL of ureteral calculi?

Historically, lithotripters were gated with the QRS complex of the electrocardiogram so as to avoid inducing cardiac arrhythmias. As a result, SW rates rarely exceeded 60–80 SW per minute. With the introduction of second- and third-generation lithotripters, nongated SWL became commonplace and treatment times were shortened.

Recent, *in vitro* and animal studies, however, have shown superior stone fragmentation when the SW rate is reduced to 30–60 SW/min [42-44]. Clinical trials have validated these experimental findings and confirmed superior stone-free rates for patients with renal calculi treated with SWL at 60 versus 120 SW/min [45]. In a meta-analysis of four RCTs comprising 589 patients treated with SWL for renal calculi at slow versus fast SW rate, Semins and co-workers found that patients treated at slow SW rate (60 SW/min) had a 10% higher likelihood of becoming stone free than those treated at fast SW rate (120 SW/min) (95% CI 3.4–16.8, p = 0.0002).

Literature search

A search of the Medline database was performed using the terms "ureteral calculi," "shock-wave lithotripsy," "shock-wave rate" and "randomized, controlled trials." The search was limited to the English-language literature published between 1948 and 2008. Owing to the paucity of data on shock-wave rate for ureteral calculi, we supplemented our search with data obtained from published abstracts from the American Urological Association (AUA) and World Congress of Endo-urology annual meetings from 2005 to 2008.

The evidence

Only a single RCT has specifically addressed slow (60 SW/min) versus fast (120 SW/min) SW rate for SWL of ureteral calculi. Pace and colleagues randomized 157 patients with ≥ 5 mm proximal ureteral calculi to 60 or 120 SW/min [46]. Slow SW delivery was associated with a higher stone-free rate (68% versus 51%, p = 0.03), reduced auxiliary procedure rate (31% versus 47%, p = 0.03) and a lower cumulative number of shock-waves (2667 versus 2938, p < 0.001), although at a cost of longer operative duration (44 versus 24.5 min, p < 0.001) compared with patients treated at 120 SW/min.

Comment

A single RCT only supports slow shock-wave delivery during SWL for ureteral calculi. Although the precise SW rate for optimal SWL treatment has not been established, slowing the SW rate to at least 60 SW/min is conditionally recommended based on low-quality evidence consisting of a single RCT (Grade 2C). This recommendation, however, is strengthened by extrapolation of high-grade evidence based on a meta-analysis of SWL trials supporting slow SW delivery for treatment of renal calculi.

Conclusion

Evidence derived from a few RCTs but primarily from case series supports both SWL and URS for the treatment of ureteral calculi. Although URS is associated with slightly higher stone-free rates and need for fewer primary procedures, the lower morbidity and acceptable stone-free rates of SWL make it a viable alternative treatment. In the setting of an uncomplicated procedure, there is moderate-quality evidence strongly suggesting that routine stenting following either SWL or URS is not mandatory. However, the definition of an uncomplicated URS procedure has not been well defined and requires further study. Low-quality evidence based on a single RCT conditionally suggests that slow SW rate (60/min) yields improved stone fragmentation and passage after SWL of ureteral calculi. Finally, adjuvant MET, using either nifedipine or tamsulosin, has shown benefit in promoting clearance of fragments after SWL and is strongly recommended based on moderate-quality evidence.

References

1. Stamatelou KK , Francis ME, Jones CA, Nyberg LM, Curhan GC. Time trends in reported prevalence of kidney stones in the United States: 1976–1994. Kidney Int 2003;63:1817-823.

2. Hollingsworth JM, Rogers MA, Kaufman SR, et al. Medical therapy to facilitate urinary stone passage: a meta-analysis. Lancet 2006;368:1171-9.

3. Dretler SP. Stone fragility – a new therapeutic distinction. J Urol 1988;139:1124-7.

4. Lee YH, Tsai JY, Jiaan BP, Wu T, Yu CC. Prospective randomized trial comparing shock wave lithotripsy and ureteroscopic lithotripsy for management of large upper third ureteral stones. Urology 2006;67:480-4.

5. Hendrikx AJ, Strijbos WE, de Knijff DW, Kums JJ, Doesburg WH, Lemmens WA. Treatment for extended-mid and distal ureteral stones: swl or ureteroscopy? Results of a multicenter study. J Endourol 1999;13:727-33.

6. `Peschel R, Janetschek G, Bartsch G. Extracorporeal shock wave lithotripsy versus ureteroscopy for distal ureteral calculi: a prospective randomized study. J Urol 1999;162:1909-12.

7. Zeng GQ, Zhong WD, Cai YB, Dai QS, Hu JB, Wei HA. Extracorporeal shock-wave versus pneumatic ureteroscopic lithotripsy in treatment of lower ureteral calculi. Asian J Androl 2002;4:303-5.

8. Pearle MS, Nadler R, Bercowsky E, et al. Prospective randomized trial comparing shock wave lithotripsy and ureteroscopy for management of distal ureteral calculi. J Urol 2001;166:1255-60.

9. Nabi G, Downey P, Keeley F, Watson G, McClinton S. Extracorporeal shock wave lithotripsy (ESWL) versus ureteroscopic management for ureteric calculi. Cochrane Database Syst Rev 2007;1:CD006029.

10. Preminger GM , Tiselius HG, Assimos DG, et al. 2007 guideline for the management of ureteral calculi. J Urol 2007;178:2418-34.

11. Preminger GM , Tiselius HG, Assimos DG, et al. 2007 Guideline for the management of ureteral calculi. Eur Urol 2007;52:1610-31.

12. Auge BK, Sarvis JA, L'Esperance JO, Preminger GM. Practice patterns of ureteral stenting after routine ureteroscopic stone surgery: a survey of practicing urologists. J Endourol 2007; 21:1287-91.

13. Haleblian G, Kijvikai K, de la Rosette J, Preminger G. Ureteral stenting and urinary stone management: a systematic review. J Urol 2008;179:424-30.

14. Borboroglu PG, Amling CL, Schenkman NS, et al. Ureteral stenting after ureteroscopy for distal ureteral calculi: a multi-institutional prospective randomized controlled study assessing pain, outcomes and complications. J Urol 2001;166:1651-7.

15. Chen YT, Chen J, Wong WY, Yang SS, Hsieh CH, Wang CC. Is ureteral stenting necessary after uncomplicated ureteroscopic lithotripsy? A prospective, randomized controlled trial. J Urol 2002;167:1977-80.

16. Cheung MC, Lee F, Leung YL, Wong BB, Tam PC. A prospective randomized controlled trial on ureteral stenting after ureteroscopic holmium laser lithotripsy. J Urol 2003;169:1257-60.

17. Damiano R, Autorino R, Esposito C, et al. Stent positioning after ureteroscopy for urinary calculi: the question is still open. Eur Urol 2004;46:381-7.

18. Grossi FS, Ferretti S, di Lena S, Crispino M. A prospective randomized multicentric study comparing stented vs non-stented ureteroscopic lithotripsy. Arch Ital Urol Androl 2006;78:53-6.

19. Ibrahim HM, Al-Kandari AM, Shaaban HS, Elshebini YH, Shokeir AA. Role of ureteral stenting after uncomplicated ureteroscopy for distal ureteral stones: a randomized, controlled trial. J Urol 2008;180:961-5.

20. Jeong H, Kwak C, Lee SE. Ureteric stenting after ureteroscopy for ureteric stones: a prospective randomized study assessing symptoms and complications. BJU Int 2004;93:1032-4.

21. Srivastava A , Gupta R, Kumar A, Kapoor R, Mandhani A. Routine stenting after ureteroscopy for distal ureteral calculi is unnecessary: results of a randomized controlled trial. J Endourol 2003;17:871-4.

22. Netto NR Jr, Ikonomidis J, Zillo C. Routine ureteral stenting after ureteroscopy for ureteral lithiasis: is it really necessary? J Urol 2001;166:1252-4.

23. Nabi G, Cook J, N'Dow J, McClinton S. Outcomes of stenting after uncomplicated ureteroscopy: systematic review and meta-analysis. BMJ 2007;334:572.

24. Makarov DV, Trock BJ, Allaf ME, Matlaga BR. The effect of ureteral stent placement on post-ureteroscopy complications: a meta-analysis. Urology 2008;71:796-800.

25. Hollenbeck BK, Schuster TG, Seifman BD, Faerber GJ, Wolf JS Jr. Identifying patients who are suitable for stentless ureteroscopy following treatment of urolithiasis. J Urol 2003;170:103-10.

26. Hendrikx AJM, Bierkens AAF, Oosterhof GON, DeBruyne FMJ. Treatment of proximal and mid ureteral calculi: a randomized trial of in situ and pushback extracorporeal lithotripsy. J Endourol 1990;4:353-64.

27. Danuser H, Ackermann DK, Marth DC, Studer UE, Zingg EJ. Extracorporeal shock wave lithotripsy in situ or after push-up for upper ureteral calculi: a prospective randomized trial. J Urol 1993;150:824-6.

28. Albala DM, Clayman RV, Meretyk S. Extracorporeal shock wave lithotripsy for proximal ureteral calculi: to stint or not to stint? J Endourol 1991;5:277-81.

29. Chang SC, Kuo HC, Hsu T. Extracorporeal shock wave lithotripsy for obstructed proximal ureteral stones. A prospective randomized study comparing in situ, stent bypass and below stone catheter with irrigation strategies. Eur Urol 1993;24:177-84.

30. Kumar A, Kumar RV, Mishra VK, Ahlawat R, Kapoor R, Bhandari M. Should upper ureteral calculi be manipulated before extracorporeal shock wave lithotripsy? A prospective controlled trial. J Urol 1994;152:320-3.

31. Chandhoke PS , Barqawi AZ, Wernecke C, Chee-Awai RA. A randomized outcomes trial of ureteral stents for extracorporeal shock wave lithotripsy of solitary kidney or proximal ureteral stones. J Urol 2002;167:1981-3.

32. El-Assmy A, El-Nahas AR, Sheir KZ. Is pre-shock wave lithotripsy stenting necessary for ureteral stones with moderate or severe hydronephrosis? J Urol 2006;176:2059-62.

33. Segura JW, Preminger GM, Assimos DG, et al. Ureteral Stones Clinical Guidelines Panel summary report on the management of ureteral calculi. The American Urological Association. J Urol 1997;158:1915-21.

34. Anderson KR, Keetch DW, Albala DM, Chandhoke PS, McClennan BL, Clayman RV. Optimal therapy for the distal ureteral stone: extracorporeal shock wave lithotripsy versus ureteroscopy. J Urol 1994;152:62-5.

35. Mobley TB, Myers DA, Jenkins JM, Grine WB, Jordan WR. Effects of stents on lithotripsy of ureteral calculi: treatment results with 18,825 calculi using the Lithostar lithotriptor. J Urol 1994;152:53-6.

36. Bhagat SK, Chacko NK, Kekre NS, Gopalakrishnan G, Antonisamy B, Devasia A. Is there a role for tamsulosin in shock wave lithotripsy for renal and ureteral calculi? J Urol 2007;177:2185-8.

37. Gravas S, Tzortzis V, Karatzas A, Oeconomou A, Melekos MD. The use of tamsulozin as adjunctive treatment after ESWL in patients with distal ureteral stone: do we really need it? Results from a randomised study. Urol Res 2007; 35:231-5.

38. Kupeli B, Irkilata L, Gurocak S, et al. Does tamsulosin enhance lower ureteral stone clearance with or without shock wave lithotripsy? Urology 2004;64:1111-15.

39. Micali S, Grande M, Sighinolfi MC, de Stefani S, Bianchi G. Efficacy of expulsive therapy using nifedipine or tamsulosin, both associated with ketoprofene, after shock wave lithotripsy of ureteral stones. Urol Res 2007;35:133-7.

40. Porpiglia F, Destefanis P, Fiori C, Scarpa RM, Fontana D. Role of adjunctive medical therapy with nifedipine and deflazacort after extracorporeal shock wave lithotripsy of ureteral stones. Urology 2002;59:835-8.

41. Resim S, Ekerbicer HC, Ciftci A. Role of tamsulosin in treatment of patients with steinstrasse developing after extracorporeal shock wave lithotripsy. Urology 2005;66:945-8.

42. Greenstein A , Matzkin H. Does the rate of extracorporeal shock wave delivery affect stone fragmentation? Urology 1999;54:430-3.

43. Weir MJ, Tariq N, Honey RJ. Shockwave frequency affects fragmentation in a kidney stone model. J Endourol 2000;14:547-50.

44. Paterson RF, Lifshitz DA, Lingeman JE, et al. Stone fragmentation during shock wave lithotripsy is improved by slowing the shock wave rate: studies with a new animal model. J Urol 2002;168:2211-15.

45. Semins MJ, Trock BJ, Matlaga BR. The effect of shock wave rate on the outcome of shock wave lithotripsy: a meta-analysis. J Urol 2008;179:194-7.

46. Honey RJ, Schuler TD, Ghiculete D, Pace KT. A randomized, double-blind trial to compare shock wave frequencies of 60 and 120 shocks per minute for upper ureteral stones. J Urol 2009;182: 1418-23.

47. Denstedt JD, Wollin TA, Sofer M, Nott L, Weir M, D'A Hone RJ. A prospective randomized controlled trial comparing nonstented versus stented ureteroscopic lithotripsy. J Urol 2001;165:1419-22.

25 Chemoprevention of prostate cancer

Amanda Beth Reed,[1] Kristin C. Reed[2] and Dipen J. Parekh[1]
[1]Department of Urology, University of Texas Health Sciences Center at San Antonio, San Antonio, TX, USA
[2] South Texas Veterans Health Care System, San Antonio, TX, USA

Introduction

In this review, we discuss the association between chemopreventive agents and prostate cancer, with a special focus on recent evidence relating to the role of 5-alpha-reductase inhibitors (5ARIs) in the prevention and diagnosis of prostate cancer.

Rationale for the chemoprevention of prostate cancer

Prostate cancer is a leading cause of cancer and cancer death in American men. For the year 2008, 186,000 prostate cancer cases were expected and 28,700 deaths due to this disease [1]. In the United States there is an overall 16.7% risk of developing prostate cancer [1] and early detection and treatment remain the primary focus for controlling the disease. More than 90% of men diagnosed with prostate cancer currently opt for treatment. This increasing incidence of prostate cancer, the morbidity and mortality of the disease and its treatments, combined with an improved insight into its biological basis and hormone dependency, have led to an increasing interest in chemoprevention strategies.

Chemoprevention refers to the use of agents to prevent cancer or the adverse outcomes of the disease. Multiple factors, including high incidence, long latency period between initial evidence of prostate cancer and the development of overt or lethal disease, and advanced age of onset and death [2,3], make prostate cancer an ideal target for chemoprevention strategies. Even a modest delay in development of symptomatic cancer may be sufficient to reduce the incidence of the disease, improve survival, and prevent the complications of the disease and the morbidity of its treatments.

This chapter reviews the evidence for the use of current chemopreventive agents in patients at risk for prostate cancer. We focus specifically on the risks and benefits of 5ARIs as there are no other effective agents that have undergone rigorous investigation with phase III randomized clinical trials with positive results. Grading of the quality of evidence and strengths of recommendations in this chapter are based on the guidelines proposed by the international Grading of Recommendations Assessment, Development, and Evaluation Working Group (Grade).

Background

As our understanding of the pathogenesis of prostate cancer improves, an increasing number of risk reduction strategies are correspondingly being developed [4]. The focus of most treatment strategies for decreasing the risk of prostate cancer (primary prevention), slowing disease progression (secondary prevention) or delaying advancement in those in whom curative therapy has failed (tertiary prevention) is the androgen axis. Androgens are essential for prostatic development, growth, and function. Testosterone, after conversion to the more potent 5-alpha-dihydrotestosterone, controls prostate mitotic activity and potentially prostate carcinogenesis. Interventions that alter circulating androgen levels or inhibit 5-alpha-reductase have proven to have the most potential as preventive agents for prostate cancer.

Two 5ARIs, finasteride and dutasteride, are currently commercially available. Finasteride is selective for the type 2 isoenzyme, which reduces the level of dihydrotestosterone (DHT) by 65–70% [5]. Dutasteride inhibits both type 1 and type 2 isoenzymes and reduces the level of DHT by approximately 90% [6]. To date, one randomized trial assessing the influence of finasteride on the prevalence of biopsy-proven prostate cancer – the Prostate Cancer Prevention Trial (PCPT) – has been completed [7]. It is expected that a second phase III trial using the dual inhibitor dutasteride – the Reduction by Dutasteride of Prostate Cancer Events (REDUCE) Trial [8] – will report its results soon. The REDUCE trial is a multicenter, international study in which subjects are randomized to receive either dutasteride or placebo for a period of 4 years. Eligibility criteria include a serum prostate-specific antigen (PSA) of 2.5–10 ng/mL and a previous negative prostate biopsy within 6 months of randomization. The protocol requires prostate biopsies to be performed after 2 and 4 years of follow-up.

Clinical question 25.1

In patients at increased risk for prostate cancer, what are the benefits of 5-alpha-reductase inhibitors in reducing the risk of prostate cancer?

Literature search

A Medline literature search was performed to identify phase III clinical trials investigating prostate cancer chemoprevention. We used the search terms "prostate cancer," "chemoprevention," "prevention," and "clinical trial." All trials that met criteria were reviewed by the authors.

The evidence

The Prostate Cancer Prevention Trial (PCPT)

The primary objective of the PCPT was to determine if finasteride could reduce the period prevalence (defined as the sum total of prostate cancers diagnosed over a period of 7 years) of prostate cancer. A total of 18,822 men at least 55 years of age, with a normal digital rectal examination (DRE) and a baseline PSA level ≤ 3 ng/mL, were enrolled and randomly assigned to finasteride (5 mg per day) or placebo. Men were asked to continue this drug regimen for 7 years. Prostate biopsy was recommended if the subsequent annual PSA level, adjusted for the finasteride effect [9], exceeded 4 ng/mL or if a DRE was suspicious. The primary endpoint of the study was the prevalence of prostate cancer diagnosed by "for cause" biopsies or "end-of-study" biopsies during the 7-year study period. Originally, the authors of the PCPT reported that there was a 24.8% reduction in the incidence of prostate cancer from 24.4% with placebo to 18.4% in men treated with finasteride. The authors also noted that magnitude of the risk reduction did not differ according to PSA level, age, race/ethnicity or family history of prostate cancer [7].

The PCPT was closed more than a year earlier than planned because the primary study endpoint, a decrease in the prevalence of biopsy-proven prostate cancer in the finasteride arm, was achieved. However, based on the dataset frozen in March 2003, high-grade tumors of Gleason grade 7–10 were more common in the finasteride group than in the placebo group. This apparent increase in the incidence of high-grade prostate cancer prompted an intense debate within the urological community regarding the benefits of finasteride-based prevention of prostate cancer and resulted in a general lack of acceptance of finasteride for prostate cancer prevention. Subsequent analyses, which included all data through the day of the trial unblinding on 23 June 2003, yielded additional information that resulted in an observed overall risk reduction of 27% [10].

Pathological characteristics of the cancers in the PCPT

A major concern about early detection of prostate cancer by PSA and prevention by finasteride is the discovery of and responsibility to treat biologically inconsequential tumors that would not require treatment during a man's lifetime. The commonly accepted pathological definition of a clinically insignificant tumor is an organ-confined, low-volume, and low-Gleason score tumor [11]. The most commonly used criteria for insignificant disease on biopsy proposed by Epstein are a combination of clinical factors (stage T1c and PSA density < 0.15 ng/mL/g), grade of tumor (Gleason score ≤ 6, with no Gleason 4 or 5), and extent of tumor (< 3 cores with tumor (no core with > 50% tumor) or < 3 mm cancer present in only 1 core) [11].

Lucia et al. [12] reviewed the pathological characteristics of prostate biopsies from men in the placebo and finasteride groups of the PCPT. These authors found that 75% of all cancers and 62% of Gleason score ≤ 6 cancers met the biopsy criteria for clinically significant tumors. In addition, surrogate measures for tumor volume, including volume of disease on biopsy, and risk of perineural invasion were lower in men who received finasteride. The risk of insignificant cancer at ranges of PSA were 51.7% (PSA 0–1.0 ng/mL), 33.7% (1.1–2.5 ng/mL), 17.8% (2.6–4 ng/mL), and 11.7% (4.1–10 ng/mL). Conversely, the risks of high-grade tumors for the same PSA strata were 15.6%, 37.9%, 49.1% and 52.4%, respectively. This study revealed that only approximately 25% of detected tumors met the criteria for insignificance, a rate similar to the findings of the contemporary series of men who undergo treatment for their disease [13]. This analysis suggests that men who developed prostate cancer on finasteride had a lower tumor volume and decrease in aggressive features across all tumor grades as compared with the placebo arm. About two-thirds of all detected tumors and half of Gleason score ≤ 6, which finasteride is known to prevent, met the definition for clinical significance. Tumors among men treated with finasteride were smaller and has less extensive characteristics.

In an analysis from 2007, Lucia assessed whether the increased risk of high-grade prostate cancer associated with finasteride in the PCPT was due to an effect of finasteride on the interpretation of tumor grade as well as the impact of a change in prostate size with finasteride on accuracy of biopsy grading [14]. Prostate biopsies with Gleason score 8–10 were examined histologically for hormonal effects, and those with Gleason score 7–10 were examined for pathological surrogates of disease extent. Prostate volumes were measured at biopsy. Samples from radical prostatectomy (N 222, finasteride; N 306, placebo) were examined for tumor grade and extent. Grades at biopsy and prostatectomy were compared between the groups. The authors found that prostate volumes were lower in the finasteride group (25.1 cm^3 versus 34.4 cm^3) and that pathological surrogates for tumor aggressiveness were lower with finasteride than with placebo. Among patients who underwent prostatectomy, patients who received placebo had a significantly higher risk of upgrading on the prostatectomy specimen than those who received finasteride. This finding suggests (and has been supported by other similar observations) that the smaller gland size that resulted from finasteride treatment facilitated diagnosis of high-grade disease while patients who received placebo were more likely to have had a biopsy that missed the high-grade tumor. These results, in combination with the biopsy data finding less extensive tumors in patients treated with finasteride, suggested that high-grade cancer was detected earlier and was less extensive in the finasteride group than in the placebo group.

Finasteride increases sensitivity of PSA and DRE

Observations made after the PCPT suggested that the increase in high-grade disease in the finasteride group may have been secondary to detection bias rather than an actual alteration in the natural history of the disease [7]. In 2006, Thompson et al. examined the impact of finasteride on the sensitivity and area under the receiver operating characteristics curve (AUC) of PSA for detecting prostate cancer [15]. They compared the placebo and finasteride groups for sensitivity and AUC of PSA for the detection of all cancers and for high-grade cancers. The AUC of PSA for all outcomes was greater for the finasteride group than the placebo group. The sensitivity of PSA was higher for men in the finasteride group than in the placebo group at all PSA cut-offs matched by specificity.

When the PCPT was designed, the authors hypothesized that finasteride could influence the detection of prostate cancer by decreasing the size of the prostate, making the DRE more sensitive. To investigate this theory, Thompson et al. again published a repeat analysis of the PCPT data in 2007 [16]. They examined sensitivity and specificity of DRE in the finasteride and placebo groups in patients who had a biopsy, PSA measurement, and DRE within 1 year prior to the biopsy, and were on treatment at the time of biopsy. They found that the sensitivity of DRE was significantly greater for cancer detection in men receiving finasteride than placebo (21.3% vs 16.7%, p = 0.015). In addition, although it did not attain statistical significance, DRE sensitivity was greater for detecting high-grade cancers in men on finasteride.

Finasteride enhances the biopsy detection of prostate cancer

Since the original publication of the PCPT data, we now know that finasteride enhances the detection of prostate cancer on "for cause" biopsies by improved sensitivity of PSA for overall and high-grade cancer detection [15,17], improved sensitivity of the DRE) [16], increased sensitivity of biopsy for high-grade cancer detection [18] and more accurate grading of high-grade prostate cancer [14,15,19].

Redman et al. [10] recently performed a series of three analyses that systematically controlled for these and other factors in estimating the true rate of cancer in the two study groups of the PCPT. They incorporated adjustments for all the aforementioned biases and showed that the cancer detection rates on biopsy in the entire PCPT of 15,990 men would have been similar, though slightly lower, than were observed in the 10,182 men who actually had an endpoint determinant. Estimated overall prostate cancer rates were 14.7% (4.8% high grade) for finasteride and 21.1% (4.2% high grade) for placebo, a 30% risk reduction in prostate cancer and a nonsignificant 14% increase in high-grade cancer with finasteride. Next, they extended to the entire PCPT population the changes from biopsy grade to prostatectomy grade, using data from the subset of 500 men who had a prostatectomy. The resulting rates, or "true" rates, of high-grade disease were 8.2% in the placebo arm and 6.0% in the finasteride arm, resulting in a 27% relative risk reduction in high-grade disease in the finasteride arm. This suggests that it was highly unlikely that finasteride actually increased the risk of high-grade cancer in the PCPT.

The third analysis examined the impact of biopsy sensitivity on the relative risk of high-grade prostate cancer and found that differential sensitivity of biopsy between the treatment arms can have a significant impact on risk ratio estimates. Biopsy sensitivity for high-grade disease is known to be lower with placebo than with finasteride, as has been shown previously [14]. Different ranges of biopsy sensitivity for high-grade cancer resulted in either a null or a reduced relative risk in the finasteride group for high-grade cancer. This final analysis revealed that as the sensitivity of prostate biopsy improves with finasteride, an even larger reduction in high-grade tumors is observed. This explains how small differences in biopsy sensitivity between the study arms could result in the apparent finasteride-associated increase in high-grade tumors on biopsy that was reported in 2003 [7].

Overall, this study suggests that the originally observed higher risk of high-grade cancer with finasteride was most likely due to facilitated diagnosis resulting primarily from increased biopsy sensitivity and that finasteride probably reduces the risk of all prostate cancers, including high-grade tumors [10].

Decreased prostate volume with finasteride increases cancer detection

Despite reduction in the total number of prostate cancers in the PCPT, the originally observed increase in the number of patients with high-grade cancer dramatically diminished interest in the use of finasteride as a chemopreventive agent [20-23]. One theory speculated that there were more high-grade tumors identified because of an alteration in the histological appearance of the tumor due to the effects of finasteride. As previously discussed, a review of the specimens from the PCPT did not support this theory and revealed that finasteride did not affect the Gleason grade assignment [14].

Further analyses indicated that the effect of finasteride on normal prostate and on low-grade prostate cancer led to biases favoring the diagnosis of high-grade disease in men treated with finasteride [10,18,24,25]. This was illustrated by the analysis of PCPT results supporting a diagnostic bias due to the effect of finasteride on prostate size [18]. Patients treated with finasteride had a significantly smaller prostate volume (median 25.1 cm^3 versus 33.5 cm^3 with placebo). The conclusion from this article is that the reduction in prostate volume with finasteride results in a disproportionate sampling of the tumor during biopsy, thereby increasing identification of high-grade tumor. When the effect of prostate size was incorporated into the analysis, the increased risk of high-grade prostate cancer with finasteride disappeared when compared to placebo. These results provide further reassurance that finasteride does not result in a clinically relevant increase in the number of high-grade prostate cancers [18].

Side effects of finasteride

A chemoprevention strategy must surmount considerable obstacles to be accepted for widespread use. It must be proven to be effective, have few side effects, and be affordable. As already detailed in this chapter, finasteride has been shown to reduce the risk of clinically significant prostate cancer, including high-grade tumors. It also has well-known efficacy in treating urinary symptoms in benign prostatic hyperplasia (BPH) as well as preventing the progression of BPH over time, making it even more attractive as a potential chemopreventive agent. The PCPT also revealed that reduced volume of ejaculate, erectile dysfunction, loss of libido, and gynecomastia were more

common in the finasteride group than in the placebo group ($p < 0.001$ for all comparisons) [7]. Various other studies have shown side effects of finasteride, with the most well-known side effect being the reported decline in sexual function associated with finasteride over relatively short study periods.

Sexual dysfunction was a prespecified secondary endpoint of the PCPT and, because of its large study population and long follow-up period, a more precise estimate of the difference between the placebo and finasteride groups could be obtained. The results of this analysis demonstrated that finasteride had only a modest effect on sexual function and its impact diminished over time [26]. As current sexual function instruments were not yet available when the PCPT began, the Sexual Activity Scale was used to gauge the effect of finasteride on sexual function. It covers four domains of sexual activity including: ability to attain an erection (5 response levels), degree of participant satisfaction with sexual activity (4 response levels), change in sexual performance (7 response levels), and frequency of sexual activity (7 response levels). Each response was converted to a 0–100 scale with the overall score being the mean of the four responses. Scores range from 0–100 with higher scores reflecting more impaired sexual function. This scale correlates quite well with currently used instruments measuring sexual function.

As men progressed through the study, the average increase in score was 8.22. Men in the finasteride arm had an average score 3.21 points higher than their counterparts in the placebo arm. This difference in sexual function score at the first assessment decreased to 2.11 points at the end of the study. After adjustment for all co-variates, mean sexual dysfunction increased in both arms from baseline (6 months after randomization) by 1.26 points per year, corresponding to a cumulative increase of 8.22 points. This study revealed that sexual dysfunction with finasteride is not clinically significant and should minimally influence the decision to treat with finasteride [27].

Implications for clinical practice

The decision on whether or not to use finasteride in individual cases needs to balance the potential benefits of finasteride against the known potential side effects of prolonged treatment. Patients must weigh the established benefits of a 25–30% reduction in prostate cancer, decreased urinary symptoms, and decreased complications of an enlarged prostate against the established side effects, which include clinically insignificant reduced sexual function and expense of medication.

After the development of an understanding of how PSA, DRE, and prostate biopsy were affected by finasteride, it appears that finasteride did not increase the risk of high-grade prostate cancer in the PCPT. With clear-cut evidence that most deaths from prostate cancer are caused by high-grade tumors, finasteride's improvement in detection of these tumors with PSA and with biopsy could be considered a major additional advantage beyond its effect on disease prevention. With an excellent safety profile and few side effects, as well as a range of benefits related to the other disease of the prostate (BPH), men aged 55 years or older should be informed of the opportunity to reduce their risk of prostate cancer with finasteride (Grade 1B).

Implications for research

It will be challenging for organized medicine to conduct future prevention trials for prostate cancer given their size, cost, complexity and duration. It should be the goal of future research to use evidence from the PCPT and other large-scale studies to identify those men who are destined to develop prostate cancer and, better still, those who are destined to suffer disease progression and, for these specific men, to institute a preventive intervention that is uniformly successful. An understanding of prostate carcinogenesis and pharmacogenomics, merged with biological samples from prospective trials, will make all of this possible.

Clinical question 25.2

Can vitamin E or selenium be recommended for chemoprevention of prostate cancer?

Literature search

A Medline literature search was performed to identify clinical trials investigating prostate cancer chemoprevention using vitamin E or selenium. We used the search terms "prostate cancer," "chemoprevention," "prevention," "vitamin E," "selenium," and "clinical trial."

The evidence: the Selenium and Vitamin E Cancer Prevention Trial (SELECT)

Vitamin E is an antioxidant and evidence suggests that it reduces androgen receptor level by transcriptional inhibition, providing a link to the androgen signaling pathway [28]. Secondary analyses from two large-scale prevention trials (one for skin cancer and one for lung cancer) suggested that vitamin E and/or selenium could reduce the risk of prostate cancer as well as disease mortality [29-33]. With this in mind, the Selenium and Vitamin E Cancer Prevention Trial (SELECT) was designed and the results recently published.

SELECT was a double-blind, randomized, placebo-controlled phase III trial designed to evaluate the value of selenium alone, vitamin E alone or the combination versus placebo in the prevention of prostate cancer, with the primary endpoint being clinical incidence of prostate cancer. Eligibility criteria included age ≥ 50 years for African Americans, age ≥ 55 years for non-African Americans, DRE not suspicious for cancer, and a PSA ≤ 4 ng/mL. Enrollment totaled 35,533 men. Prostate biopsy was performed at the recommendation of study physicians based on abnormalities in DRE or elevations of PSA based on community standards. The study was originally planned for 12 years with a minimum of 7 years of intervention depending on time of randomization. Accrual reached 32,400 men in April 2004 and was closed to further accrual with 35,533 men randomized.

The safety monitoring committee recommended early discontinuation of the study agents in September 2008 as results demonstrated no benefit from either active agent alone or in combination. The median overall follow-up was 5.46 years. Results revealed no statistically significant differences in rates of prostate cancer between the treatment groups or placebo. In addition, a nonsignificant increase in risk of prostate cancer was noted for vitamin E and a nonsignificant increase in risk of diabetes mellitus was noted for selenium.

Implications for clinical practice

With the recent publication of the SELECT results, there is Grade 1B evidence recommending against chemoprevention of prostate cancer with vitamin E and selenium supplementation. Hazard ratios and 99% CIs for prostate cancer were 1.04 for selenium (0.87–1.24), 1.13 for vitamin E (0.95–1.35), and 1.05 for the combination of selenium and vitamin E (0.88–1.25) compared with placebo. No significant differences were noted in other prespecified cancer endpoints. There was a statistically nonsignificant increase in diabetes mellitus type 2 in the selenium group and a nonsignificant increase in the risk of prostate cancer diagnosis in the vitamin E group. These data provide compelling evidence from a phase III clinical trial that neither vitamin E nor selenium will significantly reduce the risk of prostate cancer.

Implications for clinical research

The SELECT trial suggests many conclusions that will help us make advances in the chemoprevention of prostate cancer. It again proves to researchers that it is indeed possible to enroll greater than 35,000 men in a trial for disease prevention, rather than disease treatment. This trial is encouraging for ongoing research as it proves that men are interested in prevention trials, which may prove to have tremendous health benefits in the future. Chemoprevention of prostate cancer is now a proven option to reduce the burden of this disease, and men are clearly interested in helping to attain this goal. The SELECT trial also brings up the public health issue of the safety of frequently recommended supplements in the absence of large-scale trials that prove the efficacy and safety of those readily available supplements.

Conclusion

Based on the available high-quality evidence, we would recommend that a man 55 years old or older, who is undergoing regular PSA and DRE screening for prostate cancer, be informed that there is a proven method to reduce the risk of prostate cancer with finasteride. His physician should undertake a thorough discussion of his healthcare priorities, along with the benefits, risks, and cost of treatment with finasteride. A 25% risk reduction in prostate cancer will have tremendous public health consequences.

Prostate cancer prevention is now possible using finasteride, as proven in the PCPT. The results of the SELECT trial highlight the challenges with taking premature data from preclinical studies, case–control, and even population-based epidemiological studies and making them into clinical recommendations. The increased risk of prostate cancer with vitamin E and increased risk of diabetes with selenium focus serious concerns on the unknown risks of unproven agents. At the present time, men who are undergoing regular PSA testing should be informed that the only safe and proven method to reduce the risk of prostate cancer is with finasteride.

References

1. Jemal A, Siegel R, Ward E, Hao Y, Xu J, Murray T, et al. Cancer statistics, 2008. CA Cancer J Clin 2008;58(2):71-96.
2. Gronberg H. Prostate cancer epidemiology. Lancet 2003;361(9360):859-64.
3. Majeed A, Babb P, Jones J, Quinn M. Trends in prostate cancer incidence, mortality and survival in England and Wales 1971-1998. BJU Int 2000;85(9):1058-62.
4. Sarvis JA, Thompson IM. Androgens and prevention of prostate cancer. Curr Opin Endocrinol Diabetes Obes 2008;15(3):271-7.
5. McConnell JD, Wilson JD, George FW, Geller J, Pappas F, Stoner E. Finasteride, an inhibitor of 5 alpha-reductase, suppresses prostatic dihydrotestosterone in men with benign prostatic hyperplasia. J Clin Endocrinol Metab 1992;74(3):505-8.
6. Clark RV, Hermann DJ, Cunningham GR, Wilson TH, Morrill BB, Hobbs S. Marked suppression of dihydrotestosterone in men with benign prostatic hyperplasia by dutasteride, a dual 5alpha-reductase inhibitor. J Clin Endocrinol Metab 2004May;89(5):2179-84.
7. Thompson IM, Goodman PJ, Tangen CM, Lucia MS, Miller GJ, Ford LG, et al. The influence of finasteride on the development of prostate cancer. N Engl J Med 2003;349(3):215-24.
8. Andriole G, Bostwick D, Brawley O, Gomella L, Marberger M, Tindall D, et al. Chemoprevention of prostate cancer in men at high risk: rationale and design of the reduction by dutasteride of prostate cancer events (REDUCE) trial. J Urol 2004;172(4 pt 1):1314-17.
9. Etzioni RD, Howlader N, Shaw PA, Ankerst DP, Penson DF, Goodman PJ, et al. Long-term effects of finasteride on prostate specific antigen levels: results from the prostate cancer prevention trial. J Urol 2005;174(3):877-81.
10. Redman MW, Tangen C, Goodman P, Lucia MS, Coltman CA, Thompson I. Finasteride does not increase the risk of high-grade prostate cancer: a bias-adjusted modeling approach. Cancer Prev Res 2008;1:174.
11. Epstein JI, Walsh PC, Carmichael M, Brendler CB. Pathologic and clinical findings to predict tumor extent of nonpalpable (stage T1c) prostate cancer. JAMA 1994;271(5):368-74.
12. Lucia MS, Darke AK, Goodman PJ, Francisco GL, Parnes HL, Ford LG, et al. Pathologic characteristics of cancers detected in the prostate cancer prevention trial: implications for prostate cancer detection and chemoprevention. Cancer Prev Res 2008;1(3):167-73.
13. Epstein JI, Chan DW, Sokoll LJ, Walsh PC, Cox JL, Rittenhouse H, et al. Nonpalpable stage T1c prostate cancer: prediction of insignificant disease using free/total prostate specific antigen levels and needle biopsy findings. J Urol 1998;160(6 pt 2):2407-11.
14. Lucia MS, Epstein JI, Goodman PJ, Darke AK, Reuter VE, Civantos F, et al. Finasteride and high-grade prostate cancer in the Prostate Cancer Prevention Trial. J Natl Cancer Inst 2007;99(18):1375-83.
15. Thompson IM, Chi C, Ankerst DP, Goodman PJ, Tangen CM, Lippman SM, et al. Effect of finasteride on the sensitivity of PSA for detecting prostate cancer. J Natl Cancer Inst 2006;98(16):1128-33.
16. Thompson IM, Tangen CM, Goodman PJ, Lucia MS, Parnes HL, Lippman SM, et al. Finasteride improves the sensitivity of digital rectal examination for prostate cancer detection. J Urol 2007;177(5):1749-52.
17. Ankerst DP, Thompson IM. Sensitivity and specificity of prostate-specific antigen for prostate cancer detection with high rates of biopsy verification. Arch Ital Urol Androl 2006;78(4):125-9.
18. Cohen YC, Liu KS, Heyden NL, Carides AD, Anderson KM, Daifotis AG, et al. Detection bias due to the effect of finasteride on prostate volume: a modeling approach for analysis of the Prostate Cancer Prevention Trial. J Natl Cancer Inst 2007;99(18):1366-74.
19. Scardino PT. The prevention of prostate cancer – the dilemma continues. N Engl J Med 2003;349(3):297-9.
20. Unger JM, LeBlanc M, Crowley JJ, Grossman HB, Natale RB, Wozniak AJ, et al. Estimating the impact of new clinical trial proven cancer therapy and cancer chemoprevention on population mortality: the Karnofsky Memorial lecture. J Clin Oncol 2003;21(23 suppl):246s-52s.
21. Grover S, Lowensteyn I, Hajek D, Trachtenberg J, Coupal L, Marchand S. Do the benefits of finasteride outweigh the risks in the prostate cancer prevention trial? J Urol 2006;175(3 pt 1):934-8; discussion 8.
22. Zeliadt SB, Etzioni RD, Penson DF, Thompson IM, Ramsey SD. Lifetime implications and cost-effectiveness of using finasteride to prevent prostate cancer. Am J Med 2005;118(8):850-7.

23. Andriole GL, Humphrey PA, Serfling RJ, Grubb RL. High-grade prostate cancer in the Prostate Cancer Prevention Trial: fact or artifact? J Natl Cancer Inst 2007;99(18):1355-6.

24. Lucia MS, Darke AK, Goodman PJ, La Rosa FG, Parnes HL, Ford LG, et al. Pathologic characteristics of cancer detected in the Prostate Cancer Prevention Trial: implications for prostate cancer detection and chemoprevention. Cancer Prev Res 2008;1:167.

25. Pinsky P, Parnes HL, Ford L. Estimating rates of true high-grade disease in the Prostate Cancer Prevention Trial. Cancer Prev Res 2008;1(3):182-6.

26. Moinpour CM, Amy KD, Gary WD, Ian MT, Connie L, Donna Pauler A. Longitudinal analysis of sexual function reported by men in the Prostate Cancer Prevention Trial. J Natl Cancer Inst 2007;99(13):1025-35.

27. Sarvis JA, Thompson IM. Prostate cancer chemoprevention: update of the Prostate Cancer Prevention Trial findings and implications for clinical practice. Curr Oncol Rep 2008;10(6): 529-32.

28. Zhang Y, Ni J, Messing EM, Chang E, Yang CR, Yeh S. Vitamin E succinate inhibits the function of androgen receptor and the expression of prostate-specific antigen in prostate cancer cells. Proc Natl Acad Sci U S A 2002;99(11):7408-13.

29. Alpha-Tocopherol, Beta Carotene Cancer Prevention Study Group. The effect of vitamin E and beta carotene on the incidence of lung cancer and other cancers in male smokers. N Engl J Med 1994;330(15):1029-35.

30. Clark LC, Combs GF Jr, Turnbull BW, Slate EH, Chalker DK, Chow J, et al. Effects of selenium supplementation for cancer prevention in patients with carcinoma of the skin. A randomized controlled trial. Nutritional Prevention of Cancer Study Group. JAMA 1996;276(24):1957-63.

31. Duffield-Lillico AJ, Dalkin BL, Reid ME, Turnbull BW, Slate EH, Jacobs ET, et al. Selenium supplementation, baseline plasma selenium status and incidence of prostate cancer: an analysis of the complete treatment period of the Nutritional Prevention of Cancer Trial. BJU Int 2003;91(7):608-12.

32. Heinonen OP, Albanes D, Virtamo J, Taylor PR, Huttunen JK, Hartman AM, et al. Prostate cancer and supplementation with alpha-tocopherol and beta-carotene: incidence and mortality in a controlled trial. J Natl Cancer Inst 1998;90(6):440-6.

33. Blot WJ, Li JY, Taylor PR, Guo W, Dawsey S, Wang GQ, et al. Nutrition intervention trials in Linxian, China: supplementation with specific vitamin/mineral combinations, cancer incidence, and disease-specific mortality in the general population. J Natl Cancer Inst 1993;85(18):1483-92.

26 Early detection and screening for prostate cancer

Pim J. van Leeuwen, Monique J. Roobol and Fritz H. Schröder

Erasmus University Medical Centre, Rotterdam, The Netherlands

Background

The concept of screening is to identify a disease at a stage in its natural history where treatment can be applied in order to prevent death or suffering. For prostate cancer, this is challenging because the variable natural history of the disease differs markedly from slow-growing indolent tumors and highly aggressive and potentially fatal forms. Benefits of screening should be an increased but not excessive rate of early-stage detected cancers, a decrease in metastatic cancer and a reduction in cancer-specific mortality. Several authors have asked whether screening for prostate cancer is a suitable strategy to reduce prostate cancer mortality. Recently, two rando-mized prostate cancer screening trials published their final data. The European Randomized Study of Screening for Prostate Cancer (ERSPC) showed that prostate-specific antigen (PSA)-based screening lowers prostate cancer mortality while the study conducted in the United States, the Prostate, Lung, Colorectal, and Ovarian Cancer (PLCO) Screening Trial showed no benefit in prostate cancer mortality [1,2]. The ERSPC was conducted in eight European countries and enrolled 267,994 men 55–74 years of age, while the PLCO trial enrolled 155,000 women and men 55–74 years of age. The main purpose of these two trials was to evaluate whether population-based screening reduces the mortality from prostate cancer, with an acceptable level of quality-of-life aspects and associated costs. Possible disadvantages of screening are overdetection with resultant overtreatment, increased costs, side effects and complications. This chapter discusses the current evidence available on early detection and screening for prostate cancer.

Clinical question 26.1

What is the sensitivity and specificity of PSA as an early detection tool for prostate cancer?

Literature search

We searched Medline using the term "PSA" and other relevant keywords ("prostate cancer," "screening," "early detection," "sensitivity," "specificity," "randomized controlled trials," "clinical studies," "case–control cohorts"). We limited the searches to English-language articles published between January 1980 and March 2009; non-English-language studies were excluded, because their quality is difficult to evaluate.

The evidence

The main tool in screening for prostate cancer, prostate-specific antigen, was first described in 1979. It is a human protein secreted by prostate epithelial cells and is perhaps more a specific organ marker than a tumor marker since prostatitis, benign prostate hyperplasia (BPH) and other conditions can also increase PSA. PSA has a large intraindividual day-to-day variation and is influenced by bodyweight [3]. Partly due to the fact that PSA is not a cancer-specific measurement, no clear threshold level exists for PSA sensitivity and specificity [4]. In clinical practice, recommendations based on PSA vary between 2.0 and 4.0 ng/mL. Krumholtz et al. recommended a cut-off point of 2.6 ng/mL as an indicator for biopsy after they established a prostate cancer detection rate of 22% in the 2.6–4.0 ng/mL PSA range [5]. Thompson et al. demonstrated, after biopsying men in low PSA ranges, that there is no cut-point of PSA with equal sensitivity and specificity for monitoring healthy men for prostate cancer [4,6]. In this trial, after biopsying 5587 men, a prostate cancer prevalence of 15% in men with PSA 4.0 ng/mL and lower was found; 15% of those men with prostate cancer had high-grade cancer (Gleason score ≥ 7) [6]. According to these study results, a physician who requires 80% confidence in not missing a prostate cancer should apply a PSA cut-off value of 1.1 ng/mL as an indication for biopsy, which would result in 60% unnecessary biopsies.

The lack of sensitivity and specificity of PSA in low ranges is confirmed in the ERSPC tria l[7]. In Table 26.1, the continuum of prostate cancer risk for different PSA ranges is presented for the ERSPC and the Prostate Cancer Prevention Trial (PCPT) [4,7]. As shown, sensitivity decreases with increasing PSA level, while specificity increases. Besides this, Thompson et al. proved that the sensitivity and specificity of PSA are improving for high-grade cancer compared with any prostate cancer, demonstrating that PSA is a better marker of high- than of low-grade disease [4]. Considering the continuum of prostate cancer risk over different PSA ranges, one should question whether it is necessary to detect all prostate cancers present in all PSA ranges. After comparing the biopsy rates of men in the PCPT placebo arm with the cancer detection rates, interval cancers and prostate cancer deaths of three subsequent screening rounds, applying a PSA cut-off of 3.0 ng/mL as biopsy indication in the ERSPC trial, Schröder et al. concluded that if we biopsied all men regardless of PSA level, a very unfavorable balance between men biopsied and the detection of one (deadly) prostate cancer would occur [8]. This is in line with earlier publication of the ERSPC study in which was concluded that among men whose cancer was not detected at initial screening by applying a 4.0 ng/mL PSA cut-off, it was unlikely that a substantial number would progress to noncurable stages at the time of repeat screening 4 years later [9,10]. Overall, the authors concluded that, although the sensitivity and specificity of PSA are not ideal, a serum PSA cut-off of 3.0 ng/mL is not too high combined with a 4-year screening interval. Besides this, men presenting with PSA values between 2.0 and 2.9 ng/mL at initial screening might be primarily targeted [8].

Table 26.1 The continuum of prostate cancer risk for different PSA ranges, presented for the ERSPC and the PCPT

Authors	Methods	Intervention	Participants	Outcomes	Results							Notes
Thompson et al. [4]	RCT	To estimate the receiver operating characteristic (ROC) curve for PSA, PCPT	N 5587	Sensitivity and specificity of PCa detection for all PSA ranges in relation to Gleason grade	PSA, ng/mL	Prostate cancer, any grade			Prostate cancer, Gleason grade ≥ 8			N 1225 (21.9%) were diagnosed with prostate cancer
						Sen (%)	Spec (%)	LR	Sen (%)	Spec (%)	LR	
					1.1	83.4	38.9	1.4	94.7	35.9	1.5	
					2.1	52.6	72.5	1.9	86.0	65.9	2.5	
					2.6	40.5	81.1	2.1	78.9	75.1	3.2	
					3.1	32.2	86.7	2.4	68.4	81.0	3.6	
					4.1	20.5	93.8	3.3	50.9	89.1	4.7	
					6.1	4.6	98.5	3.1	26.3	97.5	10.5	
					10.1	0.9	99.7	3.0	5.3	99.5	10.6	
Schröder et al. [7]	RCT	Cancer detection rate for different PSA ranges in the ERSPC, Rotterdam section	N 9779	Distribution of PSA and prostate cancers in men aged 55–74 biopsied (2267 men) for PSA ≥ 4.0, DRE, and TRUS	PSA, ng/mL	Total biopsies (%)	Cancer (n)	Total cancer (%)	PPV	Biopsy (N) per cancer		
					0.0–0.9	36.4	4	0.8	2.2	45.8		
					1.0–1.9	31.2	45	9.5	8.8	11.4		
					2.0–2.9	12.3	30	6.3	13.6	7.4		
					3.0–3.9	7.2	44	9.3	25.3	3.9		
					4.0–9.9	10.9	241	51.0	24.5	4.1		
					≥ 10.0	2.1	109	23.0	56.5	1.8		

DRE, digital rectal examination; ERSPC, European Randomized Study of Screening for Prostate Cancer; LR, likelihood ratio; PCa, prostate cancer; PCPT, Prostate Cancer Prevention Trial; PPV, positive predictive value; PSA, prostate-specific antigen; RCT, randomized controlled trial; Sen, sensitivity; Spec, specificity; TRUS, transrectal ultrasound

In addition to Catalona et al. recommending a biopsy in men with PSA higher than 2.5 ng/mL, they suggest that prostate cancer screening should begin at age 40 years to establish a baseline PSA measurement and to assess risk for prostate cancer. Because PSA elevation at age 40–50 is more strongly associated with a later diagnosis of prostate cancer than an elevation of PSA at age 60, a primary goal of PSA testing in men ≤ 50 should be to stratify cancer risk at an early age rather than to detect prostate cancer [11–13]. In future, a risk-adjusted screening strategy based on a single baseline PSA measured at age 40–50 may be possible and prevents men receiving many unnecessary biopsies.

Clinical question 26.2

What is the additional value of digital rectal examination (DRE) and transrectal ultrasound (TRUS) in low PSA ranges for early detection and screening of prostate cancer?

Literature search

We searched Medline using the terms "digital rectal examination" and "transrectal ultrasound" with other relevant keywords ("prostate cancer," "screening," "early detection," "PSA," "sensitivity," "specificity," "randomized controlled trials," "clinical studies," "case–control cohorts"). We limited the searches to English-language articles published between January 1980 and March 2009; non-English-language studies were excluded, because the quality of these studies is difficult to evaluate.

The evidence

Although DRE is still widely used for the diagnosis of prostate cancer, its central role is superseded by the widespread application of serum PSA. DRE is possible due to the anatomical position of the prostate in the pelvis, with easy access for palpation using a finger placed per rectum. In screening and early detection programs for prostate cancer, the value of DRE remains controversial because it is not standardized and varies widely among physicians [14]. Table 26.2 provides an overview of the positive predictive value for DRE in different PSA ranges [15–21]. DRE has a low sensitivity and predictive value in men with low PSA levels where it should be most useful. At serum PSA levels below 3.0 ng/mL, 289 rectal examinations are required to find one case of clinically significant disease, and 96 rectal examinations are needed to diagnose prostate cancer of any size, grade or stage [22]. According to these results, and the fact that tumors detected by DRE had the lowest pathological stage, the ERSPC has

omitted DRE as an initial screening test [23]. In addition, Gosselaar et al. reported that an abnormal DRE was not a significant predictor for diagnosing prostate cancer on repeat screenings [24]. Although an abnormal DRE should no longer be an independent indicator for biopsy in low PSA ranges, Okotie et al. found that a substantial proportion of cancers detected by DRE alone at PSA levels < 4.0 ng/mL have clinically aggressive features; nearly 20% had a Gleason score ≥ 7 [21]. Furthermore, Gosselaar et al. point out that potentially aggressive cancers (Gleason ≥ 7) are more prevalent among men who have an abnormal DRE compared to normal DRE at PSA levels ≥ 3.0 ng/mL. Okotie et al. suggested that omission of DRE from screening protocols might compromise treatment outcomes because many of the cancers detected by DRE alone are potentially curable but may have worse outcomes by the time PSA also reaches a higher level. However, Okotie et al. conducted a univariate analysis for suspected DRE only and not a multivariate analysis with consideration of PSA. Consequently, the additional value of DRE over PSA would be small since Thompson et al. showed that 15% men with PSA ≤ 4.0 ng/mL had cancer on biopsy [6].

Transrectal ultrasound is in widespread use by urologists although less often as a primary prostate cancer screening tool. In the ERSPC, TRUS is used to guide biopsies of the prostate gland in patients with elevated serum PSA, with an additional biopsy of possible hypoechoic lesions [23]. TRUS is not useful to identify prostate cancer because of the frequent multifocality of cancer within the prostate, the variable sonographic appearance of prostate tumors, the poor specificity of focal ultrasonic abnormalities, and the substantial percentage of isoechoic prostate cancers (which cannot be differentiated from adjacent benign tissues with imaging) [25]. Some studies have shown that hypoechoic lesion-directed biopsy is as sensitive as a biopsy from an isoechoic region [26]. Table 26.3 shows the positive and negative predictive value of TRUS-guided biopsy of hypoechoic lesions in different studies [27-32]. The only studies in which sensitivity and specificity are not relative (all patients included who had a radical prostatectomy to ensure the presence of cancer) were those by Carter et al. [27]. and Terris et al. [28] who reported sensitivities of 52% and 53.3% and specificities of 68% and 75% respectively for all PSA ranges. One study determined the additional value of TRUS in low PSA ranges; they presented a low positive predictive value (9% for PSA ≤ 4.0 ng/mL) [30]. Gosselaar et al. reported the value of additional biopsies of suspicious lesions in a screening situation with systematic sextant biopsy [32]. They concluded that it would be preferable in men previously not biopsied; the additional biopsy core was statistically significantly more often positive for cancer than the random sextant biopsy cores. However, in future this value will decline because of the

Table 26.2 Positive predictive value for prostate cancer detection, DRE for different PSA ranges

Authors	Methods	Intervention	Participants	Outcomes	Results	Notes
Schröder et al. [17]	RCT	The usefulness of DRE as a stand-alone screening test and in conjunction with measured PSA. ERSPC, Rotterdam section	N 10,523	The positive predictive value and sensitivity of DRE	PSA: 0.0–0.9 PPV: 4% PSA: 1.0–1.9 PPV: 10% PSA: 2.0–2.9 PPV: 11% PSA: 3.0–3.9 PPV: 33% PSA: 4.0–9.9 PPV: 45% PSA: ≥10.0 PPV: 83%	
Crawford [16]	CCS	Methods of prostate cancer early detection, positive predictive value PSA	N 31,953	Detection rates of prostate cancer relative to PSA range and findings on DRE	PSA: 0.0–4.0 PPV: 15% PSA: 4.1–9.9 PPV: 34% PSA: ≥10.0 PPV: 72%	
Yamamoto et al. [15]	CCS	Investigate the usefulness of DRE for prostate cancer diagnosis in subjects with PSA levels of 4.0 ng/mL or less	N 90	Detection rates of prostate cancer relative to PSA range and findings on DRE	PSA: 0.0–0.9 PPV: 4% PSA: 1.0–1.9 PPV: 0% PSA: 2.0–2.9 PPV: 19% PSA: 3.0–4.0 PPV: 44%	
Bozeman et al. [18]	CCS	Men with abnormal DRE findings and a PSA level less than 4.0 ng/mL who underwent prostate biopsy	N 986	Positive predictive value DRE for PSA <4.0 ng/mL	PSA: 0.0–0.9 PPV: 2% PSA: 1.0–1.9 PPV: 6% PSA: 2.0–2.9 PPV: 13% PSA: 3.0–3.9 PPV: 21%	
Andriole et al. [20]	RCT	Diagnostic evaluation of DRE as initial screening test	N 34,115	Detection rates of prostate cancer relative to PSA range and findings on DRE	PSA: 0.0–4.0 PPV: 17% PSA: 4.1–7.0 PPV: 47% PSA: ≥10.0 PPV: 90%	
Okotie et al. [21]	CCS	Examine clinical and pathological features of men with prostate cancer detected by DRE alone, PSA level ≤4.0 ng/mL	N 36,000	Cancer detection PSA level ≤4.0 ng/mL with suspicious DRE in relation to Gleason score	303 men were diagnosed with PCa by DRE alone. 60 (20%) were nonorgan confined and 56 (20%) had a Gleason score ≥7	
Gosselaar et al. [19]	RCT	Two populations, PSA 2.0–3.9 ng/mL, were studied. Group1 was biopsied if DRE was suspicious. In group 2 all men were offered biopsy, regardless of DRE result. ERSPC, Rotterdam section	Gr 1 N 1877 Gr 2 N 801	Cancer detection rates and tumor characteristics	Gr 1: abnormal DRE prompted biopsy in 253 (13.5%) men (236 (93.3%) actually biopsied). 49 PCa detected, CDR 49/1877 = 2.6%. Gr 2: 120 cancers in 666 (83.1%) men actually biopsied, CDR = 120/801 = 15.0%. Of all PCa. 46.9% in gr 1 and 15.0% in gr 2 had biopsy Gleason score ≥7	

CCS, case–control study; CDR, cancer detection rate; DRE, digital rectal examination; Gr, group; PCa, prostate cancer; PPV, positive predictive value; PSA, prostate-specific antigen; RCT, randomized controlled trial

more common extended biopsy schemes and the decline in the percentage of men with no previous biopsy.

Comment

Although the risk of (high-grade) prostate cancer increases with the level of serum PSA, there is no serum PSA level below which there is no risk of having prostate cancer. Currently we can conclude that serum PSA is the most accurate of the three diagnostic tests. The overall findings suggest that the DRE is a poor screening tool for prostate cancer, and increasing levels of serum PSA have been demonstrated to be more important in detecting prostate cancer. Therefore DRE should not necessarily be recommended as a primary screening tool since it caused an unfavorable number of biopsies to detect one cancer in low PSA ranges. However, its role in combination with PSA for diagnosis is necessary, as it gives essential clinical information for staging and treatment decision making.

Evidence shows that TRUS has limited additional value as a screening tool, especially at low PSA ranges. Although we are aware that prostate cancer occurs in all PSA ranges, a serum PSA cut-off of 2.5 ng/mL or 3.0 ng/mL may be recommendable for prostate biopsy. Lowering the PSA cut-off

Table 26.3 Positive predictive value of TRUS for prostate cancer detection

Authors	Methods	Intervention	Participants	Outcomes	Results	Notes
Carter et al. [49]	CCS	Determine the ability of TRUS to detect early localized prostate cancer, all patients underwent radical prostatectomy	N 59	Positive predictive value TRUS for all PSA ranges	PPV: 54% and NPV: 66%	TRUS: 5 or 7 mhz
Terris et al. [28]	CCS	Determine the ability of TRUS to detect prostate cancer, all patients underwent radical cystoprostatectomy	N 51	Positive predictive value TRUS for all PSA ranges	PPV: 47% and NPV: 79%	TRUS: 7 mhz
Ellis et al. [29]	CCS	Evaluation PPV of TRUS, 6-sector prostate needle biopsies to rule out prostate carcinoma	N 1001	Positive predictive value TRUS for all PSA ranges	PPV: 17% and NPV: 75%	TRUS: 7 mhz
Ito et al. [30]	CCS	To determine the additional value of TRUS in low PSA ranges	N 297	Positive predictive value TRUS for PSA 0–4.0 ng/mL	PPV: 9% when PSA ≤4.0 ng/nL	
Gosselaar et al. [32]	RCT FU: 3 screening round	To determine the value of a hypoechoic lesion-directed biopsy in addition to a systematic sextant biopsy for detecting prostate cancer	N 10,754 in screening arm	Positive predictive value different rounds of ERSPC section Rotterdam	Round 1 PPV: 53% Round 2 PPV: 25% Round 3 PPV: 4%	TRUS: 7 mhz

CCS, case–control study; FU, follow-up; NPV, negative predictive value; PPV, positive predictive value; PSA, prostate-specific antigen; RCT, randomized controlled trial; TRUS, transrectal ultrasound

will result in an unfavorable number of unnecessary biopsies and is not required since PSA ≥ 3.0 was shown to be clinically justified when we use a 4-year screening interval. So men presenting with PSA values of < 3.0 ng/mL should not undergo biopsy but can be followed in line with the level of their initial PSA value, where men with PSA 2.0–2.9 ng/mL should be followed with increased attention. The need for a molecular marker that can distinguish aggressive cancer in low PSA ranges is crucial, especially for men with serum PSA 2.0–2.9 ng/mL.

Clinical question 26.3

What is the incidence of prostate cancer in a screened compared to a nonscreened population?

Literature search

We searched Medline using the terms "prostate cancer" and "incidence" with other relevant keywords ("screening," "early detection," "PSA," "prevalence," "randomized controlled trials," "clinical studies," "registry," "epidemiology," "case–control cohorts"). We limited the searches to English-language articles published between January 1980 and March 2009; non-English-language studies were excluded, because the quality of these studies is difficult to evaluate.

The evidence

The American Cancer Society estimates that there will be about 186,320 new cases of prostate cancer in the United States in 2008 [33]. Prostate cancer incidence differs widely between continents and from country to country. The International Association of Cancer Registries estimates that there were 679,023 cases of prostate cancer worldwide in 2002, with 513,464 (75.6%) of these occurring in developed countries [34]. This major difference is partly due to the introduction and widespread use of PSA testing for early detection of prostate cancer. From the advent of the PSA era in the early 1990s, there has been a sudden rise in prostate cancer incidence observed in Western countries. Incidence correlates with PSA testing and in the US rose by more than 20% per year during 1989–1992, when 19% of white men aged 65 years or older were being tested annually in 1992 [35]. In contrast, prostate cancer incidence in England and Wales rose by 3% per year when only 1–4% of men older than 45 years had a screening test annually in 1992 [36]. Collin et al. demonstrated that in the US age-adjusted and age-specific prostate cancer incidence rate trends were similar but consistently higher than in the United Kingdom between 1975 and 2003, with a factor of ten-difference in the frequency of PSA testing between the US (57%) and UK (6%) [36]. When interpreting incidence rates between different continents and countries, it is important to realize that variability in prostate cancer incidence can be the result of the different age structure of populations. Therefore age-adjusted and age-specific prostate cancer incidence per amount of men in the population should be used for comparison. In addition, it is essential to consider that incidence can be influenced by several risk factors other than screening, including genetic susceptibility, environmental exposure and differences in healthcare provision. Changes in prostate cancer incidence after the introduction of PSA testing for several countries in Europe, Asia and America are summarized in Table 26.4, with a reported age-standardized increase in prostate cancer of 51% between 1993 and 2001 in Europe (61.8–92.3), 61% among white men between 1989 and 1992 in the US and 5–118% in Asian countries between 1993 and 1997 [37–39].

Prostate cancer incidence differs widely between population screening studies and the general population and also in randomized screening studies (see Table 26.4) [20,23, 40–42]. After the first screening round of the ERSPC, detection rates in the screening and control arms were reported for 183,038 participants. In the screening arm 2227 prostate cancers were found, a detection rate of 3.4%, while in the control arm during the same period 891 prostate cancers were found, a detection rate of 0.9% [23]. The Swedish section of the ERSPC showed a 1.8-fold increased risk for diagnosis of prostate cancer in the screening arm compared to the control arm after 10 years of follow-up [40].

Comment

Evidence suggests that prostate cancer screening increases prostate cancer incidence, and incidence correlates positively with the amount of PSA testing in different countries all over the world. Meanwhile no molecular marker is available that can distinguish aggressive prostate cancer from that which will remain asymptomatic. Therefore overdiagnosis implies a considerable risk when applying active PSA-based screening.

Clinical question 26.4

Does screening result in prostate cancer detection at an earlier stage?

Literature search

We searched Medline using the terms "prostate cancer" and "stage" with other relevant keywords ("screening," "early detection," "incidence," "prevalence," "randomized controlled trials," "clinical studies," "registry," "epidemiology," "case–control cohorts"). We limited the searches to English-language articles published between January 1980 and March 2009; non-English-language studies were excluded, because the quality of these studies is difficult to evaluate.

The evidence

The rationale of prostate cancer screening is that, when prostate cancer is detected in a localized stage, it can be cured and the survival rate and/or the patient's quality of life can be improved. An early and expected effect of successful prostate screening therefore is a stage shift, with diagnosis occurring at earlier pathological stages that are more amenable to curative treatment.

Since the introduction of PSA screening, there has been a change in the stage distribution of newly diagnosed prostate cancer; the rate of metastatic disease decreased by 52% between 1990 and 1994 in the US [35]. Recent data from the Surveillance Epidemiology and End Results (SEER) show that in the US, 91% of prostate cancer cases are diagnosed while the cancer is still confined to the primary site or after it has spread to regional lymph nodes (localized or regional stage); 5% are diagnosed after the cancer has already metastasized (distant stage) and for the remaining 4% the staging information was unknown [35]. In comparison, these percentages were 71% and 19% for localized and distant disease respectively in 1985 [35]. In countries where prostate cancer screening is less frequent, this stage migration with reduced numbers of metastatic disease cases is less explicit. Table 26.5 displays the stage distribution after introduction of opportunistic PSA testing for the US and UK in relation to the percentage of PSA testing [37,43]. It is important to realize that these percentages are partly influenced by the simultaneously increased incidence of mainly localized disease. For instance, if the total group is made larger with mainly localized disease, then the percentage of metastatic disease will decrease. Therefore, the correct method of assessing a possible effect on stage reduction is calculating the absolute numbers.

Epidemiological data and case-control studies as well as RCTs have shown that PSA-based screening results in a favorable stage shift. The nonrandomized Tyrol trial, in which PSA-based screening became freely available to men aged 45–75 in the Federal State of Tyrol in Austria since 1993, demonstrated a significant migration to more favorable stages since the introduction of PSA screening. Labrie et al. showed in the Quebec trial that annual PSA screening results in clinically localized disease in 95% of the cases while metastatic disease almost disappeared [44]. A criticism of this study is that there was cross-over of men between the randomized groups, so that nonresponders were added to the control group, whereas patients actually screened in the control group were added to the screened group. In the Rotterdam section of the ERSPC, after comparing the intervention arm with the control arm

Table 26.4 Prostate cancer incidence trends after introduction of PSA or systematic prostate cancer screening

Authors	Methods	Intervention	Outcomes	Participants	Results	Notes
Dennis et al. [37]	CS FU: 23 yrs	Population-based incidence rates for US based on the SEER	Prostate cancer incidence trends in relation to introduction of PSA, 1973–1996	Nine regions of the SEER	Prostate cancer increase of 12.8% over period 1985–1992. Prostate cancer decrease of 9.2% over period 1992–1996	
Kvåle et al. [39]	CS FU: 24 yrs	Are the recorded incidence rates of prostate cancer associated with the introduction of PSA testing in five Nordic European countries?	Prostate cancer incidence trends in relation to introduction of PSA	Five countries: Denmark, Finland, Iceland, Norway, and Sweden	Close relation between use of PSA and cancer incidence in different countries. Increase in prostate cancer incidence in all Nordic countries except Denmark where PSA testing remained limited	
Sim et al. [38]	CS FU: 19 yrs	Are prostate cancer incidence trends changing over time in different Asian countries?	Prostate cancer incidence trends in relation to introduction of PSA	Seven countries: Philippines, Singapore, Japan, China, India, Thailand and China	Incidence of prostate cancer has risen by 5–118% in the indexed Asian countries; the incidence ratio in many Asian centers is similar to that of the high-risk countries	Incidence remains lower than in western countries
Bartsch et al. [42]	RS FU: 5 yrs	Prostate cancer incidence trends. Incidence trends in Tyrol after PSA testing became freely available	Prostate cancer incidence trends 1988–1993	More than 76,000	Prostate cancer incidence increased after introduction of PSA testing with 80% between 1988 and 1993	
Schröder et al. [9]	RCT FU: first screening round	Prostate cancer detection rate in the ERSPC after first round of screening (October 2002)	Prostate cancer detection rate	183,038	Screening arm: 2227 men diagnosed with cancer, overall detection rate 3.4% which differs 5.1% in The Netherlands and 1.6% in Italy. Control arm: 891 men diagnosed with cancer, overall detection rate 0.9% which differs from 1.3% in The Netherlands and 0.3% in Italy	
Mäkinen et al. [41]	RCT FU: first screening round	Compare prostate cancer incidence between the screening and control arm after first year post randomization in the Finnish section of ERSPC	Prostate cancer detection rate	15,685 screening arm 35,973 control arm	Prostate cancer detection rate among screeners was 2.4% (377 of 15,685) and 0.6% (40 of 7047) of nonparticipants in the screening arm. Prostate cancer detection among control arm was 0.3% (112 of 35,973)	Randomization is unequal because it is not randomized in a 1:1 pattern
Aus et al. [40]	RCT FU: 10 yrs	Evaluation whether PSA-based screening increased the risk of diagnosis of prostate cancer in the Swedish section of ERSPC	Prostate cancer incidence	9972 screening arm 9973 control arm	1.8 times more men diagnosed in the screening arm: 810 cancers detected in screening arm, 442 cancers detected in control arm	

CCS, case–control study; CS, cohort studies; FU, follow-up; PSA, prostate-specific antigen. RCT, randomized controlled trial; RS, registry study; SEER, Surveillance, Epidemiology, and End Result Program.

Table 26.5 Stage distribution after introduction of PSA or systematic prostate cancer screening

Authors	Methods	Intervention	Participants	Outcomes	Results	Notes
Dennis et al. [37]	CCS FU: 23 yrs	Relative incidence rates for prostate cancer by stage for US, based on the Surveillance, Epidemiology, and End Result Program (SEER)	Nine regions of the SEER	PCa incidence trends by stage over time 1973–1996	14.3% increase in incidence of localized disease from 1985 to 1992 15.9% decline in incidence of distant-stage prostate cancer from 1992 to 1996	19% of white men aged 65 years or older were being tested annually in 1992 in US
Mokete et al. [43]	CCS FU: 10 yrs	Evaluation of whether there is a significant tendency to a localized stage of prostate cancer diagnosis	704 men diagnosed prostate cancer UK	Change in stage at diagnosis	No significant chance in stage at diagnosis; overall, 38 (20–44)% presented with clinically localized disease, 25 (18–29)% with metastatic disease	1–4% of men >45 yrs had a screening test annually in 1992 in UK
Rietbergen et al. [45]	RCT FU: 4 yrs	Clinical stage of screen-detected compared with clinical-detected cancers, The Netherlands	N 20,632	Percentage localized and metastatic PCa	Screening arm: 459 prostate cancer: 77% localized disease, 2% metastatic Pca Clinical diagnosed 4708 Pca; 60% localized, 24% metastatic disease	
Andriole et al. [20]	CCS FU: first screening round	Prostate cancer detection by stage in the screening arm after first screening round of PLCO	N 38,350	Percentage localized and metastatic PCa	556 patients with prostate cancer within the first year of screening; 88% localized disease, 4% metastatic prostate cancer at diagnosis	
Pelzer et al. [46]	RS	Clinical stage of screen-detected compared with clinical-detected cancers, Austria	More than 76,000	Percentage diagnosed localized disease	Screening cohort Tyrol: 1208 patients cancer, 80% localized disease. Nonscreening cohort, rest of Austria: 237 cancers, 68% localized disease	
Mäkinen et al. [41]	RCT FU: first screening round	Compare prostate cancer incidence for stage between the screening and control arm in the ERSPC, Finnish section	N 15,685 screening arm N 35,973 control arm	Prostate cancer detection by stage	Detected prostate cancer 82% organ confined among screening population, 65% among the control arm was organ confined	Randomization is unequal because it is not randomized in a 1:1 pattern
Van der Cruijsen-Koeter et al. [10]	RCT FU: 4–10 yrs	Comparison of characteristics detected in the screening and control arms of the ERSPC, Rotterdam section	N 17,635 screening arm N 17,513 control arm	Prostate cancer detection by stage	1269 cancers detected in screening arm, 336 cancers detected in control arm. T1C and T2 were 5.8 and 6.0 times more often diagnosed, respectively, in the screening arm than in the control arm	
Aus et al. [40]	RCT FU: 10 yrs	Evaluation whether PSA-based screening reduces the risk of being diagnosed with metastatic prostate cancer in the ERSPC, Sweden section	N 9972 screening arm N 9973 control arm	Prostate cancer detection by stage	810 cancers detected in screening arm, 442 cancers detected in control arm. 764 T1/T2 screening arm, 370 T1/T2 control arm. 24 metastatic PCa in screening arm, 47 metastatic PCa in control arm	

CS, cohort studies; FU, follow-up; localized prostate cancer, cancer confined within prostate gland (T1–2) without extension through prostatic capsule (T3); PCa, prostate cancer; RCT, randomized controlled trial; RS, registry study and with the general population, a statistically significant migration to more favorable stages was observed in the screening arm. Mäkinen et al. confirmed these facts by presenting a statistically significant difference of 17% in localized disease in the Finish section of the ERSPC. In the Swedish section of the ERSPC, the number of men found with metastatic prostate cancer at the time of diagnosis (or who had PSA > 100 ng/mL) was 24 in the screening arm compared with 47 in the control arm (p = 0.0084) after 10-year follow-up [40]. Table 26.5 summarizes the different studies that reported a stage distribution after introduction of systematic PSA screening [10,20,40,41,45,46].

Comment

There is a substantial level of evidence that systematic prostate cancer screening causes a stage distribution to more localized disease. Besides that, a relationship is observed between the amount of opportunistic PSA testing and a stage distribution for different countries. Although this is an early effect of screening, it is not automatically predictive for a prostate cancer-specific mortality reduction. Furthermore, the distribution to a more favorable stage at diagnosis is caused by an increase in prostate cancer incidence, resulting in a recommendation of Grade 2A (i.e. weak recommendation, high-quality evidence) [47].

Clinical question 26.5

Does screening decrease prostate cancer mortality?

Literature search

We searched Medline using the terms "prostate cancer" and "mortality" with other relevant keywords ("screening," "early detection," "randomized controlled trials"). We limited the searches to English-language randomized control trials published between January 1990 and March 2009.

The evidence

Mortality data have been presented by two prostate cancer screening RCTs (Table 26.6) [1,2]. The ERSPC trial reported that PSA screening without DRE was associated with a 20% relative reduction in the death rate from prostate cancer at a median follow-up

Table 26.6 Prostate cancer mortality after the introduction of prostate cancer screening

Authors	Methods	Intervention	Participants	Outcomes	Results	Notes
Schröder et al. [1]	RCT FU: median 9 yrs	Intervention group received screening with in general interval 4 years. men were in general screened by PSA, biopsies were recommended for men with a PSA >3.0 ng/mL. Control group received usual care	Screening N 72,890 Control N 89,353	Prostate cancer-specific mortality	Significant relative reduction in PCa mortality. RR 0.80 (95% CI 0.65–0.98; p=0.04). Absolute RR 0.71 death per 1000 men. This means that 1410 men would need to be screened and 48 additional cases of PCa would need to be treated to prevent one death from PCa	Results biased by contamination in the control population
Andriole et al. [2]	RCT FU: median 11 yrs	Intervention group received annual screening. Men were screened by PSA and DRE, biopsies were recommended in men who had suspicious DRE or PSA >4.0 ng/mL. Control group received usual care	Screening N 38,343 Control N 38,350	Prostate cancer-specific mortality	No significant relative reduction in PCa mortality. RR 1.13 (95% CI 0.75–1.70)	Results biased by high level of contamination in the control population

CI, confidence interval; DRE, digital rectal examination; FU, follow-up; PCa, prostate cancer; PSA, prostate-specific antigen; RCT, randomized controlled trial; RR, relative risk of 9 years [1]. The results of the ERSPC were associated with an absolute reduction of about seven prostate cancer deaths per 10,000 men screened, 1410 men who needed to be screened and 48 men who needed treatment to prevent one death from prostate cancer death. In the US, the PLCO trial reported no mortality benefit from combined screening with PSA testing and DRE during a median follow-up of 7 years [2].

Since these trials provide contradictory outcomes, at least a few differences in the study designs have to be mentioned. First, the results of the PLCO are likely more influenced by contamination (screening in the control arm). In the PLCO the level of contamination is well established, i.e. the rate of PSA testing was 40–52% and the rate of screening by DRE ranged from 41 to 46% in the control group. In the ERSPC the level of contamination by PSA testing in the control group was estimated in the order of 20–31%. The 4.8% prostate cancers that were detected in the control population of the ERSPC after 9 years of follow-up and the 6.0% prostate cancers detected in the control population of the PLCO after 7 years of follow-up reflect this difference in level of contamination. Another explanation for the contradictory results is the difference in the compliance with the screening protocol. In the PLCO the average rate of compliance with biopsy recommendations was 40%, in the ERSPC the average rate of compliance with biopsy recommendations was 85.8% (range, 65.4 to 90.3). As a result of the difference in screening intensity and in level of contamination between the two trials, a smaller risk of excess incidence (23% versus more than 70% in the ERSPC) was observed in the PLCO trial. In essence, based on the results of the ERSPC, prostate cancer screening has the potential to reduce the prostate cancer specific mortality. However, based on the results of the PLCO trial, systematic prostate cancer screening is not effective in terms of reducing the prostate cancer specific mortality in comparison to widespread opportunistic screening and early detection.

Comment

The ERSPC has shown that prostate cancer screening results in a significant reduction in prostate cancer mortality. Although the results of the ERSPC appear favorable, men who were screened were at a significantly increased risk of being diagnosed with prostate cancer, resulting in a substantial number of men diagnosed with a disease that might have never caused symptoms or death during the patient's lifetime. For this reason, the demonstrated screening risks and benefits may not be balanced on an individual level. Therefore, later data of the ongoing randomized control trials are needed to show the cumulative results after longer follow up.

In summary, a conditional recommendation of **Grade 2B** can be offered for prostate cancer screening (i.e. weak recommendation, moderate-quality evidence) [47].

Conclusion

There is well-established evidence that prostate cancer screening is effective in terms of reducing prostate cancer mortality. Systematic prostate cancer screening increases the incidence and causes a stage distribution consisting of a significant increase in localized disease and decrease of metastatic disease. Even though there is no PSA level that allows us to identify men with no risk of prostate cancer, PSA is still the most accurate screening tool currently available. However, since the benefits of screening are associated with potential harms, a noninvasive biomarker is needed to prevent men experiencing unnecessary biopsies, overdiagnosis and overtreatment.

References

1. Schröder FH, Hugosson J, Roobol MJ, Tammela TL, Ciatto S, Nelen V, et al. Screening and prostate-cancer mortality in a randomized european study. N Engl J Med 2009;360(13):1320-8.
2. Andriole GL, Grubb RL 3rd, Buys SS, Chia D, Church TR, Fouad MN, et al. Mortality results from a randomized prostate-cancer screening trial. N Engl J Med 2009;360(13):1310-1319.
3. Baillargeon J, Pollock BH, Kristal AR, Bradshaw P, Hernandez J, Basler J, et al. The association of body mass index and prostate-specific antigen in a population-based study. Cancer 2005;103(5):1092-5.
4. Thompson IM, Ankerst DP, Chi C, Lucia MS, Goodman PJ, Crowley JJ, et al. Operating characteristics of prostate-specific antigen in men with an initial PSA level of 3.0 ng/ml or lower. JAMA 2005;294(1):66-70.
5. Krumholtz JS, Carvalhal GF, Ramos CG, Smith DS, Thorson P, Yan Y, et al. Prostate-specific antigen cutoff of 2.6 ng/mL for prostate cancer screening is associated with favorable pathologic tumor features. Urology 2002;60(3):469-73; discussion 73-4.
6. Thompson IM, Pauler DK, Goodman PJ, Tangen CM, Lucia MS, Parnes HL, et al. Prevalence of prostate cancer among men with a prostate-specific antigen level < or = 4.0 ng per milliliter. N Engl J Med 2004;350(22):2239-46.
7. Schröder FH, Carter HB, Wolters T, van den Bergh RC, Gosselaar C, Bangma CH, et al. Early detection of prostate cancer in 2007. Part 1: PSA and PSA kinetics. Eur Urol 2008;53(3):468-77.
8. Schröder FH, Bangma CH, Roobol MJ. Is it necessary to detect all prostate cancers in men with serum PSA levels < 3.0 ng/ml? A comparison of biopsy results of PCPT and outcome-related information from ERSPC. Eur Urol 2008;53(5):901-8.
9. Schröder FH, Raaijmakers R, Postma R, van der Kwast TH, Roobol MJ. 4-year prostate specific antigen progression and

diagnosis of prostate cancer in the European Randomized Study of Screening for Prostate Cancer, section Rotterdam. J Urol 2005;174(2):489-94; discussion 93-4.

10. Van der Cruijsen-Koeter IW, Roobol MJ, Wildhagen MF, van der Kwast TH, Kirkels WJ, Schroder FH. Tumor characteristics and prognostic factors in two subsequent screening rounds with four-year interval within prostate cancer screening trial, ERSPC Rotterdam. Urology 2006;68(3):615-20.

11. Lilja H, Ulmert D, Bjork T, Becker C, Serio AM, Nilsson JA, et al. Long-term prediction of prostate cancer up to 25 years before diagnosis of prostate cancer using prostate kallikreins measured at age 44 to 50 years. J Clin Oncol 2007;25(4):431-6.

12. Vickers AJ, Ulmert D, Serio AM, Bjork T, Scardino PT, Eastham JA, et al. The predictive value of prostate cancer biomarkers depends on age and time to diagnosis: towards a biologically-based screening strategy. Int J Cancer 2007;121(10):2212-17.

13. Loeb S, Roehl KA, Antenor JA, Catalona WJ, Suarez BK, Nadler RB. Baseline prostate-specific antigen compared with median prostate-specific antigen for age group as predictor of prostate cancer risk in men younger than 60 years old. Urology 2006;67(2):316-20.

14. Gosselaar C, Kranse R, Roobol MJ, Roemeling S, Schroder FH. The interobserver variability of digital rectal examination in a large randomized trial for the screening of prostate cancer. Prostate 2008;68(9):985-93.

15. Yamamoto T, Ito K, Ohi M, Kubota Y, Suzuki K, Fukabori Y, et al. Diagnostic significance of digital rectal examination and transrectal ultrasonography in men with prostate-specific antigen levels of 4 NG/ML or less. Urology 2001;58(6):994-8.

16. Crawford ED, DeAntoni EP, Etzioni R, Schaefer VC, Olson RM, Ross CA. Serum prostate-specific antigen and digital rectal examination for early detection of prostate cancer in a national community-based program. The Prostate Cancer Education Council. Urology 1996;47(6):863-9.

17. Schröder FH, van der Maas P, Beemsterboer P, Kruger AB, Hoedemaeker R, Rietbergen J, et al. Evaluation of the digital rectal examination as a screening test for prostate cancer. Rotterdam section of the European Randomized Study of Screening for Prostate Cancer. J Natl Cancer Inst 1998;90(23):1817-23.

18. Bozeman CB, Carver BS, Caldito G, Venable DD, Eastham JA. Prostate cancer in patients with an abnormal digital rectal examination and serum prostate-specific antigen less than 4.0 ng/mL. Urology 2005;66(4):803-7.

19. Gosselaar C, Roobol MJ, Roemeling S, van der Kwast TH, Schroder FH. Screening for prostate cancer at low PSA range: the impact of digital rectal examination on tumor incidence and tumor characteristics. Prostate 2007;67(2):154-61.

20. Andriole GL, Levin DL, Crawford ED, Gelmann EP, Pinsky PF, Chia D, et al. Prostate cancer screening in the Prostate, Lung, Colorectal and Ovarian (PLCO) Cancer Screening Trial: findings from the initial screening round of a randomized trial. J Natl Cancer Inst 2005;97(6):433-8.

21. Okotie OT, Roehl KA, Han M, Loeb S, Gashti SN, Catalona WJ. Characteristics of prostate cancer detected by digital rectal examination only. Urology 2007;70(6):1117-20.

22. Vis AN, Hoedemaeker RF, Roobol M, van der Kwast TH, Schroder FH. Tumor characteristics in screening for prostate cancer with and without rectal examination as an initial screening test at low PSA (0.0-3.9 ng/ml). Prostate 2001;47(4):252-61.

23. Schröder FH, Denis LJ, Roobol M, Nelen V, Auvinen A, Tammela T, et al. The story of the European Randomized Study of Screening for Prostate Cancer. BJU Int 2003;92(suppl 2):1-13.

24. Gosselaar C, Roobol MJ, Roemeling S, Schroder FH. The role of the digital rectal examination in subsequent screening visits in the European Randomized Study of Screening for Prostate Cancer (ERSPC), Rotterdam. Eur Urol 2008;54(3):581-8.

25. Vo T, Rifkin MD, Peters TL. Should ultrasound criteria of the prostate be redefined to better evaluate when and where to biopsy? Ultrasound Q 2001;17(3):171-6.

26. Onur R, Littrup PJ, Pontes JE, Bianco FJ Jr. Contemporary impact of transrectal ultrasound lesions for prostate cancer detection. J Urol 2004;172(2):512-14.

27. Carter HB, Hamper UM, Sheth S, Sanders RC, Epstein JI, Walsh PC. Evaluation of transrectal ultrasound in the early detection of prostate cancer. J Urol 1989;142(4):1008-10.

28. Terris MK, Freiha FS, McNeal JE, Stamey TA. Efficacy of transrectal ultrasound for identification of clinically undetected prostate cancer. J Urol 1991;146(1):78-83; discussion 83-4.

29. Ellis WJ, Chetner MP, Preston SD, Brawer MK. Diagnosis of prostatic carcinoma: the yield of serum prostate specific antigen, digital rectal examination and transrectal ultrasonography. J Urol 1994;152(5 pt 1):1520-5.

30. Ito K, Ichinose Y, Kubota Y, Imai K, Yamanaka H. Clinicopathological features of prostate cancer detected by transrectal ultrasonography-guided systematic six-sextant biopsy. Int J Urol 1997;4(5):474-9.

31. Littrup PJ, Bailey SE. Prostate cancer: the role of transrectal ultrasound and its impact on cancer detection and management. Radiol Clin North Am 2000;38(1):87-113.

32. Gosselaar C, Roobol MJ, Roemeling S, Wolters T, van Leenders GJ, Schroder FH. The value of an additional hypoechoic lesion-directed biopsy core for detecting prostate cancer. BJU Int 2008;101(6):685-90.

33. Joshua AM, Evans A, van der Kwast T, Zielenska M, Meeker AK, Chinnaiyan A, et al. Prostatic preneoplasia and beyond. Biochim Biophys Acta 2008;1785(2):156-81.

34. Ferlay J BF, Pisani P, Parkin DM. Cancer incidence, mortality and prevalence worldwide. IARC Cancerbase No 5, version 20. IARC Press, Lyon, 2004. Available at: www.depiarcfr/globocan/databasehtm.

35. SEER Program. SEER*Stat Database. Incidence. Available at: wwwseercancergov.

36. Collin SM, Martin RM, Metcalfe C, Gunnell D, Albertsen PC, Neal D, et al. Prostate-cancer mortality in the USA and UK in 1975-2004: an ecological study. Lancet Oncol 2008;9(5):445-52.

37. Dennis LK, Resnick MI. Analysis of recent trends in prostate cancer incidence and mortality. Prostate 2000;42(4):247-52.

38. Sim HG, Cheng CW. Changing demography of prostate cancer in Asia. Eur J Cancer 2005;41(6):834-45.

39. Kvale R, Auvinen A, Adami HO, Klint A, Hernes E, Moller B, et al. Interpreting trends in prostate cancer incidence and mortality in the five Nordic countries. J Natl Cancer Inst 2007;99(24):1881-7.

40. Aus G, Bergdahl S, Lodding P, Lilja H, Hugosson J. Prostate cancer screening decreases the absolute risk of being diagnosed with advanced prostate cancer – results from a prospective, population-based randomized controlled trial. Eur Urol 2007;51(3):659-64.

41. Makinen T, Tammela TL, Hakama M, Stenman UH, Rannikko S, Aro J, et al. Tumor characteristics in a population-based prostate cancer screening trial with prostate-specific antigen. Clin Cancer Res 2003;9(7):2435-9.

42. Bartsch G, Horninger W, Klocker H, Reissigl A, Oberaigner W, Schonitzer D, et al. Prostate cancer mortality after introduction of prostate-specific antigen mass screening in the Federal State of Tyrol, Austria. Urology 2001;58(3):417-24.

43. Mokete M, Shackley DC, Betts CD, O'Flynn KJ, Clarke NW. The increased rate of prostate specific antigen testing has not affected prostate cancer presentation in an inner city population in the UK. BJU Int 2006;97(2):266-9.

44. Labrie F, Candas B, Cusan L, Gomez JL, Diamond P, Suburu R, et al. Diagnosis of advanced or noncurable prostate cancer can be practically eliminated by prostate-specific antigen. Urology 1996;47(2):212-17.

45. Rietbergen JB, Hoedemaeker RF, Kruger AE, Kirkels WJ, Schroder FH. The changing pattern of prostate cancer at the time of diagnosis: characteristics of screen detected prostate cancer in a population based screening study. J Urol 1999;161(4): 1192-8.

46. Pelzer AE, Bektic J, Akkad T, Ongarello S, Schaefer G, Schwentner C, et al. Under diagnosis and over diagnosis of prostate cancer in a screening population with serum PSA 2 to 10 ng/ml. J Urol 2007;178(1):93-7; discussion 7.

47. Guyatt GH, Oxman AD, Kunz R, Falck-Ytter Y, Vist GE, Liberati A, et al. Going from evidence to recommendations. BMJ (Clin Res) 2008;336(7652):1049-51.

48. Otto SJ, van der Cruijsen IW, Liem MK, Korfage IJ, Lous JJ, Schroder FH, et al. Effective PSA contamination in the Rotterdam section of the European Randomized Study of Screening for Prostate Cancer. Int J Cancer 2003;105(3):394-9.

49. Carter HB, Epstein JI, Chan DW, Fozard JL, Pearson JD. Recommended prostate-specific antigen testing intervals for the detection of curable prostate cancer. JAMA 1997;277(18): 1456-60.

27 Surgical management of clinically localized prostate cancer

Daniel A. Barocas and Michael S. Cookson
Department of Urologic Surgery, Vanderbilt University Medical Center, Nashville, TN, USA

Background

The lifetime risk of being diagnosed with prostate cancer in the United States has almost doubled to 20% since the late 1980s, largely due to the widespread use of prostate-specific antigen (PSA) testing. In fact, in 2008 alone, there will be an estimated 186,320 new cases of prostate cancer diagnosed in the US [1]. In addition, an estimated 28,660 deaths from prostate cancer will occur in 2008. Consequently, prostate cancer remains the most common solid malignancy (excluding nonmelanoma skin cancers) in American men and the second leading cause of cancer deaths among American men, representing an enormous public health challenge.

Despite the fact that prostate cancer is so prevalent, many aspects of its management remain controversial. Part of the dilemma arises from the fact that while many men will be diagnosed with prostate cancer, only a small percentage will die of it. The aim of this chapter is to present the data that guide clinicians on three important questions that arise with respect to the surgical management of clinically localized (stage T1–T2NXM0) prostate cancer.

Management controversies

One of the most controversial issues in the management of a patient with a newly diagnosed, clinically localized prostate cancer is whether or not any treatment should be recommended. And, if treatment is advised, which of the available treatments is best for a particular patient. Specifically, with respect to surgery, it is debated as to whether or not radical prostatectomy offers a survival advantage over expectant management, also referred to as watchful waiting.

Evidence-Based Urology. Edited by Philipp Dahm, Roger R. Dmochowski.
© 2010 Blackwell Publishing.

At the root of this controversy are observational studies of the natural history of prostate cancer, which demonstrate that prostate cancer often manifests late in life and has a protracted clinical course [2]. The result is that up to 70% of men with prostate cancer and up to 90% of men with low-risk prostate cancer ultimately die of an unrelated cause. Another way of looking at it is that, on average, 1 in 5 or 6 men will be diagnosed with prostate cancer, while only 1 in 35 will potentially die of it. These data often fuel the debate and are even more controversial when treatment-related side effects are factored into the decision making. Despite these sobering statistics, the fact remains that the majority of American men opt for initial treatment (67%) and surgery is the most common form of treatment chosen [3].

In this chapter, we focus on three important areas involving surgical management of localized prostate cancer. We evaluate the currently available data comparing oncological efficacy of surgery versus observation strategies such as watchful waiting and active surveillance. Next, we examine whether the experience of the surgeon or the hospital has an impact on perioperative outcomes, mortality and oncological efficacy. This is an area of emerging importance and is being recognized as an independent predictor of outcomes. It too is shrouded in controversy and has practical applications given that radical prostatectomy is technically demanding, coupled with the realization that the average urologist applying for recertification logs fewer than 10 cases per year. Finally, we address the issue of neo-adjuvant hormonal therapy prior to surgery as compared to surgery alone, an area that contains multiple randomized clinical trials available for analysis.

Clinical question 27.1

In considering management for clinically localized stage T1–T2 prostate cancer, is there a benefit to surgical intervention compared to watchful waiting?

Literature search

We performed a search of PubMed for any English-language studies published prior to July 2008 pertaining to this topic. We restricted our search to studies of open radical retropubic prostatectomy and limited the results to clinical trials. We included the following search terms in the queries: "watchful waiting" or "observation" or "surveillance" and "radical prostatectomy."

The evidence

Randomized controlled trials

There are only two completed RCTs that compare survival outcomes in men with clinically localized prostate cancer who were randomized to surgery or watchful waiting [4,5]. These are presented in Table 27.1. In a high-quality randomized trial from the Scandinavian Prostate Cancer Group, Bill-Axelson et al. demonstrated advantages for radical prostatectomy over watchful waiting in a mixed population of clinically detected prostate cancer patients [4]. Whereas the earlier report with 5-year outcomes data had failed to demonstrate an overall survival advantage for surgery, the 10-year outcome data did reveal such an advantage. The absolute reduction in risk was 5% (27.0% vs 32.0%) and the corresponding relative risk of overall mortality in patients randomized to surgery was 0.74 (95% confidence interval (CI) 0.56–0.99, p = 0.04). Radical prostatectomy also proved to have advantages over watchful waiting in reducing the risk of local progression (19.2% vs 44.3%), distant metastases (15.2% vs 25.4%) and disease-specific mortality (9.6% vs 14.9%). A prespecified subgroup

analysis found that the advantage for radical prostatectomy in disease-specific mortality was limited to patients under the age of 65. However, as the authors point out, this analysis was exploratory and the study was not powered for such subgroup analyses.

This is an important landmark study because it is the first reliable evidence of a survival advantage for men with localized prostate cancer who undergo surgical treatment rather than watchful waiting. However, its applicability to the contemporary clinical presentation has been called into question. The population studied by the Scandinavian Group had clinically detected cancers (76% were palpable) that ranged from low-risk to high-risk disease, rather than screening-detected cancers that are more common in the US today. In fact, only 12% were detected based on a PSA elevation, which now constitutes the most common presentation among men in the US. Consequently, the population that was offered watchful waiting in this study is far more high risk than most patients diagnosed in contemporary series. In fact, the cohort series of conservative management in the US are largely populated with screening-detected, low-risk, low-volume prostate cancer, with characteristics suggestive of indolent disease [6].

Moreover, the trend in conservative management of low-risk clinically localized prostate cancer is toward surveillance and away from watchful waiting. In active surveillance, the aim is to spare the patient the morbidity of treatment until or unless signs of progression are detected in a fairly rigorous surveillance protocol. At that point, treatment with curative intent is initiated. By contrast, the aim of watchful waiting is to intervene with systemic palliative therapy if symptoms of advanced disease arise. Thus, while the

Table 27.1 Randomized controlled trials comparing watchful waiting with surgery for management of clinically localized prostate cancer

Author, year	Enrollment period	Criteria	Intervention	Results
Bill-Axelson et al. [4]	1989–1999	cT1 or T2 PSA <50 ng/mL	WW (N 348) RP (N 347)	10 year outcomes (median follow-up 8.2 years) RP vs WW:Disease-specific mortality: 9.6% vs 14.9% (RR 0.56, 95% CI 0.36–0.88, p=0.01) Overall mortality: 27.0% vs 32.0% (RR 0.74, 95% CI 0.56–0.99, p=0.04) Distant metastases: 15.2% vs 25.4% (RR 0.60, 95% CI 0.42–0.86, p=0.004) Local progression: 19.2% vs 44.5% (RR 0.33, 95% CI 0.25–0.44, p<0.001)
Iversen et al. [5]	1967–1975	VACURG stage I or II	Oral placebo (N 68) RP + oral placebo (N 74)	Outcomes (median follow-up 23 years) Median overall survival: RP vs WW: 10.6 vs 8.0 years, p=NS Gleason grade 7–10 vs ≤4 (RR 5.2, p<0.001)

NS, not significant; PSA, prostate-specific antigen: RP, radical prostatectomy; RR, relative risk; VACURG, Veterans Administration Co-operative Urological Research Group; WW, watchful waiting

Scandinavian study demonstrates a survival advantage for surgery over watchful waiting in a mixed population of men with prostate cancer, it remains unclear whether surgery offers advantages over active surveillance in a screening-detected population of low-risk prostate cancer patients.

The only other RCT comparing radical prostatectomy with watchful waiting was performed by the Veterans Administration Co-operative Urological Research Group (VACURG) and was reported by Iversen et al. [5]. This was a very small study, involving only 142 patients, 66 of whom had palpable disease. After 23 years of follow-up, there was no significant difference in overall survival between groups. Not surprisingly, age and grade were strongly predictive of overall mortality. As the authors point out, it is difficult to draw conclusions with regard to the efficacy of surgery compared to watchful waiting in light of the "lack of statistical power and methodological flaws."

Population-based observational studies

There are a number of population-based observational studies that demonstrate a survival advantage for surgery over conservative management of prostate cancer (Table 27.2) [3,7-9]. One of these studies failed to demonstrate an advantage for active treatments over conservative management [3]. The authors hypothesize that their appropriate use of an intention-to-treat analysis (whereby patients who had aborted prostatectomies after the discovery of positive lymph nodes were grouped with patients who had completed prostatectomies) evened

Table 27.2 Population-based observational studies comparing watchful waiting with surgery for management of clinically localized prostate cancer

Author, year	Enrollment	Criteria	Intervention	Results
Lu-Yao & Yao [3]	1983–1992 SEER database	Clinically localized disease Age 50–79	RP (N 24,257, 40.5%) RT (N 15,721, 26.3%) Conservative management (N 19,898, 33.2%)	10-year cancer-specific survival by intention-to-treat analysis: RP 83% (81–84) RT 76% (74–78) Conservative tx 82% (81–84)
Aus et al. [7]	1987–1999 National Cancer Registry of Sweden	Nonmetastatic disease (T1–T3, N0-NX, M0) Grade 1–3 PSA missing or <50 ng/mL Age ≤75	WW (N 764, 36.4%) RP (N 546, 26.0%) RT (N 289, 13.8%) ADT or other palliative tx (N 488, 23.3%) Other (N 11, 0.5%)	Active treatment vs WW after 15 years follow-up: Higher disease-specific survival for RP vs WW (HR 0.40, 95% CI 0.27–0.59, p<0.00001) No clear benefit for RT vs WW (HR 1.01, 95% CI 0.72–1.41, p=0.98)
Wong et al. [8]	1991–1999 SEER database	cT1 or T2 Gleason grade 2–7 Age 65–80	WW (N 12,608) Active treatment, either RT or RP (N 32,022)	Active treatment vs WW after 12 years of follow-up: Lower risk of death from prostate cancer (HR 0.67, 95% CI 0.58–0.77) Lower risk of death from any cause (23.8% vs 37.0%, p<0.001) Higher 5-year overall survival: 88% (87–89) vs 78% (77–79) Higher 10-year overall survival: 66% (64–66) vs 51% (49–52) Hazard ratio for death RP vs WW: 0.50 (0.47–0.53) Hazard ratio for death RT vs WW: 0.81 (0.78–0.85)
Liu et al. [9]	1992 SEER database	Local/regional disease Age 65–74 Co-morbidity score ≤1	RP (N 2567, 43.9%) RP+RT (N 302, 5.2%) RT (N 2006, 34.3%) WW (N 970, 16.6%)	Overall survival in months, adjusted HR for death: RP 127.8 mos; 0.31 (0.25–0.37) RP+RT 120.0 mos; 0.38 (0.28–0.52) RT 112.5 mos; 0.68 (0.56–0.81) WW 101.2 mos; 1.00 (reference) Disease-specific survival in months, adjusted HR: RP 139.7 mos; 0.17 (0.10–0.28) RP+RT 135.2 mos; 0.23 (0.13–0.48) RT 134.6 mos; 0.56 (0.37–0.85) WW 129.6 mos; 1.00 (reference)

HR; hazard ratio; PSA, prostate-specific antigen; RP, radical prostatectomy; RT, radiation therapy; SEER, Surveillance Epidemiology and End Results; WW, watchful waiting the playing field for comparisons with other treatments in which lymph nodes are evaluated only by clinical means. This point is valid, as using a treatment-received approach would tend to enrich the prostatectomy group with lower risk men and those with advanced disease would end up in the observation group. However, other studies, such as that by Wong et al. [8], demonstrate a survival advantage for surgery in a low-risk population, a group with a very low likelihood of aborted prostatectomy due to positive nodes.

Taken in their entirety, this group of population-based observational studies is highly suggestive of a disease-specific survival advantage for patients undergoing surgery for treatment of clinically localized prostate cancer compared to men managed conservatively. Two of the studies actually demonstrate an overall survival advantage for patients managed surgically [8,9].

Other studies

Several groups have undertaken meta-analyses of this topic. One from the Agency for Healthcare Research and Quality was published recently and drew heavily on an earlier effort by the American Urological Association [10,11]. These meta-analyses point out the paucity of high-quality evidence on which to base treatment decisions among the various management options.

There are numerous case series that describe single-institution or multi-institution experiences and pooled analyses looking at either surgery or observation [6,12-20]. While each option can be shown to have excellent long-term disease-specific survival in appropriately selected patients, these studies are not particularly useful in comparing the two management strategies. For the most part, these studies are considered low-grade evidence.

There are two nonrandomized, retrospective case–control series comparing immediate surgery to delayed surgery [21,22]. In one, a group of 38 men who were enrolled in an active surveillance protocol at Johns Hopkins went on to have delayed surgery at a median of 26.5 months after diagnosis [21]. Their pathological outcomes were compared with 150 patients with matched baseline clinical characteristics. Each group had a similar likelihood of adverse pathological findings. The other study of this type looked at 865 men with low-risk prostate cancer and examined the impact of the time between biopsy and surgery on the risk of biochemical progression [22]. The authors found no difference in the likelihood of biochemical progression between patients who delayed surgery for between 90 and 180 days compared to those who had surgery in less than 90 days (multivariable adjusted relative risk (RR) 1.10, 95% CI 0.70–1.71). However, they did find a significant trend when they included patients who delayed surgery for more than 180 days (multivariable adjusted RR 2.73, 95% CI 1.51–4.94, p = 0.002).

Comment

There is a striking paucity of high-quality evidence to help patients and clinicians determine the optimal management strategy for an individual patient with clinically localized prostate cancer. The best available evidence comes from one high-quality RCT, one underpowered RCT and a number of large population-based observational studies. Thus, by GRADE criteria, the evidence is moderate grade [23]. In comparing radical prostatectomy with watchful waiting for the treatment of clinically localized disease, the data show that patients treated with surgery have a small but measurable advantage in terms of local control, prevention of distant metastases, disease-specific survival and overall survival. This advantage may come at the cost of surgical morbidity, which must be factored into treatment decisions. The difference in survival advantage also appears to be most pronounced among younger patients in whom follow-up of a decade or more may be required before differences become apparent. In a quality of life study that accompanied the Scandinavian randomized trial, patients undergoing surgery experienced increased rates of erectile dysfunction and incontinence, but overall sense of well-being and subjective quality of life were comparable to patients on watchful waiting at a median of 4 years [24].

Implications for practice

Although radical prostatectomy appears to confer a survival advantage over watchful waiting according to one RCT and several population-based observational studies, the data are inconclusive and cannot be uniformly applied. Many factors, including patient age, risk category, patient preferences and expected morbidity of treatment, play into the decision of how to manage clinically localized prostate cancer. In the absence of a uniform consensus, the updated 2007 American Urological Association (AUA) guideline considers discussion of surgery, radiation, brachytherapy and watchful waiting as a standard [11]. The Panel also set a standard of informing the patient of the superiority of surgery compared to watchful waiting, based on the outcome of the Scandinavian randomized trial. National Comprehensive Cancer Network (NCCN) guidelines are similar, except that they do not recommend observation for intermediate-risk patients with a longer than 10-year life expectancy and high-risk patients with a longer than 5-year life expectancy [25]. European Association of Urology (EAU) guidelines call for watchful waiting and surgery as reasonable treatments for most asymptomatic men with nonmetastatic disease [26].

We agree with these recommendations, namely that men with clinically localized prostate cancer be counseled regarding both surgery and observation. Risks (including possible treatment-related and disease progression-related morbidity) and benefits of each possible management option must be explained to the patient with some neutrality on the part of the physician. However, these men must be informed that the best available evidence does show a measurable survival advantage in favor of radical prostatectomy as compared to watchful waiting. This recommendation is substantiated by only one high-quality RCT and several large population-based observational studies. Therefore, the recommendation to proceed with radical prostatectomy instead of watchful waiting for a man with clinically localized prostate cancer would be considered a weak or conditional recommendation, based on moderate-quality evidence (Grade 2B) by the GRADE criteria [23].

Implications for research

In summary, there is a paucity of high-quality data in the literature to allow for direct comparisons among different treatment modalities for patients with clinically localized prostate cancer. Given the lack of consensus on this issue, there are several studies planned. The Cochrane group has published a protocol for a systematic review of this topic [27]. There are also several randomized trials under way that plan to capitalize on the large number of men with low-risk clinically localized prostate cancer who would be candidates for observation [28]. These include the Prostate Intervention Versus Observation Trial (PIVOT) which plans to recruit approximately 2000 men [29]. They will be assigned to surgery or observation and followed for a minimum of 12 years. The primary endpoint will be all-cause mortality and secondary endpoints will include treatment-specific morbidity and mortality rates.

Another such trial is the Standard Treatment Against Restricted Treatment (START) trial, which is being spearheaded by a Canadian group. The aim is to compare standard therapies such as surgery, external beam radiation and brachytherapy with active surveillance in a group of 2000 low-risk patients. Finally, the Prostate Testing for Cancer and Treatment (PROTECT) trial is enrolling patients in Britain who will be randomized to surgery, external beam radiation or surveillance. These trials have the potential to give us greater insight into the survival outcomes of men with low-risk, clinically localized prostate cancer who undergo treatment including surgery versus active surveillance and the results will be anxiously awaited.

While surgery may prove to have a survival advantage over observation in large randomized trials, the greatest challenge may lie in individualizing therapy. Given the relatively low likelihood of dying from prostate cancer, it is clear that some men are best served by observation. To this end, we need research aimed at determining appropriate criteria for observation (perhaps based on age, co-morbidities, prostate cancer characteristics and patient preferences), appropriate trigger points for initiating therapy, and development of decision analysis tools.

Clinical question 27.2

Does surgeon or hospital volume have an impact on perioperative outcomes, mortality or oncological efficacy of radical prostatectomy?

Literature search

We performed a search of PubMed for any English-language studies published prior to July 2008 pertaining to this topic. We restricted our search to studies of open radical retropubic prostatectomy (RP) and included the following search terms in the queries: "surgeon volume," "surgical volume," "hospital volume," and "prostatectomy." Using the initial searches and the references from those articles, we identified 11 original studies that focus on the impact of hospital RP volume on surgical outcomes (including length of stay, perioperative complication rate, perioperative mortality, readmission rate, and several long-term measures of treatment effect). We found seven studies that evaluated the relationship between individual surgeon case volume and outcomes.

The evidence

There are no randomized trials comparing high-volume hospitals to low-volume hospitals or high-volume surgeons to low-volume surgeons. To answer this question, we are limited to observational studies and thus are reliant upon the power of large numbers and the efforts of investigators to design their studies to control for confounders.

Hospital volume

The data on the impact of hospital volume on radical prostatectomy outcomes are presented in Table 27.3. All seven studies addressing length of stay (LOS) found that high-volume hospitals had shorter mean LOS and a lower rate of prolonged LOS than low-volume hospitals [30-36]. Both studies addressing readmission rates found lower readmission rates at high-volume hospitals [30,33]. Four out of five studies showed lower complication rates in high-volume hospitals [30,33,36-38]. Despite a very low perioperative mortality rate for radical prostatectomy, six out of eight studies addressing this question demonstrated a significantly lower mortality rate in high-volume hospitals [30-33,36-39].

Only one study addressed oncological efficacy of radical prostatectomy with respect to hospital surgical volume. In this study, Ellison et al. demonstrated a higher rate of

Table 27.3 Population-based observational studies of radical prostatectomy outcomes, comparing low-volume and high-volume hospitals

Author, year	Population, years studied	Number of patients	Volume definition	Outcome measures and conclusions, LV hospitals vs HV hospitals
Yao & Lu-Yao [30]	Medicare 1991–1994	101,604	Quartiles by volume	Higher LOS (9% higher, p = 0.0001 for trend) Higher readmission rate (RR 1.30, 95% CI 1.21–1.39, p≤0.09) Higher complication rate (RR 1.28, 95% CI 1.24–1.32, p≤0.09) Higher mortality rate (RR 1.51, 95% CI 1.25–1.77, p≤0.09)
Ellison et al. [31]	Nationwide inpatient sample 1989–1995	66,693	Low (<25 cases/yr) Med (25–54 cases/yr) High (>54 cases/yr)	Higher rate of prolonged LOS (22% vs 6%, p<0.001) Higher mortality rate (OR 1.75, 95% CI 1.2–2.6, p<0.001)
Begg et al. [37]	SEER/Medicare 1992–1996	10,737	Quartiles by hospital case volume	No difference in 30- or 60-day mortality rate No difference in long-term incontinence Higher postoperative complication rate (32% vs 27%, p = 0.03) Higher late urinary complication rate (28% vs 20%, p<0.001)
Ellison et al. [40]	SEER/Medicare 1990–1999	12,635	Low (<34 cases/yr) Med (34–61 cases/yr) High (>61 cases/yr)	Higher risk of secondary treatments (HR 1.25, 95% CI 1.14–1.38, p<0.001)
Konety et al. [39]	Nationwide inpatient sample 1988–2002	61,039	Low (<7 cases) Med (7–20 cases) High (>20 cases)	Higher mortality rate for lower case-specific hospital volume (OR 0.22, 95% CI 0.11–0.45, p<0.05 for high volume vs low volume) Mortality rate unrelated to designation as a specialized urology center or to performance of high volume of unrelated complex procedures by Leapfrog criteria
Hollenbeck et al. [32]	National inpatient sample 1993–2003	141,052	Deciles by case volume	Higher in-hospital mortality (0.3% vs 0.04% for lowest vs highest decile; adjusted OR 3.8, 95% CI 1.8–7.9) Higher prolonged LOS rate (19.0% vs 3.9% for lowest vs highest decile; adjusted OR 4.8, 95% CI 3.5–6.7)
Judge et al. [33]	English National Health Service 1997–2004	18,027	Quintiles by case volume	No difference in adjusted odds of 30-day complications Higher rate of readmissions within 1 year (OR 1.13, 95% CI 1.01–1.26), p = 0.002 for trend) Higher mortality rate at lowest volume hospitals (0.76%); lowest rate in middle 2 tiers (0.15–0.17%); then higher for highest volume tiers (0.30%), p = 0.004 for nonlinear trend Higher LOS (6.5 vs 5.6 days for lowest vs highest volume hospitals, p<0.001 for trend)
Ku et al. [34]	National Surgical Quality Improvement Program 2001–2004	5,162	Low (<20 cases/yr) Med (21–28 cases/yr) High (>28 cases/yr)	Higher LOS (3.7 vs 3.1 days, p = 0.02) Higher transfusion rate (29.6% vs 18.2%, p = 0.02)
Alibhai et al. [38]	Canadian Institute for Health Information 1990–2001	25,404	As a continuous variable	Higher in-hospital mortality rate (OR 0.82, 95% CI 0.69–0.99, p = 0.037 for doubling of case volume) Higher in-hospital complication rate (OR 0.89, 95% CI 0.87–0.91, p = <0.001 for doubling of case volume)
Siu et al. [35]	National inpatient sample 2003	9,266	Terciles by case volume: Low (<33 cases) Med (33–82 cases) High (>82 cases)	Higher rate of prolonged LOS (OR 3.3, 95% CI 1.9–5.6) Fewer diagnostic, interventional and specialty services
Mitchell et al. [36]	University HealthSystem Consortium 2003–2007	48,086	Low (<100 cases) Med (100–499 cases) High (≥500 cases)	No difference in in-hospital mortality rate (p = 0.224) Higher LOS (3.8 vs 2.1 days, p<0.001) Higher ICU admission rate (18.6% vs 1.3%, p<0.001) Higher postoperative complication rate (15.9% vs 5.8%, p<0.001)

HV, high volume; ICU, intensive care unit; LOS, length of stay; LV, low volume; OR, odds ratio; RR, relative risk secondary procedures in patients treated at low-volume hospitals, suggesting a higher failure rate of primary therapy at these institutions [40]. While there are no randomized trials to support these findings, these studies evaluate large numbers of men and their results are quite consistent with regard to LOS, complication rates and mortality. Thus, the data are of moderate grade in support of high-volume hospitals on the basis of these parameters. Specific recommendations will be addressed below.

Surgeon volume

The data on the impact of surgeon volume on radical prostatectomy outcomes are presented in Table 27.4. Again, only observational cohort studies are available, some of which are based on large population-based databases, whereas others are single- or multiple-institution series. In general, higher surgeon volume is associated with superior complication rates (3/3 studies) [37,38,41], long-term

functional results (1/1 study) [37], lower surgical margin rates (2/2 studies) [42,43] and even superior likelihood of biochemical recurrence-free survival (1/1 study) [44]. Despite the consistency among studies, these are a mixture of population-based cohorts, multiple-institution and single-institution series. Thus, the evidence favoring high-volume surgeons is considered low grade and only weak recommendations can be made based upon it.

Comment

The evidence demonstrating more favorable perioperative outcomes in high-volume hospitals compared to low-volume hospitals is of moderate grade. The data on LOS, complication rates and mortality are particularly compelling. What is less certain is how to make use of this important information. Some have advocated regionalization of care based on these findings. However, it is unclear whether

Table 27.4 Population-based observational studies of radical prostatectomy outcomes, comparing low-volume and high-volume surgeons

Author, year	Population, years studied	Number of patients	Volume definition	Outcome measures and conclusions, LV surgeons vs HV surgeons
Begg et al. [37]	SEER/Medicare 1992–1996	10,737	Quartiles by surgeon case volume	No difference in 30- or 60-day mortality rate Higher long-term incontinence (20% vs 16%, p=0.04) Higher postoperative complication rate (32% vs 26%, p<0.001) Higher late urinary complication rate (28% vs 20%, p=0.001)
Hu et al. [41]	Center for Medicare and Medicaid Services (CMS) 1997–1998	2292	Low (<40 cases/yr) High (>40 cases/yr)	No difference in anastomotic strictures Higher complication rate (OR 0.53, 95% CI 0.32–0.89, p<0.05 for HV surgeons) Higher mean LOS (PE −0.66, 95% CI −1.26 to −0.06, p<0.05 for HV surgeons)
Eastham et al. [42]	Memorial Sloan-Kettering and Baylor 1983–2002	4629	As a continuous variable	Higher positive margin rate (p=0.01) Particular surgeon was also an independent predictor of margin status (p=0.05)
Chun et al. [43]	Single institution 1996–2004	2402	As a continuous variable	Higher positive margin rate (p<0.001)
Vickers et al. [44]	Four institutions 1987–2003	7765	Low (<50 cases) Med low (50–99 cases) Med (100–249) Med high (250–999) High (≥1000)	Higher unadjusted probability of BCR at 5 yrs (24%, 95% CI 20–29 vs 8%, 95% CI 6–10 for lowest vs highest volume surgeons) Higher adjusted probability of BCR at 5 yrs (17.9%, 95% CI 12.1–25.6 vs 10.7%, 95% CI 7.1–15.9, p<0.001 for 10 vs 250 prior cases) Probability of recurrence curve leveled out after 250 cases
Alibhai et al. [38]	Canadian Institute for Health Information 1990–2001	25,404	As a continuous variable	Higher complication rates (OR 0.84, 95% CI 0.82–0.87, p<0.001 for each doubling of surgeon volume)
Briganti et al. [62]	Single institution 2002–2007	1020	Both continuous and dichotomous (cut-off at 144 cases)	Lower lymph node yield (15.3 vs 21.1, p<0.001) Significantly lower rate of positive lymph node detection in several models (8% vs 15%, p=0.01)

BCR, biochemical recurrence; HV, high volume; LOS, length of stay; LV, low volume; OR, odds ratio; PE, parameter estimate the overall impact of such a policy would be beneficial to the patient. Potential unintended consequences could include the inconvenience of traveling long distances for appointments with the treating surgeon, having surgery away from the social support network, having difficulty maintaining an ongoing relationship with the surgeon and having fewer trained surgeons in outlying areas. It could also diminish the financial stability and preparedness for emergencies of smaller institutions [45].

Perhaps a more practical use of this information would be to determine the aspects of care at high-volume hospitals that make surgery safer and more successful. These systems could then be implemented at lower-volume hospitals in order to benefit patients on the local level. One example of this is the use of clinical care pathways, which have been shown to reduce LOS after radical prostatectomy [46]. Perhaps dissemination of systems such as clinical pathways could elevate the outcomes of lower-volume institutions to match those at busier centers.

With regard to surgeon volume, it seems to be the case that there is a learning curve. The higher the surgeon's case volume for a particular case, the better will be his or her results. This has been demonstrated in cohort studies of radical prostatectomy and robot-assisted laparoscopic prostatectomy [47,48]. However, the appropriate case volume required to achieve superior results remains to be defined and may be different for individual surgeons. In addition, case volume is just a surrogate for quality, and variations in quality among high-volume surgeons have been demonstrated [37]. Again, it may be more important to determine what makes one surgeon's results better than another's and to disseminate the techniques, rather than simply funneling patients to the busiest surgeons.

Implications for practice

To some extent hospitals, surgeons and patients are acting upon the volume–outcome relationship already. Volume data are driving hospital marketing strategies as well as patients' selection of a hospital (see, for example, the website www.healthcarechoices.org/index.html). They are prominently displayed on surgeons' websites. The federal government is effectively encouraging regionalization through its "pay for performance" program, which rewards institutions and providers for appropriate care and the Centers of Excellence Program, which designates institutions based on their track record of quality of care [45].

As mentioned above, the temptation is to utilize the volume–outcome relationship to funnel patients to high-volume centers and high-volume surgeons. However, it may have a greater overall impact to apply the lessons learned in higher-volume institutions and by higher-volume surgeons to lower-volume centers and surgeons. Although we do see an accumulation of evidence in favor of high-volume

centers and surgeons, there is as yet no strong evidence demonstrating that a regulatory or educational intervention would favorably affect outcomes. Therefore, beyond favoring additional research into this controversial topic, no specific recommendation to achieve optimal outcomes based on surgeon and hospital volume can be made at this time.

Implications for research

Future research may focus on the systems in place at the higher-volume centers that benefit patients. It is not entirely clear what aspects of care lead to improvement in outcomes in these settings. Similarly, it is not clear why higher-volume surgeons have better outcomes than lower-volume surgeons. We also do not know what is responsible for the differences in outcomes among the highest-volume surgeons. While it is not practical to randomize patients to high- versus low-volume hospitals or high- versus low-volume surgeons, some aspects of care may be amenable to study through randomized trials. For example, one could randomize patients to a pathway model versus a standard care model in a hospital where pathways are not yet in place. Similarly, experienced surgeons could randomize patients to undergo slight modifications of surgical technique versus standard technique in order to determine the elements of successful surgery. Clearly, infrequent outcomes, such as mortality, could not be tested this way, and we will continue to rely upon population-based observational studies to identify trends in these areas.

Clinical question 27.3

Does the use of neo-adjuvant androgen deprivation therapy (ADT) prior to radical prostatectomy improve outcomes over radical prostatectomy alone?

Literature search

We performed a search of PubMed for any English-language studies published prior to July 2008 pertaining to this topic. We restricted our search to studies of open radical retropubic prostatectomy and limited the results to clinical trials. We included the following search terms in the queries: "hormone therapy" or "hormonal therapy" or "androgen deprivation" and "neo-adjuvant" and "radical prostatectomy."

The evidence

There are seven RCTs comparing neo-adjuvant ADT prior to radical prostatectomy with radical prostatectomy alone (Table 27.5) [49-55]. There are also three RCTs comparing

Table 27.5 Randomized clinical trials of neo-adjuvant androgen deprivation therapy prior to radical prostatectomy.

Author, year	Inclusion criteria	Number of patients	Intervention	Median follow-up	Outcome measures and conclusions
Aus et al. [49]	T1b-3a, NX*, M0; Age <75; Life expectancy ≥10 years	126 entered; 111 evaluable	RP alone (N 55); Neo-ADT** + RP (N 56)	82 months	No difference in overall survival: 86.4% vs 83.6%, p=0.513; No difference in PSA progression-free survival: 51.5% for RP vs 49.8% for ADT, p=0.588; Lower positive margin rate in ADT group: 23.6% vs 45.5%, p=0.016
Dalkin et al. [50]	T1c, T2A, T2B; PSA >4.0 ng/mL; Life expectancy >10 years	61 entered; 56 evaluable	RP alone (N 28); Neo-ADT† + RP (N 28)		No difference in likelihood of organ-confined disease; No difference in positive margin rate
Klotz et al. [51]	T1 or T2; PSA <50 ng/mL; Negative bone scan	213 entered	RP alone (N 101); Neo-ADT‡ + RP (N 112)	69 months	No difference in overall survival: 93.9% for RP vs 88.4% for ADT+RP, p NS; No difference in PSA progression-free survival: 68.2% for RP vs 60.2% for ADT, p=0.73; Lower positive margin rate in ADT group: 27.7% vs 64.8%, p=0.001; Higher rate of organ-confined pathology: 41.6% vs 19.8%, p=0.0017
Labrie et al. [52]	Life expectancy >10 years; "Localized" prostate cancer including SV and BN invasion and ECE	161 entered	RP alone (N 71); Neo-ADT^ + RP (N 90)		Lower positive margin rate in ADT group: 7.8% vs 33.8%, p<0.001; Higher rate of organ-confined disease in ADT group: 77.7% vs 49.3%; Net staging change: 21.1% downstaged in ADT group vs 33.8% upstaged in control group
Prezioso et al. [53]	T1a-T2b; Life expectancy >5 years; WHO performance status ≤2	183 entered; 167 evaluable	RP alone (N 81); Neo-ADT§ + RP (N 86)		Lower rate of upstaging in ADT group: 67% vs 93%, p=0.001; Lower positive margin rate in ADT group: 39% vs 60%, p=0.01; Lower rate of positive lymph nodes in ADT group: 3% vs 11%, p not given
Schulman et al. [54]	T2-T3, N0; PSA <100 ng/mL	487 entered; 402 eligible; 398 evaluable	RP only (N 210); Neo-ADT† + RP (N 192)	4 years	Higher rate of downstaging in ADT group: 15% vs 7%, p<0.01; Lower positive margin rate in ADT group: p<0.01 for cT2; p=0.01 for cT3; No difference in PSA progression-free survival: 33% for RP vs 26% for ADT, p=0.18; No difference in overall survival: 95% for RP vs 93% for ADT+RP, p NS
Soloway et al. [55]	T2bNXM0; Age<75 years; PSA <50 ng/mL; Normal bone scan	303 entered; 282 eligible; 275 evaluable	RP only (N 138); Neo-ADT^f + RP (N 137)	5 years	No difference in seminal vesicle invasion: 15% vs 22%, p NS; No difference in lymph node invasion: 6% vs 6%, p NS; Lower positive margin rate in ADT group: 18% vs 48%, p<0.001; No difference in PSA progression-free survival: 67.6% for RP vs 64.8% for ADT, p=0.663

NS, not significant; Neo-ADT, neo-adjuvant androgen deprivation therapy; PSA, prostate-specific antigen; RP, radical prostatectomy

*Patients were excluded if found to have positive lymph nodes in frozen sections

**Triptorelin depot 3.75 mg intramuscular, monthly for 3 months, with cyproterone acetate 1 week before and 2 weeks after the first triptorelin injection to prevent flare phenomenon

†Goserelin acetate 3.6 mg subcutaneous, monthly for 3 months

‡Cyproterone acetate 100 mg by mouth, 3 times daily for 3 months

^Flutamide plus a luteinizing hormone-releasing hormone (LHRH) agonist for 3 months

§Leuprolide acetate 3.75 mg intramuscular, monthly for 3 months, with cyproterone acetate 1 week before and 2 weeks after the first leuprolide injection

ʲGoserelin 3.6 mg subcutaneous, monthly for 3 months, and flutamide 250 mg orally, 3 times a day for 3 months

ᶠLeuprolide acetate 7.5 mg intramuscular, monthly for 3 months, and flutamide 250 mg orally, 3 times a day for 3 months short-term versus longer-term neo-adjuvant ADT prior to radical prostatectomy [56-58]. One of these studies had a surgery-only arm and was included in the surgery alone versus neo-adjuvant ADT plus surgery analysis of margin status [57]. In addition, there is a comprehensive review and meta-analysis of the use of neo-adjuvant ADT published by the Cochrane group [59].

Impact on pathological parameters

Most studies demonstrate superior pathological parameters in patients undergoing neo-adjuvant ADT. Three out of four studies that evaluated the frequency of organ-confined disease at final pathology found that organ-confined rates were higher in patients who received neo-adjuvant ADT and this was significant in the Cochrane group's meta-analysis (overall odds ratio (OR) 2.30, 95% CI 1.72–3.08, $p < 0.00001$) [50-52,54,59]. Similarly, both studies that evaluated pathological downstaging found a higher rate of downstaging in patients who underwent neo-adjuvant ADT (overall OR 2.42, 95% CI 1.50–3.90, $p = 0.000$) [52,54,59].

Seven out of eight studies showed superior positive margin rates in patients undergoing neo-adjuvant ADT (overall OR 0.34, 95% CI 0.27–0.42, $p < 0.00001$) [49-55,57,59]. There were mixed results in the two studies that looked at seminal vesicle invasion rates [51,55]. There were also mixed results in the five studies that looked at lymph node involvement, but the overall effect favored the neo-adjuvant ADT group on the meta-analysis (overall OR 0.63, 95% CI 0.42–0.93, $p = 0.02$) [50,51,53-55,59]. A meta-analysis of the three studies that compared short-term with long-term neo-adjuvant ADT showed superior surgical margin rates (overall OR 0.56, 95% CI 0.39–0.80, $p = 0.002$ for case analysis) and higher rates of organ-confined disease (OR 1.41, 95% CI 1.05–1.89, $p = 0.02$) with longer duration of therapy [56-59].

Cancer control outcomes

Three studies compared overall survival in patients undergoing neo-adjuvant ADT prior to radical prostatectomy versus those receiving immediate radical prostatectomy [49,51,54]. None showed a statistically significant survival advantage for either group and this was confirmed on the meta-analysis (pooled OR 1.11, 95% CI 0.67–1.85, $p = 0.69$) [59]. Four studies compared disease-free survival as measured by detectable PSA [49,51,54,55]. None demonstrated a statistically significant difference between groups. However, in one study, the investigators performed a subgroup analysis that demonstrated a small but significant advantage for cT2 patients who underwent neo-adjuvant ADT (recurrence rate at 4 years was 3% vs 11%, $p = 0.03$) [54]. Another study showed that men with a baseline PSA greater than 20 ng/mL had a measurable benefit in terms of biochemical recurrence-free survival (30.5% vs 18.8%, $p = 0.015$) [51]. Despite the results of these small subset

analyses, the meta-analysis showed no benefit to neo-adjuvant ADT with regard to 5-year disease-free survival (pooled OR 1.24, 95% CI 0.97–1.57, $p = 0.13$) [59].

Comment

While neo-adjuvant ADT prior to radical prostatectomy leads to improved pathological outcomes, a benefit in terms of biochemical recurrence-free survival or overall survival has not been demonstrated. The data supporting superior pathological outcomes in patients undergoing neo-adjuvant ADT are consistent and of high grade. The cancer control outcome data are of moderate grade, owing to inconsistency, fewer studies and, potentially, insufficient follow-up to demonstrate overall survival differences. Additionally, most of these studies were designed to demonstrate pathological outcomes and were underpowered to demonstrate differences in either disease-free or overall survival. In summary, the data show that neo-adjuvant ADT prior to radical prostatectomy yields superior pathological outcomes, particularly with respect to improved margin status. However, these findings did not translate into a biochemical recurrence-free survival or overall survival benefit. Therefore, we can make a strong recommendation against the use of neo-adjuvant ADT for the purpose of improving biochemical recurrence-free survival or overall survival.

Implications for practice

Based on the available moderate- and high-quality evidence, it is our strong recommendation (**Grade 1B**) not to use neo-adjuvant ADT for the purpose of improving biochemical recurrence-free survival or overall survival. Might there be settings in which its use is appropriate? The evidence for the ability of neo-adjuvant ADT to result in downstaging, higher rates of organ-confined disease and lower rates of positive surgical margins suggests that neo-adjuvant ADT may have a role in patients with bulkier tumors. However, this concept remains to be tested.

Implications for research

Several questions about the use of neo-adjuvant ADT remain to be fully explored. First, why is there a discrepancy between the superior pathological findings and the absence of a cancer outcome or survival benefit? Some have suggested that it is due to alterations in the histological appearance of the prostate and prostate cancer induced by the hormone deprivation [60,61]. Better methods of pathological evaluation may prove revealing.

Second, is there some way in which we can exploit the known effects of neo-adjuvant ADT (decreasing the size of the prostate, the size of the tumor, improving pathological parameters) to benefit the patients? As mentioned above, perhaps neo-adjuvant ADT could improve resectability of bulky disease in patients who are limited to surgery because of contraindications to other therapies. Third, can we demonstrate a survival benefit or improvement in biochemical disease-free rates by improving the design, power or length of follow-up of these types of studies? In the study with the longest follow-up (about 7 years) by Aus et al. [49], 84.4% of radical prostatectomy alone patients were still alive and 82.6% of patients who had neo-adjuvant ADT were still living. However, given the relatively small numbers and other limitations cited, it is unlikely that any definitive improvement will be ascertained from the aforementioned studies.

References

1. Jemal A, Siegel R, Ward E, et al. Cancer statistics, 2008. CA: Cancer J Clin 2008;58:71.

2. Albertsen P, Hanley J, Fine J. 20-year outcomes following conservative management of clinically localized prostate cancer. JAMA 2005;293:2095.

3. Lu-Yao G, Yao S. Population-based study of long-term survival in patients with clinically localised prostate cancer. Lancet 1997;349:906.

4. Bill-Axelson A, Holmberg L, Ruutu M, et al. Radical prostatectomy versus watchful waiting in early prostate cancer. N Engl J Med 2005;352:1977.

5. Iversen P, Madsen P, Corle DK. Radical prostatectomy versus expectant treatment for early carcinoma of the prostate. Twenty-three year follow-up of a prospective randomized study. Scandinavian journal of urology and nephrology Supplementum, Scand J Urol Nephrol 1995;172(suppl):65.

6. Carter H, Kettermann A, Warlick C, et al. Expectant management of prostate cancer with curative intent: an update of the Johns Hopkins experience. J Urol 2007;178:2359.

7. Aus G, Robinson D, Rosell J, et al. Survival in prostate carcinoma – outcomes from a prospective, population-based cohort of 8887 men with up to 15 years of follow-up: results from three countries in the population-based National Prostate Cancer Registry of Sweden. Cancer 2005;103:943.

8. Wong Y, Mitra N, Hudes G, et al. Survival associated with treatment vs observation of localized prostate cancer in elderly men. JAMA 2006;296:2683.

9. Liu L, Coker AL, Du XL, et al. Long-term survival after radical prostatectomy compared to other treatments in older men with local/regional prostate cancer. J Surg Oncol 2008;97:583.

10. Wilt T, MacDonald R, Rutks I, et al. Systematic review: comparative effectiveness and harms of treatments for clinically localized prostate cancer. Ann Intern Med 2008;148:435.

11. Thompson I, Thrasher J, Aus G, et al. Guideline for the management of clinically localized prostate cancer: 2007 update. J Urol 2007;177:2106.

12. Chodak G, Thisted R, Gerber G, et al. Results of conservative management of clinically localized prostate cancer. N Engl J Med 1994;330:242.

13. Barry M, Albertsen P, Bagshaw M, et al. Outcomes for men with clinically nonmetastatic prostate carcinoma managed with radical prostatectomy, external beam radiotherapy, or expectant management: a retrospective analysis. Cancer 2001;91:2302.

14. Klotz L. Active surveillance with selective delayed intervention is the way to manage 'good-risk' prostate cancer. Nat Clin Pract Urol 2005;2:136.

15. Carter CA, Donahue T, Sun L, et al. Temporarily deferred therapy (watchful waiting) for men younger than 70 years and with low-risk localized prostate cancer in the prostate-specific antigen era. J Clin Oncol 2003;21:4001.

16. Zietman A, Thakral H, Wilson L, et al. Conservative management of prostate cancer in the prostate specific antigen era: the incidence and time course of subsequent therapy. J Urol 2001;166:1702.

17. Han M, Partin A, Zahurak M, et al. Biochemical (prostate specific antigen) recurrence probability following radical prostatectomy for clinically localized prostate cancer. J Urol 2003;169:517.

18. Hardie C, Parker C, Norman A, et al. Early outcomes of active surveillance for localized prostate cancer. BJU Int 2005;95:956.

19. Hull G, Rabbani F, Abbas F, et al. Cancer control with radical prostatectomy alone in 1,000 consecutive patients. J Urol 2002;167:528.

20. Desireddi N, Roehl K, Loeb S, et al. Improved stage and grade-specific progression-free survival rates after radical prostatectomy in the PSA era. Urology 2007;70:950.

21. Warlick C, Trock B, Landis P, et al. Delayed versus immediate surgical intervention and prostate cancer outcome. J Natl Cancer Inst 2006;98:355.

22. Freedland SJ, Kane CJ, Amling CL, et al. Delay of radical prostatectomy and risk of biochemical progression in men with low risk prostate cancer. J Urol 2006;175:1298.

23. Guyatt G, Gutterman D, Baumann MH, et al. Grading strength of recommendations and quality of evidence in clinical guidelines: report from an American College of Chest Physicians Task Force. Chest 2006;129:174.

24. Steineck G, Helgesen F, Adolfsson J, et al. Quality of life after radical prostatectomy or watchful waiting. N Engl J Med 2002;347:790.

25. Scherr D, Swindle PW, Scardino P, et al. National Comprehensive Cancer Network guidelines for the management of prostate cancer. Urology 2003;61:14.

26. Heidenreich A, Aus G, Bolla M, et al. EAU guidelines on prostate cancer. Eur Urol 2008;53:68.

27. Hegarty J, Beirne P, Comber H, et al. Watchful waiting versus prostatectomy for prostate cancer. Cochrane Database Syst Rev 2007;9:CD006590.

28. Barocas D, Cowan J, Smith J, et al. What percentage of newly diagnosed patients with adenocarcinoma of the prostate are candidates for surveillance? An analysis of the CaPSURE database. J Urol 2008;180(4):1330-4.

29. Wilt T, Brawer M. The Prostate Cancer Intervention Versus Observation Trial: a randomized trial comparing radical prostatectomy versus expectant management for the treatment of clinically localized prostate cancer. J Urol 1994;152:1910.

30. Yao S, Lu-Yao G. Population-based study of relationships between hospital volume of prostatectomies, patient outcomes, and length of hospital stay. J Natl Cancer Inst 1999;91:1950.

31. Ellison L, Heaney J, Birkmeyer J. The effect of hospital volume on mortality and resource use after radical prostatectomy. J Urol 2000;163:867.

32. Hollenbeck B, Dunn R, Miller D, et al. Volume-based referral for cancer surgery: informing the debate. J Clin Oncol 2007;25:91.

33. Judge A, Evans S, Gunnell D, et al. Patient outcomes and length of hospital stay after radical prostatectomy for prostate cancer: analysis of hospital episodes statistics for England. BJU Int 2007;100:1040.

34. Ku T, Kane C, Sen S, et al. Effects of hospital procedure volume and resident training on clinical outcomes and resource use in radical retropubic prostatectomy surgery in the Department of Veterans Affairs. J Urol 2008;179:272.

35. Siu W, Daignault S, Miller D, et al. Understanding differences between high and low volume hospitals for radical prostatectomy. Urol Oncol 2008;26:260.

36. Mitchell R, Lee B, Cookson M, et al. Immediate surgical outcomes for radical prostatectomy in the University HealthSystem Consortium Database: the impact of hospital case volume, hospital size and geographic region on 48,000 patients. BJU Int 2009;104(10):1442-5.

37. Begg CB, Riedel ER, Bach PB, et al. Variations in morbidity after radical prostatectomy. N Engl J Med 2002;346:1138.

38. Alibhai S, Leach M, Tomlinson G. Impact of hospital and surgeon volume on mortality and complications after prostatectomy. J Urol 2008;180:155.

39. Konety B, Allareddy V, Modak S, et al. Mortality after major surgery for urologic cancers in specialized urology hospitals: are they any better? J Clin Oncol 2006;24:2006-12.

40. Ellison L, Trock B, Poe N, et al. The effect of hospital volume on cancer control after radical prostatectomy. J Urol 2005; 173:2094.

41. Hu J, Gold K, Pashos C, et al. Role of surgeon volume in radical prostatectomy outcomes. J Clin Oncol 2003; 21:401.

42. Eastham J, Kattan M, Riedel E, et al. Variations among individual surgeons in the rate of positive surgical margins in radical prostatectomy specimens. J Urol 2003;170:2292.

43. Chun F, Briganti A, Antebi E, et al. Surgical volume is related to the rate of positive surgical margins at radical prostatectomy in European patients. BJU Int 2006;98:1204.

44. Vickers A, Bianco F, Serio A, et al. The surgical learning curve for prostate cancer control after radical prostatectomy. J Natl Cancer Inst 2007;99:1171.

45. Hollenbeck B, Miller D, Wei J, et al. Regionalization of care: centralizing complex surgical procedures. Nat Clin Pract Urol 2005;2:461.

46. Chang S, Cole E, Smith JA, et al. Safely reducing length of stay after open radical retropubic prostatectomy under the guidance of a clinical care pathway. Cancer 2005;104:747.

47. Klein E, Bianco F, Serio A, et al. Surgeon experience is strongly associated with biochemical recurrence after radical prostatectomy for all preoperative risk categories. J Urol 2008;179:2212.

48. Raman J, Dong S, Levinson A, et al. Robotic radical prostatectomy:operative technique, outcomes, and learning curve. J Soc Laparoendosc Surg 2007;11:1.

49. Aus G, Abrahamsson P, Ahlgren G, et al. Three-month neo-adjuvant hormonal therapy before radical prostatectomy: a 7-year follow-up of a randomized controlled trial. BJU Int 2002;90:561.

50. Dalkin B, Ahmann F, Nagle R, et al. Randomized study of neo-adjuvant testicular androgen ablation therapy before radical prostatectomy in men with clinically localized prostate cancer. J Urol 1996;155:1357.

51. Klotz L, Goldenberg S, Jewett M, et al. Long-term followup of a randomized trial of 0 versus 3 months of neo-adjuvant androgen ablation before radical prostatectomy. J Urol 2003;170:791.

52. Labrie F, Cusan L, Gomez J, et al. Neo-adjuvant hormonal therapy: the Canadian experience. Urology 1997;49:56.

53. Prezioso D, Lotti T, Polito M, et al. Neo-adjuvant hormone treatment with leuprolide acetate depot 3.75 mg and cyproterone acetate, before radical prostatectomy: a randomized study. Urol Int 2004;72:189.

54. Schulman C, Debruyne F, Forster G, et al. 4-Year follow-up results of a European prospective randomized study on neo-adjuvant hormonal therapy prior to radical prostatectomy in T2-3N0M0 prostate cancer. European Study Group on Neo-adjuvant Treatment of Prostate Cancer. Eur Urol 2000;38:706.

55. Soloway M, Pareek K, Sharifi R, et al. Neo-adjuvant androgen ablation before radical prostatectomy in cT2bNxMo prostate cancer: 5-year results. J Urol 2002;167:112.

56. Gleave M, Goldenberg S, Chin J, et al. Randomized comparative study of 3 versus 8-month neo-adjuvant hormonal therapy before radical prostatectomy: biochemical and pathological effects. J Urol 2001;166:500.

57. Selli C, Montironi R, Bono A, et al. Effects of complete androgen blockade for 12 and 24 weeks on the pathological stage and resection margin status of prostate cancer. J Clin Pathol 2002;55:508.

58. Van der Kwast T, Têtu B, Candas B, et al. Prolonged neo-adjuvant combined androgen blockade leads to a further reduction of prostatic tumor volume: three versus six months of endocrine therapy. Urology 1999;53:523.

59. Kumar S, Shelley M, Harrison C, et al. Neo-adjuvant and adjuvant hormone therapy for localised and locally advanced prostate cancer. Cochrane Database Syst Rev 2006;4:CD006019.

60. Murphy W, Soloway M,Barrows G. Pathologic changes associated with androgen deprivation therapy for prostate cancer. Cancer 1991;68:821.

61. Hellström,M, Häggman M, Brändstedt S, et al. Histopathological changes in androgen-deprived localized prostatic cancer. A study in total prostatectomy specimens. Eur Urol 1993;24:461.

62. Briganti A, Capitanio U, Chun FK, et al. Impact of surgical volume on the rate of lymph node metastases in patients undergoing radical prostatectomy and extended pelvic lymph node dissection for clinically localized prostate cancer. Eur Urol 2008;54(4):794-802.

28 Surgical treatment options for locally advanced prostate cancer

Lawrence L. Yeung and Charles J. Rosser
Department of Urology, University of Florida, Gainesville, FL, USA

Introduction

Prostate cancer (PCA) can be classified into three main categories: localized (confined to the gland), locally advanced (extending beyond the prostate capsule with or without nodal involvement) or metastatic. External beam radiation (EBRT), brachytherapy, cryosurgical ablation of the prostate and radical prostatectomy (RP) provide good long-term disease control in patients with pathologically localized disease [1]. The same cannot be said for locally advanced PCA. The definition of locally advanced prostate varies among experts in the field. Some restrict the definition to patients with T3 (extracapsular extension and/or seminal vesicle invasion) or T4 (invasion of surrounding organs/tissue), while others include node-positive disease [2]. Some reports include patients with high-risk features such as serum prostate-specific antigen (PSA) > 20 mg/mL or high Gleason score 8–10; still others consider patients who are status post prostatectomy with high-risk features such as positive margins, extracapsular extension, positive lymph nodes or seminal vesicle invasion [3]. In this chapter, locally advanced PCA will be defined to include pT3–4 N0–1 M0 (with or without positive margins) tumors.

Even patients with apparently clinically localized disease may be at significant risk for treatment failure. In 1998, d'Amico et al. reported on a staging system to stratify patients into groups with a low, intermediate or high risk of biochemical recurrence after definitive therapy [4]. Men at high risk for treatment failure were characterized as having ≥ clinical T2c disease or serum PSA > 20 ng/mL or Gleason score ≥ 8, and/or > 50% positive cores on biopsy [5,6]. When using single-modality treatment, these high-risk men have 5-year disease-free survival rates of 30–50%, and the optimal treatment choice remains controversial [4]. Thus, the optimal choice of treatment for locally advanced PCA remains controversial, as neither primary EBRT alone nor RP alone appears to lessen treatment failure rates in these high-risk patients.

Though the advent of PSA screening has allowed for earlier detection of PCA, 25% of patients are found to have pathological T3–4 disease [7], and the risk of biochemical recurrence is as high as 67% at 5 years in these patients [8]. Despite the advances that have been made in the treatment of PCA, there is currently no consensus on the treatment of patients who present with palpable disease outside the prostate. With this in mind, the focus of this chapter is to present the highest levels of evidence available to guide urologists with respect to the management of locally advanced PCA.

Clinical question 28.1

In men with locally advanced prostate cancer, does neo-adjuvant androgen deprivation therapy prior to RP improve clinical outcomes?

Background

Systemic hormone therapy was first combined with RP by Vallet in 1944 [9]. However, Vallet's approach, which involved depriving the prostate of androgen by means of surgical castration, received little attention until safer, reversible forms of androgen deprivation therapy became available in the 1980s [10].

Literature search

Evidence was obtained by performing a systematic literature search using PubMed. The search was performed with the terms "neo-adjuvant," "androgen deprivation," and "prostate

Evidence-Based Urology. Edited by Philipp Dahm, Roger R. Dmochowski.
© 2010 Blackwell Publishing.

cancer" combined with the clinical query filter function to limit the search to the English language. A search limit was also utilized to search for those articles categorized as a clinical trial, meta-analysis or randomized controlled trial.

The evidence

Since the 1980s several prospective randomized trials have demonstrated the efficacy of neo-adjuvant hormonal therapy (Table 28.1). Such therapy has been associated with a decreased incidence of both positive surgical margins and positive lymph node metastasis, and an increased incidence of pathological pT0 tumors [11]. The latter finding,

though promising, must be viewed with caution, however, since meticulous pathological studies suggest that at least 65% of specimens classified as pT0 after hormonal therapy still contain persistent tumor [12]. Unfortunately, no neo-adjuvant androgen deprivation therapy to date has succeeded in producing either a complete pathological response or a significant improvement in long-term biochemical disease-free survival (i.e. as determined on the basis of serum PSA level). Though an important prognostic factor in various cancers including tumors of the breast and lung [13,14], complete pathological response is difficult to achieve in prostate tumors because of their well-known refractoriness to therapy.

Table 28.1 Randomized clinical trials of neoadjuvant hormonal therapy

Study author, year	Treatment	Duration	Positive surgical margins (%)	Positive lymph node metastasis (%)	Five-year biochemical disease-free survival (%)
Labrie 1993	RP	–	38.5[*]	N/A	N/A
	Leuprolide + flutamide/RP	3 months	13		
Labrie, 1997	RP	–	33.8[*]	N/A	N/A
	LHRH agonist + flutamide/RP	3 months	7.8		
Witjes, 1997	RP	–	27[*]	12.8[*]	23[†]
	Goserelin + flutamide/RP	3 months	46	23.2	22
Homma, 1997	RP	–	81.3[*]	36.5[*]	N/A
	Leuprolide + chlormadinone/RP	3 months	63.8	20.7	
Klotz, 1999	RP	–	64.8[*]	3.2[*]	70[†]
	Cyproterone acetate/RP	3 months	27.7	6.9	62
Fair, 1999	RP	–	37[*]	3.1	66
	Goserelin acetate + flutamide/RP	3 months	21	0	69
Schulman, 2000	RP	–	41.2[*]	22.9[#]	26
	Goserelin + flutamide/RP	3 months	26.2	14.6	33
Debruyne, 2000	RP	–	47.5[*]	22.9[*]	67
	Goserelin + flutamide/RP	3 months	26.2	14.4	74
Aus, 2002	RP	–	45.5[*]	N/A	51.5
	Triptorelin + cyproterone/RP	3 months	23.6		49.8
Bono, 2001	RP	–	48.7[*]	6.25[*]	
	Goserelin + bicalutamide 3-/RP	3 months	75.6	6.1	
	Goserelin + bicalutamide 6-/RP	6 months	81	3.5	
Gleave, 2001	Leuprolide + flutamide/RP	3 months	23[*]	3.1[*]	N/A
	Leuprolide + flutamide/RP	8 months	12	0.4	
Soloway, 2002	RP	–	48[*]	6	67.6
	Leuprolide + flutamide/RP	3 months	18	6	64.8
Prezioso, 2004	RP	–	60.0[*]	11[^]	N/A
	Leuprolide + cyproterone/RP	3 months	39.0	3	

LHRH, luteinizing-hormone-releasing hormone; N/A, not assessed; RP, radical prostatectomy

[*]p<0.05

[#]p<0.05 for clinical T2 tumors, but not for clinical T3 tumors

[^]p value not reported

[†]<5-yr biochemical disease-free survival

Comment

While neo-adjuvant hormonal therapy was generally considered safe and may result in reductions in tumor size, serum PSA levels, and the incidence of positive surgical margins and positive nodal metastasis, recent studies have emphasized the potential harm associated with hormonal therapy, even when administered short term. Most importantly, though, there is no evidence that it improves biochemical disease-free or overall survival.

Recommendation

Based on high-quality and consistent evidence, we make a strong recommendation against neo-adjuvant androgen deprivation therapy prior to RP (**Grade 1A**).

Clinical question 28.2

In men with locally advanced prostate cancer, does neo-adjuvant chemotherapy prior to RP improve clinical outcomes?

Background

Chemotherapy is used today mainly in patients with metastatic, hormone-refractory prostate cancer. The Food and Drug Administration (FDA) approved mitoxantrone for use in this population after it was shown that approximately one-third of symptomatic patients had an improvement in pain, even though no survival advantage was seen [15,16]. Subsequently, the FDA approved the use of docetaxel after the results of two trials demonstrated its efficacy in this population. The first was TAX 327, which randomized 1006 men to docetaxel plus prednisone or mitoxantrone plus prednisone. The median survival of all patients treated with docetaxel was 18.2 months compared with 16.4 months for those treated with mitoxantrone [17]. The second study, SWOG 9916, randomized 770 men to docetaxel and estramustine compared with mitoxantrone and prednisone. The median survival for patients treated with docetaxel was 18.9 months compared with 16 months for mitoxantrone. Subjects in this study treated with docetaxel reported less pain and improved quality of life compared to the mitoxantrone groups [18].

To improve survival in patients with locally advanced PCA, a multimodal approach combining local and systemic therapies is likely needed. Neo-adjuvant therapies have the benefit over adjuvant therapy of potentially being able to treat micrometastatic disease that may lead to failure of local therapy, cytoreduce (downstage) locally advanced tumors, making them more amenable to a successful surgical resection with negative margins, and confirm treatment efficacy by assessing postoperative tissue specimens. Investigators in the field of breast cancer have seen improved survival rates in large, locally advanced breast cancers with the use of neo-adjuvant chemotherapy [19,20], and prostate cancer researchers have followed by studying the use of neo-adjuvant chemotherapy prior to RP.

Literature search

Evidence was obtained by performing a systematic literature search using PubMed. The search was performed with the terms "neo-adjuvant," "chemotherapy," and "prostate cancer" combined with the clinical query filter function to limit the search to the English language. A search limit was also utilized to search for those articles categorized as a clinical trial, meta-analysis or randomized controlled trial.

The evidence

There are no adequately powered randomized studies that have been completed evaluating the use of neo-adjuvant chemotherapy prior to RP. However, there have been several promising clinical trials evaluating the efficacy of these neo-adjuvant regimens (Table 28.2). In one of the larger trials, van Poppel et al. randomized 130 patients with clinical T2b and T3 disease to either 560 mg of estramustine daily for 6 weeks prior to RP, or RP alone [21]. Although the positive surgical margins rates decreased in the neo-adjuvant group, this benefit did not extend to patients with clinical T3 tumors [21].

Pettaway et al. performed a phase II study in which 33 patients with high-risk disease characterized as being clinical stage T1–2, Gleason score ≥ 8, or T2b–T2c, Gleason score of 7 and serum PSA level greater than 10 ng/mL or clinical stage T3 received 12 weeks of ketoconazole and doxorubicin alternating with vinblastine, estramustine, and androgen ablation followed by prostatectomy [22]. Due to the estrogenic effects of estramustine, a small percentage of patients (6%) developed thromboembolic events. On pathological evaluation, 33% of the patients had organ-confined disease, 63% had negative lymph nodes, and 17% had positive surgical margins. Serum PSA was undetectable postoperatively in all patients. At a median follow-up of 13 months, 61% showed no biochemical evidence of disease. However, the primary goal of achieving a 20% rate for pT0 status was not achieved in this study [22].

Konety et al. performed a phase II study of 36 patients with locally advanced (stage T3 or greater) and/or high-risk tumors (Gleason score 8–10 and/or serum PSA greater than 20 ng/mL) who received four cycles of paclitaxel, carboplatin and estramustine followed by RP [23]. Deep vein thrombosis (22%) was the most frequent complication of chemotherapy, again attributable to the estrogenic effects of estramustine. The positive surgical margin rate was 22%.

Table 28.2 Clinical trials using neoadjuvant chemotherapy

Trial	No. of patients	Therapy	Duration of therapy	Positive surgical margins (%)	Positive lymph node metastasis (%)	Biochemical disease-free survival	
						%	Follow-up
Van Poppel et al.1995 [21]	130	RP vs estramustine/RP	6 wks	N/A	N/A	84 bNED	9 mos (mean)
Pettaway et al. 2000 [22]	33	Ketoconazole/ doxorubicin/ vinblastine/ADT/RP	12 wks	17	37	61 bNED	13 mos (median)
Konety et al. 2004 [23]	36	Paclitaxel/carboplatin/ estramustine/RP	4 cycles	22	6	45 bNED	29 mos (median)
Clark et al. 2001 [24]	18	Estramustine/ etoposide/RP	3 cycles	13	13	78 bNED	14 mos (median)
Dreicer et al. 2004 [27]	29	Docetaxel/RP	6 wks	4	14	71 bNED	23 mos (median)
Febbo et al. 2005 [28]	19	Docetaxel/RP	6 mos	N/A	0	44 bNED	26.5 mos (median)
Hussain et al. 2003 [29]	21	Docetaxel/ estramustine/RP	3–6 cycles	30	10	71 bNED	13 mos (median)

ADT = androgen deprivation therapy; bNED = no biochemical evidence of disease; mos, months; N/A = not assessed; RP = radical prostatectomy; wks, weeks

The clinical stage was reduced in 39% of patients. At a median follow-up of 29 months, 45% remained free from biochemical recurrence. The clinical stage was reduced in 39% of patients [23].

Clark et al. reported on a phase II trial of 18 patients with high-risk disease (clinical stage T2b/c or T3, PSA level ≥ 15 ng/mL, and/or Gleason score ≥ 8) who received neo-adjuvant estramustine and etoposide before RP [24]. Only 16 of the patients actually underwent RP. Five patients (28%) experienced grade 3 toxicity (two with deep venous thrombosis, two with neutropenia, and one with diarrhea) and one (6%) experienced grade 4 toxicity (pulmonary embolus) before surgery. Organ-confined disease was observed in 31% and disease was confined to the prostatectomy specimen in 56%. Half of the patients achieved an undetectable PSA after neo-adjuvant therapy and prior to RP. All patients had an undetectable PSA postoperatively, and at a median follow-up of 14 months after RP, 78% had no biochemical evidence of disease [24].

Since the approval of the use of docetaxel in hormone-refractory PCA, trials have been performed demonstrating its safety in a neo-adjuvant setting [25,26]. Dreicer et al. performed a phase II trial consisting of 29 men with high-risk disease (clinical stage T2b–T3, PSA > 15 ng/mL, and/or Gleason score ≥ 8) who received six doses of docetaxel 40 mg/m^2 intravenously administered weekly for 6 weeks followed by RP. On pathological review, only

11% had organ-confined disease, 89% had extracapsular extension, 14% had lymph node metastasis, and there were no pathological complete responders to docetaxal. While 79% of patients experienced some reduction in PSA level post chemotherapy, 24% of patients had more than a 50% reduction in PSA level in response to docetaxel alone. Postoperatively, 71% of the subjects are free from biochemical recurrence at 23 months follow-up. No unexpected toxicities or intraoperative complications occurred [27].

Febbo et al. performed a trial utilizing docetaxel in a neo-adjuvant fashion prior to RP in 19 patients with high-risk PCA (clinical stage T3, PSA ≥ 20 ng/mL, and/or Gleason score 4 + 3 = 7 or greater) [28]. The patients received weekly docetaxel (36 mg/m^2) for 6 months, followed by RP. A reduction of at least 25% and 50% of tumor volume was seen in 68% and 21% as measured by endorectal MRI, respectively. Sixteen of the 19 patients completed the chemotherapy regimen and underwent RP. On pathological evaluation, 38% had organ-confined disease, 62% had extracapsular extension, and none had lymph node metastasis. As with all the other neo-adjuvant chemotherapy trials, there were no pathological complete responders. Toxicity consisted of mostly grade 1 and 2 fatigue and mild gastrointestinal effects such as taste disturbance, nausea, and diarrhea. At a median follow-up of 26.5 months, 7 out of 16 (44%) patients remained free of biochemical recurrence [28].

Hussain et al. combined the use of estramustine, which alters androgen metabolism, with docetaxel in 21 patients with high-risk PCA (clinical stage T2b or greater, PSA $\geq$ 15 ng/mL, and/or Gleason score $\geq$ 8) [29]. The chemotherapy regimen consisted of docetaxel (70 mg/m^2) and estramustine (280 mg three times daily) for 3–6 courses. Ten patients underwent RP, with negative surgical margins in seven patients (70%). There was one episode of grade 4 neutropenia, with the remainder of toxicities being mainly grade 3 neutropenia and deep venous thrombosis (DVT). Despite the use of aspirin, three of the first seven patients developed DVTs due to the use of estramustine. Low-dose warfarin was subsequently given to the remaining patients and no further DVTs occurred. At a median follow-up of 13 months, 71% of patients remained free of biochemical recurrence [29].

The success of docetaxel in hormone-refractory prostate cancer, along with the results of the aforementioned phase II neo-adjuvant chemotherapy studies, led to the development of a phase III trial by the Cancer and Leukemia Group B (CALGB 90203), randomizing patients with clinical T1–T3a NX M0 PCA to either RP alone or a chemohormonal therapy regimen consisting of leuprolide acetate or goserelin for 18–24 weeks as well as six cycles of docetaxel followed by RP [30]. The entry criteria also stipulated that the patients have high-risk disease with either a Gleason score of 8–10 or a probability of biochemical progression-free survival at 5 years after surgery less than 60% by Kattan nomogram prediction [31]. The goal of the trial is to enroll 750 patients, with the primary outcome being the 3-year biochemical progression-free survival rate. The trial was opened in July 2007 and as of 30 June 2008, it had accrued only 35 patients [32].

Comment

The use of neo-adjuvant chemotherapy prior to RP is tolerated reasonably well and is associated with a decrease in both serum PSA levels and positive surgical margins. However, none of the agents studied to date has resulted in a pathologic complete response. The median follow-up in these neo-adjuvant trials was at most 29 months. As researchers have learned from the neo-adjuvant hormonal trials, a decrease in positive surgical margins does not necessarily translate into an improvement in biochemical disease-free survival [33,34]. Further randomized control trials are necessary to evaluate the efficacy of these neo-adjuvant agents. It is critical that urologists work in conjunction with oncologists to enroll patients into these neo-adjuvant chemotherapy protocols to substantiate these trials and prevent them from closure due to lack of accrual. Therefore, longer-term follow-up data are necessary to determine if these patients are free of disease in the long term and if there is an impact on overall survival.

Recommendation

The studies reviewed were either of very low quality or were early phase trials that were not designed to compare neo-adjuvant chemotherapy to the standard of care. Therefore, the authors can make no recommendation for the use of neo-adjuvant chemotherapy prior to RP.

Clinical question 28.3

In men with pathological T3 disease or pathological T2 with positive margins after RP, does adjuvant radiation therapy improve clinical outcomes?

Background

As previously noted, patients with adverse pathological features, such as extracapsular extension, seminal vesicle invasion or positive margins, after RP have up to a 67% chance of biochemical recurrence at 5 years [35]. Failure is thought to be due to occult local or systemic disease not eradicated by surgery. The purpose of adjuvant radiation is to sterilize any residual tumor cells in the prostate bed following RP, with the ultimate goal of decreasing local and biochemical recurrence and improving overall survival.

Literature search

Evidence was obtained by performing a systematic literature search using PubMed. The search was performed with the terms "adjuvant," "radiation therapy," and "prostate cancer" combined with the clinical query filter function to limit the search to the English language. A search limit was also utilized to search for those articles categorized as a clinical trial, meta-analysis or randomized control trial.

The evidence

Several RCTs have been performed [36-39] comparing RP followed by immediate adjuvant radiation therapy to RP alone in men with pathological T3 disease or pathological T2 with positive margins (Table 28.3). In addition, Morgan et al. performed a meta-analysis of EORTC 22911 and SWOG 8794 trials [40].

EORTC 22911 reported by Bolla et al. was a multi-institutional RCT designed to compare RP followed by immediate adjuvant radiation (N 502) to RP alone (N 503) for patients with positive surgical margins or pT3 prostate cancer [36]. Immediate postoperative radiotherapy

Table 28.3 Randomized trials comparing adjuvant radiation to observation after RP for advanced pathological features

Trial	Inclusion criteria	Number randomized	Time to initiation of adjuvant RT	Median follow-up	Primary endpoint	Outcomes
EORTC 22911 [36,41]	EPE, SVI, and/or PSM; age ≤75	1005	<16 weeks	5 yrs	BPFS	Improved BPFS (HR 0.48, 98% CI 0.37–0.62, p<0.0001)
SWOG 8794 [32,42]	EPE, SVI, and/or PSM; SWOG PS 0-2	431	<18 weeks	12.7 yrs	MFS	Improved MFS (HR 0.71, 95% CI 0.54–0.94, p = 0.016) Improved BPFS (HR 0.43, 95% CI 0.31–0.58, p<0.001) Decreased disease recurrence (HR 0.62, 95% CI 0.46–0.82, p = 0.001) Decreased need for ADT (HR 0.45, 95% CI 0.29–0.68, p<0.001)
German Cancer Society ARO 96-02 and AUO AP 09/95 [39]	EPE or SVI with or without PSM; undetectable PSA after RP	307	8–12 weeks	4.5 yrs	BPFS	Improved BPFS (HR 0.53, p = 0.0015)

ADT, androgen deprivation therapy; BPFS, biochemical progression-free survival; EORTC, European Organization for the Research and Treatment of Cancer; EPE, extraprostatic extension; MFS, metastasis-free survival; NR, not reported; PS, performance status; PSM, positive surgical margin; RT, radiotherapy; SVI, seminal vesicle invasion; SWOG, Southwest Oncology Group

consisted of 60 Gy conventional radiation delivered over 6 weeks. Radiotherapy was instituted within 16 weeks of surgery irrespective of PSA level and only after patients recovered from surgery and were without major voiding complaints. Patients were eligible for the trial if they were ≤ 75 years of age and had pN0M0 tumors with one or more high-risk pathological risk factors including extracapsular extension, positive surgical margins or seminal vesicle invasion. The primary endpoint was biochemical progression-free survival. After a median follow-up of 5 years, the patients in the irradiated group had a significantly improved freedom from biochemical progression compared to RP alone (hazard ratio (HR) 0.48, 98% confidence interval (CI) 0.37–0.62, p < 0.0001). Clinical progression-free survival was also significantly improved (p = 0.0009). A separate analysis of the EORTC 22911 trial demonstrated that patients with positive surgical margins benefited the most from postoperative radiotherapy [41]. Postoperative radiation was found to prevent 291 biochemical recurrences per 1000 patients compared to 88 biochemical recurrences per 1000 patients with negative surgical margins. However, there was no significant difference in overall survival. Grade 2 or 3 late toxicities were more frequent in the irradiated group (p = 0.0005), and severe toxicities (≥ grade 3) were rare in ether group and not significantly different. The authors concluded that immediate postoperative radiotherapy

might not be indicated in patients with negative surgical margins, but further investigation is necessary [41].

SWOG 8794 was a randomized control trial designed to determine if adjuvant radiotherapy after RP improves metastasis-free survival in patients with stage pT3N0M0 PCA [37]. After undergoing RP, 214 patients were randomized to receive 60–64 Gy of external beam radiotherapy in 30–32 fractions to the prostatic fossa and another 211 patients to receive observation. Of those men randomized to observation, 70 (33%) ultimately crossed over to receive salvage radiation. Radiotherapy was administered within 18 weeks of surgery, and an undetectable PSA level was not required at enrollment. Patients were eligible for the trial if they had pN0M0 tumors with one or more high-risk pathological risk factors including extracapsular extension, positive surgical margins or seminal vesicle invasion. Patients were excluded from randomization for total urinary incontinence, rectal injury, persistent urinary extravasation or pelvic infection. The primary endpoint of the study was metastasis-free survival defined as time to first occurrence of metastatic disease or death due to any cause. An interim analysis of the trial with a median follow-up of 10.6 years demonstrated no statistical difference in metastasis-free survival between radiation and observation arms (HR 0.75, 05% CI 0.55–1.02, p = 0.06) or in overall survival (HR 0.80, 95% CI 0.58–1.09, p = 0.16) [37]. However, there was a significant improvement in PSA relapse with adjuvant radiotherapy with a median biochemical recurrence-free interval of 10.3 years versus 3.1 years for observation (HR 0.43, 95% CI 0.31–0.58, p < 0.001). Disease recurrence was also significantly reduced with radiotherapy with a median recurrence-free survival of 13.8 years versus 9.9 years for observation (HR 0.62, 95% CI 0.46–0.82, p = 0.001). Additionally, adjuvant radiation was found to reduce the risk of initiation of hormonal treatment (HR 0.45, 95% CI 0.29–0.68, p < 0.001) [37]. Similar to EORTC 22911, a subset analysis demonstrated that patients who had positive surgical margins benefited the most from adjuvant radiation therapy compared to others who received adjuvant radiation therapy [42].

In a recent update of the SWOG 8794 trial with a median follow-up of 12.7 years in the radiation arm and 12.5 years in the observation arm, an additional 40 patients reached the primary endpoint of metastatic disease or death [43]. Of the patients randomized to observation, 54% have died or have metastatic disease (median metastasis-free survival 12.9 years) compared to 43% who received adjuvant radiation therapy (median metastasis-free survival 14.7 years) (HR 0.71, 95% CI 0.54–0.94, p = 0.016). A significant difference was also detected in the primary endpoint of overall survival, where death from any cause occurred in 52% of the patients randomized to radiation (median overall survival 15.2 years) compared to 41% in the observation group (median overall survival 13.3 years) (HR 0.72, 95% CI 0.55–0.96, p = 0.023) [43]. It was noted that more rectal complications, urethral strictures, and total urinary incontinence were encountered in patients who received adjuvant radiation [37].

The multi-institutional German Cancer Society ARO 96-02/AUO AP 09/95 trial randomized 307 patients with pT3N0M0 PCA with or without positive surgical margins after RP to observation or 60 Gy of adjuvant radiotherapy given in 30 fractions [38,39]. Information on this trial is limited at the time of this publication as it is available only in abstract format. Similar to SWOG 8794, patients in the EORTC 22911 were eligible for enrollment irrespective of postoperative PSA level. However, patients in the German Cancer Society trial were only eligible for randomization if they achieved an undetectable PSA postoperatively. The primary endpoint of the study was biochemical progression-free survival. At a median follow-up of 4.5 years, the HR for biochemical progression-free survival in the adjuvant radiation arm was 0.53 (p = 0.0015). Toxicities were only reported in the adjuvant radiotherapy arm in this trial. Acute grade 3 bladder toxicity occurred in 3%, while late grade 2 and 3 bladder toxicities occurred in 16% and 2%, respectively. Acute grade 2 rectal toxicities occurred in 12% and there were no grade 3 acute rectal toxicities, while late grade 2 rectal toxicities occurred in 10% [38,39].

Comment

Based on the aforementioned studies, adjuvant radiotherapy after RP given to men with pT3N0M0 PCA significantly reduces the risk of PSA recurrence, metastasis and need for hormonal therapy, and resulted in an improvement in overall survival compared to observation alone. While these trials addressed the question of whether patients with pT3 PCA with or without positive margins after RP benefit from immediate adjuvant radiotherapy compared to observation, perhaps the more relevant question to clinical practice is the timing of the administration of the radiotherapy, either when PSA is undetectable (adjuvant radiotherapy) or when it becomes detectable or surpasses a certain threshold (salvage radiotherapy).

Recognizing the inherent limitations of subgroup analyses for the subset of patients in the SWOG 8794 trial who were initially observed and then received salvage radiation at the time of PSA failure, metastasis-free survival was inferior to that of those who received radiotherapy when PSA was still undetectable [43]. Several retrospective studies have also shown the superiority of adjuvant radiotherapy compared to salvage radiotherapy [44]. Radiotherapy and Androgen Deprivation in Combination after Local Surgery (RADICALS) is a phase III trial currently accruing patients that is designed to address the optimal timing of the administration of postoperative radiation as well as determining the optimal duration of hormonal therapy with adjuvant radiation to the prostate bed after RP. This trial randomizes patients with high-risk features such as pT3, positive margins, Gleason score > 6 or PSA > 10 ng/mL to either adjuvant radiation or salvage radiation at the time of biochemical failure (defined as two consecutive rises in PSA and PSA > 0.1 ng/mL or three consecutive rises in PSA) radiotherapy. A second randomization attempts to determine the optimal duration of hormonal therapy with adjuvant radiotherapy by randomizing patients to radiotherapy alone, radiotherapy plus 6 months of androgen deprivation therapy or radiotherapy plus 2 years of androgen deprivation therapy. The RADICALS trial aims to recruit greater than 4000 patients, so widespread support from urologists, medical oncologists, and radiation oncologists will be required for successful completion of this trial to answer these important clinical questions [45].

Recommendation

Based on moderate-quality evidence, the authors make a conditional recommendation for the use of adjuvant radiation therapy to improve clinical outcomes in men with pathological T3 disease or pathological T2 disease with positive margins after RP (**Grade 2B**). However, the timing of administration of the radiation, either when the PSA remains undetectable or at the first sign of PSA recurrence, remains under investigation.

Clinical question 28.4

In men with locally advanced prostate cancer, does adjuvant hormonal therapy after RP improve clinical outcomes?

Background

Patients with high-risk pathological features after RP have up to a 67% chance of biochemical recurrence at 5 years [8]. Failure in these patients is thought to be due to local disease not removed at the time of surgery or undetected systemic disease. The rationale behind adjuvant hormonal therapy after RP is to eliminate micrometastatic disease, thereby reducing local recurrences and distant metastasis.

Literature search

Evidence was obtained by performing a systematic literature search using PubMed. The search was performed with the terms "adjuvant," "androgen deprivation," and "locally advanced prostate cancer" combined with the clinical query filter function to limit the search to the English language. A search limit was also utilized to search for those articles categorized as a clinical trial, meta-analysis or randomized controlled trial.

The evidence

There are two RCTs [46,47] and a report of pooled results for three RCTs [48] evaluating the use of adjuvant hormonal therapy after RP in men with locally advanced disease (Table 28.4). Messing et al. [46] aimed to determine whether immediate androgen deprivation therapy (ADT) extends survival in men with node-positive PCA. In the study, 98 node-positive men who were status post RP were randomized to immediate ADT (3.6 mg goserelin subcutaneously every 28 days or bilateral orchidectomy, by choice of the patient) or to observation with ADT to be given upon detection of distant metastasis or symptomatic recurrences. The primary endpoint was progression-free survival, with secondary endpoint being overall and disease-specific survival. With a median follow-up of 11.9 years, men who received immediate ADT had improved overall survival (HR 1.84, 95% CI 1.01–3.35, p = 0.04), prostate cancer-specific survival (HR 4.09, 95% CI 1.76–9.49, p = 0.0004), and progression-free survival (HR 3.42, 95% CI 1.96–5.98, p < 0.0001) [37].

Table 28.4 Randomized trials comparing immediate androgen deprivation after RP to observation

Trial	Inclusion criteria	Number randomized	Treatment arms	Median follow-up	Primary endpoint	Outcomes
Messing et al. 2006	≤ cT2 disease who had RP + BPLND with nodal disease; negative BS + CXR; no hormonal tx before randomization	98	3.6 mg goserelin subcutaneously every 28 days or bilateral orchidectomy vs observation	11.9 yrs	PFS	Improved: OS (HR 1.84, 95% CI 1.01–3.35, p = 0.04) PCSS (HR 4.09, 95% CI 1.76–9.49, p = 0.0004) PFS (HR 3.42, 95% CI 1.96–5.98, p<0.0001)
Wirth et al. 2004 [47]	≤75 yo; stage pT3–4N0M0	309	Flutamide 250 mg oral tid vs observation	6.1 yrs	PFS, OS	Improved PFS (HR 0.51, 95% CI 0.32–0.81, p = 0.0041) No difference in OS (HR 10.4, 95% CI 0.53–2.02, p = 0.92)
McLeod et al. 2006 [49]	Clinically or pathologically localized (T1–2N0/X) or locally advanced (T3–4, any N, or any T, N+) PCA; negative BS	8113	Bicalutamide 150 mg oral daily vs placebo	7.4 yrs	PFS, OS	Improved PFS in all patients (HR 0.69, 95% CI 0.58–0.82, p<0.001) For patients who underwent RP, no OS benefit seen (HR 1.09, 95% CI 0.85–1.39, p = 0.51)

BPLND, bilateral pelvic lymph node dissection; BS, bone scan; CXR, chest x-ray; OS, overall survival; PCA, prostate cancer; PCSS, prostate cancer-specific survival; PFS, progression-free survival; RP, radical prostatectomy; tid, three times daily; tx, treatment

In the RCT by Wirth et al. [47], 309 men with locally advanced, lymph node-negative PCA (defined as pT3-4N0M0) were randomized to receive either flutamide 250 mg three times daily or no adjuvant treatment. The primary endpoints of the study were recurrence-free survival and overall survival. Recurrence was defined as a PSA value > 5 ng/mL, two values > 2 ng/mL more than 3 months apart, three values > 1 ng/mL more than 3 months apart or any clinical recurrence. With a median follow-up of 6.1 years, patients who received flutamide had a better recurrence-free survival (HR 0.51, 95% CI 0.32–0.81, $p = 0.0041$). However, there was no difference in overall survival (HR 10.4, 95% CI 0.53–2.02, $p = 0.92$). Although there was a significant improvement in recurrence-free survival, this advantage was not without significant side effects as 43% of the patients in the flutamide arm withdrew from the trial due to toxicities such as nausea, vomiting, and hepatotoxicity [47].

The largest of the adjuvant hormonal therapy trials was the Early Prostate Cancer Trial reported on by McLeod et al. [49]. This was an international, randomized, double-blinded, placebo-controlled study designed for a combined analysis. The three trials randomized a total of 8113 men with clinically or pathologically localized (T1–2, N0/X) or locally advanced (T3–4, any N, or any T, N +) PCA with negative bone scans for metastatic disease to either bicalutamide 150 mg oral daily or placebo following standard care (watchful waiting, radical prostatectomy or radiotherapy). Approximately one-third of the patients in the study had T3–T4 disease and approximately one-third had a Gleason score ≥ 7. The primary endpoints of the trials were progression-free survival and overall survival.

The North American trial, known as Trial 23, differed from the other two trials in that patients with positive lymph nodes and those who were candidates for watchful waiting were excluded from the study [50]. At a median follow-up of 7.4 years, patients who received bicalutamide for locally advanced disease had significant improvement in progression-free survival (HR 0.69, 95% CI 0.58–0.82, $p < 0.001$), irrespective of whether they underwent RP, watchful waiting or radiotherapy. When all patients with locally advanced disease were combined and evaluated with regard to overall survival, there was no difference between the watchful waiting, RP, and radiotherapy groups (HR 0.95, 95% CI 0.77–1.16, $p = 0.59$). However, in the subgroup of patients who had locally advanced disease and underwent radiotherapy, there was an overall survival benefit with adjuvant bicalutamide (HR 0.65, 95% CI 0.44–0.95, $p = 0.03$). This significant benefit was not seen in the subgroup of patients who underwent RP and received adjuvant bicalutamide (HR 1.09, 95% CI 0.85–1.39, $p = 0.51$). Patients who received adjuvant bicalutamide reported that the most common side effects of treatment were breast pain (73.6%) and gynecomastia (68.8%), which

were mild to moderate in greater than 90% of cases, but caused 16.8% of patients to withdraw from treatment. Other infrequent side effects included impotence (9.3%), decreased libido (3.6%), hot flushes (9.2%), and abnormal liver function tests (3.1%) [50].

A meta-analysis of the Messing and Wirth studies demonstrated that adjuvant androgen deprivation therapy following RP did not significantly improve overall survival at 5 years (OR 1.50, 95% CI 0.79–2.85, $p = 0.2$) or at 10 years (OR 0.53, 95% CI 0.33–0.84, $p = 0.008$). However, it did show a significant improvement in disease-free survival at 5 (OR 3.73, 95% CI 2.30–6.03, $p < 0.00001$) and 10 years (OR 2.06, 95% CI 1.34–3.15, $p = 0.0009$) [48].

Comment

While the Messing et al. trial did demonstrate an overall survival advantage with adjuvant ADT, this study has been criticized because of the small sample size, noncentralized pathology review in the original report, and imbalanced randomization [37]. When analyzed in the meta-analysis, the overall survival advantage was not evident. In addition, ADT is associated with significant acute and long-term complications such as impotence, hot flushes, metabolic and cognitive changes, changes in bone mineral density, gynecomastia, and breast pain [51]. Lastly, the initiation of ADT in this setting has a significant cost to the patient. Therefore, the decision to use adjuvant hormone therapy must be made between physician and patient after a thorough discussion is held with regard to efficacy, side effect profile and cost of the treatment.

Recommendation

Based on moderate-quality evidence, the authors make a conditional recommendation for the use of adjuvant hormonal therapy after RP to improve clinical outcomes in men with locally advanced PCA (**Grade 2B**).

Clinical question 28.5

In men with locally advanced prostate cancer, does adjuvant chemotherapy after RP improve clinical outcomes?

Background

Chemotherapy has been mainly used in patients with hormone-refractory disease, but this paradigm is changing as improved outcomes are being observed with newer drugs and drug combinations [52]. Despite years of research, the most effective current forms of therapy for locally advanced

PCA continue to provide only marginal improvements in clinical outcomes. These factors have led to an interest in introducing systemic chemotherapy earlier in the treatment course of patients with locally advanced disease.

The evidence

There are three phase III trials evaluating the use of adjuvant chemotherapy with or without ADT after RP. The Southwest Oncology Group (SWOG) 9921 trial was designed to compare ADT (bicalutamide 50 mg daily plus goserelin acetate 10.8 mg subcutaneously every 12 weeks for 2 years total) to ADT plus chemotherapy (mitoxantrone 12 mg/m^2 every 21 days for six cycles with prednisone 5 mg twice daily for six cycles) in patients with locally advanced disease, defined as Gleason score $\geq$ 8, pT3b–T4 or N1 disease, Gleason score 7 with positive surgical margin, preoperative PSA level $\geq$ 15 ng/mL or PSA level > 10 ng/mL with Gleason score $\geq$ 8 [53]. A total of 983 patients were enrolled in the trial, which was short of the goal of 1360 patients. However, due to three reported cases of acute myelogenous leukemia (AML) in the mitoxantrone treatment arm consisting of 487 patients (0.6%), the trial was closed to further accrual in January 2007. The prevalence of AML in this cohort (0.6%) was similar to the prevalence in subjects with breast cancer treated with mitoxantrone. Despite termination of the trial, these subjects will continued to be followed closely to monitor for latent development of AML, with the possibility of still being able to detect a difference between treatment arms [53].

TAX 3501 is an ongoing phase III trial of adjuvant chemotherapy in men who have undergone radical prostatectomy. Participants are being randomly assigned to one of the following three treatment groups: observation; leuprorelin acetate for 18 months or leuprorelin acetate plus docetaxel 75 mg/m^2 every 3 weeks for six cycles. A second round of randomization is planned for when patients in the observation group show evidence of disease progression, at which time they will be randomly assigned to receive 18 months of either ADT or ADT plus docetaxel. Target accrual is 2172 men and the primary endpoint is progression-free survival [54].

The Veterans Affairs Co-operative Studies Program (CSP) recently opened the Veterans Affairs CSP 553 trial called Chemotherapy After Prostatectomy for High-Risk Prostate Carcinoma [55]. This trial is designed to prospectively compare early adjuvant chemotherapy after RP using docetaxel 75 mg/m^2 every 3 weeks plus prednisone 5 mg twice daily for a total of six cycles to observation alone for patients who are potentially cured by RP but who are at high risk for relapse (defined as greater than 50% risk of biochemical relapse at 5 years after RP). This phase III study was started in June 2006 and has the goal of accruing and randomizing 636 patients who had

clinically localized (cT1-T2) PCA and were subsequently found to have poor prognostic features after RP and pelvic lymph node dissection including stage pT3b–T4 tumors, stage pT3a tumors with Gleason score $\geq$ 7, stage pT2 tumors with Gleason score 8–10 and positive surgical margins or preoperative PSA > 20 ng/mL. The primary endpoint of the trial is progression-free survival. Secondary outcomes include metastasis-free survival, cancer-specific survival, overall survival, quality of life and toxicity, and the interval to the initiation of ADT. The CSP 553 trial is the only study to date to evaluate the efficacy of chemotherapy alone, sparing patients the toxicities associated with ADT. The anticipated trial closure date is June 2012 [55].

Comment

A multimodal approach for the treatment of patients with locally advanced prostate cancer appears to be the key to successful clinical outcomes. Enrollment of patients into prospective clinical trials is paramount in determining the effectiveness of these chemotherapeutic regimens.

Recommendation

After a thorough review, there appears to be insufficient evidence to make a recommendation for the use of adjuvant chemotherapy after RP in patients with locally advanced PCA. Therefore, no recommendation can be made at this time.

Conclusion

Despite the prevalence of PCA, there remains no consensus on the optimal treatment methods for the disease. A summary of the evidence-based clinical questions that were posed in this chapter can be summarized in the following statements. No evidence exists reporting inferiority of RP compared to EBRT in the treatment of patients with locally advanced PCA. The use of neo-adjuvant hormone therapy was not of any benefit to men with locally advanced PCA undergoing RP. Though some preliminary reports are encouraging for the use of neo-adjuvant chemotherapy in men with locally advanced PCA undergoing RP, it is still investigational. In a select group of patients, the use of adjuvant radiotherapy after RP significantly reduces the risk of PSA recurrence, metastasis, and need for hormonal therapy, and even improves overall survival. The use of adjuvant ADT may improve disease-free survival at 5 and 10 years, but it is associated with significant acute and long-term complications and an absence of improvement in overall survival. Several large randomized trials utilizing chemotherapy in the adjuvant settings are ongoing, and it is anticipated that these studies will help to determine whether their use results in improved clinical outcomes. An integrated approach combining local and systemic therapies is likely necessary in the management of locally advanced PCA. Enrollment of patients into clinical trials is crucial in determining the efficacy of these therapies.

References

1. Gjertson C, Asher K, Sclar J, Goluboff E, Olsson C, Benson M, et al. Local control and long-term disease-free survival for stage D1 (T2-T4N1-N2M0) prostate cancer after radical prostatectomy in the PSA era. Urology 2007;70(4):723-7.

2. Royal College of Radiologists' Clinical Oncology Information Network, British Association of Urological Surgeons. Guidelines on the management of prostate cancer. Clin Oncol 1999;11(2):S53-88.

3. Kibel AS, Nelson JB. Adjuvant and salvage treatment options for patients with high-risk prostate cancer treated with radical prostatectomy. Prostate Cancer Prostat Dis 2007;10(2):119-26.

4. D'Amico AV, Whittington R, Malkowicz SB, Schultz D, Blank K, Broderick GA, et al. Biochemical outcome after radical prostatectomy, external beam radiation therapy or interstitial radiation therapy for clinically localized prostate cancer. JAMA 1998;280(11):969-74.

5. Lee A, Schultz D, Renshaw A, Richie J, d'Amico A. Optimizing patient selection for prostate monotherapy. Int J Radiat Oncol Biol Phys 2001;49(3):673-7.

6. Lieberfarb M, Schultz D, Whittington R, Malkowicz B, Tomaszewski J, Weinstein M, et al. Using PSA, biopsy Gleason score, clinical stage, and the percentage of positive biopsies to identify optimal candidates for prostate-only radiation therapy. Int J Radiat Oncol Biol Phys 2002;53(4):898-903.

7. Mettlin C, Murphy GP, Lee F, Littrup PJ, Chesley A, Babaian R, et al. Characteristics of prostate cancer detected in the American Cancer Society-National Prostate Cancer Detection Project. J Urol 1994;152(5 pt 2):1737-40.

8. Han M, Partin AW, Zahurak M, Piantadosi S, Epstein JI, Walsh PC. Biochemical (prostate specific antigen) recurrence probability following radical prostatectomy for clinically localized prostate cancer. J Urol 2003;169(2):517-23.

9. Akakura K, Isaka S, Akimoto S, Ito H, Okada K, Hachiya T, et al. Long-term results of a randomized trial for the treatment of Stages B2 and C prostate cancer: radical prostatectomy versus external beam radiation therapy with a common endocrine therapy in both modalities. Urology 1999;54(2):313-18.

10. Tolis G, Ackman D, Stellos A, Mehta A, Labrie F, Fazekas A, et al. Tumor growth inhibition in patients with prostatic carcinoma treated with luteinizing hormone-releasing hormone agonists. Proc Natl Acad Sci USA 1982;79(5):1658-62.

11. Köllermann J, Feek U, Müller H, Kaulfuss U, Oehler U, Helpap B, et al. Nondetected tumor (pT0) after prolonged, neo-adjuvant treatment of localized prostatic carcinoma. Eur Urol 2000;38(6):714-20.

12. Köllermann J, Hopfenmüller W, Caprano J, Budde A, Weidenfeld H, Weidenfeld M, et al. Prognosis of stage pT0 after prolonged neo-adjuvant endocrine therapy of prostate cancer: a matched-pair analysis. Eur Urol 2004;45(1):42-5.

13. Jones RS, Richards K, Russell T. Relative contributions of surgeons and decision support systems. Surg Clin North Am 2006;86(1):169-79, xi.

14. Milleron B, Westeel V, Quoix E, Moro-Sibilot D, Braun D, Lebeau B, et al. Complete response following preoperative chemotherapy for resectable non-small cell lung cancer: accuracy of clinical assessment using the French trial database. Chest 2005;128(3):1442-7.

15. Tannock I, Osoba D, Stockler M, Ernst D, Neville A, Moore M, et al. Chemotherapy with mitoxantrone plus prednisone or prednisone alone for symptomatic hormone-resistant prostate cancer: a Canadian randomized trial with palliative end points. J Clin Oncol 1996;14(6):1756-64.

16. Kantoff P, Halabi S, Conaway M, Picus J, Kirshner J, Hars V, et al. Hydrocortisone with or without mitoxantrone in men with hormone-refractory prostate cancer: results of the cancer and leukemia group B 9182 study. J Clin Oncol 1999;17(8):2506-13.

17. Tannock IF, de Wit R, Berry WR, Horti J, Pluzanska A, Chi KN, et al. Docetaxel plus prednisone or mitoxantrone plus prednisone for advanced prostate cancer. N Engl J Med 2004;351(15):1502-12.

18. Petrylak D, Tangen C, Hussain M, Lara PJ, Jones J, Taplin M, et al. Docetaxel and estramustine compared with mitoxantrone and prednisone for advanced refractory prostate cancer. N Engl J Med 2004;351(15):1513-20.

19. Eastham P. Reimbursement policies discourage off-label drug use. Oncol Times 2005;27(20):8-10.

20. Shannon C, Smith I. Is there still a role for neo-adjuvant therapy in breast cancer? Crit Rev Oncol Hematol 2003;45(1):77-90.

21. Van Poppel H, de Ridder D, Elgamal AA, van de Voorde W, Werbrouck P, Ackaert K, et al. Neo-adjuvant hormonal therapy before radical prostatectomy decreases the number of positive surgical margins in stage T2 prostate cancer: interim results of a prospective randomized trial. The Belgian Uro-Oncological Study Group. J Urol 1995;154(2 pt 1):429-34.

22. Pettaway C, Pisters L, Troncoso P, Slaton J, Finn L, Kamoi K, et al. Neo-adjuvant chemotherapy and hormonal therapy followed by radical prostatectomy: feasibility and preliminary results. J Clin Oncol 2000;18(5):1050-7.

23. Konety B, Eastham J, Reuter V, Scardino P, Donat S, Dalbagni G, et al. Feasibility of radical prostatectomy after neo-adjuvant chemohormonal therapy for patients with high risk or locally advanced prostate cancer: results of a phase I/II study. J Urol 2004;171(2 pt 1):709-13.

24. Clark P, Peereboom D, Dreicer R, Levin H, Clark S, Klein E. Phase II trial of neo-adjuvant estramustine and etoposide plus radical prostatectomy for locally advanced prostate cancer. Urology 2001;57(2):281-5.

25. Berger A, Niescher M, Fischer-Colbrie R, Pelzer A, Bartsch G, Horninger W. Single-agent chemotherapy with docetaxel significantly reduces PSA levels in patients with high-grade localized prostate cancers. Urol Int 2004;73(2):110-12.

26. Oh W, George D, Kaufman D, Moss K, Smith M, Richie J, et al. Neo-adjuvant docetaxel followed by radical prostatectomy in patients with high-risk localized prostate cancer: a preliminary report. Semin Oncol 2001;28(4 suppl 15):40-4.

27. Dreicer R, Magi-Galluzzi C, Zhou M, Rothaermel J, Reuther A, Ulchaker J, et al. Phase II trial of neo-adjuvant docetaxel before radical prostatectomy for locally advanced prostate cancer. Urology 2004;63(6):1138-42.

28. Febbo P, Richie J, George D, Loda M, Manola J, Shankar S, et al. Neo-adjuvant docetaxel before radical prostatectomy in patients with high-risk localized prostate cancer. Clin Cancer Res 2005;11(14):5233-40.

29. Hussain M, Smith D, El-Rayes B, Du W, Vaishampayan U, Fontana J, et al. Neo-adjuvant docetaxel and estramustine chemotherapy in high-risk/locallyadvanced prostate cancer. Urology 2003;61(4):774-80.

30. CALGB. Phase III randomized study of radical prostatectomy with versus without neo-adjuvant chemohormonal therapy comprising docetaxel and androgen-deprivation therapy with leuprolide acetate or goserelin in patients with high-risk, clinically localized prostate cancer. Available from: www.cancer.gov/clinicaltrials/CALGB-90203.

31. Ohori M, Abbas F, Wheeler TM, Kattan MW, Scardino PT, Lerner SP. Pathological features and prognostic significance of prostate cancer in the apical section determined by whole mount histology. J Urol 1999;161(2):500-4.

32. SWOG. A randomized phase iii study of neo-adjuvant docetaxel and androgen deprivation prior to radical prostatectomy versus immediate radical prostatectomy in patients with high-risk, clinically localized prostate cancer. Available from: https://www.swogstat.org/ROS/ROSBooks/Fall%202008/Genitourinary.pdf.

33. Debruyne F, Witjes W, Schulman C, van Cangh P, Oosterhof G. A multicentre trial of combined neo-adjuvant androgen blockade with Zoladex and flutamide prior to radical prostatectomy in prostate cancer. The European Study Group on Neo-adjuvant Treatment. Eur Urol 1994;26(suppl 1):4.

34. Debruyne F, Witjes W. Neo-adjuvant hormonal therapy prior to radical prostatectomy: the European experience. Mol Urol 2000;4(3):251-6; discussion 257.

35. Epstein JI, Carmichael M, Walsh PC. Adenocarcinoma of the prostate invading the seminal vesicle: definition and relation of tumor volume, grade and margins of resection to prognosis. J Urol 1993;149(5):1040-5.

36. Bolla M, van Poppel H, Collette L, van Cangh P, Vekemans K, da Pozzo L, et al. Postoperative radiotherapy after radical prostatectomy: a randomised controlled trial (EORTC trial 22911). Lancet 2005;366(9485):572-8.

37. Thompson IM Jr, Tangen CM, Paradelo J, Lucia MS, Miller G, Troyer D, et al. Adjuvant radiotherapy for pathologically advanced prostate cancer: a randomized clinical trial. JAMA 2006;296(19):2329-35.

38. Wiegel T, Hinkelbein W, Bottke D, Willich N, Piechota H, Souchon R. Adjuvant RT versus wait and see in patients with pT3 prostate cancer after radical prostatectomy – 5 year results (slide presentation). Available from: media.asco.org/player/default.aspx.

39. Wiegel T, Bottke D, Willich N, Semjonov J, Siegmann A, Stoeckle M, et al. Phase III results of adjuvant radiotherapy versus "wait and see" in patients with pT3 prostate cancer following radical prostatectomy (ARO 96-02/AUO AP 09/95). Int J Radiat Oncol Biol Phys 2007;69(3):S172-3.

40. Morgan S, Waldron T, Eapen L, Mayhew L, Winquist E, Lukka H. Adjuvant radiotherapy following radical prostatectomy for pathologic T3 or margin-positive prostate cancer: a systematic review and meta-analysis. Radiother Oncol 2008;88(1):1-9.

41. Van der Kwast T, Bolla M, van Poppel H, van Cangh P, Vekemans K, da Pozzo L, et al. Identification of patients with prostate cancer who benefit from immediate postoperative radiotherapy: EORTC 22911. J Clin Oncol 2007;25(27):4178-86.

42. Swanson G, Hussey M, Tangen C, Chin J, Messing E, Canby-Hagino E, et al. Predominant treatment failure in postprostatectomy patients is local: analysis of patterns of treatment failure in SWOG 8794. J Clin Oncol 2007;25(16):2225-9.

43. Thompson I, Tangen C, Paradelo J, Lucia M, Miller G, Troyer D, et al. Adjuvant radiotherapy for pathological T3N0M0 prostate cancer significantly reduces risk of metastases and improves survival: long-term followup of a randomized clinical trial. J Urol 2009;181(3):956-62.

44. Anscher M. Adjuvant radiotherapy following radical prostatectomy is more effective and less toxic than salvage radiotherapy for a rising prostate specific antigen. Int J Cancer 2001;96(2):91-3.

45. Parker C, Sydes M, Catton C, Kynaston H, Logue J, Murphy C, et al. Radiotherapy and androgen deprivation in combination after local surgery (RADICALS): a new Medical Research Council/National Cancer Institute of Canada phase III trial of adjuvant treatment after radical prostatectomy. BJU Int 2007;99(6):1376-9.

46. Messing EM, Manola J, Sarosdy M, Wilding G, Crawford ED, Trump D. Immediate hormonal therapy compared with observation after radical prostatectomy and pelvic lymphadenectomy in men with node-positive prostate cancer. N Engl J Med 1999;341(24):1781-8.

47. Wirth MP, See WA, McLeod DG, Iversen P, Morris T, Carroll K. Bicalutamide 150 mg in addition to standard care in patients with localized or locally advanced prostate cancer: results from the second analysis of the early prostate cancer program at median followup of 5.4 years. J Urol 2004;172(5 pt 1):1865-70.

48. Kumar S, Shelley M, Harrison C, Coles B, Wilt T, Mason M. Neo-adjuvant and adjuvant hormone therapy for localised and locally advanced prostate cancer. Cochrane Database Syst Rev 2006;4:CD006019.

49. McLeod D, Iversen P, See W, Morris T, Armstrong J, Wirth M. Bicalutamide 150 mg plus standard care vs standard care alone for early prostate cancer. BJU Int 2006;97(2):247-54.

50. McLeod D, See W, Klimberg I, Gleason D, Chodak G, Montie J, et al. The bicalutamide 150 mg early prostate cancer program: findings of the North American trial at 7.7-year median followup. J Urol 2006;176(1):75-80.

51. Schröder F. Early versus delayed endocrine therapy for prostate cancer. Endocr Relat Cancer 2007;14(1):1-11.

52. Oh W, Kantoff P. Management of hormone refractory prostate cancer: current standards and future prospects. J Urol 1998;160(4):1220-9.

53. Flaig T, Tangen C, Hussain M, Stadler W, Raghavan D, Crawford E, et al. Randomization reveals unexpected acute leukemias in Southwest Oncology Group prostate cancer trial. J Clin Oncol 2008;26(9):1532-6.

54. Oh W. High-risk localized prostate cancer: integrating chemotherapy. Oncologist 2005;10(suppl 2):18-22.

55. Montgomery B, Lavori P, Garzotto M, Lee K, Brophy M, Thaneemit-Chen S, et al. Veterans Affairs Cooperative Studies Program study 553: chemotherapy after prostatectomy, a phase III randomized study of prostatectomy versus prostatectomy with adjuvant docetaxel for patients with high-risk, localized prostate cancer. Urology 2008;72(3):474-80.

29 Radiation therapy for clinically localized prostate cancer

Michael Myers, Priya Mitra, Mitchell Anscher, Anthony Addesa and Michael Hagan

Department of Radiation Oncology, Virginia Commonwealth University, Richmond, VA, USA

Background

Radiation therapy (RT) has been considered one of the standard therapeutic approaches for the treatment of prostate cancer since the 1950s. It was believed that RT offered comparable results to the standard radical perineal prostatectomy, with less morbidity. Since that time there have been substantial advances in both surgical and RT techniques. With regard to RT, technological advances in both treatment planning and delivery have resulted in significant improvements in efficacy with a corresponding reduction in morbidity, particularly in the last 20 years.

Treatment options

Standard therapeutic approaches to localized prostate cancer include radical prostatectomy (retropubic or perineal), robot-assisted laparoscopic prostatectomy, external beam radiotherapy (EBRT), high dose rate and low dose rate brachytherapy and combinations of external beam radiotherapy with brachytherapy. Several factors should be considered when selecting a treatment option. One would be risk of failure based on clinical stage, prostate-specific antigen (PSA) level, and Gleason score. Specific initial therapies are recommended according to whether the risk category is low, intermediate or high, referring to the patient's risk of recurrence after therapy. Low risk is defined by the National Comprehensive Cancer Network (NCCN) as men with stage T1–T2a prostate cancer, a Gleason score between 2 and 6, and a PSA value $\leq$ 10 ng/mL. Intermediate risk is defined as any T2b–T2c cancer or any Gleason 7 score or PSA value between 10 and 20 ng/mL.

Evidence-Based Urology. Edited by Philipp Dahm, Roger R. Dmochowski.
© 2010 Blackwell Publishing.

High risk is defined as those with T3a–T3b prostate cancer, a Gleason score of 8–10 or a PSA value > 20 ng/mL. Other factors to consider when recommending treatment options include patient's life expectancy, underlying medical conditions, and patient preference.

This chapter aims to present evidence available on several topics in which there has been a reasonable degree of consensus achieved. The topics included in the chapter will address external beam radiotherapy dose, intensity-modulated radiation therapy (IMRT) versus three-dimensional conformal radiotherapy (3D-CRT), as well as patient selection for pelvic lymph node irradiation, brachytherapy and androgen deprivation therapy.

Clinical question 29.1

What is the optimal dose for the treatment of localized prostate cancer with external beam radiotherapy?

Literature search

We performed a literature search using PubMed and Medline. Search terms included combinations of the following: "prostate cancer," "IMRT," "three-dimensional conformal radiation therapy," "dose escalation," "randomized controlled trials." No time frame limitations were applied.

The evidence

The advent of 3D-CRT and subsequently IMRT provided the capability to deliver higher doses, with an acceptable risk of toxicity, for the treatment of prostate cancer. There have been several single-institution prospective phase I/II trials confirming the benefits of dose escalation as well as a small number of phase III randomized controlled trials (Table 29.1).

A prospective RCT reported by Pollack et al. enrolled 301 patients with T1–T3 prostate cancer to receive 70 Gy

Table 29.1 Effect of dose escalation trials for localized prostate cancer

Authors	Methods	Eligibility	Intervention	Participants	Outcomes	Disease-free survival	Toxicity	Notes
Zelefsky et al. [7]	Phase I prospective trial, Median F/U 36 mos	T1c–T3	Dose escalation: 64.8 v 70.2 v 75.6 v 81 Gy	64.8 Gy – 96 pts; 70.2 Gy – 266 pts; 75.6 Gy – 320 pts; 81.0 Gy – 61 pts	Initial response to treatment; Relapse toxicity; Effect of neo-adjuvant androgen deprivation on local outcome	Stat sig improvement in local control in 81 Gy v 75.6 Gy group (p=.005); Stat sig improvement in PSA relapse-free outcome in the intermediate (p=.04) and unfavorable (p=.03) risk groups	Stat sig increase in grade II GI toxicity in 75.6 and 81 Gy groups (p<.001); Stat sig increase in grade II GU toxicity in 75.6 and 81 Gy groups (p=.002)	Neoadjuvant androgen blockade for large-volume prostates; Prostate biopsy at 2.5 yrs if NED; only 36% eligible pts underwent biopsy; Identified factors which sig affect PSA relapse-free survival: -PSA<10 (p<.01) -stage T1–2 (p<.01) -GS<7 (p<.01)
Zelefsky et al. [8]	Phases I and II, prospective trial, Median F/U 60 mos	As above	Dose escalation: 64.8 v 70.2 v 75.6 v 81 v 86.4 Gy	64.8 Gy – 96 pts; 70.2 Gy – 269 pts; 75.6 Gy – 445 pts; 81.0 Gy – 250 pts; 86.4 Gy – 40 pts	PSA relapse-free survival; Post-irradiation prostate biopsy; Late toxicity	Stat sig improvement in PSA relapse-free survival with dose of at least 75.6 Gy (p<.001); Stat sig improvement in PSA relapse-free survival with dose of at least 75.6 Gy for each prognostic risk group: -Favorable (p=.04) -Intermediate (p=.008) -Unfavorable (p=.006)	Stat sig increase in 5-yr grade II rectal toxicity with dose ≥75.6 Gy; Stat sig decreased incidence of late grade II and III rectal toxicity with IMRT v 3DCT (p<.01); Stat sig decrease in late grade II rectal toxicity at 3 yrs in IMRT v 3DCT for pts treated with 81 Gy (p=.005) Stat sig increase in grade II GU toxicity at five yrs when dose ≥75.6 Gy; No stat sig difference in GU toxicity with IMRT v 3DCT (p=.32); No ≥ grade III toxicity in pts treated with 86.4 Gy	229 of 290 pts receiving 81 or 86.4 Gy treated with IMRT; remaining 871 pts treated with 3DCT; 39% pts were treated with neoadjuvant androgen deprivation, those with large volume prostates; Patients classified into low, intermediate, and unfavorable prognostic risk groups based on PSA, GS, and T stage
Michalski et al. [9]	Prospective dose escalation study, Median F/U 79 mos	As above	Dose escalation: 66–86.4 Gy	Low-risk: 446 pts; Intermediate-risk: 849 pts; High-risk: 752 pts	PSA relapse-free survival; DMFS	Stat sig improvement in PSA relapse-free survival for intermediate (p<.0001) and high-risk* (p=.023) groups treated with ≥ 75.6 Gy *most apparent when comparing 86.4 go 75.6 Gy subgroups	N/A	48% pts received neo-adjuvant androgen deprivation; Patients treated with either 3DCT or IMRT

Study	Design / Follow-up	Inclusion criteria	Arms / Dose	No. of patients	Endpoints	Outcome	Toxicity	Comments
Dearnaley et al. [12]	RCT, Median F/U 63 mos	T1b-T3aN0M0 PSA <50	Standard-dose (64 Gy) v Escalated-dose (74 Gy) Conformal Radiation therapy	Std Dose – 422 pts; Escalated – 421 pts	bPFS; Freedom from local progression; Mets-free survival OS; Late toxicity	Hazard ratio (Esc:Std dose) 0.67 (stat sig better, p = .0007) At 5 years, bPFS 71% vs 60% (Esc vs Std dose)	Rate of at least grade 2 rectal toxicity at 6 mo (Esc:Std): 185 vs 142 No difference in trial groups regarding urinary toxicity	All patients received neoadjuvant androgen suppression (3–6 mo)
Peeters et al. [3]	RCT, Median F/U 51 mos	All T stages, some except- ions PSA <60	Conventional dose (68 Gy) v Experimental dose (78 Gy)	Conventional – 332 pts; Experimental – 337 pts	FFF (biochemical or clinical); FFCF; OS; Toxicity	Significantly higher FFF in experimental arm (p = .01) Stat sig lower biochemical failure at five years (p = .02) No stat sig difference in FFCF at five years	Higher incidence of at least grade 2 GI toxicity but not stat sig (p=.2) No stat sig difference for at least grade 3 GI toxicity (p = .4) No difference in GU toxicity	Allowed use of hormonal therapy 41 pts treated with IMRT 36 pts in experimental arm treated with dose between 68–76 Gy Not powered for subgroup analysis
Peeters et al., 2005 (39)	RCT, Median F/U 31 mos	All T stages, some except- ions PSA <60	Standard arm (68 Gy) v Experimental arm (78 Gy)	Standard – 331 pts; Experimental – 333 pts	Acute toxicity; Late toxicity	N/A	No stat sig difference between the two arms regarding acute GI or GU toxicity No stat sig difference between the two arms regarding late GI toxicity (≥grade II or ≥III) except for rectal bleeding (p = .005) No stat sig difference between the two arms for late GU toxicity (≥ grade II or ≥III) except for nocturia (p = .05)	Hormonal therapy (HT) allowed, commonly used in high-risk pts Stratified for hospital, HT, age, and dose- volume groups 41 pts in high-dose arm received simul- taneous integrated boost using IMRT 36 pts in high-dose arm received <78 Gy Adapted toxicity scoring scales
Pollack et al. [13]	RCT, Median F/U 40 mos	T1-3, Nx0M0	Standard arm (70 Gy) v Experimental arm (78 Gy)	Std Arm – 150 pts; Experimental – 151 pts	FFF (biochemical or clinical); Freedom from distant mets; OS; Prostate bx positivity at 2 yrs	Borderline significant improved FFF with higher dose (p=.058) Pts had a significantly higher 5-yr FFF with 78 Gy if PSA>10 (p=.011), T3 disease (p=.047), or Gleason score 2–6 (p=.05)	No significant side effects related to dose noted	Hormonal therapy not allowed unless high-risk

(Continued on p. 282)

Table 29.1 (Continued)

Authors	Methods	Eligibility	Intervention	Participants	Outcomes	Disease-free survival	Toxicity	Notes
Pollack et al. 2002 (1)	RCT, Median F/U 60 mos	As above	As above	As above	As above	Stat sig improvement in 6-yr FFF with 78 Gy (p = .03) Stat sig improvement in FFF at 60 mo follow-up in pts with pre-treatment PSA>10 ng/mL (p = .012)	Stat sig increase in ≥ grade 2 rectal toxicity in 78 Gy arm Stat sig increased chance of ≥ grade II rectal toxicity if >25% of rectum received ≥70 Gy No significant difference in bladder toxicity	Patients stratified by pretreatment PSA into: ≥10, >10–20, and >20 ng/mL The largest difference between the two arms regarding FFF is before five years
Zietman et al. 2005 (5)	RCT, Median F/U 66 mos	T1b-T2b PSA<15	Conventional arm (70.2 Gy) v High-dose arm (79.2 Gy)	Conventional – 197 pts High-dose – 196 pts	Biochemical failure Local control OS Morbidity	5-yr Freedom from biochemical failure significantly higher in high-dose arm (p<.001) Above holds for low and intermediate-risk disease (p<.001, p=.02, respectively), not high risk (p=.8)	Stat sig increase in acute (p=.004) and late (p=.005) grade 2 GI morbidity No stat sig difference in acute or late GU morbidity	No hormonal therapy Proton boost (19.8 v 20.8 GyE) Near 90% of each arm received planned dose

3DCT, three-dimensional conformal therapy; bPFS, biochemical progression-free survival; DMFS, distant metastasis-free survival; EBRT:external beam radiation therapy; Esc, escalated; FFCF, freedom from clinical failure; FFF, freedom from failure; GI, gastrointestinal; GS, Gleason score; GU, genitourinary; GyE, Gray equivalent; HT, hormonal therapy; IMRT, intensity-modulated radiation therapy; NED, no evidence of disease; OS, overall survival; PPI, permanent seed implant; PSA, prostate-specific antigen; RP, radical prostatectomy; Std, standard versus 78 Gy [1]. The 6-year PSA relapse-free survival (RFS) for the 70 vs 78 Gy arms were 64% vs 70% (p = 0.03), respectively. Subgroup analysis detected no significant benefit when patients had PSA levels < 10. Recently, the update to this study reported by Kuban et al. found the benefit of dose escalation remained significant with maturation of the study [2]. The difference in PSA RFS outcomes between the two study arms increased with time (78% vs 59% at 8 years, and 73% vs 50% at 10 years). With the longer follow-up, a benefit was now seen for the first time in patients with low-risk disease (8-year PSA RFS of 63% vs 88% for those treated with 70 Gy vs 78 Gy, respectively, p = 0.042).

A multicenter RCT from The Netherlands, reported by Peeters et al., enrolled 664 patients with stage T1b–4 prostate cancer to receive either 64 Gy or 74 Gy [3]. Eligibility criteria were adenocarcinoma of the prostate including all T stages with PSA less than 60 ng/mL, except T1a and well-differentiated (Gleason score < 5) T1b–c tumors with PSA < 4 ng/mL. They reported a significant benefit in freedom from failure (FFF) at 5 years of 54% versus 64% for the groups receiving 64 Gy and 74 Gy, respectively. FFF was defined as no clinical evidence of disease or biochemical recurrence by ASTRO definition (three consecutive increases in PSA level after a nadir).

A RCT from the United Kingdom, reported by Dearnaley et al., studied 843 men with localized prostate cancer treated with 3D-CRT to a dose of 64 Gy versus 74 Gy [4]. Eligibility criteria included histological confirmed T1b–T3aN0M0 prostate cancer. All patients received androgen suppression consisting of a luteinizing hormone-releasing analog accompanied by antiandrogen treatment at first to prevent disease flare. They reported a 71% vs 60% biochemical progression-free survival (bPFS) at 5 years in the escalated vs standard groups, respectively (hazard ratio (HR) 0.67 95% confidence interval (CI) 0.53–0.85). Subgroup analysis found a significant bPFS for dose escalation in the high-risk group (HR 0.60, 95% CI 0.44–0.81), but no statistically significant benefit in the intermediate- or low-risk groups.

Zietman et al. conducted a RCT of dose escalation employing a combination of proton therapy as a boost following conventional photon external beam therapy [5]. They studied 393 patients with stage T1b through T2b prostate cancer and PSA levels less than 15 ng/mL who received either 70.2 cobalt gray equivalents (CGE) or 79.2 CGE. The treatment was delivered using a conformal photon dose of 50.4 Gy with a proton beam boost dose of either 19.8 Gy or 28.8 Gy, for total doses of either 70.2 CGE or 79.2 CGE. The 5-year freedom from biochemical failure was 61.4% for conventional-dose and 80.4% for high-dose therapy (p < 0.001). When subgroup analysis was performed the authors observed a significant benefit in both low-risk and intermediate-risk patients, but no benefit in the high-risk group.

Hanks et al. reported the phase I/II experience from Fox Chase in which they confirmed the direct relationship between dose and PSA outcome in patients when comparing doses from 70 Gy up to 78 Gy [6]. This study also divided the group into six subgroups based on PSA value (< 10, 10–19.9, ≥ 20) as well as favorable (stage T1–T2a, GS < 7) and unfavorable (stage T2b–T3, GS 7–10) risk groups. There was a significant 5-year PSA RFS in three of the six subgroups including PSA < 10 unfavorable, PSA 10–19.9 unfavorable and PSA ≥ 20 favorable. The authors concluded that a dose between 70 and 80 Gy is absolutely critical except for the most favorable and the most unfavorable subsets. Dose below 70 Gy may be acceptable for the most favorable subgroup.

The phase I/II experience from the Memorial Sloan Kettering Cancer Center (MSKCC), reported by Zelefsky et al., looked at both post-treatment biopsy and PSA failure in patients treated with dose-escalated EBRT [7]. In this study the radiation dose was systematically increased from 64.8 to 86.4 Gy by increments of 5.4 Gy in consecutive groups of patients. A positive biopsy at > 2.5 years after treatment was observed in only 1/15 (7%) of patients receiving 81.0 Gy, compared with 12/25 (48%) after 75.6 Gy, 19/42 (45%) after 70.2 Gy, and 13/23 (57%) after 64.8 Gy (p = 0.05). An update to this study evaluated clinical outcome according to risk group based on T-stage, pretreatment PSA and Gleason score [8]. Low-risk patients were considered those with PSA < 10 ng/mL, T-stage < T2b and Gleason score < 7. Those patients meeting all three criteria, two criteria or 0–1 criterion were considered favorable risk, intermediate risk and high risk, respectively. The 5-year actuarial PSA RFS rate for favorable risk disease receiving 64.8–70.2 Gy was 77% compared to 90% for those treated with 75.6–86.4 Gy (p = 0.05). The corresponding rates were 50% versus 70% in intermediate-risk cases (p = 0.001), and 21% versus 47% in unfavorable risk cases (p = 0.002).

The main limitation to dose escalation for prostate cancer has been the surrounding normal tissue tolerance, most importantly that of the rectum and bladder. Michalski et al. reported the toxicity outcome for 173 patients enrolled on RTOG 9406, a prospective phase I dose escalation study conducted to determine the maximally tolerated radiation dose in men treated with 3D-CRT for localized prostate cancer [9]. They found that despite a nearly 20% dose escalation (81.6 Gy vs 68.5Gy), compared to the historical RTOG trials, significantly fewer long-term bowel or bladder complications were noted. Storey et al. reported on the toxicity of the M.D. Anderson hospital experience and found that the group receiving 78 Gy had a significantly higher late grade 2 rectal toxicity than the group receiving 70 Gy [10]. However, if less than 25% of the rectum received 70 Gy or less, only 13% of patients experienced grade 2 rectal complications as compared to a 37% risk with a greater volume treated. They also reported that bladder complications were no different for the 70 Gy and 78 Gy arms.

Comment

Computed tomography-guided 3D-CRT and IMRT have enabled safe delivery of higher radiation doses to the prostate. For patients with low-risk disease, a minimum dose of 70 Gy is recommended (conditional recommendation **Grade 2B**). For intermediate- and high-risk disease, a dose of 75 Gy or greater appears to offer improved local control and disease specific survival (conditional recommendation **Grade 2B**).

Clinical question 29.2

Is IMRT better than 3D-CRT for treating localized prostate cancer?

Literature search

A literature searched was performed using PubMed and Medline. Search terms included combinations of the following: "prostate cancer," "IMRT," "three-dimensional conformal radiation therapy," "dose escalation," "randomized controlled trials." No time frame limitations were applied.

The evidence

There are no randomized controlled trials that directly compare IMRT to 3D-CRT in localized prostate cancer. Instead, the shift in treatment modality to IMRT has stemmed from dose escalation studies and associated toxicity analyses; see Table 29.2.

The MSKCC has several large prospective phase I/II dose escalation studies that address this issue [7,8,11]. The first two publications demonstrated a statistically significant improvement in PSA RFS and local control with increased dose [7,8]. The most recent publication suggests that intermediate- and high-risk patients are the key patients to target with a higher dose [11].

Five RCTs comparing a standard dose arm to an escalated dose consistently demonstrate improved biochemical disease-free survival with the higher dose for locally advanced prostate cancer [1,2,4,12,13].

As dose escalation was validated with 3D-CRT, one problem remained: toxicity. Despite the improved control of prostate cancer, the majority of the studies revealed a statistically significant increase in gastrointestinal toxicity [7,8,12]. With the implementation of IMRT, however, it was theorized that patients would be spared the toxicity while allowing for dose escalation. Dose constraints could

be applied to limit the amount of radiation delivered to nearby normal tissue structures, specifically the rectum and bladder. Phase I/II studies have confirmed a reduction in gastrointestinal toxicity using IMRT, compared to historical controls (see Table 29.2).

Comment

Dose escalation is necessary to adequately control localized prostate cancer. In order to limit toxicity, a more conformal treatment technique is necessary. IMRT is the most effective tool currently available to accomplish these objectives (strong recommendation **Grade 1B**).

Clinical question 29.3

Which patients should have the pelvic lymph nodes irradiated?

Literature search

A literature search was performed using PubMed and Medline. Search terms included combinations of the following: "prostate cancer," "pelvic lymph node irradiation," "pelvic lymph nodes," "elective nodal irradiation," "radiation therapy," "randomized controlled trials." No time frame limitations were applied.

The evidence

The first randomized study addressing pelvic irradiation was published in 1977 [14]. The data offered support for extended-field radiotherapy in prostate cancer to improve disease-free survival. Several other studies were subsequently performed; however, the majority of these took place prior to the development of PSA and its influence on risk stratification as well as prior to advanced imaging [37,38].

There is one large RCT that has focused on the differences in progression-free survival (PFS) between whole-pelvic (WP), which included pelvic lymph nodes, and prostate-only (PO) radiation therapy – RTOG 9413 [15]. Patients in this study were estimated to have a risk of pelvic lymph node metastases of at least 15%, based on the Roach formula (2/3(PSA) + ((Gleason score 6) × 10)). A subset analysis was performed to determine whether there was a difference in PFS for WP, "mini-pelvis," and PO radiation therapy [16]. These studies demonstrate a significant improvement in PFS with WP or lymph node irradiation. Despite the change in PFS, these data suggest significantly increased toxicity with WP radiation therapy [16]. However, the authors note that, as the study began in 1994, the modern techniques of 3D-CRT and IMRT were not routinely used.

Table 29.2 Effect of pelvic irradiation for localized prostate cancer

Authors	Methods	Eligibility	Intervention	Participants	Outcomes	Results	Toxicity	Notes
Asbell et al. [37]	RCT, Median F/U 84 mos	Clinical stage A2 or B prostate cancer without evidence of LN involvement	PO RT v Prostate + Pelvic RT	PO RT 225 pts Prostate + Pelvic RT 220 pts	LC DM NED-Survival Survival	No stat sig difference at 5yrs: Survival- 78 v 80% LC- 88 v 90% DM- 84 v 83% NED-survival- 67 v 64%	Prostate + Pelvic RT pts with ability to have an erection: ~89% on at least 1 f/u ~47% at last f/u	Prostate RT dose = 65 Gy in 6.5 - 7 wks Pelvic LN RT dose = 45-50 Gy in 4.5 - 6.5 wks Evidence of LN involvement based on surgical or radio- graphic (i.e. LAG) staging Patients with prior HT: 5% (PO) v 6% (Prostate + Pelvic RT)
Ploysong-sang et al. [38]	Retrospective review, Median F/U 78 mos	Prostate adenoca, stage A-C	Prostate RT (P) v WP + Prostate boost	P RT 116 pts WP + P 126 pts	LR DM DFS OS Treatment-related morbidity	Stat sig decrease in LR for stage C patients (34 v 16%) No stat sig difference in DM for any or all stages Stat sig improved 3-yr DFS for Stage C pts treated with WP + P (30 v 63%) Stat sig improved OS for stage B and C pts treated with WP + P (70 v 90%, 40 v 72% respectively) Stat sig improvement in 5-yr DFS with WP + P for WD and MD cancers (45 v 63%); not stat sig for PD cancers (24 v 35%)	Stat sig increased acute toxicity with WP + P (61 v 41%) No stat sig difference in late toxicity	WP+ P RT dose = 46-50 + 20 Gy P RT dose = 70-75 Gy PSA not available until last few years 19% (WP + P) v 25% had hormonal manipulation prior to RT
Roach et al. [15]	RCT, Median F/U 59.5 mos	Any T stage, PSA ≥100, Estimated LN involvement of ≥15%	WP RT + N & CHT v PO RT + N & CHT v WP RT + AHT v PO RT + AHT	WP RT + N & CHT: 322 pts (Arm 1) PO RT + N & CHT: 323 pts (Arm 2) WP RT + AHT: 322 pts (Arm 3) PO RT + AHT: 325 pts (Arm 4)	PFS OS LF DM PSA failure	Stat sig improvement in 4-yr PFS for pts treated with WP vs PO RT, p =.02 No stat sig difference in OS between WP and PO RT, but trend toward lower rate of PSA failure with WP RT (p=0.065) Stat sig increase in PFS with WP RT + N & CHT arm for intermediate to high-risk pts (p=.014); no difference in low- risk groups	No stat sig difference in acute or late GI/GU toxicity between WP and PO pts	Total RT dose = 70.2 Gy, regardless of WP v PO radiation Arms 1 and 2 treated with HT for 4 mos; arms 3 and 4 received HT for 6 mos

(Continued on p. 286)

Table 29.2 (Continued)

Authors	Methods	Eligibility	Intervention	Participants	Outcomes	Results	Toxicity	Notes
Roach et al. [16]	RCT subset analysis, Median F/U not listed	Any T stage, PSA ≥100, Estimated LN involvement of ≥15%	WP RT + N & CHT v PO RT + N & CHT	WP RT + N & CHT: 309 pts (Arm 1) PO RT + N & CHT: 301 pts (Arm 2) dichotomized into: –MP: 170 pts –PO: 131 pts	PFS Biochemical failure OS Toxicity	Stat sig improvement in PFS in WP v MP+PO pts (p=.02) Stat sig decrease in biochemical failure with WP RT v MP or PO RT (p=.022 and p=.029, respectively) No difference in OS	Acute GI/GU Toxicity (≥grade 2): Stat sig increase with WP RT (p<.001, p=.016, respectively) Late GI Toxicity (≥grade 3): Stat sig increase with WP RT (p=.006)	MP represents a field size less than the median (10 x 11 cm); PO is field size above the median 3DCT and IMRT were not routinely used
Seaward et al. [17]	Retrospective review Median F/U 35 mos for WPRT group 30 mos for PORT group	Clinically localized prostate cancer pts with high risk of LN involvement (≥15%)	WPRT v PORT	WPRT – 196 pts PORT – 310 pts Number of high-risk pts dependent on formula used: –2-variables: 201 pts –3 variables: 240 pts	PFS	Stat sig improvement in PFS with WPRT v PORT, regardless of which equation was used –2-variable: p<.0001 –3-variable: p=.02 No stat sig difference in PFS for pts with low risk of LN involvement	No significant difference in GI/GU toxicity between the two groups	49% of all pts treated with 3DCT as part of therapy (nearly 50% in each group) 20% pts received neo-adjuvant or adjuvant HT
Pan et al. [19]	Retrospective review, Median F/U 42 mos for PRT group, 24 mos for No PRT group	Clinically localized prostate cancer treated with definitive 3DCT	PRT v No PRT	PRT – 693 pts No PRT – 588 pts Patients stratified by risk of pelvic LN involvement: –Low: 709 pts –Intermed: 263 pts –High: 309 pts	bNED	Stat sig improvement in bNED with PRT in pts with inter-mediate risk for LN involvement (p=.02) Stat sig relative risk reduction with PRT on multivariate analysis (RR 0.72, CI 0.54–0.97) –no stat sig difference between the three groups of LN risk	N/A	Approximately 20% of each group received neoadjuvant androgen suppression Mean total dose 71.4 Gy (PRT) and 73.2 (no PRT) Pelvic LN risk groups defined by updated Partin tables: –Low: 0–5% –Intermed: >5–15% –High: >15%

3DCT, three-dimensional conformal therapy; AHT, adjuvant hormonal therapy; bNED, freedom from biochemical recurrence; CHT, concurrent hormonal therapy; CI, confidence interval; DM, distant metastases; f/u, follow-up; GI, gastrointestinal; GU, genitourinary; HT, hormonal therapy; IMRT, intensity-modulated radiation therapy; Intermed, intermediate; LAG, lymphangiogram; LC, local control; LF, local failure; LN, lymph node; LR, local recurrence; MD, moderately differentiated; MP, mini-pelvis; N, neo-adjuvant; NED, no evidence of disease; OS, overall survival; PD, poorly differentiated; PFS, progression-free survival; PO, prostate only; PRT, pelvic irradiation; PSA, prostate-specific antigen; RR, relative risk; RT, radiation therapy; WD, well-differentiated; WP, whole pelvic

There are two large retrospective studies that address which patients will benefit most from pelvic lymph node irradiation [17]. In addition to the equation used in RTOG 9413, the first study used a modified version of the Roach formula to estimate the risk of lymph node positivity [17]. Regardless of the equation used, there was a statistically significant improvement in PFS with the use of WP irradiation; however, there was no significant difference in PFS for patients with a low risk of lymph node involvement [17]. An update of this retrospective study noted an improved freedom from PSA failure in intermediate-risk patients receiving WP radiation (p < 0.0001) but not for high-risk patients [18]. The explanation for the difference between these two groups of patients is the presence of distant micrometastases in the high-risk patients. The second retrospective study, however, demonstrated a significant relative risk reduction with pelvic irradiation across all groups of lymph node risk [19]. See Table 29.1 for a summary of the above-mentioned studies.

Comment

The evidence suggests that pelvic lymph node irradiation is an effective method in treating patients with prostate cancer, if the risk of lymph node involvement is estimated to be at least 15%. Modern techniques should be used in an effort to reduce the likelihood of side effects (conditional recommendation Grade 2C evidence).

Clinical question 29.4

Which patients with localized prostate cancer should receive androgen deprivation (AD) in conjunction with RT?

Literature search

A literature search was performed using PubMed and Medline. Search terms included combinations of the following: "prostate cancer," "androgen deprivation," "androgen suppression," "randomized controlled trials." No time frame limitations were applied.

The evidence

There are several RCTs evaluating whether hormonal therapy influences the survival of any subgroups of patients with localized prostate cancer. The studies also focused on whether short- or long-term androgen deprivation therapy was required for improved outcome.

For patients with a low-risk prostate cancer, there has been no Level 1 evidence demonstrating benefit with the addition of androgen deprivation therapy to radiation

therapy. Although Pilepich et al. found that a subset of patient with Gleason scores of 2–6 had improved outcomes, including survival, the patients enrolled in this study had bulky disease, placing them into at least the intermediate-risk category based on clinical stage [20]. A large retrospective analysis of 1586 men reported by D'Amico et al. found no significant difference in biochemical recurrence (p = 0.09, RR = 0.5) with the addition of AD to EBRT in the treatment of low-risk prostate cancer [21].

There is considerable controversy regarding the optimal radiotherapeutic management of patients with intermediate-risk prostate carcinoma. The current recommendations advocate short-term AD + RT for patients with intermediate-risk disease. One RCT supporting this recommendation was reported by D'Amico et al.; the study involved 206 patients with intermediate- or high-risk disease randomized to receive EBRT with or without 6 months AD therapy [22]. The authors found a 5-year overall survival (OS) benefit of 88% versus 78% (p = 0.04) with the addition of AD. Although this study did not report a subgroup analysis, the majority of patients included would be classified as intermediate risk. Another RCT reported by Laverdiere et al. evaluated the benefits and sequencing of androgen deprivation administered with EBRT in localized prostate cancers [23]. In this study, the majority of patients had intermediate-risk disease. The 7-year biochemical disease-free survival was significantly different between the group receiving no hormones and the group receiving 3 months of neo-adjuvant AD – 42% vs 66% (p = 0.009), respectively. They also compared the group receiving no hormones with a group receiving neo-adjuvant, concurrent and adjuvant AD for a total of 10 months and found a biochemical disease-free survival benefit of 42% versus 69% (p = 0.003), respectively. There was no significance difference in overall survival between the two groups receiving hormones. A criticism raised regarding the D'Amico and Laverdiere studies was that the total radiation dose was 64 Gy in the latter study and 70 Gy in the former, both lower than typically used today. With evidence that the benefits seen with androgen deprivation in combination with lower doses of radiation (64–70 Gy) might be obtained with dose escalation alone in patients with intermediate-risk prostate cancer, the role of AD in combination with high-dose radiation remains a question for future studies.

The benefit from adjuvant androgen deprivation for high-risk prostate cancer was established in the first generation of the Radiation Therapy Oncology Group (RTOG) studies (Table 29.3) [20,24-28]. The first three studies included hormonal therapy but did not compare treatment with and without hormone therapy (RTOG 75-06, RTOG 77-06, RTOG 83-07). The subsequent studies evaluated the benefit of adjuvant hormonal therapy as well as the timing and duration of HT. A study reported by Roach et al., RTOG 94-13, evaluated the use of adjuvant AD and pelvic radiation

Table 29.3 Effect of adjuvant hormone therapy for localized prostate cancer

Authors	Methods	Eligibility	Intervention	Participants	Results	Toxicity	Notes
Lawton et al. RTOG 8531 [27]	RCT, Median F/U 5.6 years	T3 or N1	Lifetime Zoladex vs. none	977 enrolled	OS benefit for GS 8-10 with the addition of hormones (p = 0.036)	Not evaluated in this study	A statistically significant benefit with the addition of hormone therapy was also found with local failure, distant metastasis and disease free survival
Pilepich et al. RTOG 8610 [28]	RCT, Median F/U 6.7 years	T2-T4 bulky tumors	4 months CAB vs. none	471 enrolled	OS benefit for GS 2-6 with the addition of hormones (p = 0.015)	Not evaluated in this study	In patients with GS 7-10 there was no statistical improvement in locoregional control, distant metastasis or survival
Hanks et al. RTOG 9202 [29]	RCT, Median F/U 5.8 years	T2c-T4	CAB for 4 months then randomized to zoladex for 24 months vs. none	1554 enrolled	OS benefit for GS 8-10 with the addition of hormones (p = 0.044)	Late radiation grades 3, 4, and 5 gastrointestinal toxicity ascribed to the LTAD-RT arm (2.6% v 1.2% at 5 years, P .037),	All other efficacy end points, including CSS, showed a significant advantage for the LTAD-RT arm
D' Amico et al. [21]	Retrospective cohort study, Median F/U 4.2 years	Intermediate and high risk	CAB for 6 months vs. none	206 enrolled	OS benefit with the addition of hormones (p = 0.04)	Not evaluated in this study	The majority of patients on this study had intermediate risk disease according to NCCN classification
Bolla et al. [30]	RCT, Median F/U 3.9 years	92% T3-T4 > 70% GS 7-10 > 80% PSA > 10	Zoladex for 3 years vs. none	415 enrolled	OS benefit with the addition of hormones (p = 0.002)	Hot flashes: 62% Late grade 1–3 incontinence (29% vs. 16%, P = 0.002) Late grade 1–3 urethral stricture (20% vs. 13%(P = 0.09)	Although patients with Stage T1/2 with grade 3 disease were included, patients with stage T3–T4 disease were the majority (367 patients compared to 17 patients)

CAB, combined androgen blockade; CSS, cause-specific survival;.GS, Gleason score; LTAD-RT, long-term androgen deprivation with radiation therapy; NCCN, National Comprehensive Cancer Network; OS, overall survival

in patients with a risk of pelvic lymph node disease [15]. They evaluated 1292 patients with at least a 15% risk of lymph node involvement according to the equation: + LN risk = (2/3) PSA + ((GS − 6) × 10). The study contained four arms comparing WP radiation to PO radiation with either receiving neo-adjuvant and concurrent AD (4 months) or adjuvant AD (4 months). There was no overall survival benefit between cohorts but the group receiving WP radiation and neo-adjuvant and concurrent AD had a significantly improved progression-free survival.

The RTOG 92-02, reported by Hanks et al., studied the benefit of long-term adjuvant AD (24 months) after initial AD (4 months) with EBRT in patients with locally advanced prostate cancer [29]. They reported a significant benefit in all endpoints including distant metastasis but not overall survival. With subgroup analysis, they found improved overall survival when the Gleason score was 8–10. A similar European study reported by Bolla et al. randomized 415 men to received EBRT with or without 3 years of AD starting on the first day of treatment [30]. They reported a benefit in all endpoints in the combined treatment group compared to the radiotherapy-alone group, including a 5-year OS improvement of 78% versus 62%, respectively (p = 0.002).

Comment

The combination of AD and EBRT for the treatment of high-risk prostate cancer results in an apparent increase in local control and disease-free survival, as supported by several prospective, randomized trials (strong recommendation Grade 1B). The benefit for intermediate-risk disease is still controversial, especially with the advent of technological advances allowing for dose escalation. No recommendations can be made. Future studies comparing dose escalation with and without AD will hopefully clarify this issue. For patients with low-risk disease, there has been no compelling evidence for the addition of AD in their management (conditional recommendation Grade 2B).

Clinical question 29.5

Which patients with prostate cancer can be treated with brachytherapy alone?

Literature search

A literature search was performed using PubMed and Medline. Search terms included combinations of the following: "prostate cancer," "permanent prostate brachytherapy," "interstitial radiation," "randomized controlled trials." No time frame limitations were applied.

The evidence

The selection of patients who would benefit from prostate brachytherapy relies on the probability of organ-confined disease. Although there is no randomized phase III evidence comparing brachytherapy with EBRT, there are several reports from single institutions comparing EBRT, prostatectomy and brachytherapy seed implant based on prognostic risk groups (Table 29.4) [23-27]. Kupelian et al. studied 2991 consecutive patients treated with low-dose rate brachytherapy, EBRT, both brachytherapy and EBRT or radical prostatectomy (RP) [31]. For patients with unfavorable risk factors including stage T2b, PSA > 10 or Gleason score $\geq$ 7, both RP and brachytherapy alone had a significantly worse biochemical relapse-free survival (p = 0.042) when compared to EBRT. D'Amico et al. reported the outcome of 1872 patients treated with EBRT, low-dose rate brachytherapy + /- HT and RP [32]. They found no significant difference in outcomes for low-risk patients. However, for patients with intermediate and high risk, the outcomes for brachytherapy alone were inferior to either EBRT or RP (p = 0.003). A third study reported by Beyer & Brachman compared 2222 patients with T1–T2 disease receiving either interstitial brachytherapy or

EBRT [33]. They reported an improved biochemical RFS for patients with PSA 10–20 (p = 0.001) and Gleason score 8–10 (p = 0.04).

However, there have been studies that have shown no difference in outcome when comparing combination EBRT and brachytherapy with brachytherapy alone. The Seattle experience, reported by Blasko et al., studied 403 patients who received brachytherapy alone vs brachytherapy combined with external beam radiotherapy for early-stage prostate carcinoma [34]. After subgroup analysis, the intermediate-risk disease group showed no benefit in biochemical RFS with the addition of EBRT, 84% vs 85%, respectively. Within the intermediate-risk group, patients receiving combination therapy presented with a higher mean PSA (17.2 vs 14.9 ng/mL), and a greater proportion with Gleason scores of 7 (55 vs 45%). However, these differences were not statistically significant. Merrick et al. evaluated 668 consecutive patients for the impact of supplemental EBRT and/or AD therapy after permanent prostate brachytherapy [35]. Their classification of intermediate-risk disease included patients with one of the following risk factors: clinical stage T2c or greater, Gleason score $\geq$ 7 or PSA > 10 ng/mL. High-risk disease included two or more risk factors. Subgroup analysis of the 146 intermediate-risk patients who did not receive hormone therapy revealed the 8-year biochemical progression-free survival to be 95% versus 99% for those receiving monotherapy and combination therapy, respectively (p = 0.21).

In a report by Frank et al., a panel of experts were surveyed on the management of intermediate-risk prostate cancer with interstitial implant as monotherapy [36]. In the absence of perineural invasion (PNI), all of those surveyed would perform monotherapy for intermediate-risk patients, Gleason score 7 (3 + 4) or PSA 10–20, with cT1c and < 30% cores positive. Up to 80% would perform monotherapy for patients with cT1c, Gleason score 7 (4 + 3), and < 30% cores positive. Eighty to 90% of physicians would perform an implant alone with cT2a and either a PSA of 10–20 or Gleason score of 7 (3 + 4) and < 30% cores positive. Fifty to 60% of those surveyed stated that they would treat a patient with cT2b disease, Gleason score 7 (3 + 4), or PSA 11–20, with less than two-thirds of the biopsy cores positive in the absence of PNI.

The NCCN guidelines currently recommend brachytherapy as the sole modality of treatement for patients with low-risk disease. For patients with intermediate-risk disease, interstitial brachytherapy is recommended in combination therapy with EBRT. For high-risk patients, brachytherapy is generally not recommended but may be considered in conjunction with both EBRT and hormone therapy.

While no definite conclusions can be reached using nonrandomized retrospective data, these studies have provided the basis on which prospective RCTs can be designed. One such study by the Radiation Therapy

Table 29.4 Trials comparing brachytherapy with or without external beam radiotherapy

Authors	Methods	Eligibility	Intervention	Participants	Results	Toxicity	Notes
Kupelian et al. [31]	Phases I and II, prospective trial, Median F/U 56 mos	T1-T2	RP vs. EBRT < 72 Gy vs. EBRT > 72 Gy vs. PPI + EBRT vs. PPI	2991	PPI inferior to EBRT and PPI + EBRT (p = .042) with unfavorable risk factors (Stage T2b, PSA > 10, GS ≥ 7)	Not evaluated in this study	BF defined as PSA levels > 0.2 for RP cases. 3 consecutive rising PSA levels for all other cases
D'Amico et al. [32]	Retrospective cohort study, Median F/U 38 months	T1-T2	RP vs. EBRT vs. PPI vs. PPI with HT	1872	PPI +/- HT inferior to EBRT (p < 0.01) for high risk disease (Stage T2c, PSA > 20, GS ≥ 8) PPI without HT inferior to EBRT and RP (p < 0.003) for intermidiate risk disease (Stage T2b, PSA 10 - 20, GS 7)	Not evaluated in this study	No difference in outcome between groups for low risk disease HT consisted of 3 months neoadjuvant LHRH
Beyer et al. [33]	Retrospective cohort study, Median F/U EBRT 41.3 months PPI 51.3 months	T1-T2	EBRT vs. PPI	2222	PPI inferior to EBRT for PSA 10-20 (p = .001) GS 8-10 (p = 0.04)	Not evaluated in this study	Median EBRT dose was 66.6 Gy. No hormone therapy with either treatment
Blasko et al.[34]	Phases I and II, prospective trial, Median F/U 58 mos	T1-T3	PPI +/- EBRT	634	No significant benefit with the addition EBRT for all risk groups	RTOG grade 2 rectal toxicity: PPI + EBRT 6% PPI alone 2% RTOG grade 3 rectal toxicity: PPI + EBRT 2% PPI alone 0	Patients treated with combination therapy had significantly more advanced disease. EBRT consisted of 45 Gy to the whole pelvis
Merrick et al. [35]	Phases I and II, prospective trial, Median F/U 58.6 mos	T1b-T3a	PPI +/- EBRT	668	No significant benefit with the addition EBRT for low and intermediate risk groups	Not evaluated in this study	Only 14 of the 190 high risk patients did not receive EBRT

BF, biochemical failure; EBRT, external beam radiation therapy; GS, Gleason score; PPI, prostate permanent seed implant; HT, hormone therapy; LHRH, luteinizing hormone-releasing hormone; PSA, prostate-specific antigen; RP, radical prostatectomy.

Oncology Group will be comparing EBRT and brachytherapy versus brachytherapy alone for patients with intermediate-risk disease. The study, RTOG 0232, is currently open and will hopefully offer some insight as to whether patients with intermediate-risk factors have an acceptable outcome with brachytherapy as a sole therapy.

Comment

At present, there is general agreement that brachytherapy is appropriate as monotherapy for low-risk patients (conditional recommendation **Grade 2B**), and inappropriate for high-risk patients (conditional **Grade 1B** evidence). Its role as monotherapy for intermediate-risk patients remains undetermined and is the subject of a randomized controlled trial. No recommendation can be made according to Grade.

References

1. Pollack A, Zagars G K, Starkschall G, et al. Prostate cancer radiation dose response: results of the M D Anderson phase III randomized trial. Int J Radiat Oncol Biol Phys 2002;53:1097-105.
2. Kuban D, Tucker S, Dong L, et al. Long-term results of the M.D. Anderson randomized dose-escalation trial for prostate cancer. Int J Radiat Oncol Biol Phys 2008;70:67-74.

3. Peeters S, Heemsbergen WD, Koper P, et al. Dose–response in radiotherapy for localized prostate cancer: results of the Dutch multicenter randomized phase III trial comparing 68 Gy of radiotherapy with 78 Gy. J Clin Oncol 2006;24:1990-6.

4. Dearnaley P, Hall E, Lawrence D, et al. Phase III pilot study of dose escalation using conformal radiotherapy in prostate cancer: PSA control and side effects. Br J Cancer 2005;92:488-98.

5. Zietman AL, DeSilvio ML , Slater JD, et al. Comparison of conventional-dose vs high-dose conformal radiation therapy in clinically localized adenocarcinoma of the Prostate. JAMA 2005;294: 1233-9.

6. Hanks GE, Hanlon AL, Pinover WH, et al. Dose selection for prostate cancer patients based on dose comparison and dose response studies. Int J Radiat Oncol Biol Phys 2000;46:823-32.

7. Zelefsky MJ, Leibal SA, Gaudin PB, et al. Dose escalation with three-dimensional conformal radiation therapy affects the outcome in prostate cancer. Int J Radiat Oncol Biol Phys 1998;41:491-500.

8. Zelefsky MJ, Fuks C, Hunt M, et al. High dose radiation delivered by intensity modulated conformal radiotherapy improved the outcome of localized prostate cancer. Int J Radiat Oncol Biol Phys 2001;166: 871-81.

9. Michalski JM, Purdy JA, Winter K, et al. Preliminary report of toxicity following 3D radiation therapy for prostate cancer on 3DOG/RTOG 9406. Int J Radiat Oncol Biol Phys 2000;46:391-402.

10. Storey MR, Pollack A, Zagars GK, et al. Complications from dose escalation in prostate cancer: preliminary results of a randomized trial. Int J Radiat Oncol Biol Phys 2000;48:635-42.

11. Zelefsky M, Yamada Y, Fuks Z. Long-term results of conformal radiotherapy for prostate cancer: impact of dose escalation on biochemical tumor control and distant metastases-free survival outcomes. Int J Radiat Oncol Biol Phys 2008;71:1028-33.

12. Dearnaley D, Sydes M, Graham J. Escalated-dose versus standard-dose conformal radiotherapy in prostate cancer: first results from the MRC RT01 randomised controlled trial. Lancet Oncol 2007;8: 475-87.

13. Pollack A, Zagars G, Smith L. Preliminary results of a randomized radiotherapy dose-escalation study comparing 70 Gy with 78 Gy for prostate cancer. J Clin Oncol 2000;18:3904-11.

14. Bagshaw M, Pistenma D, Ray G. Evaluation of extended-field radiotherapy for prostatic neoplasm: 1976 progress report. Cancer Treat Rep 1977;61:297-306.

15 Roach M, DeSilvio M, Lawton C. Phase III trial comparing whole-pelvic versus prostate-only radiotherapy and neoadjuvant versus adjuvant combined androgen suppression: Radiation Therapy Oncology Group 9413. J Clin Oncol 2003;21:1904-11.

16. Roach M, DeSilvio M, Valicenti R. Whole-pelvis, "mini-pelvis," or prostate-only external beam radiotherapy after neoadjuvant and concurrent hormonal therapy in patients treated in the Radiation Therapy Oncology Group 9413 Trial. Int J Radiat Oncol Biol Phys 2006;66:647-53.

17. Seaward S, Weinberg V, Lewis P. Improved freedom from PSA failure with whole pelvic irradiation for high-risk prostate cancer. Int J Radiat Oncol Biol Phys 1998;42:1055-62.

18. Seaward S, Weinberg V, Lewis P. Identification of a high-risk clinically localized prostate cancer subgroup receiving maximum benefit from whole-pelvic irradiation. Cancer J 1998;4:370-7.

19. Pan C, Kim K, Taylor J. Influence of 3D-CRT pelvic irradiation on outcome in prostate cancer treated with external beam radiotherapy. Int J Radiat Oncol Biol Phys 2002;53: 1139-45.

20. Pilepich MV, Caplan R, Byhardt RW, et al. Phase III trial of androgen suppression using goserelin in unfavorable-prognosis carcinoma of the prostate treated with definitive radiotherapy: report of radiation oncology group protocol 85-31. J Clin Oncol 1997;15:1013-21.

21. D'Amico AV, Schultz D, Loffredo M, et al. Biochemical outcome following external beam radiation therapy with or without androgen suppression therapy for men with clinically localized prostate cancer. JAMA 2000;284:1280-3.

22. D'Amico AV, Manola J, Loffredo M, et al. 6-month androgen suppression plus radiation therapy vs radiation therapy alone for patients with clinically localized prostate cancer. JAMA 2004;292:821-8.

23. Laverdière J, Nabid A, de Bedoya LD, et al. The efficacy and sequencing of a short course of androgen suppression on freedom from biochemical failure when administered with radiation therapy for T2-T3 prostate cancer. J Urol 2004;171: 1137-40.

24. Pilepich MV, Krall J, Sause WT, et al. Prognostic factors in carcinoma of the prostate: analysis of RTOG study 75-06. Int J Radiat Oncol Biol Phys 1987;13:339-49.

25. Pilepich MV, Asbell SO, Krall JM, et al. Correlation of radiotherapeutic parameters and treatment related morbidity: analysis of RTOG study 77-06. Int J Radiat Oncol Biol Phys 1987;13:1007-12.

26. Pilepich MV, Krall JM, John MJ, et al. Hormonal cytoreduction in locally advanced carcinoma of the prostate treated with definitive radiotherapy: preliminary results of RTOG 83-07. Int J Radiat Oncol Biol Phys 1989;16:813-17.

27. Lawton CA, Winter K, Murray K, et al. Updated results of the phase III RTOG trial 85-31. Evaluating the potential benefit of androgen suppression following standard radiation therapy for unfavorable prognosis carcinoma of the prostate. Int J Radiat Oncol Biol Phys 2001;49:937-46.

28. Pilepich MV, Winter K, John MJ, et al. Phase III Radiation Therapy Oncology (RTOG) Trial 86-10 of androgen deprivation before and during radiotherapy in locally advanced carcinoma of the prostate. Int J Radiat Oncol Biol Phys 2001;50: 1243-52.

29. Hanks GE, Pajak TF, Porter A, et al. Phase III trial of long-term adjuvant androgen deprivation after neoadjuvant hormonal cytoreduction and radiotherapy in locally advanced carcinoma of the prostate: the Radiation Therapy Oncology Group Protocol 92–02. J Clin Oncol 2003;21:3972-8.

30. Bolla M, Gonzalez D, Warde P, et al. Improved survival in patients with locally advanced prostate cancer treated with radiotherapy and goserelin. N Engl J Med 1997;337:295-300.

31. Kupelian PA, Potters L, Khuntia D, et al. Radical prostatectomy, external beam radiotherapy < 72 Gy, external beam radiotherapy ≥ 72 Gy, permanent seed implantation, or combined seed/external beam radiotherapy for stage T1–T2 prostate cancer. Int J Radiat Oncol Biol Phys 2004;58:25-33.

32. D'Amico AV, Whittington R, Malkowicz SB, et al. Biochemical outcome after radical prostatectomy, external beam radiation therapy, or interstitial radiation therapy for clinically localized prostate cancer. JAMA 1998;280:969-74.

33. Beyer CB, Brachman DG. Failure free survival following brachytherapy alone for prostate cancer: comparison with external beam radiotherapy. Radiother Oncol 2000;57:263-7.

34. Blasko JC, Grimm PD, Sylsvester JE, et al. The role of external beam radiotherapy with I-125/Pd-103 brachytherapy for prostate carcinoma. Radiother Oncol 2000;57:273-8.

35. Merrick GS, Butler WM, Wallner KE, et al. Impact of supplemental external beam radiotherapy and/or androgen deprivation therapy of biochemical outcome after permanent prostate brachytherapy. Int J Radiat Oncol Biol Phys 2005;61:32-43.

36. Frank SJ, Grimm SD, Sylvester JE, et al. Interstitial implant alone or in combination with external beam radiation therapy for intermediate-risk prostate cancer: a survey of practice patterns in the United States. Brachytherapy 2007;6:2-8.

37. Asbell S, Krall J, Pilepich M. Elective pelvic irradiation in stage A2, B carcinoma of the prostate: analysis of RTOG 77-06. Int J Radiat Oncol Biol Phys 1988;6:1307-16.

38. Ploysongsang S, Aron B, Shehata W. Radiation therapy in prostate cancer: whole pelvis with prostate boost or small field to prostate? Urology 1992;40:18-26.

39. Peeters S, Heemsbergen WD, van Putten WL, et al. Acute and late complications after radiotherapy for prostate cancer: results of a multicenter randomized trial comparing 68 Gy to 78 Gy. Int J Radiat Oncol Biol Phys 2005;61:1019–34.

30 Metastatic prostate cancer

Mike D. Shelley and Malcolm D. Mason

Cochrane Urological Cancers Unit, Velindre NHS Trust, Cardiff, UK

Background

Approximately 10% of men with newly diagnosed prostate cancer present with metastases. In addition, 3–41% of patients with localized (T1–T2) and 12–55% with locally advanced prostate cancer (T3–T4) fail primary therapies and develop metastatic disease at 10 years [1]. When prostate cancer has progressed to this advanced stage, it is incurable. Deaths per year from metastatic prostate cancer are estimated to be 204,000 globally and account for 4–15% of all cancer-related deaths, depending on the proportion of elderly men in the population [2-4].

The main site of metastatic disease is bone and autopsy studies have indicated that 85–100% of men who die of prostate cancer have bone metastases [1]. Factors that are associated with an increased risk of developing metastatic disease include clinical stage, Gleason score > 8, and a pre-therapy PSA of > 20 ng/mL. These factors may allow stratification of patients for treatment selection.

The standard first-line therapy for symptomatic metastatic prostate cancer is androgen suppression therapy which has a response rate of about 85%. Patients who fail first-line therapy may benefit from androgen withdrawal with response rates of 30–40% and duration of about 6 months. Second-line hormone manipulation may also be used but nearly all patients will eventually become refractory to androgen deprivation therapy. At this stage, treatment options are palliative and include chemotherapy, external beam radiotherapy, bisphosphonates and radio-isotopes.

This chapter will present evidence on some of the major issues regarding the treatment of metastatic prostate cancer.

Literature search

Medline, EMBASE and the Cochrane Library were searched for randomized studies, systematic reviews and meta-analyses of treatment interventions in metastatic prostate cancer. Databases were searched from 1966 to 2008 with no language restrictions.

Clinical question 30.1

What is the most effective timing of hormone therapy: immediate or deferred?

The evidence

Androgen suppression is effective in delaying tumor progression in men with prostate cancer. In patients with locally advanced or asymptomatic metastatic prostate cancer, controversy exists concerning the ideal time to initiate hormone therapy. Patients with symptomatic disease should be treated immediately, but for asymptomatic disease the situation is less clear. Due to the protracted course of well-differentiated prostate cancer, many men with asymptomatic disease may die of other causes before disease progression requires intervention, and treating such patients with immediate hormone therapy would expose them to unnecessary treatment-related side-effects such as gynecomastia, cardiotoxicity, osteoporosis, and erectile impotence. In addition, early hormone therapy could theoretically select for androgen-independent cells and prematurely develop a condition which has no viable treatment options. However, early androgen suppression may be more effective when the tumor burden is low and may delay the development of serious complications. Alternatively, delaying hormone treatment could provide an effective treatment when disease progression occurs rather than being palliative to asymptomatic disease. A number of randomized

Evidence-Based Urology. Edited by Philipp Dahm, Roger R. Dmochowski.
© 2010 Blackwell Publishing.

trials have compared the clinical value of giving immediate or delayed androgen deprivation therapy in patients with advanced prostate cancer (Table 30.1).

Between 1960 and 1975, the Veterans Administration Co-operative Urological Research Group (VACURG) conducted a series of randomized trials of various treatments for patients with newly diagnosed prostate cancer [5,6]. In these studies, men with advanced prostate cancer were randomized to various doses of diethylstilbestrol (DES) or to placebo. Those patients in the placebo group received hormone therapy when the disease had progressed, and can thus be considered as receiving deferred hormone therapy. In one trial there was no significant difference in overall

survival between immediate or deferred treatment although only 44% of patients assigned to placebo progressed and actually had their treatment changed. However, a separate study indicated that immediate androgen deprivation (DES 1 mg), beginning at diagnosis, increased overall survival in stages III and IV compared to deferred treatment. However, no statistical p values were reported.

Another study by the Medical Research Council trial randomized 934 men with histologically confirmed adenocarcinoma of the prostate to receive either immediate (N 469) or deferred (N 465) androgen deprivation hormone therapy [7]. Patients had either local disease considered too far advanced for curative treatment (T2–T4) or asymptomatic

Table 30.1 Randomized trials and meta-analyses of immediate versus delayed hormone therapy in metastatic prostate cancer

Authors	Methods	Interventions	Participants	Outcomes	Results
Byar [5]	RCT, single blind, placebo-controlled. Randomization method not stated	Patients randomized to one of the following: placebo (N 485), DES 5 mg (N 476), orchidectomy plus placebo (N 469), orchidectomy plus DES (N 473)	1903 men with confirmed stage III or IV (local spread or distant metastases) prostate cancer	Overall survival (OS) Toxicity	Stage III: 177 deaths with delayed and 184 on immediate HT Stage IV: 189 deaths with delayed and 182 on immediate HT DES arm more cardiotoxicity
Byar & Corle [6]	RCT, placebo-controlled. Randomization method not stated	Patients randomized to one of the following: 0.2 mg DES, 1 mg DES (immediate) 5 mg DES, placebo (delayed)	508 men stage III or IV prostate cancer	Overall survival. Toxicity	0.2 mg DES inactive 5 mg DES very toxic Stage III: 37 of 75 deaths with delayed and 35 of 73 on immediate HT Stage IV: 40 of 53 deaths with delayed and 31 of 55 on immediate HT
MRC [7]	RCT Double-blind, placebo-controlled. Centrally randomized	Immediate treatment: orchidectomy or LHRH analog (N 469) Deferred treatment: the same when progression evident (N 465)	938 men with incurable T2–T2 prostate cancer (500) or asymptomatic metastatic disease (438)	Disease-specific survival (D-SS) Overall survival	Overall survival: 328 deaths in immediate group, 361 in deferred (p<0.01) 203 died of prostate cancer in immediate group, 257 in deferred (p = 0.001)
AHRQ [9]	Systematic review and meta-analysis	Immediate and deferred androgen suppression	Men with clinically confirmed advanced prostate cancer, who were not previously treated with hormonal therapy. 3 trials, 1209 patients	Overall survival	HR 0.914 (95% CI 0.815–1.026) no significant difference No quality of life data available in the trials
Nair [10]	Systematic review and meta-analysis	Immediate and deferred androgen suppression	Men with advanced prostate cancer. 4 trials, 2167 patients	Overall survival	At 10 years the pooled OR (95% CI) was 1.50 (1.04–2.16) significantly in favor of immediate therapy

HR, hazard ratio; HT, hormone therapy; OR, odds ratio; RCT, randomized controlled trial metastatic disease and a life expectancy of 12 months or more. Hormone therapy either commenced immediately at the time of diagnosis or was deferred until the disease had progressed sufficiently to warrant clinical intervention. A significant improvement in overall survival was reported for immediate treatment when all patient groups were pooled. However, when individual groups were analyzed, only men with nonmetastatic disease had a significant improvement in overall survival. In men with metastatic disease at randomization, there was no significant difference in survival between the two arms. Overall, significantly more men receiving deferred hormone therapy developed complications. A more recent review of the data after a longer follow-up indicates that there is no significant difference in overall survival between patients treated immediately and those receiving deferred hormone therapy [8].

A meta-analysis of the three trials discussed above [9] utilized a random effect model that reduced to a fixed effect model when the studies were homogeneous. The combined hazard ratio (95% confidence interval (CI)) was 0.91 (0.815–1.026) where a ratio of less than 1 indicates that immediate therapy is superior, although statistical significant was not reached. A second meta-analysis published by the Cochrane Library [10] included an additional study of immediate versus deferred therapy after radical prostatectomy and pelvic lymphadenopathy in men with node-positive prostate cancer [11]. This analysis concluded that early androgen suppression may provide a small but statistically significant improvement in overall survival at 10 years.

Comment

Although only one trial of men with metastatic prostate cancer documented an improvement in overall survival with immediate treatment (VACURG II), another study reported a reduced rate of severe complications when hormone therapy is given early (MRC). These findings tend to support the use of immediate androgen suppression therapy in metastatic prostate cancer. Evidence and recommendation **Grade 1B**.

Clinical question 30.2

Do data on nonsteroidal antiandrogens support the use of combined androgen blockage?

The evidence

Androgen suppression (AS), either by orchidectomy or medical castration with a luteinizing-hormone releasing-hormone (LHRH) agonist, is the standard first-line treatment

for advanced prostate cancer. This treatment reduces circulating testicular-derived testosterone, thereby minimizing androgen-induced growth stimulation of prostate tumors. However, residual testosterone, secreted by the adrenal glands, may still induce some stimulatory activity on prostate tumor growth. This can be theoretically overcome by blocking androgen receptors in the tumor using antiandrogens. This combined therapeutic approach of using androgen suppression and antiandrogens is termed combined androgen blockage (CAB) or maximum androgen blockage (MAB). Antiandrogens may be steroidal in structure, such as cyproterone acetate, or nonsteroidal, such as nilutamide or flutamide. Both these classes of antiandrogens have been incorporated into randomized trials comparing the efficacy of CAB with AS. It is clinically important to determine whether one class of antiandrogens is superior when used in a CAB regime.

There have been no randomized trials comparing CAB using a nonsteroidal antiandrogen with CAB using a steroidal antiandrogen. However, a large meta-analysis undertaken by the Prostate Cancer Trialists Collaborative Group compared 27 randomized trials of CAB versus AS and provided a separate analysis of trials incorporating nonsteroidal and steroidal antiandrogens [12].

Individual patient data were collected from the 27 trials and included information on stage, age, assigned treatment, last follow-up, date of death and cause of death. In the CAB regimes orichidectomy or an LHRH agonist was combined with nilitamide in eight trials, flutamide in 12 trials and cyproterone acetate in seven trials, with a total number of patients of 8275. At the end of the study 72% of men had died, of whom 80% had died of prostate cancer. The pooled analysis indicated a 5-year overall survival rate of 25.4% for CAB and 23.6% for AS alone, which was not statistically significant (p = 0.11). When a subgroup analysis was preformed, cyproterone acetate studies, which contributed 20% of the evidence, favored AS alone, with 5-year overall survival rates of 15.4% for CAB and 18.1% for AS (p = 0.04). However, the studies using the nonsteroidal antiandrogens in the CAB regime were significantly in favor of CAB, with 5-year overall survival rates of 27.4% for CAB and 24.7% for AS alone (p = 0.005).

Comment

The evidence suggests that the administration of CAB using nonsteroidal antiandrogens appears to be superior in terms of overall survival compared to the use of steroidal antiandrogens. However, the absolute difference in 5-year overall survival rates between CAB when using nonsteroidal antiandrogens and AS is only 2.9%. Evidence and recommendation **Grade 2B**.

Clinical question 30.3

Does intermittent androgen deprivation therapy reduce the side effects compared to continuous treatment?

The evidence

Continuous androgen suppression (CAS) produces excellent short-term results for advanced prostate cancer but the long-term outcome is limited by treatment-related side effects and the development of disease unresponsive to androgen manipulation. Intermittent androgen suppression (IAS) may inhibit metabolic pathways associated with the onset of androgen-independent disease and is a relatively recent area of research. With IAS, patients are treated with androgen deprivation for a period of time until a clinical or biochemical response is achieved, at which point the treatment is stopped. Active monitoring is continued until there is evidence of disease progression, when androgen deprivation therapy is started again and this cycle is repeated. The major aims of IAS are to maintain androgen responsiveness and to reduce the toxicity associated with continuous hormone therapy, in particular restoration of sexual function between treatment cycles.

Five randomized trials have compared IAS with CAS in patients with metastatic prostate cancer (Table 30.2). One small study reported that fewer patients developed hormone resistance when receiving IAS compared to CAS (10% versus 38%) [13]. Potency was maintained in 96% of men during the intervals between IAS cycles

Table 30.2 Randomized trials comparing intermittent versus continuous hormone therapy in metastatic prostate cancer

Authors	Methods	Interventions	Participants	Outcomes	Results
Hering [13]	RCT, single center. Randomization method not stated	200 mg/day cyproterone acetate in both arms. IAS stopped when PSA nadir reached and restarted at pretreatment PSA	43 men with confirmed stage D2 prostate cancer. T3–T4 M+ with or without nodal disease	Toxicity response Disease progression	No difference in toxicity (p = 0.39) (gastrointestinal, gynecomastia, asthenia, vomiting). No difference in impotence rate (p = 0.62) 39% on CAS and 16% on IAS became hormone resistant
Langenhuijsen [16]	Multicenter RCT Randomization method not stated	All had 24-week induction of MAB (busurelin plus nilutamide), then randomized to IAS or CAS	97 IAS, 96 CAS 155 T2–4,NxM1, 38 T2–4N1–3M0, PSA <4 ng/mL	Progression Overall survival Toxicity Quality of life	Median TTP: 18 months IAS, 24 months CAS. Withdrawals for adverse events: 20 CAS, 6 IAS No significant difference in QOL No difference in overall survival at 66 months follow-up
De Leval [15]	RCT Randomization method not stated	Initial flutamide 25 mg × 3 daily. Then 3–6 months MAB flutamide plus goserelin (3.6 mg monthly) × 3–6. Then randomized to IAS or CAS. IAS restarted at PSA 10 ng/mL	77 men with advanced prostate cancer. T3 or T4 and/or metastatic, or relapsed with PSA >4 ng/mL	Toxicity	Toxicity: hot flushes, loss of libido, erectile dysfunction – less with IAS (no p value)
Calais [14]	Multicenter RCT Randomization method not stated	Three-month induction MAB (cyproterone acetate (CPA) 200 mg for 2 weeks then monthly decapeptyl plus 200 mg CPA daily). Then randomized to IAS or CAS	626 randomized. T3–T4 M0 and M1 PSA >4 ng/mL	Toxicity Quality of life Survival	Side effects minor (hot flushes most common) – no difference QOL scores similar in each arm No difference in overall survival (p = 0.84)
Miller [19]	Prospective, multicenter RCT	Goserelin plus bicalutamide for IAS and CAS. All had 24-week induction of MAB	335 men with advanced prostate cancer. Stages T1–4,N1–3 or T1–4N0–3,M1	Progression Survival Quality of life Toxicity	Median TTP: 16.6 months IAS, 11.5 months CAS (log rank p = 0.1758) Median time to death (any cause): 51.4 months IAS, 53.8 months CAS (p = 0.658) No difference in adverse events

and post treatment in 40% on IAS and 25% on CAS [14]. Three studies reported no difference in toxicities between patients groups although one observed the frequency of hot flushes, loss of libido and erectile function was less with IAS [15]. Quality of life was improved with IAS in one study [13] and similar in both arms in two trials [14,16]. There was no significant improvement in overall survival [14,16].

A systematic review of these four studies, plus an additional randomized trial on men with nonmetastatic disease but locally advanced prostate cancer [17], concluded that IAS has a slightly reduced adverse event rate compared to CAS and appears more favouable in controlling impotence [18].

A more recent randomized trial, not included in the above systematic review, reported a reduction in the time to disease progression with IAS compared to CAS but the difference was not statistically significant [19]. Although the incidence of adverse events was similar in both arms of the trial, self-assessment of quality of life and sexual activity favored IAS. In addition, the off-treatment periods with IAS were > 40%, contributing to an overall improvement in quality of life.

Comment

The evidence suggests that IAS appears to be as effective as CAS in terms of overall survival. In addition, IAS has shown encouraging results with a trend towards an improvement in treatment-related side effects and quality of life. Evidence and recommendation **Grade 1B**.

Clinical question 30.4

How effective is docetaxel chemotherapy in metastatic prostate cancer?

The evidence

For many years, metastatic prostate cancer was considered to be unresponsive to chemotherapy. However, the last decade has seen a major turnaround in this concept and now chemotherapy is an important treatment option for men with this condition. Recent randomized studies of docetaxel [20-23] were pivotal in changing medical opinion on the use of chemotherapy because they were the first to suggest that an improvement in overall survival was attainable with chemotherapy (Table 30.3).

Two of these studies were particularly important. In the first, overall survival was the primary endpoint when comparing mitoxantrone plus prednisone, considered to be the standard palliative treatment, with two schedules of docetaxel plus prednisone [22]. Docetaxel was administered

using a weekly or 3-weekly schedule. When compared to the mitoxantrone arm, the hazard ratio for death in the 3-weekly docetaxel arm was 0.76 (95% CI 0.62–0.94, p = 0.009) and that for the weekly schedule was 0.91 (95% CI 0.75–1.11, p = 0.36). This indicates a statistically significant improvement in overall survival with the 3-weekly docetaxel regime, with a 24% reduction in the risk of death. In addition, a significant reduction in pain was observed in patients receiving the 3-weekly docetaxel regimen compared to the mitoxantrone arm (35% versus 22%, p = 0.01) but not with the weekly schedule (31%), although the median duration of pain response (3.5–5.6 months) was not significantly different between groups. The quality of life assessment also showed a significant improvement with the 3-weekly schedule of docetaxel compared to those treated with mitoxantrone (22% versus 13%, p = 0.009). Grade 3/4 neutropenia was significantly more common with the 3-weekly docetaxel (32%) than for those patients receiving weekly docetaxel or mitoxantrone (2% and 22%), although the frequency of febrile neutropenia was less than 4% in all arms. Nausea and vomiting were common with all regimens (38–42%) and diarrhea was significantly more frequent with both docetaxel schedules. Discontinuation of treatment with docetaxel was due to fatigue, musculoskeletal events, nail changes, sensory neuropathy, and infection whereas for mitoxantrone, cardiac dysfunction was the major reason.

The second randomized trial compared mitoxantrone plus prednisone with docetaxel plus estramustine in patients with hormone-refractory prostate cancer, with overall survival as the primary endpoint [23]. The results indicated a significant improvement in overall survival, median time to disease progression, and the percentage of patients achieving a PSA response for the docetaxel-estramustine arm. However, this regime was significantly more toxic in terms of gastrointestinal side effects (p = 0.001), nausea and vomiting (p = 0.001), infection (p = 0.004), metabolic toxicity (p < 0.001) and neurological dysfunction (p = 0.001). It should also be noted that there was no significant difference in pain relief between the two groups as assessed by the patients.

Comment

These randomized studies have established the efficacy of docetaxel in combination with prednisone for the treatment of metastatic prostate cancer and should be considered the chemotherapeutic regime of first choice for men with this disease. Evidence and recommendation **Grade 1A**.

Clinical question 30.5

What is the role of bisphosphonates in metastatic prostate cancer?

Table 30.3 Randomized studies of docetaxel in metastatic hormone-refractory prostate cancer

Randomized trial	Interventions compared	Dose and schedule	Patients randomized	% PSA response	Median time to progression (months)	Median overall survival (months)
Dahut [20]	1. Docetaxel	30 mg/m^2 IV weekly × 3	25	37	3.7	14.7
	2. Docetaxel halidomide	As above 200 mg orally daily	50	53	5.9	28.9
Oudard [21]	1. Docetaxel Estramustine Prednisone	70 mg/m^2 on day 2 every 21 days 280 mg twice daily (max 840 mg) 10 mg/day	44	67*	8.8*	18.6
	2. Docetaxel Estramustine Prednisone	35 mg/m^2 days 2 & 9 every 21 days 280 mg twice daily (max 840 mg) 10 mg/day	44	63*	9.3*	18.4
	3. Mitoxantrone Prednisone	12 mg/m^2 every 21 days 10 mg/day	42	18	17.0	13.4
Tannock [22]	1. Docetaxel Prednisone	75 mg/m^2 every 3 weeks 5 mg twice daily	335	45*	38	18.9*
	2. Docetaxel Prednisone	30 mg/m^2 weekly 5 mg twice daily	334	48*	35	17.4
	3. Mitoxantrone Prednisone	12 mg/m^2 every 3 weeks 5 mg twice daily	337	32	56	16.5
Petrylak [23]	1. Docetaxel Estramustine	60 mg/m^2 days 2 & 6 280 mg days 1–5	386	50*	6.3*	17.5*
	2. Mitoxantrone Prednisone	12 mg/m^2 day 1 5 mg twice daily	384	27	3.2	15.6

*Significantly different, p<0.05

The evidence

Between 35% and 85% of men with advanced prostate cancer will have bone metastases. The invasion of metastatic malignant cells into the bone marrow is thought to induce abnormal ostoeblastic bone formation which is preceded by osteoclastic activation. Bone resorption and synthesis may become uncoupled and unbalanced, leading to inappropriate new bone formation and loss of bone integrity. This leads to the clinical syndrome of bone pain, an increased susceptibility to fracture and spinal cord compression. Whilst radiotherapy and chemotherapy are clinically useful for men with this condition, the side effects limit their use. Bisphosphonates are a relatively recent therapy that has shown activity in the treatment of bone metastases from prostate cancer.

Early clinical trials using bisphosphonates such as etidronate failed to show significant evidence of activity. More encouraging results were reported by a randomized MRC study, which showed a reduction in time to bone progression-free survival with clodronate compared to placebo [24]. However, there are now several bisphosphonates

available, and the second-generation, nitrogen-containing bisphosphonates, such as zoledronate, pamidronate, alendronate and risedronate, appear to be more potent.

Zoledronate was evaluated in a double-blind trial in which 435 men with hormone-refractory prostate cancer and bone metastases were randomized to 8 mg (reducing to 2 mg) zoledronate or placebo [25]. Skeletal-related events were significantly reduced with 4 mg zoledronate (33.2% and 44.2%, p = 0.021). In addition, the median time to the first skeletal event was significantly increased with zoledronate (p = 0.01). The 4 mg dose appeared to be well tolerated. An update of this study confirmed that zoledronate reduced the risk of skeletal-related events by 36% (risk ratio 0.64, 95% CI 0.485–0.845, p = 0.002) [26].

A more recent systematic review and meta-analysis of bisphosphonates for advanced metastatic prostate cancer analyzed data from 10 randomized trials including 1955 men with advanced prostate cancer [27]. This review reported that pain response rates were improved with bisphosphonates compared to controls (27.9% versus 21.1%, p = 0.07). In addition, the rate of skeletal-related events was significantly reduced with bisphosphonates (37.8%

versus 43%, p = 0.05). Although nausea and vomiting were significantly increased with bisphosphonates, no other increase in adverse events was observed.

Bisphosphonates have also been evaluated for their role in reducing bone mineral loss associated with androgen deprivation therapy for advanced prostate cancer. In a randomized trial, pamidronate has been shown to reduce bone loss in hip and lumbar spine in men receiving leuprolide for the treatment of advanced or recurrent prostate cancer [28]. Similarly, zoledronic acid is reported to increase bone mineral density in hip and spine during androgen deprivation therapy for prostate cancer [29].

Comment

Bisphosphonates, especially the more potent ones, have a clinical role in alleviating bone pain from metastatic prostate cancer that is refractory to other pain-controlling therapies. In addition, clinical benefits can be achieved in controlling skeletal-related events as well as limiting bone density loss due to androgen suppression therapy. Evidence and recommendation **Grade 2B**.

Clinical question 30.6

How effective are radio-isotopes in alleviating pain in metastatic prostate cancer?

The evidence

Radio-isotopes are used to treat prostate cancer that has metastasized to the bone. They are administered intravenously and follow a similar distribution pattern to that of calcium. Consequently, radio-isotopes tend to localize in bone, especially in the metastatic lesions. Two radio-isotopes, strontium-89 (^{89}Sr) and samarium-153 (^{153}Sm), have been approved in the USA and Europe for the palliation of pain associated with bone metastases in advanced prostate cancer. Extensive observational studies have shown that radio-isotopes are effective in inducing pain relief, with response rates between 45% and 95% [30]. However, randomized trials are needed to establish whether elemental strontium has an effect itself or whether there is a placebo effect.

^{89}Strontium has been compared to placebo in two randomized studies (Table 30.4). The first was a double-blind study of 49 patients receiving either 3 injections at monthly intervals of 75 Mbq ^{89}Sr or saline as the placebo [31]. Pain relief was similar in both groups although the 2-year survival rate was significantly superior in those patients receiving ^{89}Sr. The second study recruited 32 patients and compared ^{89}Sr to stable strontium as the placebo [32]. Response was assessed at 5 weeks post therapy and was

scored according the patient's general condition, mobility, analgesic consumption and pain analysis. There was a significantly better therapeutic response with ^{89}Sr compared to placebo (p < 0.01) and complete pain relief was only observed on the active treatment arm.

The therapeutic value of ^{89}Sr as an adjunct to external beam radiotherapy in endocrine-resistant metastatic prostate cancer bone pain has been assessed in a Canadian phase III trial [33]. Patients received local field radiotherapy to the painful site at doses of either 30 Gy over 14 days or 20 Gy over 7 days. They were then randomized to either ^{89}Sr or saline placebo. Although there was no significant difference in pain relief and survival between patient groups, there was a significant reduction in analgesic consumption (p < 0.05) with ^{89}Sr and progression of pain, as measured by new sites of pain (p < 0.002). A randomized study conducted by the EORTC directly compared ^{89}Sr with palliative local field radiotherapy [34]. Overall survival was better with local field radiotherapy although this was of borderline significance (p = 0.048). However, there was no difference in progression-free survival, subjective response or biochemical response (see Table 30.3). An additional study randomized men to radiotherapy (local or hemi-body) or ^{89}Sr and showed similar rates for pain response and overall survival, but with fewer new pain sites for ^{89}Sr [35].

In an attempt to enhance the activity of radio-isotope therapy for painful bone metastases, the effect of low-dose cisplatin plus ^{89}Sr has been assessed by an Italian group [36]. Patients were randomized to ^{89}Sr plus cisplatin or ^{89}Sr plus placebo. Pain response was significantly greater and longer in those men receiving cisplatin, with significantly fewer new pain sites. In addition, bone disease progression was less in the cisplatin arm. There was no difference in toxicity or survival.

Recently, a randomized placebo-controlled trial assessed the efficacy and toxicity of ^{153}Sm in men with painful metastatic prostate cancer [37]. At 4 weeks analgesic consumption was significantly reduced (p < 0.05) and pain assessment was significantly improved (p = 0.004) in those men receiving ^{153}Sm compared to placebo. Mild and reversible myelosuppression was the only clinically important side effect observed with ^{153}Sm. There was no difference in overall survival between the ^{153}Sm and placebo groups.

The alpha-emitter radium 223 (^{223}Ra) has also shown promise in symptomatic hormone-refractory prostate cancer [38]. In this placebo-controlled, randomized phase II study, bone alkaline phosphatase, a marker of bone turnover, was significantly reduced in men receiving ^{223}Ra. The time to PSA progression was significantly increased in the treatment arm, as was the time to the first skeletal-related event. Toxicities were similar in both arms of the trial.

Toxicities associated with systemic radio-isotopes are mainly hematological and generally mild and reversible (see Table 30.3). In addition, some studies have observed

Table 30.4 Randomized trials of systemic radio-isotopes for the palliation of hormone-refractory prostate cancer

Authors	Methods	Interventions	Participants	Outcomes	Results
Buchali [31]	RCT, double-blind, placebo-controlled Randomization method not stated	Comparison of ^{89}Sr (3 doses 75 MBq – monthly; or placebo (saline)	49 men with advanced prostate cancer and multiple metastases 45 were either T3 or T4	Pain – reports at 9 & 12 weeks, scintigraphy, radiography, hematology	41 had pain requiring analgesics. 7/19 (37%) and 11/22 (50%) had pain relief with ^{89}Sr and placebo respectively (NS) Scintigraphy (26 evaluable) – regression or stable assessment in 8/15 (33%) ^{89}Sr and 5/11 (45%) placebo (NS) Survival – rate at 2 yrs 46% ^{89}Sr vs 4% placebo (p<0.05) Thrombocytopenia 11/22 in ^{89}Sr (50%) (irreversible in 5), 4/17 in placebo (24%)
Lewington [32]	RCT, double-blind, placebo-controlled Randomization method not stated	Randomized to either stable strontium (placebo N 12) or Sr^{89} 150 MBq (N 14). Cross-over at 6 weeks	26 of 32 evaluable pts with prostate cancer and refractory painful bone metastases. 64–79 years All had increasing requirement for analgesics	Response evaluated after 1st and 2nd injections combined: performance status, analgesic use, extent of disease (bone imaging), and pain (sites scored)	^{89}Sr more effective than placebo 1st injection p<0.01 2nd injection p<0.03 1st assessment for ^{89}Sr and placebo: CR in 4 (33%) and 0, substantial in 1 (8%) and 1 (7%), some in 3 (25%) and 2 (14%), no relief in 4 (33%) and 11(78%) 3 pts had Gr. 4 platelet (1 had placebo, 2 had ^{89}Sr)
Porter [33]	RCT, placebo-controlled, Randomization method unclear	All pts received local field RT (30 Gy/d × 14 d or 20 Gy × 5/7 d). Then randomized to placebo (saline) or Sr^{89} 10.8 mCi	126 men with HRPC from 8 Canadian cancer centers Both groups 71 yrs (48–86 ^{89}Sr, 57–82 placebo) PS 72.3 ^{89}Sr, 78.2 placebo	PS. Pain – RTOG system used – severity (0–4) & frequency (0–4) of pain Analgesic intake scored 0–4 (potency + frequency). Quality of life	Overall median survival 30.5 wks (^{89}Sr 27, placebo 34 wks, p = 0.6) At 3 months 17.1% on ^{89}Sr stopped analgesics compared to 2.4% on placebo (p<0.05) At 6 months, CR and PR 40% & 40% (^{89}Sr) vs 30% & 20% (placebo) More patients on placebo had new active pain sites (1.2 vs 0.59, p<0.002) >50% ↓ in PSA – 50% (^{89}Sr), 10% (placebo) (p<0.01), QOL superior with ^{89}Sr (p<0.05) ^{89}Sr vs placebo – WBC: Gr.3–4, 8 (11%) vs 0; platelets: Gr.3–4, 22 (24%) vs 2 (3.5%)
Oosterhof [34]	RCT, multicenter No randomization method stated	Sr^{89} 150 MBq (4 mCi) IV (N 101) or RT = median 20 Gy/5 (4 Gy/1 – 43 Gy/24) (N 102), with 6-weekly follow-up	203 HRPC (71 yrs, 44–86) with painful bone metastases	Response rate: subjective – progression Survival Toxicity PSA response ↓ ≥50%	Subjective response rate: 34.7% ^{89}Sr, 33.3% RT. PSA response: 13% ^{89}Sr, 10% RT. TTP 3.0 months ^{89}Sr, 3.3 months RT. PFS 3.0 months ^{89}Sr, 3.3 months RT Survival shorter with Sr^{89} (7.2 & 11.0 months, p = 0.0457). % surviving 1 year; ^{89}Sr 33.7 (24.4–42.9), RT 44.6% (34.9–54.3) Gr. 3/4 NV and diarrhea in 4% & 2% Sr^{89}, 1% & 8.3% RT. Gr. 3–4 hematol 0% ^{89}Sr & 2% RT

Study	Design/method	Intervention	Patients	Outcomes	Results
Quilty [35]	RCT, multicenter. Centrally held randomization schedule	^{89}Sr 200 MBq (5.4 mCi) or RT (HB 6 Gy upper half or 8 Gy lower half, or local field RT 20 Gy daily × 5) Median follow-up 12 weeks	305 men with prostate cancer and painful bone metastases. N 76 ^{89}Sr/72 RT N 77 ^{89}Sr/80 HB	Pain response, Toxicity, Survival	Pain relief: 63.6% HB vs 66.1% ^{89}Sr 61% RT vs 65.9% ^{89}Sr Fewer new sites with ^{89}Sr ($p<0.05$) No difference in survival ($p = 0.01$). Median survival: 33 and 28 weeks for ^{89}Sr and RT ($p = 0.1$) Platelets Gr. 3–4 11 (7%) ^{89}Sr and 5 (3.4%) RT. Gr 3 WBC with ^{89}Sr in 5 (3%). GIT toxicities 10% ^{89}Sr, 27% RT, 43% HB
Sciuto [36]	RCT, placebo-controlled trial Method used random numbers	Randomized to ^{89}Sr 148 MBq + 50 mg/m^2 cisplatin or ^{89}Sr + placebo Follow-up until death	70 men with HRPC and painful bone metastases (69 yrs, 51–89 yrs)	Survival, Pain response at 2 months, Toxicity	Overall response: 32/35 (91%) cisplatin, 22/35 (63%) placebo ($p<0.01$). Respective durations: 120 days and 60 days ($p = 0.002$). New sites: 14% cisplatin, 30% placebo ($p = 0.18$) Median overall survival: 9 months cisplatin, 6 months placebo ($p = 0.3$) Gr. 3–4 anemia 9% cisplatin, 11% placebo
Sartor [37]	RCT, double-blind, placebo-controlled Centrally randomized	Randomized to ^{153}Sm EDTMP (Lexidronam) 1 mCi/kg (N 101) or placebo (nonradio-active ^{153}Sm) (N 51)	152 with HRPC and painful bone metastases	Analgesic use, Pain – measured by patient-derived VAS and PDS, Toxicity	Opioid use reduced with ^{153}Sm ($p<0.028$) VAS and PDS improved with ^{153}Sm ($p<0.05$)
Nilsson [38]	RCT, multicenter, placebo-controlled Centrally randomized	Randomized to ^{223}Ra 50 KBq/kg every 4 weeks (N 33) or placebo (saline) every 4 weeks (N 31)	64 patients from 12 European centers. All had confirmed prostate cancer and at least one painful bone lesion	Alkaline phosphatase (AP), Skeletal-related events (SRE), PSA response, Overall survival (OS)	Median change in AP: 65% ^{223}Ra and 9.3% placebo ($p<0.001$) HR for first SRE: 1.75 (0.96–3.19, $p = 0.065$) Median time to PSA progression: 26 weeks ^{223}Ra and 8 weeks placebo ($p = 0.048$) Median OS: 65.3 weeks ^{223}Ra and 46.4 weeks placebo ($p = 0.02$)

CR, complete response; HB, hemi-body radiation; HR, hazard ratio; HRPC, hormone-refractory prostate cancer; NS, not significant; NV, nausea and vomiting; PDS, Pain Descriptor Scales; PFS, progression-free survival; PS, performance status; PSA, prostatic-specific antigen; QOL, quality of life; RCT, randomized controlled trial; RT, radiotherapy; TTP, time to progression; VAS, visual analog scales an antitumor activity of radio-isotopes as measured by a fall in serum PSA and reduced evidence of tumor on post-treatment bone scans.

Comment

External beam radiotherapy offers excellent palliation of focal painful bone lesions in metastatic prostate cancer but may require repeated treatment when multiple sites are evident. Bone-seeking radio-isotopes provide an effective alternative therapy for pain relief. Combining chemotherapy with radio-isotopes may improve efficacy. Repeated doses appear to be safe and may provide sustained pain relief compared to a single treatment. Evidence and recommendation Grade 1A.

Implications for practice

It is strongly recommended that men with symptomatic metastatic prostate cancer should be offered immediate androgen suppression therapy. This may be achieved by bilateral orchidectomy or by use of a LHRH analog. Combined androgen blockade appears to be only marginally better in terms of survival but is more toxic, and the decision to use additional antiandrogens requires informed discussion. Intermittent androgen suppression therapy should be considered as an alternative to continuous androgen suppression therapy, especially in men experiencing severe side effects from androgen suppression. In patients whose disease has become unresponsive to androgen suppression therapy, docetaxel-based chemotherapy is recommended. When painful bony metastases develop, radiotherapy, using either external beam radiotherapy or systemic radio-isotopes (^{89}Sr or ^{153}Sm), should be offered as palliative therapy.

Implications for research

Men with metastatic prostate cancer currently receive androgen suppression therapy for an indefinite period but it is unclear how long therapy should last. Prolonged androgen suppression therapy leads to many complications such as loss of bone and osteoporosis and this affects quality of life. More studies are needed to establish clear guidelines to identify those men who are experiencing severe side effects of androgen suppression therapy and who would not benefit from continued therapy. Limited evidence suggests that in some men, testosterone remains low following several years of androgen suppression therapy, possibly due to destruction of Leydig cells by continued gondotropin deprivation. Studies should address whether measuring testosterone levels aids in identifying these men to help justify continued withdrawal of therapy.

Although the results for intermittent androgen suppression therapy are encouraging, the conclusions are limited by few studies, with small sample size and short duration. Further randomized trials are needed to establish the full potential benefits of intermittent androgen suppression therapy. Such trials should establish whether survival and quality of life for men with metastatic prostate cancer are significantly improved. Newer hormonal agents, such as abiraterone acetate, may be promising, but the results of the ongoing phase III trials should be awaited before making further recommendations.

The precise role of bisphosphonates in the treatment of metastatic bone disease needs further evaluation. The next generation of clinical trials should address the complementary activity of bisphosphonates with radiotherapy and chemotherapy as this would probably reflect the clinical setting under which bisphosphonates may be administered. The relative benefits of bisphosphonates and radiotherapy are being evaluated in the RIB UK study which should report in the near future. Additional studies are needed to establish the role of bisphosphonates, supplemented with calcium and vitamin D in the prevention of bone loss during hormone therapy.

The development of new treatments requires the identification of novel target sites for intervention. Several new potential therapies for advanced and metastatic prostate cancer are being investigated and include epothilones, antiangiogenic agents, vaccines, cyclo-oxygenase inhibitors, EGFR inhibitors, and endothelin antagonists. These may provide new opportunities in the near future to improve on the management of this debilitating disease.

References

1. Carlin BI, Andriole GL. The natural history, skeletal complications, and management of bone metastases in patients with prostate carcinoma. Cancer 2000;88:2989-94.
2. Jemal A, Siegel R, Ward E, Murray T, Xu J, Tham MJ. Cancer statistics 2007. Ca Cancer J Clin 2007;57:43-66.
3. Parkin DM. Global cancer statistics in the year 2000. Lancet Oncol 2001;2:533-43.
4. Quin M, Babb P. Patterns and trends in prostate cancer incidence, survival, prevalence and mortality. Part 1: International comparisons. BJU Int 2002;90(2):162-73.
5. Byar DP. Proceedings: The Veterans Administration Cooperative Urological Research Group's studies of cancer of the prostate. Cancer 1973;32(5):1126-30.
6. Byar DP, Corle DK. Hormone therapy for prostate cancer: results of the Veterans Administration Cooperative Urological Research Group studies. NCI Monographs 1988;7:165-70.
7. Medical Research Council Prostate Cancer Working Party Investigators Group. Immediate versus deferred treatment for advanced prostatic cancer: initial results of the Medical Research Council trial. BJU 1997;79:235-46.

8. Kirk D, for the Medical Research Council Prostate Cancer Working Party Investigators Group. Immediate vs deferred hormone treatment for prostate cancer: how safe is androgen deprivation? BJU Int 2000;86(suppl 3):220.

9. Agency for Health Care Research and Quality (AHRQ). Relative effectiveness and cost-effectiveness of methods of androgen suppression in the treatment of advanced prostate cancer. Report No. 4. Rockville, MD: Agency for Health Care Research and Quality, 1999.

10. Nair B, Wilt T, MacDonald R, Rutks I. Early versus deferred androgen suppression in the treatment of advanced prostate cancer. Cochrane Library. Oxford: Update Software, 2002.

11. Messing EM, Manola J, Sarsody M, Wilding G, Crawford ED, Trump D. Immediate hormone therapy compared with observation after radical prostatectomy and pelvic lymph adenopathy in men with node-positive prostate cancer. N Engl J Med 1999;341:1781-8.

12. Prostate Cancer Trialists Collaborative Group. Maximum androgen blockade in advanced prostate cancer: an overview of the randomized trials. Lancet 2000;355:1491-8.

13. Hering F, Rodrigues PRT, Lipay MA, Nesrallah L, Srougi M. Metastatic adenocarcinoma of the prostate: comparison between continuous and intermittent hormone treatment. Braz J Urol 2000;26(3):276-82.

14. Calais F, Bono A, Whelan, P, et al. Phase III study of intermittent MAB versus continuous MAB – an international cooperative study – quality of life. Eur Urol 2006 5(2):209.

15. De Leval J, Boca P, Yousef E, Nicolas H, Jeukenne M, Seidel M. Intermittent versus continuous total androgen blockade in the treatment of patients with advanced hormone-naive prostate cancer: results of a prospective randomized multicentre trial. Clin Prostate Cancer 2002:1(3):163-7.

16. Langenhuijsen JF, Schasfoort EMC, Heathcote P, et al. Intermittent androgen suppression in patients with advanced prostate cancer: an update of the TULP survival data. Proceedings of the European Association of Urology Conference, Milan, 2008, Abstract No. 538.

17. Yamanaka H, Ito K, Naito S, Tsukamoto T, Usami M, Fujimoto H. Effectiveness of adjuvant intermittent endocrine therapy following neoadjuvant endocrine therapy and external beam radiation therapy in men with locally advanced prostate cancer. Prostate 2005;63(1):56-64.

18. Conti PD, Atallah AN, Arruda H, Soares BGO, Dib EL, Wilt TJ. Intermittent versus continuous androgen suppression for prostate cancer. Cochrane Database Syst Rev 2007;4:CD005009.

19. Miller K, Steiner U, Lingnau A, et al. Randomized prospective study of intermittent versus continuous androgen suppression in advanced prostate cancer. ASCO Annual Meeting Proceedings, Chicago, 2007, Abstract No. 5015.

20. Dahut DD, Gulley J, Arlem P, et al. Randomized phase II trial of docetaxel plus thalidomide in androgen-independent prostate cancer. J Clin Oncol 2004;22(13):2532-9.

21. Oudard S, Banu E, Beuzeboc P, et al. Multi-centre randomized phase II study of two schedules of docetaxel, estramustine, and prednisone versus mitoxantrone plus prednisone in patients with metastatic hormone-refractory prostate cancer. J Clin Oncol 2005;23(15):3343-51.

22. Tannock IF, de Wit R, Berry WR, et al. Docetaxel plus prednisone or mitoxantrone plus prednisone for advanced prostate cancer. N Engl J Med 2004;352:1502-12.

23. Petrylak DP, Tangen CM, Hussain MH, et al. Docetaxel and estramustine compared with mitoxantrone and prednisone for advanced refractory prostate cancer. N Engl J Med 2004;35:1513-20.

24. Dearnaley D, Sydes M, Mason M, et al. A double-blind, placebo-controlled randomized trial of oral sodium chlodronate for metastatic prostate cancer (MRC PRO5 trial). J Nat Cancer Inst 2003;95(17):1300-11.

25. Saad F, Gleason DM, Murray R, et al. A randomized placebo controlled trial of zoledronic acid in patients with HRPC. J Nat Cancer Inst 2002;94:364-9.

26. Saad F, Gleason D, Murray R, et al. Long-term efficacy of zoledronic acid for the prevention of skeletal complications in patients with metastatic hormone-refractory prostate cancer. J Nat Cancer Inst 2004;96(11):879-82.

27. Yuen KK, Shelley MD, Sze WM, Wilt T, Mason M. Bisphosphonates for advanced prostate cancer. Cochrane Database Syst Rev 2006;4:CD006250.

28. Smith MR, McGoven FJ, Zietman A, et al Pamidronate to prevent bone loss during androgen-deprivation therapy for prostate cancer. N Engl J Med 2001;345:948-55.

29. Smith MR, Eastman J, Gleason D, Shasha D, Tchekmedyian S, Zinner N. Randomized controlled trial of zoledronic acid to prevent bone loss in men receiving androgen deprivation therapy for nonmetastatic prostate cancer. J Urol 2003;169:2008-12.

30. Finlay IG, Mason MD, Shelley M. Radio-isotopes for the palliation of metastatic bone cancer: a systematic review. Lancet Oncol 2005;6:392-400.

31. Buchali K, Correns HJ, Schuerer M, Schnorr D, Lips H, Sydow K. Results of a double blind study of 89-strontium therapy of skeletal metastases of prostatic carcinoma. Eur J Nucl Med 1988;14(7-8):349-51.

32. Lewington VJ, McEwan AJ, Ackery DM, et al. A prospective, randomized double-blind crossover study to examine the efficacy of strontium-89 in pain palliation in patients with advanced prostate cancer metastatic to bone. Eur J Cancer 1991;27(8):954-8.

33. Porter AT, McEwan AJ, Powe JE, et al. Results of a randomized phase-III trial to evaluate the efficacy of strontium-89 adjuvant to local field external beam irradiation in the management of endocrine resistant metastatic prostate cancer. Int J Rad Oncol Biol Phys 1993;25(5):805-13.

34. Oosterhof GO, Roberts JT, de Reijke TM, et al. Strontium(89) chloride versus palliative local field radiotherapy in patients with hormonal escaped prostate cancer: a phase III study of the European Organisation for Research and Treatment of Cancer, Genitourinary Group. Eur Urol 2003;4(5):519-26.

35. Quilty PM, Kirk D, Bolger JJ, etal. A comparison of the palliative effects of strontium-89 and external beam radiotherapy in metastatic prostate cancer. Radiother Oncol 1994;31:33-40.

36. Sciuto R, Festa A, Rea S, et al. Effects of low-dose cisplatin on 89Sr therapy for painful bone metastases from prostate cancer: a randomized clinical trial. J Nucl Med 2002;43(1):79-86.

37. Sartor O, Reid RH, Hoskin PJ, et al. Samarium-153-Lexidronam complex for treatment of painful bone metastases in hormone-refractory prostate cancer. Urology 2004;63(5):940-5.

38. Nilsson S, Franzen L, Parker C, et al. Bone targeted radium-223 in symptomatic HRPC. Lancet Oncol 2007;8:587-94.

31 Treatment of superficial bladder cancer

Alexander Karl[1,2] *and Badrinath R. Konety*[2]

[1]Department of Urology, School of Medicine, University of California-San Francisco, San Francisco, CA, USA
[2]Department of Urology, University of Munich LMU, Munich, Germany

Background

In the Western world, transitional cell carcinoma (TCC) of the bladder represents the fourth most frequently diagnosed malignancy. In 2008, an estimated 68,810 new incidences of TCC of the bladder will be diagnosed in the US [1]. Of the patients newly diagnosed with bladder cancer, approximately 75–85% present with a nonmuscle-invasive (superficial) tumor. A wide range of recurrence and progression rates has been reported among patients with bladder cancer, and these rates depend largely on the number of tumors initially identified, tumor size, prior recurrence rate, T category, grade and concomitant carcinoma *in situ* (CIS). According to data from the European Organization for Research and Treatment of Cancer (EORTC), the probability of recurrence 5 years after the initial diagnosis is 31–78%, and the probability of progression at 5 years is < 1–45% [2]. These high recurrence and progression rates necessitate long-term surveillance and various adjuvant therapeutic strategies in patients with bladder cancer.

Treatment options

Depending on the estimated aggressiveness of the disease, therapeutic options range from a single transurethral resection of bladder tumor (TURBT) with early post transurethral resection (TUR) instillation therapy over TURBT followed by multiple cycles of intravesical chemo- or immunotherapy (bacille Calmette–Guerin: BCG) to radical cystectomy.

The aim of the initial TURBT or biopsy is to obtain tissue for the correct diagnosis and to remove all visible lesions. The resection strategy depends on the size and number of the lesions. A complete and correct TUR has been reported to be essential for optimizing response [3].

Generally, after TURBT of nonmuscle-invasive bladder cancer, one immediate postoperative instillation of chemotherapy is recommended. The need for further adjuvant intravesical therapy depends on the calculated aggressiveness of the detected tumor. Different chemotherapeutic agents are used in a variety of application schedules. BCG as intravesical immunotherapy has shown the ability to reduce recurrence and even progression rates in high-grade superficial tumors. Finally, there is the option of immediate cystectomy in those patients who present with nonmuscle-invasive tumor but may have a high risk of progression based on pathological features. Reported indicators for a higher risk of progression are multiple recurrent high-grade tumors, high-grade T1 tumors, and high-grade tumors with concomitant CIS. In such patients, a delayed cystectomy could lead to decreased disease-specific survival [4].

Clinical question 31.1

What is the benefit from a single immediate postoperative intravesical instillation of a chemotherapeutic agent?

Literature search

We searched for systematic reviews, meta-analyses, randomized trials and observational studies in the Cochrane Library (2008) and Medline (1966–Jan 2009) using the search terms: "bladder cancer," "instillation therapy," "early intra-vesical chemotherapy," "immediate instillation," "early instillation," "urothelial carcinoma."

The evidence

A meta-analysis of seven randomized trials involving 1476 patients with a median follow-up of 3.4 years found that one immediate instillation of chemotherapy within 6–24

Evidence-Based Urology. Edited by Philipp Dahm, Roger R. Dmochowski.
© 2010 Blackwell Publishing.

hours post TURBT has the ability to decrease the recurrence rate by 12% and the odds of recurrence by 39% [5]. Other studies demonstrate that immediate chemo-instillation after TURBT reduces the risk of recurrence by about 50% at 2 years and ≥ 15% at 5 years [6-9]. Mitomycin C, epirubicin and doxorubicin have been shown to be comparably beneficial [5]. Another randomized prospective study demonstrates that a delayed instillation therapy (between 7 and 15 days after the initial resection) is associated with a significantly higher recurrence rate compared to an immediate instillation therapy if no maintenance therapy is applied [7] (see Table 31.1). Immediate instillation therapy has no reported influence on the progression rate or overall survival of patients with superficial bladder cancer.

Comment

The presented studies indicate that a single intravesical instillation of chemotherapy immediately following TURBT (< 24 hours) significantly decreases the risk of recurrence in patients with nonmuscle-invasive bladder cancer. Therefore it should be administered to all patients following TURBT of presumably nonmuscle-invasive

bladder cancer. No single chemotherapeutic drug has been shown to be superior. In terms of the optimal timing for immediate instillation therapy, a meta-analysis could not detect *significant* differences in efficacy as long as the instillation is given within 24 hours; however, instillation in the first 6 hours seems preferable [5].

In general, one immediate instillation is considered to be safe, as long as there is no evident bladder perforation or known allergies to the applied substance. Known prior reaction to an intravesically instilled chemotherapeutic agent should be considered a relative contraindication to such instillation with a different agent (**Grade 1B**).

Clinical question 31.2

BCG treatment – is maintenance therapy the standard of care?

Literature search

We searched for systematic reviews, meta-analyses, randomized trials and observational studies in the Cochrane

Table 31.1 Immediate postoperative intravesical instillation of a chemotherapeutic agent

Authors	Participants	Purpose	Results	OR/p-value	level of evidence
Cai [57]	n = 161 n = 80 immediate epirubicin plus delayed BCG treament n = 81 delayed BCG treatment only	Immediate instillation of epirubicin to improve BCG efficacy in high risk superf. TCC	No statistical difference was observed between the 2 groups: in terms of recurrence rate in terms of time to first recurrence	p = 0.82 p = 0.095	Ib no statistical improvement detected if epirubicin is given immediately in addition to delayed BCG
Barghi [6]	n = 43 n = 22 immediate instillation of MMC n = 21 placebo arm	Single immediate instillation vs. placebo low risk superficial TCC	1 (4.5%) recurrence at 12 and 24 months with immediate MMC instil. 8 (38.1%) recurrence at 12 and 24 months in placebo group 95% – 9-month tumor free survival rate in MMC group 71%- 9 month tumor free survival rate in placebo group	p = 0.007 p = 0.007	Ib immediate instillation superior to no instil. therapy
Sylvester [5]	n = 1476	Immediate instillation in single and multiple bladder cancer (Ta/T1) followup 3.4 years	Recurrence in 362 patients (48.4%) on TUR alone Recurrence in 267 patients (36.7%) receiving chemotherapy	OR 0.61, p < 0.0001	Ia immediate instillation superior to no instil. therapy
Solsona [18]	n = 121 n = 57 MMC group n = 64 control group	Immediate instillation in low risk superficial bladder cancer	Early recurrence: immediate MMC superior over control Late recurrence: MMC group superior over control at the limit of stat. sign. Early + late recurrence: MMC group and controlgroup no stat sign. diff.	p = 0.019 p = 0.575 p = 0.734	Ib single MMC instillation significantly decreased recurrence rates and tumor per year rates at short term followup

(Continued on p. 306)

Table 31.1 (Continued)

Authors	Participants	Purpose	Results	OR/p-value	level of evidence
Bouffioux [7]	n = 965 n = 483 (early treatment arm) n = 482 (delayed treatment arm)	Early versus delayed instillations (time to first recurrence, average follow-up of 2.75 years)	At least 1 rec.: 161 of 374 patients (43%) on early treatment At least 1 rec.: 187 of 378 patients (49%) on delayed treatment	p = 0.18	early instilliation superior to delayed instil. therapy
Oosterlink [8]	n = 431 prim. or rec. stages Ta-T1 TCC	Single immediate instillation vs. placebo Recurrence rate after a follow up of 2 years	Reduction of recurrence rate by immediat instil. around 50%		lb immediate instillation superior to no instil. therapy

Library (2008) and Medline (1966–Jan 2009) using the search terms: "bladder cancer," "urothelial carcinoma," "BCG," "bacille Calmette–Guerin," "intravescial therapy," "maintenance."

The evidence

Based on meta-analysis of published data involving 2658 patients from 24 trials, maintenance intravesical BCG therapy appears to reduce recurrence and progression rates [10]. In this meta-analysis, four trials were analyzed in which no maintenance therapy was given. In these cases no reduction in progression (p = 0.27) was observed. In the other 20 trials that used some form of BCG maintenance therapy, a reduction of 37% in the odds of progression was demonstrated (p = 0.00004). However, at least 1 year of maintenance BCG therapy was required to demonstrate its superiority in preventing recurrence or progression [11]. In a second meta-analysis involving nine clinical trials, only those patients receiving BCG maintenance demonstrated statistically significant reduction in tumor progression compared to mitomycin C (MMC) (p = 0.02) [12]. Lamm et al. conducted a prospective multicenter study that also supports the concept of maintenance BCG therapy [13]. The median recurrence-free survival was found to be 35.7 months in the group not receiving any maintenance therapy compared to 76.8 months in the group receiving maintenance therapy (p < 0.001). Based on current literature, the optimal maintenance BCG regimen is still unclear due to lack of data.

Comment

Based on the presented studies, maintenance intravesical instillation of BCG is associated with reduced risk of recurrence and progression from nonmuscle-invasive bladder cancer [10-12,13,14] and should be regarded as the standard of care. Although a variety of different maintenance regimens have reported efficacy, the optimal regimen is still unclear. Based on data from one randomized trial [13], the regimen commonly used has been induction BCG instillations once a week for 6 weeks. Additional 3-weekly instillations are performed 12 weeks following the first BCG instillation as long as there is no evidence of disease recurrence. Additional 3-weekly instillations are performed at 6-monthly intervals thereafter for a total of 2–3 years. According to Decobert et al., at least three cycles of BCG seem to be needed to achieve optimum results [15]. It has to be taken into account that BCG maintenance therapy may be associated with an increased risk of side effects, which was reflected by the relatively low percentage of patients who completed all recommended BCG cycles in the largest randomized trial of BCG maintenance therapy [13] (see Table 31.2). In general, more adverse reactions are reported in BCG-treated patients than in MMC-treated patients. The possible risk of BCG treatment should be balanced for every patient individually (**Grade 2B**).

Clinical question 31.3

What treatment is recommended for BCG-refractory nonmuscle-invasive TCC?

Literature search

We searched for systematic reviews, meta-analyses, randomized trials and observational studies in the Cochrane Library (2008) and Medline (1966–Jan 2009) using the search terms: "bladder cancer," "urothelial carcinoma," "BCG refractory," "BCG failure," "bacille Calmette–Guerin," "BCG long term," "treatment."

The evidence

Definition of a BCG failure
A BCG treatment is considered to have failed either if a tumor progresses to a muscle-invasive stage or if a tumor

Table 31.2 BCG maintenance therapy

Authors	Participants	Purpose	Results	p value	level of evidence
Decobert [15]	n = 40 no BCG maint. n = 24 one maint. cycle n = 16 two maint. cycles n = 31 at least 3 maint. cycles	Outcome according to the number of recieved BCG cycles	rec. free survival after 12 months: 41% one cycle 67% two cycles 89% at least 3 cycles		IIb at least 3 cycles of BCG seem needed
Han [58]	n = 1070 BCG maint. n = 2072 no BCG maint.	Comparison BCG maint. subgroup/ no BCG maint. subgroup	Odds ratio (OR) was used as the effect size estimate: OR = 0.47 for BCG maint. therapy OR = 0.90 for no BCG maint. therapy	p = 0.004 p = 0.71	Ia BCG maint. – superior over non maint.
Sylvester [10]	n = 2065 BCG maint. n = 593 no BCG maint.	Influence of BCG maint. on the risk of progression	BCG maint.: reduction of 37% in the odds of progression No BCG maint.: reduction in odds of progression (OR 1.28)	p = 0.00004 p = 0.27	Ia BCG maint. – superior over non maint.
Lamm [13]	n = 192 no BCG maint. n = 192 BCG maint.	Comparison BCG maint./no maint. therapy	median rec. free survival no BCG maint. – 35.7 months median rec. free survival with BCG maint. – 76.8 months	p < 0.001	Ib BCG maint. – superior over non maint.

BCG, bacille Calmette-Guerin; maint., maintenance; MMC, mitomycin C; OR, odds ratio; rec., recurrence; RR, relative risk

of higher grade and/or stage, even if nonmuscle invasive, is identified at either 3 or 6 months after initiation of induction BCG instillation therapy [16].

According to Herr & Dalbagni, a BCG failure should not be declared until after at least 6 months of BCG therapy [16]. In patients with tumor detected at 3 months, an additional course of BCG for 6 weeks has yielded a complete response in more than 50% of patients with papillary tumors and CIS [16,17]. On the other hand, Solsona et al. suggest that presence of tumor at the first cystoscopy following completion of induction BCG therapy for 6 weeks, i.e. at 3 months after commencement of instillation of BCG, indicates lack of response and a significantly worse outcome [18]. Lerner et al. found that a failure to achieve a complete response after BCG induction therapy is associated with a significant risk of a worsening event and death for patients with CIS or Ta–T1 bladder cancer [19].

The EAU guidelines strongly advocate immediate cystectomy upon BCG failure, because of the high risk of development of muscle-invasive tumor in these patients.

Alternative approaches such as the use of BCG plus interferon in patients with BCG failure have been shown to be effective in phase II studies, with 44–59% recurrence-free survival at 2 years [20,21].

Also promising seems the combination of BCG and electromotive MMC. A randomized study involving 212 patients showed significant improvement of BCG plus electromotive MMC over BCG treatment alone in terms of recurrence rate, progression rate and even disease-specific mortality [22]. Despite these promising results, these strategies are still considered experimental and should not be performed outside clinical trials.

The intravesical instillation of valrubicin represents the only FDA-approved treatment in this special setting [23]. In the randomized controlled trial conducted prior to FDA registration, obtained response rates were as low as 21% in the salvage setting (see Table 31.3).

Comment

In case of a BCG failure defined after 3 or 6 months of intravesical therapy, the actual recommendation is immediate cystectomy, if patients are suitable for surgery. A variety of alternative strategies are reported which are deemed experimental and therefore lack high-level evidence to support their use.

Even though BCG in combination with alpha-interferon or the combination of BCG and electromotive MMC show promising results, patients who have received repeat cycles of intravesical BCG or have BCG-refractory CIS are unlikely to respond in the long term and may be better advised to undergo cystectomy.

While a clear recommendation on the optimal timing of radical cystectomy cannot be made, Level II evidence suggests that at least in high-risk patients such as those with T1 disease, cystectomy performed within 2 years of diagnosis can yield better survival rates [24] (**Grade 1C**).

Table 31.3 Treatment of BCG-refractory nonmuscle-invasive TCC

Authors	Participants	Purpose	Results	p-value	level of evidence
Lerner [19]	n = 593	Induction BCG ± maintenance BCG	Patients with complete response during induction BCG: 5-year survival probability of 77% Patients without complete response during induction BCG: 5-year survival probability of 62%	p = 0.0008	IIb superior: complete response during induction BCG
Joudi [20]	n = 1007 n = 536 BCG naive group n = 467 BCG failure group	IFN-alfa with BCG IFN-alfa (50 million units) plus standard dose BCG (naive group) IFN-alfa (50 million units) plus reduced dose BCG (failure group)	Disease free at 24 months 59%-BCG naive group Disease free at 24 months 45%-BCG failure group		IIb IFN-alfa with BCG seems efficient and safe
Di Stasi [22]	n = 212 n = 105 BCG alone n = 107 BCG plus electromotive MMC	BCG alone compared to sequential BCG plus electromotive MMC median follow up 88 months	Disease free intervall - BCG alone: 21 months Disease free intervall - BCG plus electromotive MMC: 69 months Progression – BCG alone: 21.9% Progression – BCG plus electromotive MMC: 9.3% Disease specific mortality – BCG alone:16.2% Disease specific mortality – BCG plus electromotive MMC:5.6%	p = 0.0012 p = 0.004 p = 0.01	Ib BCG plus electromotive MMC seems superior to BCG treatment alone
O'Donnell [21]	n = 490 n = 259 BCG naive group n = 231 BCG failure group	BCG IFN alfa-2b for BCG naive and previous BCG failure median of 24 months follow up	Disease free at 24 months BCG naive group: 57% Disease free at 24 months BCG failure group: 42%		IIb IFN-alfa with BCG seems efficient and safe
Steinberg [23]	n = 90	Intravesical valrubicin for the treatment of CIS with failure or recurrence after BCG median follow up 30 months	Complete response in 19 (21%) patients 7 patients remained disease-free at the last evaluation Median time to failure and/or last followup > 18 months Recurrence detected in 79 patients		IIb Valrubicin seems effective and well tolerated

BCG, bacille Calmette-Guerin; IFN, interferon; maint., maintenance; MMC, mitomycin C; OR, odds ratio; RR, relative risk

Clinical question 31.4

When should a second TURBT be performed?

Literature search

We searched for systematic reviews, meta-analyses, randomized trials and observational studies in the Cochrane Library (2008) and Medline (1966–Jan 2009) using the search terms: "bladder cancer," "urothelial carcinoma," "second transurethral resection," "second-look resection," "repeat resection," "TUR."

The evidence

In patients with superficial bladder cancer, a second TURBT has been shown to be beneficial in terms of staging and recurrence rates. Miladi et al. present in their systematic literature review different aspects of the performance of a second-look TURBT [25]. Repeat TURBT has been shown to provide more precise clinical staging in 9–49% of analyzed cases, a detection of residual tumors in 26–83% of cases and an upstaging from T1 to muscle-invasive disease in 24–28% of cases.

Two other studies report that a second-look TURBT detects an understaging of Ta–T1, high-grade tumors which are actually found to be muscle invasive in up to 10% of patients [26,27]. Persistent disease after resection of a T1 tumor has been observed in as many as 33–53% of patients [27]. As the treatment of a Ta–T1, high-grade tumor and a T2 tumor differs substantially, precise disease staging is essential. It has been demonstrated that a repeat TURBT can increase recurrence-free and progression-free survival [28,29] as well as response to BCG [30] (see Table 31.4). There is no consensus about the strategy and timing of a second TURBT. Most authors recommend a resection 2–6 weeks after the initial TURBT.

Comment

Most of the reviewed studies indicate that a repeat TURBT should always be performed when the initial resection was incomplete or when multiple and/or large tumors are present. A second resection is also recommended when there is no muscle tissue contained in the pathological specimen. Furthermore, a second TUR should be performed when a high-grade, nonmuscle-invasive tumor or a T1 tumor has been detected at the initial TURBT (**Grade 1C**).

Clinical question 31.5

Does fluorescence cystoscopy influence recurrence rates?

Literature search

We searched for systematic reviews, meta-analyses, randomized trials and observational studies in the Cochrane Library (2008) and Medline (1966–Jan 2009) using the search terms: "bladder cancer," "urothelial carcinoma," "fluorescence endoscopy," "photodynamic diagnosis," "recurrence rate," "5-ALA," "hexyl aminolevulinate," "blue light cystoscopy," "photosensitizer."

The evidence

The clinical relevance of fluorescence cystoscopy (FC) in terms of prevention of tumor recurrence has been addressed by several authors. In prospective randomized

Table 31.4 Second TURBT

Authors	Participants	Purpose	Results	p-value/log rank	level of evidence
Divrik [29]	n = 74 MMC plus second TURBT n = 68 MMC only	Second TURBT after 2-6 weeks	Recurrence free survival in MMC with second TURBT: after 1 year 86.35%, 2 years 77.67%, 3 years 68.72% Recurrence free survival in MMC only arm: after 1 year 47.08%, 2 years 42.31%, 3 years 37.01% Progression for MMC plus second TURBT: 4.05% Progression for MMC only: 11.76%	log rank 0.0001 log rank 0.0974	Ib second TURBT superior
Herr [30]	n = 132 single TURBT n = 215 second TURBT	Comparison BCG treatment – with/without second TURBT	single TURBT: 57% recurrence or residual tumor at first cystoscopy single TURBT: 34% later progression second TURBT: 29% recurrence or residual tumor at first cystoscopy second TURBT: 7% later progression	p = 0.001	III second TURBT superior
Jakse [27]		Second TURBT after 4-8 weeks	Detection of residual tumor in 27-62% Upstaging to muscle invasive disease in 0-10%		I second TURBT optimized staging
Miladi [25]		Second TURBT after 2-6 weeks	Correction of staging failure in 9-49% Detection of residual tumor in 26-83% T1 tumor proved to be muscle invasive in second resection in 24-28%		I second TURBT optimized staging
Grimm [28]	n = 83 second TURBT n = 41 no second TURBT	Long-term outcome	Residual tumor: 33% of all ReTURBT cases (27% of Ta and 53% of T1) Tumor detection at the initial resection site: 81% Recurrence overall: 53% Recurrence without second TURBT: after 1 year 21%, 2 years 57%, 3 years 61% Recurrence with second TUR-B: after 1 year 18%, 2 years 29%, 3 years 32%	p < 0.03	III second TURBT superior

OR, odds ratio; MMC, mitomycin C; RR, relative risk

trials, patients with suspected bladder carcinoma were stratified and TURBT performed either by white light cystoscopy (WL) only or under white light and fluorescent cystoscopy. Riedl et al. [31] investigated 102 patients, showing a significant reduction of 59% in residual tumor on repeat resection 2–6 weeks later in those undergoing TURBT with WL and FC compared to those patients resected using WL alone (p = 0.005).

Other randomized trials have also demonstrated similar findings [32,33]. To prove whether the additional lesions detected and the decreased rate of residual tumor affect the recurrence rate, Filbeck et al. [34] conducted a randomized trial comparing TURBT guided by either FC or WL. The patients were followed up every 3 months with WL and cytology in both groups. The median follow-up of the 191 patients available for analysis was 43 months for the FC arm and 42 months for the WL arm. There was no statistical difference in the patient risk profiles or intravesical therapy. The recurrence-free survival rate after 12, 24 and 48 months was 90.9%, 90.9% and 85% in the FC arm, and 78.6%, 69.9% and 60.7% in the WL arm, respectively (p < 0.001). The superiority of FC to guide tumor detection and resection was an independent prognostic variable and the adjusted hazard ratio for FC-TUR versus WL-TUR was 0.29.

These findings were confirmed by the updated results of this study published with 8 years of follow-up data [35] reporting a recurrence-free survival rate after 2, 4, 6, and 8 years of 73%, 64%, 54%, and 45% in the WL group and 88%, 84%, 79%, and 71% in the FC group, respectively, revealing a statistically significant difference in favor of TUR performed with FC visualization (= 0.0003) (see Table 31.5).

Comment

The complete resection of all tumors in the bladder is one of the crucial factors in preventing disease recurrence [36]. FC appears to be superior to conventional WL TURBT with respect to the completeness of resection and recurrence-free survival. This advantage of decreased bladder tumor recurrence appears to be maintained over a long period of follow-up. The differences in recurrence-free survival imply that FC offers a clinically relevant procedure to reduce the incidence of tumor recurrence (**Grade 2B**).

Clinical question 31.6

Is the use of urine markers other than cytology supported by currently available data?

Literature search

We searched for systematic reviews, meta-analyses, randomized trials and observational studies in the Cochrane

Table 31.5 Fluorescence cystoscopy and residual tumor/recurrence rate

Authors	Participants	Purpose	Results	p value	level of evidence
Denzinger [35]	n = 103 WL n = 88 FC	Recurrence rate after 1 to 8 years Influence of FC on recurrence /residual tumor	FC: recurrence free survival after 2 years 88%, 4 years 84%, 6 years 79%, 8 years 71% WL: recurrence free survival after 2 years 73%, 4 years 64%, 6 years 54%, 8 years 45%	p = 0.0003	Ib FC reduces recurrence rate
Filbeck [34]	n = 103 WL n = 88 FC	Influence of FC on recurrence /residual tumor second look TURBT after 6 weeks Recurrence rates after 1 to 4 years	Second look TURBT FC: tumor detection in 4.5% WL: tumor detection in 25.2% FC: recurrence free survival after 1 year 90.9%, 2 years 90.9, 4 years 85% WL: recurrence free survival after 1 year 78.6%, 2 years 69.9, 4 years 60.7%	p < 0.0001 p = 0.0005	Ib FC reduces recurrence rate
Kriegmair [33]	n = 64 WL n = 65 FC	Tumor-free resected cases in FC and WL second look TURBT after 10-14 days	Second look TURBT FC: tumor free at second look 67.3% WL: tumor free at second look 46.9%	p = 0.031	Ib FC-higher tumor free rate at second look TURBT
Riedl [31]	n = 51 FC n = 51 WL	Influence of FC on recurrence rates second look TURBT after 6 weeks	Second look TURBT FC: tumor detection in 8 of 51 (16%) WL: tumor detection in 20 of 51 patients (39%) Significant reduction of residual tumor in FC	p = 0.005	Ib FC-reduction of residual tumor

FC, fluorescence-guided TURBT; WL, white light-guided TURBT

Library (2008) and Medline (1966–Jan 2009) using the search terms: "bladder cancer," "urothelial carcinoma," "urinary markers," "cytology," "marker," "diagnosis."

The evidence

A variety of urine markers are currently available for the diagnosis of bladder cancer, but only a few have received FDA approval [37]. Many of these markers appear to be more sensitive than urine cytology, especially for the detection of low-grade Ta tumors. On the other hand, some of these markers are also less specific than cytology which implies a higher rate of false-positive results [38-51]. Especially in patients with bladder inflammation, stone disease or other benign bladder conditions, reduced

marker specificity can be observed. The sensitivities and specificities of a variety of urine-based markers are listed in Table 31.6.

Comment

Currently it is not clear whether urine marker tests offer additional information that is influential in changing patient management in terms of follow-up or therapeutic decisions [37,52,53]. Also, the additional costs to the healthcare system have to be taken into account. Further studies involving larger numbers of patients are required to determine their accuracy and widespread applicability in guiding treatment of bladder cancer. Data from ongoing randomized, controlled studies are awaited in this

Table 31.6 Urine markers

Author	Participants	Compared markers	Test with best sensitivity/study	Test with best specificity/study	Test with best negative predictive value/study
Hautmann [43]	n = 94	ImmunoCyt, HA, HAase, Cytology	HA-HAase (83.3%)	Cytology (79.7%)	HA-HAase (90.9%)
Schroeder [47]	n = 115	HA-HAase, BTA stat, UBC, dipstick, cytology	HA-HAase (88.1%)	HA-HAase, cytology (81%)	HA-HAase (90.1%)
Bhuiyan [38]	n = 232	NMP22, BTA stat, cytology, Telomerase, Hb dipstick, chemiluminescent hemoglobin	Telomerase (77%)	Telomerase (98%)	Telomerase (91%)
Friedrich [51]	n = 103	FISH, NMP22, BTA stat, Lewis X, 486p3/12	Lewis X (91%)	FISH (89%)	Lewis X (90%)
Halling [42]	n = 265	BTA stat, dipstick, UroVysion, Telomerase	UroVysion (81%)	UroVysion (96%)	NS
Toma [48]	n = 126	ImmunoCyt, BTA stat, UroVysion, NMP22, Lewis X	Lewis X (95.5%)	FISH (89.1%)	Lewis X (90%)
Boman [39]	n = 92	NMP22, BTA stat, UBC, dipstick, RBC flow cytometry, cytology	BTA stat (78%)	Fixed for all at 73%	BTA stat (70%)
Giannopoulos [41]	n = 234	NMP22, BTA stat, UBC, cytology	UBC (80.5%)	UBC (80.2%)	UBC (80.2%)
Sanchez-Carbayo [46]	n = 267	NMP22, UBC, CYFRA 21–1, Tissue polypeptide antigen, cytology	CYFRA 21–1 (83.8%)	All fixed at 95%	CYFRA 21–1 (95.8%)
Ramakumar [45]	n = 196	NMP22, BTA, Telomerase, FDP, dipstick, cytology, chemiluminescent hemoglobin	BTA stat (74%)	Telomerase (99%)	NS
Landman [44]	n = 47	NMP22, BTA, cytology, telomerase	NMP22 (81%)	Cytology (94%)	NS
Wiener [49]	n = 291	BTA stat, NMP22, Quanticyt™, cytology	Quanticyt™ and cytology (59%)	Cytology (100%)	Cytology (84%)

regard. Lower level evidence in the form of observational and cohort studies suggests that urine-based markers can lead to the enhanced diagnosis of new and recurrent bladder tumors as well as diagnose recurrent tumors following intravesical chemo- or immunotherapy [54-56] (Grade 2C).

References

1. Bladder Cancer. National Cancer Institute. Available at: www.cancer.gov/cancertopics/types/bladder. 2007.

2. Sylvester R, van der Meijden A, Oosterlinck W, et al. Predicting recurrence and progression in individual patients with stage Ta T1 bladder cancer using EORTC risk tables: a combined analysis of 2596 patients from seven EORTC trials. Eur Urol 2006;49:466.

3. Brausi M, Collette L, Kurth K, et al. Variability in the recurrence rate at first follow-up cystoscopy after TUR in stage Ta T1 transitional cell carcinoma of the bladder: a combined analysis of seven EORTC studies. Eur Urol 2002;41:523.

4. Raj G, Herr H, Serio A, et al. Treatment paradigm shift may improve survival of patients with high risk superficial bladder cancer. J Urol 2007;177:1283.

5. Sylvester R, Oosterlinck W, van der Meijden A. A single immediate postoperative instillation of chemotherapy decreases the risk of recurrence in patients with stage Ta T1 bladder cancer: a meta-analysis of published results of randomized clinical trials. J Urol 2004;171:2186.

6. Barghi M, Rahmani M, Hosseini Moghaddam S, Jahanbin M. Immediate intravesical instillation of mitomycin C after transurethral resection of bladder tumor in patients with low-risk superficial transitional cell carcinoma of bladder. Urol J 2006;3:220.

7. Bouffioux C, Kurth K, Bono A, et al. Intravesical adjuvant chemotherapy for superficial transitional cell bladder carcinoma: results of 2 European Organization for Research and Treatment of Cancer randomized trials with mitomycin C and doxorubicin comparing early versus delayed instillations and short-term versus long-term treatment. European Organization for Research and Treatment of Cancer Genitourinary Group. J Urol 1995;153:934.

8. Oosterlinck W, Kurth K, Schroder F, et al. A prospective European Organization for Research and Treatment of Cancer Genitourinary Group randomized trial comparing transurethral resection followed by a single intravesical instillation of epirubicin or water in single stage Ta, T1 papillary carcinoma of the bladder. J Urol 1993;149:749.

9. Oosterlinck W, Kurth K, Schroder F, Sylvester R, Hammond B. A plea for cold biopsy, fulguration and immediate bladder instillation with Epirubicin in small superficial bladder tumors. Data from the EORTC GU Group Study 30863. Eur Urol 1993;23:457.

10. Sylvester R, van der Meijden, A, Lamm D. Intravesical bacillus Calmette–Guerin reduces the risk of progression in patients with superficial bladder cancer: a meta-analysis of the published results of randomized clinical trials. J Urol 2002;168:1964.

11. Bohle A, Jocham D, Bock P. Intravesical bacillus Calmette–Guerin versus mitomycin C for superficial bladder cancer: a formal meta-analysis of comparative studies on recurrence and toxicity. J Urol 2003;169:90.

12. Bohle A, Bock P. Intravesical bacille Calmette–Guerin versus mitomycin C in superficial bladder cancer: formal meta-analysis of comparative studies on tumor progression. Urology 2004;63:682.

13. Lamm D, Blumenstein B, Crissman J, et al. Maintenance bacillus Calmette–Guerin immunotherapy for recurrent TA, T1 and carcinoma in situ transitional cell carcinoma of the bladder: a randomized Southwest Oncology Group Study. J Urol 2000; 163:1124.

14. Pawinski A, Sylvester R, Kurth K, et al. A combined analysis of European Organization for Research and Treatment of Cancer, and Medical Research Council randomized clinical trials for the prophylactic treatment of stage TaT1 bladder cancer. European Organization for Research and Treatment of Cancer Genitourinary Tract Cancer Cooperative Group and the Medical Research Council Working Party on Superficial Bladder Cancer. J Urol 1996;156:1934.

15. Decobert M, LaRue H, Harel F, et al. Maintenance bacillus Calmette–Guerin in high-risk nonmuscle-invasive bladder cancer: how much is enough? Cancer 2008;113:710.

16. Herr H, Dalbagni G. Defining bacillus Calmette–Guerin refractory superficial bladder tumors. J Urol 2003;169:1706.

17. Sylvester R, van der Meijden A, Witjes J, et al. High-grade Ta urothelial carcinoma and carcinoma in situ of the bladder. Urology 2005;66:90.

18. Solsona E, Iborra I, Dumont R, et al. The 3-month clinical response to intravesical therapy as a predictive factor for progression in patients with high risk superficial bladder cancer. J Urol 2000;164:685.

19. Lerner S, Tangen C, Sucharew H, Wood D, Crawford E. Failure to achieve a complete response to induction BCG therapy is associated with increased risk of disease worsening and death in patients with high risk non-muscle invasive bladder cancer. Urol Oncol 2009;27(2):155

20. Joudi F, Smith B, O'Donnell M. Final results from a national multicenter phase II trial of combination bacillus Calmette–Guerin plus interferon alpha-2B for reducing recurrence of superficial bladder cancer. Urol Oncol 2006;24:344.

21. O'Donnell M, Lilli K, Leopold C. Interim results from a national multicenter phase II trial of combination bacillus Calmette–Guerin plus interferon alfa-2b for superficial bladder cancer. J Urol 2004;172:888.

22. Di Stasi S, Giannantoni A, Giurioli A, et al. Sequential BCG and electromotive mitomycin versus BCG alone for high-risk superficial bladder cancer: a randomised controlled trial. Lancet Oncol 2006;7:43.

23. Steinberg G, Bahnson R, Brosman S, et al. Efficacy and safety of valrubicin for the treatment of Bacillus Calmette–Guerin refractory carcinoma in situ of the bladder. The Valrubicin Study Group. J Urol 2000;163:761.

24. Herr HW, Sogani PC. Does early cystectomy improve the survival of patients with high risk superficial bladder tumors? J Urol 2001;166:1296.

25. Miladi M, Peyromaure M, Zerbib M, Saighi D, Debre B. The value of a second transurethral resection in evaluating patients with bladder tumours. Eur Urol 2003;43:241.

26. Brauers A, Buettner R, Jakse G. Second resection and prognosis of primary high risk superficial bladder cancer: is cystectomy often too early? J Urol 2001;165:808.

27. Jakse G, Algaba F, Malmstrom P, Oosterlinck W. A second-look TUR in T1 transitional cell carcinoma: why? Eur Urol 2004;45:539.

28. Grimm M, Steinhoff C, Simon X, et al. Effect of routine repeat transurethral resection for superficial bladder cancer: a long-term observational study. J Urol 2003;170:433.

29. Divrik R, Yildirim U, Zorlu F, Ozen H. The effect of repeat transurethral resection on recurrence and progression rates in patients with T1 tumors of the bladder who received intravesical mitomycin: a prospective, randomized clinical trial. J Urol 2006;175:1641.

30. Herr H. Restaging transurethral resection of high risk superficial bladder cancer improves the initial response to bacillus Calmette–Guerin therapy. J Urol 2005;174:2134.

31. Riedl C, Daniltchenko D, Koenig F, et al. Fluorescence endoscopy with 5-aminolevulinic acid reduces early recurrence rate in superficial bladder cancer. J Urol 2001;165:1121.

32. Filbeck T, Pichlmeier U, Knuechel R, et al. Do patients profit from 5-aminolevulinic acid-induced fluorescence diagnosis in transurethral resection of bladder carcinoma? Urology 2002;60:1025.

33. Kriegmair M, Zaak D, Rothenberger K, et al. Transurethral resection for bladder cancer using 5-aminolevulinic acid induced fluorescence endoscopy versus white light endoscopy. J Urol 2002;168:475.

34. Filbeck T, Pichlmeier U, Knuechel R, Wieland W, Rossler W. [Reducing the risk of superficial bladder cancer recurrence with 5-aminolevulinic acid-induced fluorescence diagnosis. Results of a 5-year study.] Urologe A 2003;42:1366.

35. Denzinger S, Burger M, Walter B, et al. Clinically relevant reduction in risk of recurrence of superficial bladder cancer using 5-aminolevulinic acid-induced fluorescence diagnosis: 8-year results of prospective randomized study. Urology 2007;69:675.

36. Kurth K, Denis L, Sylvester R, et al. The natural history and the prognosis of treated superficial bladder cancer. EORTC GU Group. Prog Clin Biol Res 1992;378:1.

37. Lokeshwar V, Habuchi T, Grossman H, et al. Bladder tumor markers beyond cytology: International Consensus Panel on bladder tumor markers. Urology 2005;66:35.

38. Bhuiyan J, Akhter J, O'Kane D. Performance characteristics of multiple urinary tumor markers and sample collection techniques in the detection of transitional cell carcinoma of the bladder. Clin Chim Acta 2003;331:69.

39. Boman H, Hedelin H, Jacobsson S, Holmang S. Newly diagnosed bladder cancer: the relationship of initial symptoms, degree of microhematuria and tumor marker status. J Urol 2002;168:1955.

40. Fernandez-Gomez J, Rodriguez-Martinez J, Barmadah S, et al. Urinary CYFRA 21.1 is not a useful marker for the detection of recurrences in the follow-up of superficial bladder cancer. Eur Urol 2007;51:1267.

41. Giannopoulos A, Manousakas T, Gounari A, et al. Comparative evaluation of the diagnostic performance of the BTA stat test, NMP22 and urinary bladder cancer antigen for primary and recurrent bladder tumors. J Urol 2001;166:470.

42. Halling K, King W, Sokolova I, et al. A comparison of BTA stat, hemoglobin dipstick, telomerase and Vysis UroVysion assays for the detection of urothelial carcinoma in urine. J Urol 2002;167:2001.

43. Hautmann S, Toma M, Lorenzo Gomez M, et al. Immunocyt and the HA-HAase urine tests for the detection of bladder cancer: a side-by-side comparison. Eur Urol 2004;46:466.

44. Landman J, Chang Y, Kavaler E, et al. Sensitivity and specificity of NMP-22, telomerase, and BTA in the detection of human bladder cancer. Urology 1998;52:398.

45. Ramakumar S, Bhuiyan J, Besse J, et al. Comparison of screening methods in the detection of bladder cancer. J Urol 1999; 161:388.

46. Sanchez-Carbayo M, Herrero E, Megias J, Mira A, Soria F. Comparative sensitivity of urinary CYFRA 21-1, urinary bladder cancer antigen, tissue polypeptide antigen, tissue polypeptide antigen and NMP22 to detect bladder cancer. J Urol 1999;162:1951.

47. Schroeder G, Lorenzo-Gomez M, Hautmann S, et al. A side by side comparison of cytology and biomarkers for bladder cancer detection. J Urol 2004;172:1123.

48. Toma M, Friedrich M, Hautmann S, et al. Comparison of the ImmunoCyt test and urinary cytology with other urine tests in the detection and surveillance of bladder cancer. World J Urol 2004;22:145.

49. Wiener H, Mian C, Haitel A, et al. Can urine bound diagnostic tests replace cystoscopy in the management of bladder cancer? J Urol 1998;159:1876.

50. Konety B. Molecular markers in bladder cancer: a critical appraisal. Urol Oncol 2006;24:326.

51. Friedrich M, Toma M, Hellstern A, et al. Comparison of multi-target fluorescence in situ hybridization in urine with other non-invasive tests for detecting bladder cancer. BJU Int 2003;92:911.

52. Glas A, Roos D, Deutekom M, et al. Tumor markers in the diagnosis of primary bladder cancer. A systematic review. J Urol 2003;169:1975.

53. Lotan Y, Roehrborn C. Sensitivity and specificity of commonly available bladder tumor markers versus cytology: results of a comprehensive literature review and meta-analyses. Urology 2003;61:109.

54. Grossman H, Messing E, Soloway M, et al. Detection of bladder cancer using a point-of-care proteomic assay. JAMA 2005;293:810.

55. Grossman H, Soloway M, Messing E, et al. Surveillance for recurrent bladder cancer using a point-of-care proteomic assay. JAMA 2006;295:299.

56. Kipp BR, Karnes R, Brankley S, et al. Monitoring intravesical therapy for superficial bladder cancer using fluorescence in situ hybridization. J Urol 2005;173:401.

57. Cai T, Nesi G, Tinacci G, et al. Can early single dose instillation of epirubicin improve bacillus Calmette–Guerin efficacy in patients with nonmuscle invasive high risk bladder cancer? Results from a prospective, randomized, double-blind controlled study. J Urol. 2008 Jul;180(1):110-5. Epub 2008 May 15.

58. Han RF, Pan JG. Can intravesical bacillus Calmette-Guérin reduce recurrence in patients with superficial bladder cancer? A meta-analysis of randomized trials. Urology. 2006 Jun;67(6):1216-23.

32 Treatment of muscle-invasive bladder cancer

James Thomasch and Sam S. Chang
Department of Urologic Surgery, Vanderbilt University Medical Center, Nashville, TN, USA

Background

There were more than 67,000 new cases of urothelial carcinoma of the bladder and nearly 14,000 deaths from the disease in the United States in 2007 [1]. The majority of new cases of urothelial carcinoma of the bladder are diagnosed when the disease is not muscle invasive. However, 20–40% of new cases are muscle invasive at time of diagnosis and a significant proportion of patients diagnosed with noninvasive disease will eventually progress to muscle-invasive disease [2]. The current gold standard for treatment of muscle-invasive urothelial carcinoma is radical cystectomy with pelvic lymphadenectomy. In one large single-institution contemporary series of radical cystectomy outcomes, 5- and 10-year recurrence-free survival rates after surgery were 68% and 66% respectively. Overall 5- and 10-year survival rates in this series were 60% and 43% respectively, with 3% perioperative mortality [3]. However, the question remains: can we improve on these numbers with adjuvant/neo-adjuvant chemotherapy or perhaps spare the bladder altogether?

Clinical question 32.1

Does adjuvant chemotherapy after radical cystectomy for muscle-invasive urothelial carcinoma of the bladder confer a survival advantage?

Literature search

A systematic search was conducted using the PubMed database from 1990 to 2008 using the terms: "muscle invasive," "urothelial carcinoma," "radical cystectomy," "transitional cell carcinoma," "bladder cancer," "neo-adjuvant" and "adjuvant chemotherapy."

The evidence

There have been a total of 11 RCTs investigating adjuvant chemotherapy after radical cystectomy for bladder cancer, but only six of these trials had individual patient data available for subsequent review (Table 32.1). Two meta-analyses of these data have since been performed. All these studies compared cisplatin-based chemotherapy regimens with localized extirpative therapy alone (in the form of radical cystectomy). One of these trials investigated cisplatin therapy alone [4]; the other five used cisplatin-based combination therapy [5-9]. Individually, these trials enrolled a small number of patients, with total accrual ranging from 50 to 108 patients. Furthermore, interpreting and then subsequently utilizing these data in the clinic

Table 32.1 Randomized controlled trials of adjuvant chemotherapy following radical cystectomy versus radical cystectomy alone

Study	Patients (N)	Disease-free survival (adjuvant chemo/vs cystectomy alone)	Overall survival (adjuvant chemo/ vs cystectomy alone)
Studer et al. [4]	77	NS	NS
Skinner et al. [5]	91	51% vs 34%	70% vs 46%
Stockle et al. [6]	49	42% vs. 17%	27% vs 17%
Freiha et al. [7]	50	50% vs 22%	NS
Bono et al. [8]	83	NS	NS
Otto et al. [9]	108	NS	NS

NS, not significant

Evidence-Based Urology. Edited by Philipp Dahm, Roger R. Dmochowski.
© 2010 Blackwell Publishing.

setting has been virtually impossible due to methodological flaws in their design and execution [10].

Inadequacies have been identified in each of the six aforementioned RCTs. These include major problems such as insufficient sample sizes, early cessation of patient entry, premature interim analyses, incorrect statistical methods, and failure to report important endpoints [11]. These shortcomings notwithstanding, a benefit of adjuvant chemotherapy was demonstrated in three out of the six trials.

Skinner et al. demonstrated benefit for patients receiving adjuvant chemotherapy in time to progression, cancer-specific survival, and overall survival [5]. However, major criticisms of this trial include the fact that there was inadequate accrual of potentially eligible participants and therapy during the study was nonuniform. Moreover, the maximum benefit was observed in a subgroup that was not prospectively identified at the outset of the study [11].

Similarly, the study by Stockle et al. demonstrated increased time to progression as well as improved cancer-specific and overall survival for patients who were randomized to adjuvant chemotherapy versus radical cystectomy alone [6]. Interestingly and importantly, patients in the cystectomy-alone arm were not offered the option of chemotherapy at time of recurrence, which may have affected the differences in survival.

Freiha and colleagues reported a benefit of adjuvant chemotherapy with regard to relapse-free survival but not overall survival [7]. Participants who recurred were offered the same chemotherapy regimen as patients who received adjuvant chemotherapy at the outset. The authors suggest that the lack of difference in overall survival may be attributable to the salvage of patients with metastatic disease who began chemotherapy only after recurrence was documented.

It should be emphasized that each of these three previously discussed studies that support the use of adjuvant chemotherapy was terminated early due to interim analyses that showed marked benefit in the chemotherapy arm [5-7]. A fourth RCT was stopped early after interim analysis revealed less benefit than anticipated [4]. Of note, the study by Studer et al. was the only trial that used cisplatin monotherapy [4]. Early cessation of RCTs is one of many recognized potential sources of bias and therefore calls into question the validity of the data reported in these studies [12].

In an attempt to address the many concerns about these individual studies and make use of the available data, two meta-analyses of these RCTs have been conducted [13,14]. The meta-analysis by the Advanced Bladder Cancer Meta-Analysis Collaboration (ABC) is the stronger of these two because it utilized individual patient data (IPD) analysis as opposed to pooled analysis. Therefore, the ABC meta-analysis will be the focus of the remainder of this discussion.

The ABC meta-analysis focused on the six previously mentioned RCTs. IPD was retrieved for a total of 493 patients. This represents 90% of all patients randomized in adjuvant chemotherapy trials comparing cisplatin combination therapy to cystectomy alone and 66% of patients randomized in all known bladder cancer adjuvant chemotherapy trials. Follow-up data on two patients from the Bono et al. study were not available [8]. Therefore, final analysis consisted of 491 patients [13].

Overall survival and disease-free survival were the two primary outcome measures of this meta-analysis. There was a 25% relative decrease in the risk of death for patients treated with adjuvant chemotherapy (95% confidence interval (CI) 0.60–0.96). This equates to a 9% (95% CI 1–16%) absolute reduction in the risk of death for patients given chemotherapy at 3 years. However, further statistical analysis revealed that the study was underpowered to detect an absolute risk reduction for death below approximately 15% [13].

Disease-free survival was measured in 383 patients because data regarding recurrence were not available for one trial [9]. The reduction in relative risk of recurrence was 32% (95% CI 0.53–0.89) with an absolute risk reduction of 12% (95% CI 4–19%) at 3 years [13].

Comment

Proponents of adjuvant chemotherapy claim that patients with favorable surgical pathological findings at the time of radical cystectomy could be spared the toxicity and possible adverse effects of antineoplastic drugs. Indeed, subgroup analyses of both adjuvant and neo-adjuvant chemotherapy trials have revealed that patients with pT3–T4 disease are most likely to benefit from chemotherapy compared to patients with organ-confined disease. Furthermore, in studies of metastatic urothelial carcinoma, only 40–60% of tumors prove to be chemosensitive. Therefore, a counter-argument to the use of neo-adjuvant chemotherapy is that a significant percentage of patients who would not benefit from treatment (either because their disease would not need chemotherapy or they harbor tumor that is in fact resistant to chemotherapy) are not only being exposed to these potentially toxic drug regimens, but will also have potentially curative local therapy delayed. An adjuvant chemotherapy approach attempts to maximize individualization of treatment by assimilating the pathological findings at cystectomy.

There exist six RCTs investigating adjuvant chemotherapy after radical cystectomy for urothelial carcinoma of the bladder for which data were available for meta-analysis. Unfortunately, each of these trials has significant methodological flaws and the total number of patients is still small. A careful meta-analysis by the ABC group has yielded results that favor adjuvant chemotherapy after radical cystectomy. However, despite these encouraging numbers, the meta-analysis was underpowered to substantiate the reported survival benefits. More importantly, the underlying suboptimal quality of each individual study included in the meta-analysis makes it impossible to endorse the universal use of adjuvant chemotherapy in patients undergoing radical cystectomy for muscle-invasive bladder cancer. There are currently several large RCTs in progress attempting to answer this question. Treating physicians await the findings and should be encouraged to enroll patients in adjuvant chemotherapy trials.

Clinical question 32.2

Does neo-adjuvant chemotherapy for patients undergoing local treatment (either radical cystectomy or radiotherapy) for muscle-invasive bladder cancer result in a survival advantage?

Literature search

A systematic search was conducted using the PubMed database from 1990 to 2008 using the terms: "muscle-invasive," "urothelial carcinoma," "radical cystectomy," "transitional cell carcinoma," "bladder cancer," "neo-adjuvant" and "adjuvant chemotherapy."

The evidence

There are 11 RCTs comparing neo-adjuvant chemotherapy to localized therapy alone (Table 32.2). Three of these trials

involved cisplatin monotherapy and the others utilized cisplatin-based combination chemotherapy. Four of the trials included radiation therapy in some form as the means for local tumor control. Total patient accrual in each trial ranged from 99 to 976 patients. Individually, only the largest of the trials [18] demonstrated a significant overall and disease-specific survival benefit for patients receiving neo-adjuvant chemotherapy. In addition, two large meta-analyses of the data from these 11 RCTs have been performed and have confirmed a survival benefit for patients receiving neo-adjuvant chemotherapy for muscle-invasive bladder cancer prior to local treatment [26,27].

The largest RCT investigating neo-adjuvant chemotherapy was conducted by the European Organization for Research and Treatment of Cancer (EORTC) [18]. This study of 976 patients compared neo-adjuvant cisplatin-based combination chemo-therapy (CMV) and local therapy (either radical cystectomy or radiotherapy) versus localized therapy alone. The original analysis of this data that was published in 1999 did not demonstrate a significant difference in survival. After 7.4 years of follow-up, a 5.5% overall survival benefit (p = 0.048) was noted in the group of patients who had received neo-adjuvant chemotherapy. However, as the investigators performing this study pointed out, their study was not powered to detect a difference in overall survival of less than 10%.

A similar trial was performed in the United States by the Southwest Oncology Group (SWOG) [19]. This was a smaller trial (298 patients) and also utilized cisplatin-based combination neo-adjuvant chemotherapy. Patients in the control arm underwent radical cystectomy alone. After

Table 32.2 Randomized controlled trials of neo-adjuvant chemotherapy prior to radiotherapy and/or radical cystectomy

Study	Patients (N)	Local therapy	Disease-free survival (neo-adjuvant chemo/vs local therapy alone)	Overall survival (neo-adjuvant chemo/vs local therapy alone)
Wallace et al. [15]	255	RT	NS	NS
Coppin et al. [16]	99	RT or preop RT + RC	NS	NS
Martinez et al. [17]	121	RC	30.3 vs 13.1 mos	NS
EORTC/MRC [18]	976	RT or RC	46% vs 39%	55.5% vs 50%
SWOG 8710 [19]	298	RC	Not reported	57% vs 43% (p = 0.06)
Bassi et al. [20]	206	RC	NS	NS
GISTV [21]	171	RC	NS	NS
Orsatti et al. [22]	104	RC	NS	NS
Malmstrom et al. [23]	311	RT then RC	NS	NS
Sherif et al. [24]	317	RC	NS	NS
Abol-Enein et al. [25]	194	RC	NS	NS

NS, not significant; RC, radical cystectomy: RT, radiotherapy

5 years, overall survival was 57% in the chemotherapy group versus 43% in the surgery-alone group. The original analysis of this data was performed using a single-sided t-test and the results were statistically significant (p = 0.04). However, when a two-sided analysis was performed, the overall survival benefit in the neo-adjuvant chemotherapy group did not prove to be statistically significant (p = 0.06).

The Advanced Bladder Cancer Meta-Analysis Collaboration (ABC) performed a meta-analysis of 11 neo-adjuvant chemotherapy RCTs [26]. IPD from 3005 patients was included in the analysis. This represents 98% of patients from all eligible RCTs investigating neo-adjuvant chemotherapy for muscle-invasive bladder cancer. When all trials were considered together, overall survival at 5 years was superior in the neo-adjuvant chemotherapy group (4% absolute benefit, p = 0.022). Disease-free survival was also improved (8% absolute benefit, p = < 0.0001).

Interestingly, subgroup analysis revealed that for patients receiving cisplatin combination neo-adjuvant chemotherapy, there was improved absolute overall and disease-free survival (5% and 9% respectively). Patients receiving cisplatin monotherapy exhibited a trend toward worsening overall and disease-free survival (approximately –5%), but there were too few patients in this subgroup for the results to achieve significance. It should be noted that the results of this meta-analysis mirror the results from the EORTC trial. This is almost certainly explained by the fact that this was the largest trial included and therefore contributed a disproportionately large number of patients compared to the other trials that were analyzed.

A Canadian meta-analysis performed in 2004 revealed similar results to the ABC data [27]. In an analysis of 2605 patients from 11 RCTs, the authors reported that overall survival was improved (absolute benefit of 6.5%, p = 0.006) in patients receiving cisplatin-based combination neo-adjuvant chemotherapy.

Comment

The significant rate of bladder cancer recurrence after definitive local therapy for muscle-invasive disease is clear evidence that a significant proportion of patients likely harbor micrometastatic disease at the time of initial diagnosis. Advocates of neo-adjuvant chemotherapy believe that this approach is optimal for treating distant disease when the possible extravesical tumor burden is at its smallest, thereby providing the likeliest chance of long-term cure. Response can be evaluated during treatment, and nonresponders can stop chemotherapy and proceed directly to surgery or radiation. Additionally, patient performance status is typically at its peak prior to undergoing surgery or radiation and patients are more likely to be able to tolerate the negative effects of chemotherapy.

There have been 11 RCTs and two meta-analyses evaluating the effect of neo-adjuvant chemotherapy prior to local therapy for patients with muscle-invasive bladder cancer. Individually, each of these trials was underpowered and only the EORTC trial demonstrated a significant survival benefit for the neo-adjuvant chemotherapy group. However, both meta-analyses confirmed a statistically significant survival benefit associated with neo-adjuvant chemotherapy of approximately 5% at 5 years.

Morbidity of neo-adjuvant chemotherapy in these trials was low, but there is a lack of validated quality of life data to assess its ultimate impact on patients. Moreover, the patients in these trials tended to be younger with better renal function than many patients currently presenting with muscle-invasive urothelial carcinoma. Thus, although the data are convincing, the modest survival benefit associated with neo-adjuvant chemotherapy in this setting may not be generalizable to all patients presenting with muscle-invasive bladder cancer. However, some believe that the benefit of neo-adjuvant chemotherapy may in fact be understated by the current data. Reasons for this supposition include the use of perhaps suboptimal radiotherapy (when compared to surgery) for local control and the inadequacy of chemotherapy regimens employed in some of these studies. Indeed, cisplatin monotherapy is clearly inferior to combination therapy based on multiple trials and three of the RCTs included in the meta-analyses utilized cisplatin monotherapy.

Clinical question 32.3

Is there any role for bladder preservation in patients presenting with muscle-invasive urothelial carcinoma of the bladder?

Literature search

A systematic search was conducted using the PubMed database from 1990 to 2008 using the terms: "muscle-invasive," "urothelial carcinoma," "radical cystectomy," "transitional cell carcinoma," "bladder cancer," "neo-adjuvant" and "adjuvant chemotherapy."

The evidence

There are currently no RCTs comparing bladder-sparing therapy to radical cystectomy. However, there have been prospective studies evaluating transurethral resection (TUR) or partial cystectomy (alone or in combination with chemotherapy) as well as studies evaluating radiotherapy combined with chemotherapy after TUR.

Herr prospectively compared outcomes of 151 patients undergoing radical TUR alone versus radical cystectomy in a cohort of patients initially diagnosed with muscle-invasive urothelial carcinoma of the bladder [28]. Requirements for entry into the study included a restaging TUR demonstrating absence of muscle invasion. Patients with residual tumor < T2 were allowed to enter the trial. All 151 eligible patients were offered the option of immediate cystectomy or conservative management consisting of TUR alone with close follow-up (cystoscopy every 3–6 months). Fifty-two patients chose cystectomy and 99 chose the bladder-sparing approach. Patients who progressed to muscle-invasive disease during the course of the study underwent radical cystectomy. After 10 years of follow-up, 76% of patients in the bladder-sparing group were alive versus 71% in the immediate cystectomy group (p = 0.3). Of patients who initially elected conservative therapy, 57% survived > 10 years with a functioning bladder. Subgroup analysis revealed that patients in the bladder-sparing group who were T0 at time of entry into the trial were more likely to survive with their bladder when compared to patients who had evidence of disease at the time of restaging TUR (68% vs 27%, p = 0.001).

Solsona and colleagues performed a similar study that prospectively followed 133 patients with muscle-invasive urothelial carcinoma who underwent TUR alone versus a control group of 76 patients who underwent immediate radical cystectomy [29]. In order to be eligible for the bladder-sparing approach in this trial, patients had to have no evidence of residual tumor at time of restaging TUR. Mean follow-up in this series was 81.6 months. Disease-specific survival rates at 5 and 10 years in the bladder-sparing group were 80.5% and 74.5% respectively. These did not differ significantly from patients who underwent cystectomy. Bladder preservation rates at 5 and 10 years were 82.7% and 79.6% respectively. Of note, associated CIS was an independent predictor of progression in this study.

A prospective study of 104 patients by Sternberg et al. evaluated patients with muscle-invasive urothelial carcinoma of the bladder (T2–T4) who received three cycles of M-VAC chemotherapy prior to undergoing TUR alone, partial cystectomy or radical cystectomy [30]. Patients who were T0 after restaging TUR following chemotherapy were considered for bladder-sparing therapy. In order to qualify for partial cystectomy, patients were required to have a solitary lesion in a favorable anatomical location, no associated CIS, and at least a partial response to chemotherapy. Overall, 52 patients were in the TUR alone group, 13 patients underwent partial cystectomy, and 39 patients received radical cystectomy. For patients undergoing TUR alone after chemotherapy, overall survival was 67% and disease-free survival was 38% (with 44% maintaining an intact bladder) after a median follow-up of 56 months. In the partial cystectomy group, overall survival was 69%

and disease-free survival was 31% after median follow-up of 88 months. Of patients who underwent radical cystectomy, overall and disease-free survival were 46% and 38% respectively after median follow-up of 45 months.

Several studies investigating trimodality therapy for muscle-invasive urothelial carcinoma of the bladder have been performed. The effectiveness of concomitant TUR, chemotherapy, and radiotherapy has been investigated by the Radiation Therapy Oncology Group (RTOG) and others. In the largest and most recent trial performed by RTOG, 190 patients with T2–T4a bladder cancer were enrolled and underwent TUR followed by M-VAC chemotherapy and concurrent induction radiotherapy with 40 Gy [31]. One hundred and twenty-one complete responders then underwent consolidation with chemotherapy and radiotherapy for a total dose of 65 Gy. Forty-one patients who did not achieve a complete response after induction underwent radical cystectomy. Thirty-four patients who did not complete the protocol were excluded from the final analysis. During the course of the study, 25 patients in the bladder-sparing group developed recurrent invasive tumors and underwent salvage cystectomy. The 5- and 10-year overall survival rates for patients in the bladder-sparing group were 54% and 36% respectively. Disease-specific survival rates at 5 and 10 years in this group were 63% and 59% respectively. Forty-five percent of patients maintained an intact bladder at 5 years. The disease-specific survival rate for patients with an intact bladder was 46% at 5 years. The authors note that although approximately one-third of patients in the bladder-sparing group ultimately required salvage cystectomy, overall survival in this group was not inferior to patients who had proceeded to immediate cystectomy.

Most recently, Herr performed a unique analysis of a cohort of patients with muscle-invasive urothelial carcinoma of the bladder who refused cystectomy altogether after achieving a complete response to neo-adjuvant cisplatin-based combination chemotherapy [32]. This prospective study included 63 patients and overall survival after a median of 86 months was 64%, with 54% of survivors maintaining a functioning native bladder. All patients in this cohort who died succumbed to bladder cancer (36%). Nineteen of these patients experienced relapse first in the bladder only, leading the author to conclude that refusing radical cystectomy led to an added mortality risk of 30% (if one assumes that radical cystectomy would have resulted in cure for these patients).

Comment

There have been no RCTs comparing bladder-sparing therapy to radical cystectomy for muscle-invasive urothelial carcinoma of the bladder. The prospective data that exist primarily examine TUR alone, TUR in combination with chemotherapy or trimodality therapy with TUR, chemotherapy, and radiotherapy. Although prospective, the lack of randomization and associated selection biases make valid interpretations difficult. Proponents of bladder-sparing therapy espouse the improved quality of life associated with this approach and maintain that survival rates reported from these trials are similar to those of contemporary radical cystectomy series. Adequate quality of life studies, however, are lacking. Cumulatively, these factors make it extremely difficult to objectively and fairly compare survival rates for patients undergoing radical cystectomy to patients receiving bladder-sparing therapy even within individual trials. This is because the patients who undergo immediate radical cystectomy in these studies often have more advanced disease at the outset. Therefore, their survival would be expected to be inferior if given the same treatment modality as patients who are allowed to enter bladder-sparing protocols.

For all the reported studies, patients with organ-confined disease, unifocal tumors, and absence of residual tumor at time of restaging TUR had better survival when undergoing bladder-sparing regimens. What these studies suggest is that there may be a role for bladder-sparing therapy for patients with favorable prognostic indicators such as these. However, without a well-designed RCT comparing a bladder-sparing approach to radical cystectomy, one cannot make an evidence-based endorsement of bladder-sparing therapy at this time as superior or even equivalent to radical cystectomy for muscle-invasive disease. Until we have better data, a patient who refuses radical cystectomy for muscle-invasive bladder cancer must do so at his/her own risk.

Implications for practice

Adjuvant chemotherapy after radical cystectomy

Conditional recommendation FOR use based on moderate-quality evidence, **Grade 2B**. There are several large RCTs currently in progress investigating the effectiveness of adjuvant chemotherapy after radical cystectomy. In the meantime, clinicians should examine the risks/benefits of chemotherapy in the adjuvant setting on an individual basis. In particular, patients with nonorgan-confined disease are most likely to benefit from this modality. Patients should be counseled that previous studies suggest that there may in fact be a benefit, but that Level 1 evidence is not currently available on this matter.

Neo-adjuvant chemotherapy prior to radical cystectomy

Conditional recommendation FOR use based on high-quality evidence, **Grade 2A**. Meta-analysis of RCTs has confirmed an approximate 5% overall survival benefit at 5 years for patients undergoing neo-adjuvant chemotherapy prior to radical cystectomy. This benefit is modest and patients included in the trials were younger and had better renal function than many patients who present with muscle-invasive bladder cancer. Therefore, clinicians should carefully evaluate the fitness of patients being considered for this approach and counsel them about the risks/benefits of delaying definitive local therapy while receiving chemotherapy.

Bladder-sparing therapy as an alternative to radical cystectomy

Strong recommendation AGAINST use based on low-quality evidence, **Grade 1C**. Studies of bladder-sparing therapies have been small and widely disparate in terms of patients enrolled and types of therapy offered. Although many of these studies report that overall survival for patients on bladder-sparing protocols is similar to radical cystectomy series, patients should be counseled that all studies of bladder-sparing protocols have been nonrandomized. Thus, they are hampered by multiple biases that make valid interpretation nearly impossible. A RCT of bladder-sparing therapy for patients with good-risk tumor features versus radical cystectomy is needed before this approach can be safely recommended to patients.

References

1. Barocas DA, Clark PE. Bladder cancer. Curr Opin Oncol 2008; 20:307-14.
2. Huang GJ, Stein JP. Open radical cystectomy with lymphadenectomy remains the treatment of choice for invasive bladder cancer. Curr Opin Urol 2007;17:369-75.
3. Stein JP, Skinner DG. Radical cystectomy for invasive bladder cancer: long term results of a standard procedure. World J Urol 2006;24:296-304.
4. Studer, UE et al. Adjuvant cisplatin chemotherapy following radical cystectomy for bladder cancer: results of a prospective randomized trial. J Urol 1994;152:81-4.
5. Skinner, DG et al. Adjuvant chemotherapy following cystectomy benefits patients with deeply invasive bladder cancer. Semin Urol 1990;8:279-84.
6. Stockle, et al. Adjuvant polychemotherapy of non-organ confined bladder cancer after radical cystectomy revisited: long term results of a controlled prospective study and further clinical experience. J Urol 1995;153:47-52.
7. Freiha, F. et al. A randomized trial of radical cystectomy versus radical cystectomy plus cisplatin, vinblastine, and methotrexate chemotherapy for muscle invasive bladder cancer. J Urol 1996;155:495-9.
8. Bono, AV et al. Adjuvant chemotherapy in locally advanced bladder cancer: final analysis of a controlled multicentre study. ActaUrol Ital 1997;11:5-8.

9. Otto, T. et al. Adjuvant chemotherapy in locally advanced bladder cancer (pT3/ pN1-1, M0): a Phase III study. Eur Urol 2001;39(suppl 5):147.

10. Sternberg CN,Collette L. What has been learned from meta-analyses of neo-adjuvant and adjuvant chemotherapy in bladder cancer? BJU 2006;98:487-96.

11. Sternberg, CN et al. Chemotherapy for bladder cancer: treatment guidelines for neo-adjuvant chemotherapy, bladder preservation, adjuvant chemotherapy, and metastatic cancer. Urology 2007;69(suppl 1A):62-79.

12. Lewis SC, Warlow CP. How to spot bias and other potential problems in randomized controlled trials. J Neurol Neurosurg Psychiatry 2004;75:181-7.

13. Ruggeri, EM et al. Adjuvant chemotherapy in muscle-invasive bladder carcinoma: a pooled analysis from phase III studies. Cancer 2006;106:783-8.

14. Advanced Bladder Cancer (ABC) Meta-Analysis Collaboration. Adjuvant chemotherapy in invasive bladder cancer: a systematic review and meta-analysis of individual patient data. Eur Urol 2005;48:189-201.

15. Wallace, DM et al. Neo-adjuvant cisplatin therapy in invasive transitional cell carcinoma of the bladder. BJU 1991;67:608-15.

16. Coppin, CM et al. Improved local control of invasive bladder cancer by concurrent cisplatin and preoperative or definitive radiation. J Clin Oncol 1996;14:2901-7.

17. Martinez Piniero, JA et al. Neo-adjuvant cisplatin chemotherapy before radical cystectomy in invasive transitional cell carcinoma of the bladder: a prospective randomized phase III study. J Urol 1995;153(pt 2):964-73.

18. International Collaboration of Trialists. Neo-adjuvant cisplatin, methotrexate, and vinblastine chemotherapy for muscle-invasive bladder cancer: a randomised controlled trial. Lancet 1999;354:533-40.

19. Natale, RB et al. SWOG 8710 (INT-0080): randomized phase III trial of neo-adjuvant M-VAC and cystectomy versus cystectomy alone in patients with locally advanced bladder cancer. Proc Am Soc Clin Oncol 1995;20:2a.

20. Bassi, P et al. Neo-adjuvant M-VAC of invasive bladder cancer: the G.U.O.N.E. multicenter phase III trial. Eur Urol 1998;33 (suppl 1):142.

21. GISTV (Italian Bladder Cancer Study Group). Neo-adjuvant treatment for locally advanced bladder cancer: a randomized prospective clinical trial. J Chemother 1996;8(suppl 4):345-6.

22. Orsatti, M et al. Altering chemo-radiotherapy in bladder cancer: a conservative approach. Int J Radiat Oncol Biol Phys 1995;33:173-8.

23. Malmstrom, PU et al. Five year followup of a prospective trial of radical cystectomy and neo-adjuvant chemotherapy. J Urol 1996;155:1903-6.

24. Sherif, A. et al. for the Nordic Urothelial Cancer Group. Neo-adjuvant cisplatin-methotrexate chemotherapy of invasive bladder cancer: Nordic Cystectomy Trial 2. Scand J Urol Nephrol 2002;36:419-25.

25. Abol-Enein, H. et al. Neo-adjuvant chemotherapy in treatment of invasive transitional bladder cancer: a controlled, prospective, randomized study. BJU 1997;80(suppl 2):49.

26. Advanced Bladder Cancer Meta-Analysis Collaboration. Neo-adjuvant chemotherapy in invasive bladder cancer: a systematic review and meta-analysis. Lancet 2003;361: 1927-34.

27. Winquist, et al. Genitourinary Cancer Disease Site Group of Cancer Care Ontario Program in Evidence-Based Care Practice Guidelines Initiative: neo-adjuvant chemotherapy for transitional cell carcinoma of the bladder: a systematic review and meta-analysis. J Urol 2004;171:561-9.

28. Herr HH. Transurethral resection of muscle-invasive bladder cancer: 10-year outcome. J Clin Oncol 2001;19:89-93.

29. Solsona, et al. Feasibility of transurethral resection for muscle infiltrating carcinoma of the bladder: long-term followup of a prospective study. J Urol 1998;159:95-9.

30. Sternberg, C. N. et al. Can patient selection for bladder preservation be based on response to chemotherapy? Cancer 2003;97:1644-51.

31. Shipley, W.U. et al. Selective bladder preservation by combined modality protocol treatment: long-term outcomes of 190 patients with invasive bladder cancer. Urology 2002;60: 62-6.

32. Herr, H.W. et al. Outcome of patients who refuse cystectomy after receiving neo-adjuvant chemotherapy for muscle-invasive bladder cancer. Eur Urol 2007;54:126-32.

33 Metastatic bladder cancer

Mike D. Shelley and Malcolm D. Mason

Cochrane Urological Cancers Unit, Velindre NHS Trust, Cardiff, UK

Background

In the United States of America and Europe, between 50,000 and 70,000 new cases of bladder cancer are diagnosed each year. It is the second most common urogenital cancer and predominantly affects elderly men and women with a ratio of 3:1. Early-stage superficial bladder cancer, confined to the urothelium, can often be managed with serial resection and intravesical therapy, whist the standard treatments for invasive bladder cancer are cystectomy or radiotherapy, often combined with neo-adjuvant chemotherapy. Overall 5-year survival rates for muscle-invasive disease are between 10% and 40% depending on the depth of tumor penetration and the extent of visceral involvement. For patients who fail these primary therapies and develop metastases or those who are diagnosed with metastatic bladder cancer, the prognosis is poor, with less than 5% alive at 5 years. For patients with metastatic bladder cancer, systemic chemotherapy is the standard treatment.

This chapter will review the evidence on the efficacy and toxicity of chemotherapeutic regimes in the treatment of metastatic bladder cancer.

Literature search

A search strategy was developed using the Cochrane search strategy for randomized trials combined with thesaurus and text words for chemotherapeutic regimes and metastatic bladder cancer. Initially Medline was searched from 1966 to 2008. The search strategy was then modified to search EMBASE, Web of Science and the Cochrane Library.

Evidence-Based Urology. Edited by Philipp Dahm, Roger R. Dmochowski.
© 2010 Blackwell Publishing.

Clinical question 33.1

Is cisplatin alone as effective as cisplatin in combination with methotrexate, cyclophosphamide or adriamycin?

The evidence

Four randomized trials have compared cisplatin alone with cisplatin plus methotrexate, cyclophosphamide or adriamycin (Table 33.1) [1-4]. A randomized trial of 53 patients receiving either cisplatin alone or in combination with methotrexate reported no difference in clinical response or survival [1]. In another study of 109 patients randomized to either cisplatin alone or combined with cyclophosphamide, no significant difference in response rate was seen between the two arms [2]. Similarly, when cisplatin alone was compared to cisplatin plus adriamycin and cyclophosphamide, there was no significant difference in response rate, response duration or survival [3]. Notably, the combination regime in this study was more toxic, with 27% of patients having granulocytopenia compared to none with cisplatin alone. In a study of 135 patients with disseminated transitional cell carcinoma [4], 17% of evaluable patients had a partial or complete remission with cisplatin alone compared to 33% for those receiving a combination of cisplatin, doxorubicin plus cyclophosphamide (p = 0.09). Crude median survival was slightly better with the combination regime (6 months versus 7.3 months, p = 0.17), but was significantly more toxic; 34% developed grade 3 or 4 hematological toxicity compared to 3% for cisplatin alone.

Comment

In small randomized trials, single-agent cisplatin induces similar response rates and overall survival estimates when

Table 33.1 Effect of cisplatin alone or in combination with methotrexate, cyclophosphamide or adriamycin on clinical outcomes

Authors	Methods	Interventions	Participants	Outcomes	Results
Hillcoat et al. [1]	RCT – method not stated. 4 patients lost to follow-up	Randomized to cisplatin 80 mg/m^2 day 1 every 4 weeks or cisplatin 80 mg/m^2 day 2 plus methotrexate 50 mg/m^2 days 1 and 15 every 4 weeks	110 patients with measurable metastatic urothelial tumors	Response rates Toxicity Survival	53 patients randomized to combination arm and 55 to cisplatin. Maximum follow-up 2–5 years CR 9% in each arm, overall (CR plus PR) 24/53 (45%) for combination and 17/55 (31%) for cisplatin, p=0.18 Hematological toxicity and mucositis more frequent on combination arm (p=0.01 and 0.0005, respectively) N/V greater in combination arm (p=0.06). Two deaths on combination arm, one with cisplatin Median survival combination 8.7 months, 7.2 months for cisplatin (log-rank p=0.7). No difference in relapse-free survival (log-rank p=0.8)
Soloway et al. [2]	RCT – randomized by contacting the Statistical Co-ordinating Centre of Collaborative Group	Cisplatin (DDP) at a dose of 70 mg/m^2 in arm 1 and cisplatin and cyclophosphamide at an initial dose of 750 mg/m^2 in arm 2	109 patients with biopsy-proven advanced bladder cancer. Metastatic or regionally advanced disease Tumor confined to the bladder alone	Duration of response (complete clinical response (CR) and partial response (PR)). Disease progression	50 randomized to arm 1 (DDP alone), 59 to arm 2 (DDP plus cyclophosphamide). Arm 1 – response 20% (5 CR and 5 PR, 32% disease stabilization) Arm 2 – response 11.9% (3 CR and 4 PR, 33.9% disease stabilization) No statistical significance in response between arms At 6 months: 64.8% in the DDP arm progressed, 57.1% in the combination arm N/V moderate in 25% and severe in 8%, caused 9 withdrawals 27% in the combination arm required dose reduction
Troner et al. [3]	RCT – method not stated	Randomized to cisplatin (DDP) 60 mg/m^2 or (DDP) plus cyclophosphamide 400 mg/m^2 plus doxorubicin 40 mg/m^2 every 21 days	116 patients with inoperable or metastatic carcinoma of the bladder, ureters or renal pelvis. 91 evaluable	Response (Southeastern Group criteria) Toxicity Survival	DDP response 15% (median duration 12.7 weeks), combination 21% (12.4 weeks) DDP 47/57 died (median survival 21 weeks), combination 43/53 died (29 weeks) DDP 2 deaths from renal failure, 1 in combination arm. 27% granulocytopenia and cardiotoxicity in 2 patients with combination. None with DDP
Kandekar et al. [4]	RCT – method not stated	Randomized to cisplatin (DDP) 60 mg/m^2 or (DDP) plus cyclophosphamide 400 mg/m^2 plus doxorubicin 40 mg/m^2 every 21 days	135 patients with disseminated transitional cell carcinoma	Response (ECOG criteria) Toxicity Survival	93 evaluable. Response DDP 17% (median duration 9 months), combination 33% (7 months) DDP 21% severe N/V, 3% hemotoxicity, combination 63% severe N/V, 34% grade 2–6 hemotoxicity, 1 death

CR, complete response; N/V, nausea and vomiting; PR, partial response; RCT, randomized controlled trial compared to cisplatin combined with methotrexate or cyclophosphamide, although the combination of cisplatin, adriamycin and cyclophosphamide appears to be more active. The combination regimes were significantly more toxic (evidence and recommendation Grade 1A).

Clinical question 33.2

Does the combination of cisplatin, methotrexate and vinblastine (CMV) induce higher response rates than methotrexate plus vinblastine (MV)?

The evidence

Only one study has addressed this issue. A multicenter, Medical Research Council study enrolled 214 patients with poor performance status and metastatic bladder cancer and randomized 108 to receive CMV and 106 to VM [5]. At 2 years post randomization, a total of 204 patients had died – 101 allocated to CMV and 103 allocated to VM. Statistical analysis revealed a hazard ratio of 0.68 (95% CI 0.51–0.90, p = 0.0065) indicating a 32% reduction in the relative risk of dying with CMV. This translates into an overall improvement in median survival of 2.5 months (from 4.5 to 7 months). CMV was considerably more toxic, with five treatment-related deaths (cardiovascular toxicity N 2, septicemia N 2, renal failure N 1) compared to none with VM. CVM resulted in grade 3 neutropenia or thrombocytopenia in five patients compared to none with VM. Hospitalization with systemic antibiotics was required for neutropenic fever in 11 and two patients receiving CMV or MV, respectively. Long-term toxicity presented as neurotoxicity in nine patients on CMV and one on MV.

Comment

The combination of CMV for the treatment of metastatic bladder cancer in poor performance status patients is associated with a small improvement in overall survival, but more toxicity compared to MV. No recommendations can be made.

Clinical question 33.3

Are response rates and survival superior with methotrexate, vinblastine, adriamycin and cisplatin (MVAC) compared to single-agent or combination chemotherapy?

The evidence

Three prospective randomized studies have established MVAC as a standard chemotherapeutic regime for metastatic

bladder cancer (Table 33.2). In a study by Loehrer et al. [6], 246 assessable patients were randomized to either cisplatin alone or to MVAC. The combination regime significantly increased complete and partial response rates, with respective levels of 13% and 25% for MVAC and 3% and 8% for cisplatin alone. The median progression-free survival was superior with MVAC (10 versus 4.3 months) with five complete responders to MVAC still free of disease at 8.5–39.5 months. Overall survival was also significantly improved with MVAC compared to cisplatin alone (median times 12.5 versus 8.2 months, p = 0.0002). However, MVAC was more toxic, inducing significantly more severe leukopenia and fever. In an update of this study, overall survival remained significantly better with MVAC compared to cisplatin alone (log rank p = 0.00015) [7]. At 6 years, 11 patients were alive, two treated with cisplatin alone and nine with MVAC.

Logothetis et al. [8] compared MVAC with another cisplatin-based regime, CisCA (cisplatin, cyclophosphamide, adriamycin), in a randomized study of 110 patients with metastatic bladder cancer. Overall response was significantly better for MVAC (46% versus 65%, p = 0.05) and median survival (44.4 weeks vs 36.1 weeks).

MVAC has also been evaluated against the triplet 5-fluorouracil, interferon alpha-2b and cisplatin (FAP) in a randomized setting [9]. The objective response rate for those assigned to FAP was 42% (complete response in 10%). This compared to 59% for those receiving MVAC (complete response in 24%). The Kaplan–Meier estimate of median survival was 12.5 months for both groups (no p value given).

Comment

The evidence suggests that, in terms of response rates and overall survival, MVAC is superior to single-agent cisplatin, CisCA and FAP (evidence and recommendation Grade 1A).

Clinical question 33.4

Does increasing the dose-intensity of MVAC improve overall survival?

The evidence

The standard dose regime of MVAC was compared to high-dose intensity MVAC plus granulocyte colony-stimulating factor (HD-MVAC) in an international randomized EORTC phase III study [10]. Two hundred and sixty-three patients with advanced bladder cancer were randomized. An objective response (complete and partial)

Table 33.2 Comparison of methotrexate, vinblastine, adriamycin and cisplatin (MVAC) combination chemotherapy with other chemotherapy regimes

Authors	Methods	Interventions	Participants	Outcomes	Results
Loehrer et al. [6]	RCT – patients stratified according to Karnofsky performance score and previous radiotherapy.No randomization method stated	Patients randomized to receive either single-agent cisplatin 70 mg/m² on day 1(N 126) or MVAC (N 120) (methotrexate 30 mg/m² on days 1, 15 and 22, vinblastine 3 mg/m² on days 2 , 15 and 22, doxorubicin 30 mg/m² on day 2 and cisplatin 70 mg/m² on day 2) Courses were repeated every 28 days	269 patients with advanced urothelial carcinoma, 246 assessable	Response Progression-free survival Overall survival Toxicity	MVAC superior in terms of response (39% vs 12%, p<0.0001), progression-free survival (median times 4.3 vs 10 months) and overall survival (median times 12.5 vs 8.2 months, p<0.0002). Grade 3 or 4 leukopenia 1% for cisplatin and 24% MVAC (p<0.0001), granulocytic fever 0% and 10% (p<0.0002), sepsis 1% and 6% (p = 0.04), mucositis 0% and 17% (p<0.0001), N/V 1% and 12% (p = 0.0004)
Saxman et al. [7]	Update of Loehrer 1992 [6]	As above	255 assessable patients with histologically proven advanced bladder cancer	Survival	Minimum follow-up 6 years, MVAC significantly better survival (p = 0.00015) Transitional cell tumors significantly longer survival than adenocarcinomas or squamous cell tumors (p = 0.0078) and worse with liver metastasis (p = 0.0022) or bone metastasis (p = 0.0032) 6 year follow-up: 2 patients (1.6%) alive in the cisplatin group and 9 (6.8%) in the MVAC arm (4.3% of total population) 5 patients (3.7%) in the MVAC arm and 2 (1.6%) in the cisplatin arm were alive and continuously free of urothelial cancer at >6 years
Logothetis et al. [8]	RCT – stratified by histology and extent of dissemination Randomization method not stated	Patients were randomized to receive either CisCA (cyclophosphamide 650 mg/m² day1, doxorubicin 50 mg/m² day 2, cisplatin 100 mg/m² day 2) or MVAC (methotrexate 30 mg/m² days 1, 15 and 22, vinblastine 3 mg/m² days 2 , 15, and 22, doxorubicin 30 mg/m² day 2, and cisplatin 70 mg/m² day 2)	110 patients with measurable metastatic urothelial tumors	Clinical response Toxicity Survival	Overall responses (complete and partial) were 46% (32–62%) for CisCA and 65% (52–77%) for MVAC, p<0.05 Toxicities include leukopenic fever, neuropathy, renal, hepatic and gastrointestinal bleeding. There was no significant difference in the frequency of toxic reactions although renal toxicity occurred in 41% on CisCA compared to 17% on MVAC The survival duration with MVAC (mean 62.6 weeks; median 48.35; range 5.0 to 162.3) was significantly superior to CisCA (mean 40.4 weeks; median 36.1; range 7 to 147.1)
Siefker-Radtke et al. [9]	RCT – method of randomization not stated	Patients were randomized to receive either MVAC (methotrexate 30 mg/m² day 1, vinblastine 3 mg/m², doxorubicin 30 mg/m² and cisplatin 70 mg/m² day 2 repeated every 28 days) or FAP (5-fluorouracil 500 mg/m²/d continuous 5-day infusion in weeks 1 and 4, interferon-alpha 5 MIU/m²/d for 5 days in week 1 and 4, cisplatin 25 mg/m² on days 1, 8, 15, 22). Repeated 6 weekly	122 patients with locally advanced or metastatic bladder cancer	Response rate Progression Survival Toxicity	MVAC 59% objective response (24% CR) FAP 48% (10% CR) Median time to progression 9.9 months in both arms MVAC 48% had at least grade 3 nonhematological toxicity FAP 83% (mainly mucositis with 8 deaths) Myelosuppression was main toxicity with MVAC

CR, complete response; RCT, randomized controlled trial

was seen in 72% of patients on HD-MVAC compared to 58% with the standard MVAC. Median time to progression was significantly improved with the HD-MVAC regime (hazard ratio (HR) 0.73, 95% CI 0.56–0.95, p = 0.017). At a median follow-up of 7.3 years, the median overall survival was 15.1 months with HD-MVAC versus 14.9 months for MVAC (no p value given). The 5-year survival rate was 21.8% (95% CI 18.4--34.0) and 13.5% (95% CI 7.4–19.6) for the HD-MVAC and MVAC regimes, respectively. There was one toxic death in both arms of the study. Grade 4 leukopenia was worse with MVAC (16% versus 8%), as was neutropenic fever (26% versus 10%), although grade 4 thrombocytopenia was more evident with HD-MAVAC (6% versus 11%).

Comment

The evidence suggests that the addition of G-CSF to the standard MVAC regime enables a higher dose intensity of MVAC to be offered with an improvement in time to progression and some survival advantage (evidence and recommendation **Grade 2B**).

Clinical question 33.5

How effective is the combination gemcitabine plus cisplatin (GC) compared to other chemotherapeutic regimes?

The evidence

Three randomized trials have evaluated the combination of GC in patients with advanced or metastatic bladder cancer. The first compared GC with the standard MVAC regime in 405 patients (GC N 203, MVAC N 202) [11]. Overall response rates were 54.3% for GC and 55% for MVAC. The respective time to progressive disease was similar (HR 1.05, 95% CI 0.82–1.32, p = 0.75) as was overall survival (HR 1.04, 95% CI 0.82–1.32, p = 0.75). MVAC resulted in more grade 3 and 4 neutropenia, mucositis, infection and diarrhea. An update of this study [12] indicated that the 5-year overall survival rates for GC and MVAC were similar (13.0% and 15.3%, p = 0.53).

The second study compared GC with paclitaxel, gemcitabine and cisplatin (PGC) as first-line therapy in advanced transitional cell carcinoma of the urothelium [13]. Forty-three patients were randomized to receive GC and 42 to receive PGC and the observed response rates were respectively 44% and 43%. Progressive disease was seen in 29% of patients on PGC and 33% on GC with corresponding median times to progression of 32 weeks and 26 weeks. Overall survival was similar in both groups with median survival times of 61 weeks (PGC) and

49 weeks (GC) although no p values were quoted. PGC was more myelotoxic with grade 3 and 4 leukopenia observed in 49% compared to 35% for GC (p = 0.053). Thrombocytopenia was also more common with PGC (36% versus 21%, p = 0.018). There were two treatment-related deaths in the PGC group due to sepsis.

A phase II study randomized 110 chemo-naive patients (55 per arm) to receive GC or gemcitabine plus carboplatin (GCb) [14]. The main objective of this study was to compare the toxicity of these two regimes. Grade 3–4 hematological toxicities were recorded in 16–34% of patients on GC and 25–50% with GCb. Grade 3–4 neutropenia was the most common toxicity reported, with 34.6% occurring with GC and 45.5% with GCb. No statistical evaluation was reported. Grade 3–4 nonhematological toxicities for GC and GCb included nausea and vomiting (75% and 65%), diarrhea (14.5% and 20%), infection (11% and 15%) and nephrotoxicity (25% and 16%). Overall response on 80 evaluable patients was 49% and 40% for GC and GCb respectively. The corresponding median time to progression was similar for both regimes, although in favor of GC (8.3 and 7.7 months), as was median overall survival (12.8 and 9.8 months).

Comment

Gemcitabine plus cisplatin appears to be equivalent to the combinations of MVAC and PGC in terms of response and survival but is less toxic. GC appears to have a similar toxicity profile to GCb with slightly superior activity (evidence and recommendation **Grade 2B**).

Clinical question 33.6

What is the role of new chemotherapeutic regimes and systemic agents in metastatic bladder cancer?

The evidence

Several novel drug combinations and new agents have shown activity in metastatic bladder cancer. A number of studies have investigated promising combinations of gemcitabine and paclitaxel (Taxol) as both first-line and second-line therapy.

An Italian phase II study [15] administered gemcitabine and paclitaxel every 2 weeks to patients who had received prior treatment with cisplatin-based chemotherapy. This group reported an overall response rate of 60%, and a median overall survival of just over 14 months. In another study, a Spanish group reported on the addition of cisplatin to this combination and achieved an overall response rate of 78% and a median overall survival of 15.6 months [16]. Comparable results have been reported when carboplatin has been substituted for cisplatin [17]. This triplet of gemcitabine, paclitaxel and carboplatin induced a response rate of 68% and a median overall survival of 14.7 months. A similar response rate, but an extended median overall survival of 20 months has been seen with the combination of paclitaxel, cisplatin and ifosfamide [18]. It remains to be seen whether new combinations can continue to improve response rates and overall survival in metastatic bladder cancer and they should be evaluated in randomized trials.

A number of new agents have been evaluated as second-line therapy. Disappointing results have been reported for ixabepilone, a novel epothilone B analog which promotes tubulin polymerization. This agent has only modest activity (response rate 12%, median overall survival 8 months) as second-line therapy for metastatic bladder cancer, with significant toxicity [19].

Methotrexate has demonstrated activity in advanced bladder cancer and this has prompted the assessment of newer antifolate analogs. Single-agent premetexed has reported activity (response rate 28%) as a second-line treatment option [20]. Response rates for trimetexate [21] and piritrexim [22] are reported to be between 17% and 23% in patients who have had prior chemotherapy.

A multicenter randomized trial has recently reported on the efficacy of the microtubule inhibitor vinflunine in patients following cisplatin-based therapy [23]. Three hundred and seventy patients were randomized to receive vinflunine (280–320 mg/m^2) plus best supportive care versus best supportive care alone. There was significant grade 3–4 hematological toxicity with one fatal pancytopenia in the vinflunine arm. Constipation, fatigue and abdominal pain were also significant side effects. No data were presented for the best supportive care arm. Multivariate analysis adjusting for prognostic factors indicated a significant overall survival advantage with vinflunine (p = 0.035) with a 23% reduction in the risk of dying compared to best supportive care alone (HR 0.77, 95% CI 0.60–0.98).

A recent phase II study assessed the activity of sunitinib, a novel vascular endothelial growth factor (VEGF)-targeted agent in patients with relapsed or refractory urothelial carcinoma [24]. Sunitinib was administered orally as a single agent in 6-week cycles of 50 mg daily for 4 weeks. Of the 45 patients, 41 were evaluable for response and three had a partial response, one had a 30% reduction in tumor volume and 11 had stable disease. Regression was seen in liver, bone, lung, bladder, soft tissue and lymph node lesions. Grade 3–4 toxicities included fatigue, hand and foot syndrome, hemorrhage, hypertension and mucositis, with one treatment-related fatality. The study was too immature to report on response duration and overall survival.

Trastuzumab, a humanized monoclonal antibody that binds to Her/neu, has recently been assessed in metastatic or recurrent bladder cancer [25]. In a multicenter phase II trial, patients received trastuzumab, paclitaxel, carboplatin and gemcitabine with the primary endpoint of determining cardiac toxicity, which was seen in 27% of patients. The most common grade 3–4 toxicity was myelosuppression, with two therapy-related deaths. Seventy percent of patients responded with a median time to progression and survival of 9.3 and 14.1 months, respectively. A randomized trial is needed to determine the true contribution of trastuzumab in this combination. No recommendation can be made at present.

Comment

New combinations of chemotherapeutics, with single-agent activity, are providing encouraging results in first- and second-line settings. Vinflunine is the first agent to show a survival advantage as second-line therapy and warrants further study. Sunitinib also has activity as a second-line treatment but induces significant toxicity.

Implications for practice

There is now a wealth of evidence to indicate that advanced or metastatic bladder cancer is a chemosensitive tumor and that combination chemotherapy has a role in the management of this condition. The combination MVAC is an active chemotherapeutic regime for patients with metastatic bladder cancer which may be supplemented with G-CSF to reduce hematological and gastrointestinal toxicity. However, this regime has not been compared to best supportive care in a randomized trial, so its exact contribution to overall survival is unclear.

The combination of gemcitabine and cisplatin appears to be better tolerated than MVAC and of comparable efficacy and is now considered the standard chemotherapeutic strategy for patients with metastatic bladder cancer.

Although chemotherapy is active in metastatic bladder cancer, the recommendation to use this modality should take into account not only the effectiveness but also the toxicity associated with this therapy. Patients with advanced or metastatic disease are elderly and generally in poor health with a poor outlook. Chemotherapy is always associated with side effects ranging from mild to severe (grade 3–4) and in many studies presented in this review, treatment-related fatalities have been reported. The recommendation for the use of chemotherapy has to be balanced against the improvement in clinical symptoms and the potential gain in survival, which appears to be improving. In the latter stages of the patient's life, quality of life is a prime consideration, assessment of which is sadly lacking in the majority of studies. Taking these factors into account, the use of chemotherapy in metastatic bladder cancer is strongly recommended and should be a treatment option available to patients.

Implications for research

Although advances in chemotherapy for advanced or metastatic bladder cancer have been made in recent years, long-term survivors are rare. The results are still unsatisfactory and newer regimes should be investigated in randomized trials.

Cisplatin-based chemotherapy appears to be one of the most active of chemotherapeutics regimes studied but is associated with side effects, including nephrotoxicity. Many elderly patients with advanced urothelial cancer have poor renal function and are not good candidates for cisplatin therapy. In these patients, alternatives to cisplatin need to be evaluated including carboplatin [26] and the use of dose-dense sequential chemotherapy with this agent [27]. Other cisplatin alternative regimes such as gemcitabine and oxaliplatin have been shown to be active and tolerable in unfit patients [28] and should be investigated further in this patient group.

All future studies should include an assessment of quality of life. A major aim of new studies of chemotherapy should be to improve this important endpoint. If this were achieved then the recommendation to use this modality would be greatly strengthened.

The available evidence on prognostic or predictive markers to predict response to chemotherapy in patients with advanced bladder cancer is scant and should be the topic of further investigation. Overexpression of p53, a cell cycle regulatory protein in bladder cancer, has been reported to correlate with resistance to MVAC chemotherapy. Other biological prognostic markers such as bcl-2, Her/neu, p-glycoprotein, glutathione and metalloproteinase may have a role in determining outcome in response to chemotherapy in bladder cancer patients [29]. The determination of factors that accurately predict those patients who would benefit from chemotherapy would therefore be a significant advancement in the management of metastatic disease.

References

1. Hillcoat BL, Raghavan D, Matthew J, et al. Randomized trial of cisplatin versus cisplatin plus methotrexate in advanced cancer of the urothelial tract. J Clin Oncol 1989;7:706-9.
2. Soloway MS, Einstein A, Corder MP, et al. A comparison of cisplatin and the combination of cisplatin and cyclophosphamide in advanced urothelial cancer. Cancer 1983;52;767-72.
3. Troner M, Birch R, Omura GA, Williams S. Phase III comparison alone versus cisplatin, doxorubicin and cyclophosphamide in the treatment of bladder (urothelial) cancer: a South Eastern Cancer study Group Trial. J Urol 1987;137;660-2.
4. Kandekar JD, Elson PJ, DeWys WD, Slayton RE, Harris DT. Comparative activity and toxicity of cis-diaminedichloroplatinum (DDP) and a combination of doxorubicin, cyclophosphamide, and DDP in disseminated transitional cell carcinoma of the urinary tract. J Clin Oncol 1985;3:539-45.
5. Mead GM, Russell M, Clark P, et al. A randomized trial comparing methotrexate and vinblastine (MV) with cisplatin, methotrexate and vinblastine (CVM) in advanced transitional cell carcinoma: results and a report on prognostic factors in a Medical Research Council study. Br J Cancer 1998;78:1067-75.
6. Loehrer PJ, Einhorn LH, Elson PJ, et al. A randomized comparison of cisplatin alone or in combination with methotrexate, vinblastine, and doxorubicin in patients with metastatic urothelial carcinoma: a Cooperative Group study. J Clin Oncol 1992;10:1066-73.
7. Saxman SB, Propert KJ, Einhorn LH, et al. Long-term follow-up of a phase III intergroup study of cisplatin alone or in combination with methotrexate, vinblastine and doxorubicin in patients with metastatic urothelial carcinoma: a Cooperative Group study. J Clin Oncol 1997;15:2564-9.
8. Logothetis C, Dexeus FH, Fin L, et al. A prospective randomized trial comparing MVAC and CISCA chemotherapy for patients with metastatic urothelial tumours. J Clin Oncol 1990;8:1050-5.
9. Siefket-Radtke AO, Millikan RE, Tu S-M, et al. Phase III trial of fluorouracil, interferon alfa-2b, and cisplatin versus methotrexate, vinblastine, doxorubicin and cisplatin in metastatic or unresectable urothelial cancer. J Clin Oncol 2002;20:1361-7.
10. Sternberg CN, de Mulder P, Schornagel JH, et al. Seven year update of an EORTC phase III trial of high-dose intensity M-VAC chemotherapy and G-CFS versus classic M-VAC in advanced urothelial tract tumours. Eur J Cancer 2006;42:50-4.
11. Von der Masse H, Hansen SW, Roberts TJ, et al. Gemcitabine and cisplatin versus methotrexate, vinblastine, doxorubicin, and cisplatin in advanced or metastatic bladder cancer: results of a large randomized, multinational, multicentre, phase III study. J Clin Oncol 2000;17:3068-77.
12. Von der Masse H, Sengolov L, Roberts TJ, et al. Long-term survival results of a randomized trial comparing gemcitabine plus cisplatin, with methotrexate, vinblastine, doxorubicin, and cisplatin in advanced or metastatic bladder cancer. J Clin Oncol 2005;23:4602-8.
13. Lorusso V, Crucitta E, Silvestris N, et al. Randomized, open-label, phase II trial of paclitaxel, gemcitabine and cisplatin versus gemcitabine and cisplatin as first-line chemotherapy in advanced transitional cell carcinoma of the urothelium. Oncol Rep 2005;13:283-7.
14. Doglotti L, Carteni G, Siena S, et al. Gemcitabine plus cisplatin versus gemcitabine plus carboplatin as first-line chemotherapy in advanced transitional cell carcinoma of the urothelium: results of a randomized phase I trial. Eur Urol 2007;52 (1):134-41.
15. Sternberg CN, Calabro F, Pizzocaro G, Marini L, Schnetzer S, Sella A. Chemotherapy with an every-2-week regimen of gemcitabine and paclitaxel in patients with transitional cell

carcinoma who have received prior cisplatin-based therapy. Cancer 2001;92:2993-8.

16. Bellmunt V, Guillem V, Paz-Ares L, et al. Phase III study of paclitaxel, cisplatin and gemcitabine in advanced transitional cell carcinoma of the urothelium. J Clin Oncol 2000;18:3247- 55.

17. Hussain M, Vaishampayan U, Du W, et al. Combination paclitaxel, carboplatin and gemcitabine is an active treatment for advanced urothelial cancer. J Clin Oncol 2000;19(9);2527-33.

18. Bajorin DF, McCarffrey JA, Dodd PM, et al. Ifosfamide, paclitaxel and cisplatin for patients with advanced transitional cell carcinoma of the urothelial tract: final report of a phase II trial evaluating two dosing schedules. Cancer 2000;88(7):1671-8.

19. Dreicer R, Li S, Manola J, Haas NB, Roth BJ, Wilding G. Phase 2 trial of epothilone B analog BMS-247550 (ixabepilone) in advanced carcinoma of the urothelium (E3800). Cancer 2007;110:759-63.

20. Sweeny CJ, Roth B, Kabbinavar F, et al. Phase II study of premetrexed for second-line treatment of transitional cell carcinoma of the urothelium. J Clin Oncol 2006;24:3451-6.

21. Witte RS, Elson P, Khandakar J, et al. An Eastern Cooperative Oncology Group phase II trial of trimetrexate in treatment of advanced urothelial carcinoma. Cancer 2004;73:688-91.

22. Khorsand M, Lange J, Feun L, et al. Phase II trial of oral piritrexim in advanced previously treated transitional cell cancer of the bladder. Invest New Drugs 1997;15:157-63.

23. Bellmunt J, Molins H, von der Masse C, et al. Randomized phase III trial of vinflunine (V) plus best supportive care (B) vs B alone as 2nd line therapy after platinum-containing regimen in advanced transitional cell carcinoma of the urothelium (TCCU). Proc Am Soc Clin Oncol 2008;26:5028.

24. Gallagher DJ, Milowsky MI, Gerst A, et al. Final results of a phase II study of sunitinib in patients with relapsed or refractory urothelial carcinoma. Proc Am Soc Clin Oncol 2008;26:5082.

25. Hussein MH, MacVicar GR, Petrylak DP, et al. Trastuzumab, paclitaxel, carboplatin and gemcitabine in advanced human epidermal growth factor recptor-2/neu-positive urothelial carcinoma: results of a multinational phase II National Cancer Institute trial. J Clin Oncol 2007;25:2218-24.

26. Petrrioli R, Frediani B, Manganelli A, et al. Comparison between a cisplatin containing regimen and a carboplatin containing regimen for recurrent or metastatic bladder cancer patients. Cancer 1996;77:344-51.

27. Galsky MD, Iasonos A, Mironov S, Scattergood J, Boyle MG, Bajorin DF. Phase II trial of dose-dense doxorubicin plus gemcitabine followed by paclitaxel plus carboplatin in patients with advanced urothelial carcinoma and impaired renal function. Cancer 2007;109:549-55.

28. Carles J, Esteban E, Climent M, et al. Gemcitabine and oxaliplatin combination: a multi-centre phase II trial in unfit patients with locally advanced or metastatic urothelial cancer. Ann Oncol 2007;18:1359-62.

29. Al-Sukhum S, Hussain M. Current understanding of the biology of advanced bladder cancer. Cancer 2003;97(8):2064-75.

34 Treatment of localized kidney cancer

Frédéric Pouliot, Jeffrey C. LaRochelle and Allan J. Pantuck

Institute of Urologic Oncology and Department of Urology, David Geffen School of Medicine, University of California, Los Angeles, CA, USA

Introduction

The annual number of patients with renal cell carcinoma (RCC) has increased in the last decade, due in part to an increase in incidentally found tumors, but studies suggest that this increase is not due to lead time bias alone [1]. This increasing incidence of RCC has occurred across all clinical stages, but the highest increase has been observed for the incidence of localized tumors, with an average annual increase of 3.7% between 1973 to 1998 based on the SEER database [2,3]. Similarly, the incidental detection of RCC has increased, being 7% in a series from 1935 to 1965, whereas it increased to 61% in a series from 1998 [4,5].

Since the outcome of patients surgically treated for localized RCC of less than 4 cm is very good (96% 5-year disease-free survival), the management of localized RCC has more recently also focused on outcomes other than just oncological ones [6]. Of those, the perioperative outcomes and renal functional outcomes have been studied to optimize the treatment of localized RCC. Furthermore, new management strategies such as laparoscopy, cryotherapy, radiofrequency and active surveillance have emerged in the last two decades with the common goal of providing better quality of life and functional outcomes while preserving oncological success associated with more radical techniques. The interest in studying oncological outcomes together with perioperative and renal function outcomes has led to a substantial number of good-quality publications that can allow us to give recommendations on various aspects of the treatment of localized RCC. From a surgical standpoint, the role of partial nephrectomy, laparoscopic radical nephrectomy and lymph node dissection has been studied sufficiently to allow us to provide recommendations using the Grade level of evidence.

Comparing open and laparoscopic radical nephrectomy

Background

Radical nephrectomy (RN) is indicated for the treatment of renal tumors suspicious for RCC with the goal of surgically curing the patient and preventing metastasis. Traditionally, RN includes the *en bloc* removal of the tumor, kidney, adrenal, perirenal fat and Gerota's fascia, which can be done through many surgical approaches. Most approaches have been developed for open radical nephrectomy (ORN). Depending on the tumor location, size and invasion of the venous system, thoracoabdominal, transabdominal, flank or lumbotomy approaches have been described. These can be performed by both transperitoneal or extraperitoneal approaches.

In the last 20 years, however, laparoscopic surgery has emerged as an alternative to the open approach in urology. The first laparoscopic radical nephrectomy (LRN) was described by Clayman et al. in 1991 [7]. Since then, techniques and approaches of LRN have evolved, and this technique is now widely used in urological practice. One of these further evolutions is the use of a hand-port that allows surgeons to assist laparoscopic manipulation with one hand in the patient without compromising the pneumoperitoneum. This technique has been named hand-assisted laparoscopic nephrectomy (HALN). Like RN, laparoscopic nephrectomy can also be performed by the transperitoneal or retroperitoneal approaches. Several postulated advantages of laparoscopic surgeries include reduction in the length of hospital stay, less requirement for opioid pain relief, faster recuperation, and better cosmetic results. Opponents of LRN initially raised questions regarding the risk of trauma to intra-abdominal organs, the inability to palpate intra-abdominal organs and lymph nodes, and the inability to perform adequate lymph node dissection (LND). During the same period, simple

Evidence-Based Urology. Edited by Philipp Dahm, Roger R. Dmochowski.
© 2010 Blackwell Publishing.

laparoscopic nephrectomy (LN) has also been developed for living donor nephrectomy, which has allowed prospective randomized study to compare open nephrectomy (ON) and laparoscopic approaches for perioperative morbidity [8-11]. Many of these studies are now published, and a meta-analysis is available [12].

In this section, we will summarize the literature regarding two questions related to radical nephrectomy approaches. What are the differences in perioperative outcomes between open and laparoscopic nephrectomy? What are the differences in oncological outcomes between open and laparoscopic radical nephrectomy?

Clinical question 34.1

What is the role of laparoscopic nephrectomy in the management of RCC?

Literature search

Potentially relevant studies were identified by a search of the Medline electronic database (source PubMed, 1966 to December 2008) using relevant keywords in combination, as follows: nephrectomy AND laparoscopy AND open (163 articles retrieved) OR nephrectomy AND laparoscopy AND open AND review (24 articles retrieved). Original and review articles were selected based on language (English only) and revelance of their title. A total of 112 articles were kept for abstract analysis.

We have included in our analysis studies performed to analyze differences between ORN and LRN for RCC. Prospective and retrospective studies were included. Studies including nephroureterectomy, nephrectomy for known benign lesions, and noncontemporary comparisons between ORN and LRN were excluded. When two studies were from the same cohort and/or center, only the most recent update was included. Since relatively few studies were randomized and/or prospective, we extended our analysis to randomized prospective studies that were done in the context of living donor nephrectomy and that have compared open and laparoscopic approaches to study the perioperative outcomes or the two approaches. We also included the results of a recent meta-analysis that combined all the studies comparing the perioperative outcomes of open and laparoscopic living donor nephrectomy.

The evidence

Perioperative outcomes

We identified two prospective, nonrandomized studies and nine retrospective studies that addressed perioperative outcomes after radical nephrectomy for RCC (Table 34.1)

[13-23]. Five of the 11 studies compared HALN with ORN. The perioperative factors that were reviewed included: operative time, blood loss, transfusions, complications, morphine equivalent requirements and hospital stay. Regarding operating room (OR) time, one prospective and four retrospective studies reported statistically significantly (SS) less OR time for ORN. Three studies reported less, but not SS less, OR time for ORN. Two other studies reported a SS increased OR time with ORN, but those two studies had extraordinary long ORN OR time when compared to other series [17,20]. Average OR time among studies was 166 minutes for ORN and 223 minutes for LRN (excluding the Malaeb and Kawauchi studies). Blood loss was consistently less with the LRN approach in all studies. Only two out of the 11 studies did not show a SS difference [14,21]. Average blood loss was 431 mL for ORN and 190 mL for LRN. Similarly, transfusion rates were 0–20% for the RN. Two out of four studies reported SS more, one less, and one no difference in the transfusion rate with ORN. Complication rates where similar when comparing the two approaches (range was 3–55% for ORN and 0–37% for LRN). Only one retrospective study reported SS fewer complications with LRN [13]. Pain, which is reflected by consumption of morphine equivalents, was SS less in all the LRN studies that looked at this outcome. Finally, average hospital stay was 3.6 days for LRN and 5.8 days for ORN (excluding the Kawauchi study which had an extraordinarily long hospital stay that might reflect surgeon preference rather than the effect of surgery). Of note, three studies have also shown than LRN was associated with a shorter time to return to normal activities [14,21,22].

Since no randomized controlled trial (RCT) was available to assess perioperative outcomes to compare ON and LN, we included in our analysis four RCTs that were published in the living donor kidney transplant literature (Table 34.2) [8-11]. A fifth study by Oyen et al. was not included since the same group published their updated results in 2005 [9,24]. Regarding OR time, all the RCTs showed that LN was SS longer than ON. In the two studies that assessed blood loss, no SS difference was observed. Only one study statistically analyzed the complications, and no difference was observed between the two techniques [11]. Pain assessed by morphine equivalent was higher in the ON group in two of the three studies that reported statistics on this outcome. Finally, hospital stay was not SS different in two RCTs while SS less for LN in one study. Of note, the Oyen study had a prolonged hospital stay with an average of more than 6 days for both techniques.

In a meta-analysis, Nanidis et al. analyzed all the published studies comparing open and laparoscopic living donor nephrectomy [12]. A total of 6594 patients were included from 73 studies. Overall, the meta-analysis revealed that ON was associated with less OR and warm ischemia times, while LN was associated with a decrease

Table 34.1 Studies comparing perioperative and oncological outcomes between open (ORN) and laparoscopic radical nephrectomy (LRN)

Author	Year	Ref#	Type of study	N	OR time (min)		Hospital stay (day)		Blood loss (ml)		Complications (%)		Pain[1]		RFS(%)[3]		DSS (%)[4]		Follow-up
					ORN	LRN	ORN	LRN	ORN	LRN	ORN	LRN	ORN	LRN	ORN	LRN	ORN	LRN	LRN/ORN
Ono et al.	1999	22	Retrospective	100	198	312	na	na	512	215	8	13	68	31	98	96	na	na	24/24
Dunn et al.	2000	15	Retrospective	94	168	330	5.2	3.4	451	172	55	37	na	na	91	90	na	na	25/25
Nakada et al.	2001	21	Retrospective	36	118	221	4.7	3.9	238	171	na	na	na	na	na	na	na	na	na
Kawauchi et al.	2003	17	Retrospective	44	234	204	21.5	11.5	495	170	18	9	36	16	na	na	na	na	na
Lee et al.	2003	18	Retrospective	104	181	195	8.9	6.8	263	183	8	6	na	na	na	na	na	na	na
Baldwin et al.	2003	13	Retrospective	47	150	168	3.8	1.3	467	125	27	0	98	23	na	na	na	na	7.8/6.0
Busby et al.	2003	14	Retrospective	44	153	265	4.8	3.4	299	186	14	14	46	11	na	na	na	na	na
Makhoul et al.	2004	19	Retrospective	65	133	134	8.8	5.5	357	133	3	8	3	2	0	0	100	100	12.4/20.4
Shuford et al.	2004	23	Retrospective	74	na[2]	na	3.6	1.5	256	232	10	12	na	na	na	na	na	na	na
Malaeb et al.	2005	20	Prospective	19	341	205	6.2	2.9	870	261	na	na	95	16	na	na	na	na	na
Hemal et al.	2007	16	Prospective	112	165	181	6.6	3.6	537	245	16	12	na	na	90	90	94	95	51/57

Advantage ORN, statistically significant (p < 0.05)
Advantage LRN, statistically significant (p < 0.05)
No statistically significant advantage for any technique
[1] mg equivalent of morphine
[2] Not available
[3] Recurrence-free survival
[4] Disease-free survival

Table 34.2 Randomized controlled studies comparing perioperative outcomes between open (ON) and laparoscopic nephrectomy (LN) for living donor transplant

Author	Year	Ref#	Type of study	N	OR time (min)		Hospital stay (Day)		Blood loss	complications (%)		Pain[1]		Return to normal activities (day)	
					ORN	LRN	ORN	LRN		ORN	LRN	ORN	LRN	ORN	LRN
Wolf et al.	2001	11	RCT	70	125	206	2.6	1.7	see note[3]	15	17	111	59	22	15
Oyen et al	2005	9	RCT	122	140	180	6.7	6.2	na	0	8	36	28	na	na
Brook et al.	2005	8	RCT	60	135	186	na[2]	na	na	na	na	na	na	na	na
Simforoosh et al.	2005	10	RCT	200	152	271	2.2	2.3	see note[4]	9	17	11	12	57	34
Nanidis et al.	2008	12	Meta-analysis	6594	less by 52 min		less by 1.6 days		74 ml less	17	13	70.2 mg less		less by 24 weeks	

■ Advantage ORN, statistically significant (p < 0.05)
■ Advantage LRN, statistically significant (p < 0.05)
■ No statistically significant advantage for any technique
[1]mg equivalent of morphine
[2]not available
[3]156 ml for LRN vs 216 ml for ORN
[4]Evaluated with hematocrit

in hospital stay, analgesic use, complications and a faster return to normal activity. However, when pooling the RCTs, the decrease in OR time associated with ON was the only difference between the two groups. Surprisingly, no difference in hospital stay, analgesic use or time to normal activity was observed. This is an unexpected result since the two studies that looked at time to normal activity did show a statistical difference between the two groups [10,11].

Oncological outcomes

Only four series out of 11 compared the oncological outcomes between LRN and ORN (see Table 34.1) [16,19,22]. None of these have shown a SS difference in recurrence-free (RFS) or disease-specific (DSS) survivals. Ono et al. compared 40 ORN to 60 LRN performed between 1992 and 1998 [22]. Clinical T1 disease represented 10% of the ORN cases, while it represented 28% of cases for LRN. The remaining patients were cT2 preoperatively. RFS after 24 months of follow-up was 98% and 96% for ORN and LRN, respectively. Makhoul et al. compared 133 ORN with 134 LRN with similar tumor size and Fuhrman nuclear grades (p = 0.2 and 0.68, respectively) [19]. Mean tumor sizes were 4.8 and 3.9 cm for ORN and LRN while mean Fuhrman nuclear

grades were 1.5 and 1.6, respectively. After a mean follow-up of 12 and 20 months (LRN and ORN), no recurrences were observed in either group. Finally, Hemal et al. compared the two approaches for T2-only tumors [16]. RFS and DSS were not SS between ORN and LRN (RFS = 90% both appro-ach, DSS = 94% (ORN) and 95% (LRN)). Of note, follow-up was longer by 6 months for ORN compared to LRN.

Comment

The advent of laparoscopy in urology has changed the surgical management of RCC. The initial enthusiasm for LRN was mainly related to its shorter hospital stay and reduced narcotic requirements after surgery. Early studies comparing the laparoscopic and open approaches for radical nephrectomy were biased by the comparison of laparoscopic to historical open series. Of note, most series have compared perioperative characteristics between the two approaches in a retrospective manner, rendering definitive conclusions difficult for a number of outcomes. In our opinion, subjective outcomes like hospital stay, complications, and transfusion rates are not valid if the criteria for discharge, complications or transfusions are not collected prospectively. For instance, ORN hospital stay varied from 3.6 to 21 days depending on the study chosen (see Table 34.1). Since laparoscopy was still in development and had to find its place as a new technique during the period of many of these studies, surgeons might have used different criteria to discharge their patients from hospital after one surgery versus another. On the other hand, some outcomes are less likely to be biased by subjective interpretation even if they are collected in a retrospective manner. For OR time and blood loss, we believe that conclusions regarding these specific outcomes are stronger. Another important factor to consider is that the size of the tumor in each group was not always compared in some studies [21,23]. This could have had an effect on factors like OR time or blood loss.

Despite these relative limitations in our analysis, certain conclusions can be drawn from the highest quality studies performed and the trends in the others. In our opinion, the study by Hemal et al. is the single best study to assess the perioperative and oncological outcomes comparing ORN with LRN because it was prospective and included only clinical T2 tumors [16]. In this study, it was shown that LRN was associated with a SS increase in OR time, but a SS decrease in hospital stay, blood loss, pain and transfusion rate. No SS differences in complications, RFS or DSS were observed between the two groups. All these conclusions are in agreement with most of the retrospective studies included in the analysis as well as the meta-analysis performed from the living donor kidney transplant literature. We believe that the combination of these studies is sufficient to draw conclusions on the aforementioned outcomes (see next section).

It is worth pointing out that, in addition to oncological outcome, another important outcome to assess when evaluating a patient candidate for RN is renal function. Even if LRN demonstrates advantages compared to ORN on many perioperative outcomes, there may be additional reasons to consider an open partial nephrectomy rather than a LRN. Increasingly, it is these two alternatives between which a decision must be made. Furthermore, when preclinical imaging shows enlarged lymph nodes or thrombus in the vena cava, management might be better suited to an open approach.

Implications for practice

Based on studies selected from the oncological and renal transplant literature, we believe there is sufficient evidence to show that LRN should be the first treatment option in patients with uncomplicated clinical T1 or T2 RCC not amenable to partial nephrectomy. The combined studies from radical nephrectomy series as well as those from living donor nephrectomy series have shown that LN is associated with a decrease in blood loss, transfusion rates, pain, time to normal activity and hospital stay (see Tables 34.2, 34.3). The decrease in OR time associated with ORN does not counterbalance the advantages of LRN when it is an option.

Oncological outcomes appear to be similar for the two techniques, but the evidence for this is weaker. ORN should be considered for individual cases where an advantage is expected for the patient regarding oncological outcomes. The advantages might be a decrease in waiting time for surgery, removal of extensive lymph nodes, venous extension or concomitant metastasis.

Recommendation

Laparoscopic radical nephrectomy should be strongly considered as the first option for patients with uncomplicated clinical T1 or T2 RCC not amenable to partial nephrectomy based on its reduced perioperative morbidity and equivalent oncological outcomes (strong recommendation, moderate-quality evidence, **Grade 1B**).

Implications for research

Research should now focus on prospective, randomized studies with oncological outcomes as the primary endpoint since evidence on perioperative outcomes is already strong.

Role of lymph node dissection in the treatment of localized renal cell carcinoma

Background

Lymph node metastasis may occur in up to 20% of cancers. In a recent review of the literature by Godoy et al., prevalence of LN metastasis was found in 3.3–66% of patients, depending on the extent of LN dissection or clinical cancer stage [25]. However, when considering only series that included nephrectomy for localized RCC, positive LNs were found less frequently, between 3.3% and 14.1% [26-30]. Primary landing zones of RCC metastasis are the interaortocaval nodes on the right and the para-aortic nodes on the left, though lymphatic spread from RCC is notoriously variable and unpredictable [25]. Advocates for LND propose it for two reasons: staging and/or therapeutic purposes. The initial template for RCC LND was described by Robson, and included paracaval, precaval, interaortocaval, pre-aortic and retro-aortic LNs, extending caudally from the iliac bifurcation to the crus of the diaphragm cephalad [31]. Since then, the template has been modified through the years to include fewer lymph nodes, with the goal of decreasing morbidity. Limited LND was defined as including the pre-, retro-, and para-aortic and interaortocaval nodes on the right side and the para-, pre- and retro-aortic nodes on the left side [27]. However, since the therapeutic benefit of LND has been debated, it has been difficult to recommend what would be the best LN dissection from a therapeutic perspective.

Table 34.3 Studies comparing perioperative and oncological outcomes of localized renal cell carcinoma treated with or without lymph node dissection (LND)

Author	Year	Ref#	N	Type of study	Groups	Outcome 5y DSS[2]	Outcome 10y DSS[2]	p value	Complications LND −	Complications LND +	Conclusions from the authors
Herrlinger et al.	1991	33	511	Prospective	LND[1] limited (overall RCC)	58	41	p < 0.01	3.5%	1%[7]	Systematic and extended lymphadenectomy improves the prognosis of patients with renal cell carcinoma
					LND full (overall RCC)	66	56				
					LND limited (confined RCC)	92	80				
					LND full (confined RCC)	81	54				
Schafhauser et al.	1999	29	1035	Retrospective	LND full	70	58	p < 0.01	2.5%	0.4 %[7]	Al least 4% of patients benefit from LND
					LND limited	62	50				
					LND none	66	45				
Minervini et al.	2001	27	167	Retrospective	LND limited	78	na	p = 0.91	na	na	There is no clinical benefit in terms of overall outcome in undertaking regional LND in the absence
					LND none	79	na				
Pantuck et al.	2003	28	495	Retrospective	LND none, clinically localized RCC	75[4]	na	p = 0.42[5]	23%	17%[6]	Regional lymph node dissection is unnecessary in patients with clinically negative lymph nodes
					LND + any, clinically localized RCC	70[4]	na				
Joslyn et al.	2005	32	4453	Retrospective	#nodes examined = 0	96	na	p = 0.07	na	na	More extensive lymphadenectomy does not appear to increase further the probability of CSS
					#nodes examined = 4–6	85	na				
					#nodes examined = 7–9	83	na				
					#nodes examined > 10	87	na				
Blom et al.	2008	26	732	RCT	LND full	80[4]	na	p = 0.87[5]	22%	26%[6]	No survival advantage of a complete lymph-node dissection in conjunction with a radical nephrectomy could be demonstrated
					LND none	80[4]	na				

[1]Lymph node dissection
[2]Disease-specific survival
[3]Abbreviations: IMA = inferior mesenteric artery, RCC = renal cell carcinoma
[4]Extrapolation from the Kaplan–Meier graphs
[5]Statistics from the Kaplan–Meier graphs
[6]Not statistically significant
[7]Perioperative mortality only

In this section, we will summarize the literature regarding some questions related to LND. The main question we have tried to answer is: Is there a therapeutic effect of LND in localized kidney cancer? We will also discuss the morbidity of LND for localized RCC.

Clinical question 34.2

What is the role of lymphadenectomy in localized RCC?

Literature search

Potentially relevant studies were identified by a search of the Medline electronic database (source PubMed, 1966 to December 2008) using relevant keywords in combination, as follows: renal cell carcinoma AND lymphadenectomy (313 articles retrieved), lymph node AND renal cell carcinoma OR kidney cancer (157 articles retrieved), lymphadenectomy AND kidney cancer (40 articles retrieved), lymph node dissection AND renal cell carcinoma OR kidney cancer (18 articles retrieved). Original and review articles were selected based on language (English only) and revelance of their title. A total of 268 articles were kept for abstract analysis. Only studies from which we could distinguish outcomes for localized RCC to those from metastatic RCC were included. Studies evaluating the role of LND for metastatic RCC or preoperative enlarged nodes on imaging were not included.

The evidence

Oncological outcomes

We identified one randomized prospective trial, one prospective nonrandomized trial, and four retrospective trials that address this question. Table 34.3 enumerates the studies that we will discuss. We identified two studies that suggest that LND in RCC may increase survival and four studies that suggest that LND does not increase survival.

Studies showing that lymphadenectomy does not increase survival in RCC Recently, Blom et al. published the final results regarding the overall survival of patients included in the EORTC prospective multicenter randomized trial of LND in localized RCC [26]. Patients having a localized resectable RCC based on preoperative imaging were randomized to radical nephrectomy alone or radical nephrectomy with limited LND. Extent of LND was protocol defined, and was limited to pre-aortic, para-aortic and peridiaphragmatic LN on the left side and pre-, para-, and retro-aortic and interaortocaval LN on the right side, both from the bifurcation of the iliac vessels to the crus of the diaphragm. Approximately 85% of their patients

had pT2 or pT3 diseases and none had metastastic or suspicious lymph nodes. At a median follow-up of 12.6 years, there was no difference between the two groups in overall survival (OS), regional or distant progression. The authors concluded that there is no benefit to performing LND in patients with localized RCC.

This study, due to its randomized, propective and multicentric design as well as systematized follow-up, is difficult to criticize from a methodological standpoint. It is certainly the best study to answer the question raised in this chapter. Three other studies, despite being retrospective, offer the same conclusions. Pantuck et al. reported an absence of benefit when performing LND for DSS in localized RCC [28]. This study has the limitations of being retrospective and including patients for whom the extent of LND was not systematized. Moreover, no comparison of tumor characteristics of patients with and without LND is available. In another retrospective study with similar results, Minervini et al. compared 5-year survival of patients with (N = 49) and without (N = 108) LND [27]. LND was regional and included pre-, para- and retrocaval or aortic LN ipsilateral to the tumor. Cephalocaudal extension of the LND was from the inferior mesenteric artery to the renal pedicle. Pathological tumor characteristics of the patients with and without LND as well as 5-year DSS were not statistically different between the two groups. The limitations of this study are the lower percentage of pT3–T4 tumors (approximately 20%) when compared to the Pantuck and Blom studies (between 30% and 40%) and the limited nature of the LND. Finally, using the large SEER database, Joslyn et al. analyzed the cancer-specific survival of patients who had nephrectomy for RCC relative to the number of lymph node retrieved [32]. They concluded that the extent of LND was not associated with better DSS survival. Again, this retrospective study did not correlate the pathology report of the nephrectomy with the number of lymph nodes retrieved, which could be an important selection biais against patients who had more lymph nodes retrieved.

Studies that show that lymphadenectomy increases survival in RCC Only nonrandomized studies have suggested that LND could improve survival in combination with nephrectomy for RCC. Schafhauser et al. retrospectively compared three groups of patients who had nephrectomy: patients who underwent extended LND, patients with limited LND performed only for suspicious LN, patients without LND [29]. Despite a significant difference in pathological tumor characteristics between the groups favoring the group without LND (lower grades and stages), the authors observed an improved 5-year cancer-specific survival advantage for the extended lymphadenectomy group. They calculated that 4% of their patients would benefit from extended LND in terms of survival. It is noteworthy that 50% of the patients included in this study were pT3 stage, which is much higher than the previous negative studies. If those higher risk patients included would benefit more from LND than lower risk patients, this difference in tumor characteristics might explain the difference of conclusions when compared to the previously described negative studies. However, a possible bias in this retrospective study is the 6.3-fold increased perioperative mortality in the limited LND group. If statistical analysis would correct for those patients, the difference in DSS might have been nonsignificant.

In a prospective nonrandomized study, Herrlinger et al. reported a SS difference between patients who had a limited versus an extended LND [33]. All patients had a transabdominal approach with or without a regional lymphadenectomy. Metastatic patients and those older than 72 years old were excluded. A significant difference in survival between the two groups was found for pT1–2N0M0, pT3aN0M0 and pT1–3N + M0 diseases but not in the pT3bN0M0 subgroup. However, there was no table comparing the pathological characteristics of patients with and without LND. The reported threefold higher perioperative mortality in the group without LND is again counterintuitive. This might reflect a selection bias with patients with more advanced stages or decreased performance status in the facultative LND group. Finally, although the author states that the study was prospective, no detail is provided to describe how the patients were assigned to each group or how the sample size, treatment effect size or study power was calculated. Further, it is not clear whether the decision to perform LND was determined preoperatively.

Complications of lymphadenectomy

To assess this question, we analyzed the reported morbidity in the same studies used to determine the effect of LND on survival. Perioperative mortality was between 0% and 3.5%. All studies reached the same conclusion that LND does not increase the risk of complication when compared to nephrectomy performed without LND. Two types of outcomes have been reported: complications and mortality. In their studies, Herrlinger and Schafhauser reported their perioperative mortality, and did not find an increased risk of mortality in patients undergoing LND. In fact, for an unknown reason, both studies have shown an increased risk of perioperative mortality in the group without LND which is likely explained by selection bias. No statistics were provided to determine if this difference was statistically significant. In the UCLA series, Pantuck et al. did not find any SS difference in complication rate, transfusion or perioperative mortality between the patients with or without LND . Complications were 23% in the LND group and 17% in the group without LND [28]. The EORTC phase III 80811 trial prospectively evaluated the complications of

LND when combined with nephrectomy alone [26]. The authors reported a nonstatistically significant difference in the complication rates. Twenty-six percent of patients with LND had complications compared to 22% of those without LND. Blood loss, lymph fluid drainage and embolism were higher in the LND group but none of these complications was statistically significant [29,33].

Taken together, these results show that LND does not increase the morbidity of nephrectomy in patients with localized RCC.

Comment

The emergence of minimally invasive technologies such as laparoscopic partial and radical nephrectomy (see next section) has rendered the question of lymphadenectomy in RCC of prime importance, since in most surgeons' hands these approaches do not permit extended LND to be performed. Considering the importance of nephron-sparing surgery for small renal tumors, the reduced morbidity of laparoscopic renal surgery when compared to the open approach (see preceding section) and the recently published EORTC randomized phase III trial, it seems clear that there is no benefit for lymphadenectomy in clinically localized RCC. One could certainly argue that there is a staging benefit in performing LND, particularly since no study has shown an increased complication rate of LND. However, we believe that this benefit would be only for a limited number of patients since contemporary series show that positive lymph nodes are found in only 3–7% of patients [26-28]. Moreover, in the presence of positive lymph nodes, there is no adjuvant treatment recommended in the absence of systemic metastasis. In our opinion, the staging advantage of performing an extended open LND would not exceed the benefit provided by laparoscopy.

However, it is worth noting that this opinion regarding LND applies only to localized RCC. In the presence of enlarged lymph nodes or metastatic disease, the role of LND might be important, though there is no randomized trial that has assessed this question. In the context of preoperative enlarged lymph nodes on CT scan, Pantuck et al. showed that patients who had LND did better than patients without LND, with an improvement in survival of approximately 5 months [28]. Similarly, Canfield et al. have reported a RFS of 30% at a median follow-up of 17 months in patients with positive lymph nodes preoperatively and who underwent lymphadenectomy and nephrectomy [34]. These results provide support for LND in the setting of abnormal lymph nodes. However, urologists should be aware that the specificity of enlarged lymph nodes on preoperative CT-scan is low. Studer reported that of 43 patients with retroperitoneal lymphadenopathy by CT criteria (lymph nodes 1.0–2.2 cm), only 18 (42%) had LN metastases while CT scans missed positive nodes in only five of 163 patients [35].

Finally, LND in the context of cytoreductive nephrectomy also merits discussion. LND was shown to be pronostic in the context of cytoreductive nephrectomy for metastatic disease. Survival was statistically better in metastatic patients with LND [28]. Moreover, it was also associated with improved survival in patients treated with immunotherapy [36]. Whether positive lymph node resection is part of the cytoreductive aspect of nephrectomy by decreasing the tumor burden or if lymph node metastasis by itself confers resistance to immunotherapy is unknown and merits further study. With the advent of new therapeutic drug regimens such as tyrosine and mTOR kinase inhibitors, the finding of a positive lymph node may help the clinician to orient the patient to treatments other than immunotherapy. However, the significance of a positive lymph node in the mTOR kinase inhibitor era is presently unknown.

Recommendations

- Lymphadenectomy provides no clinical benefit in patients with localized RCC (weak recommendation, moderate-quality of evidence, **Grade 2B**).
- Lymphadenectomy is not associated with an increased morbidity (strong recommendation, moderate-quality evidence, **Grade 1B**).
- There is some evidence that lymphadenectomy may provide benefit in the setting of metastatic disease (weak recommendation, low-quality evidence, **Grade 2C**).

Implications for research

Recently, much has been learned to explain the molecular mechanisms behind the clinical patterns of observed metastatic spread. For example, it is well established that angiogenesis, the formation of new blood vessels, is necessary for the growth and metastatic spread of solid tumors. The vascular endothelial growth factor (VEGF) family of genes encompasses unique isoforms, each capable of binding to unique receptors. Evidence is accumulating that different VEGF family members are important in determining the route of metastatic spread, through either classic angiogenesis via blood vessels or through lymphangiogenesis. The factors that promote regulation of different VEGF gene expressions are not entirely clear. It is possible that individual tumor genetics and risk factor exposure may lead to differential tumor gene expression, resulting in unique tumor biologies with unique patterns of spread and responses to treatment. Future research needs to elucidate why some tumors disseminate early through the lymphatics, why some disseminate through both lymphatic and visceral spread, and why some tumors never spread.

Role of partial nephrectomy in the treatment of localized renal cell carcinoma

Background

The proportion of renal masses discovered incidentally, before the tumor has enlarged and compromised the entire kidney, has been steadily increasing [37]. This trend, due in large part to widespread use of improved noninvasive imaging, has led to the more frequent utilization of partial nephrectomy (PN). Initially restricted to imperative cases such as those involving a solitary kidney or pre-existing renal insufficiency, encouraging results prompted many to expand the indications for elective PN. Recent years have seen a steady increase in the use of PN for renal masses [37]. PN has now become the standard if not preferred treatment for smaller renal masses in the setting of a normal contralateral kidney.

One obvious advantage offered by PN is its ability to preserve renal function by sparing normal renal tissue. Accumulating evidence from population-based analyses is demonstrating that impaired renal function, as measured by glomerular filtration rate (GFR), has effects on several health outcomes. Go et al. reported the results of an analysis of over 1 million subjects in a large health maintenance organization [38]. They found that incremental decreases in GFR were associated with increased rates of hospitalizations, cardiovascular events, and all-cause mortality, with the increased morbidity and mortality rising more dramatically when GFR falls below 45 mL/min. Evidence such as this heightens the interest in techniques that can potentially preserve renal function.

There are, however, additional rationales for the use of PN over RN for small renal masses. First, a relatively high percentage of benign lesions are found when small lesions are resected. In tumors < 4 cm, the rate of benign lesions found at operation has been reported to be approximately 20% [39,40]. Second, there is the risk for the metachronous development of contralateral tumors in patients with RCC. Rabbani et al. found that patients with a diagnosis of RCC remained at a significantly elevated risk for contralateral RCC beyond 10 years [41].

In this section, we will review the role of PN by comparing its oncological, renal functional, and perioperative outcomes to those of RN.

Clinical question 34.3

What is the role of partial nephrectomy in the treatment of localized renal cell carcinoma?

Literature search

A PubMed search was conducted using the search terms: "radical nephrectomy," "partial nephrectomy," "complications," and "renal function," alone or in combination. After title review of retrieved articles, a total of 193 articles were retained for abstract analysis. With respect to laparoscopic and open approaches for PN, open PN is currently the standard while laparoscopic PN is performed primarily in specialized centers and is subject to considerable variability in technique. Therefore, in gathering data on complications, open PN was the focus, with one large-scale comparison between open and laparoscopic PN mentioned for completeness.

The evidence

Oncological outcomes

Studies that show that PN is equivalent to RN for oncological outcomes There is one small prospective study in the literature comparing PN and RN, and several other retrospective studies with larger numbers of patients [42-49]. The prospective study reported by D'Armiento reported equivalent DSS (96%) after a median follow-up of 70 months for 40 patients randomized to PN (N = 19) or RN (N = 21) for lesions < 4 cm [46]. One of the earliest series directly comparing the outcome of RN and PN for small renal masses with a normal contralateral kidney was a retrospective analysis by Butler et al. [47]. The 5-year DSS for 42 patients undergoing RN and 46 patients undergoing PN was 97% and 100%, respectively. In a somewhat larger series, Lerner et al. reported that for 177 patients with tumors ≤ 4 cm, progression-free survival did not differ by technique (92% for PN vs 97%, p = 0.28) [44]. Additionally, 16% of the patients undergoing PN in that series had either a synchronous or metachronous contralateral renal tumor, which could have resulted in poorer outcomes of the PN group. Additional studies with similar outcomes are included in Table 34.4.

Several series have challenged the previously accepted limit of 4 cm as the cut-off for lesions amenable to PN. Patard et al. reported a multi-institutional study of 379 patients with lesions < 7 cm undergoing PN compared to 1075 patients undergoing RN for similar sized tumors [42]. There was no difference in cancer-specific deaths for the cohort as a whole (2.2% vs 2.6%, p = 0.8) and for the subset of tumors 4–7 cm (6.2% vs 9%, p = 0.6). Leibovich et al. also showed that patients undergoing PN for tumors 4–7 cm did not fare worse than those undergoing RN [45]. DSS at 5 years for PN was 98% vs 86% for RN. After adjusting for grade, T stage, subtype, and necrosis, PN and RN did not demonstrate an actual survival advantage. Additional studies with similar conclusions regarding PN for tumors 4–7 cm are listed in Table 34.5.

Studies that show that PN is not equivalent to RN in oncological outcomes We could find no study demonstrating an inferior outcome for PN compared to RN for lesions smaller than 4 cm. The report by Lerner et al. described an advantage for RN for tumors greater than 4 cm,

Table 34.4 Oncological outcomes after radical (RN) or partial nephrectomy (PN) for renal cell carcinoma

Author	Year	Ref#	Tumor size (cm)	N (PN/RN)	F/U[1](Yrs) Median	DSS[2] (PN/RN,%)	Comments
Butler et al.	1995	47	< 4	46/42	4.0	100/97	Retrospective. Normal contralateral kidney required
Lerner et al.	1995	44	< 4	113/64	4.3	92/96	Retrospective. Pts with tumors > 4 cm had worse DSS
D'Armiento et al.	1997	46	< 4	19/21	5.7	95/95	Prospective. Normal contralateral kidney required
Barbalias et al.	1999	49	< 5	41/49	NA[3]	97.5/98.4	Retrospective. All pts included
Belldegrun et al.	1999	48	< 7	98/79	4.7	100/97.5	Retrospective. All pts included. Pts with tumors > 7 cm had worse DSS
Leibovich et al.	2004	45	4 to 7	91/844	7.4	98/96	Retrospective. Normal contralateral kidney required
Patard et al.	2004	42	< 4	314/499	4.3	97.8/97.4	Retrospective. All pts included
			4 to 7	65/576	4.3	93.8/91	
Mitchell et al.	2005	43	> 4	33/66	3.4	93.5/83.3	Retrospective. Bilateral RCC excluded

[1]F/U = follow-up
[2]DSS = disease specific survival
[3]NA = Not available

Table 34.5 Renal outcomes after radical (RN) or partial nephrectomy (PN) for renal cell carcinoma

Author	year	Ref#	Outcome	N (PN/RN)	Loss in outcome (PN/RN,%)	ESRD[1] (PN/RN)	Comments
Mc Kiernan et al.	2002	51	Serum Cr[2] > 2.0	117/173	0/15	0/0	NI[3]contralateral kidney,preop cr < 1.5 mg/dL
Zorn et al.	2007	52	SerumCr > 1.5	42/55	0/36	0/0	NI contralatera kidney,preop cr < 1.5. mg/dL
				SerumCr > 2.0	0/15		
Huang et al.	2007	53	GFR[4] < 60 at 3 y	287/204	20/65	0/0	NI contralateral kidney,perop cr < 1.5 mg/dL
				GFR[4] < 60 at 3 y	385/26	5/36	
Snow et al.	2008	54	Final GFR	48/37	79/555	0/0	NI contralateral kidney,peroep cr < 2 mg/dL
Clark et al.	2008	55	%change in CrCl	26/37	−6/−32	0/1	NI contralateral kidney.No exclusion for Cr levels

[1]ESRD-endstage renal disease
[2]Cr-creatinine
[3]NI-Normal
[4]GFR-Glomerular filtration rate
[5]GFR (ml/min/1,73m[2],not loss)

though the degree of improvement was not described [44]. However, in this series RN showed improved survival for the cohort as a whole, but failed to show a difference for the subset of tumors 4 cm or less. Further, this report did not exclude patients with imperative indications for PN (e.g. solitary kidney or bilateral RCC) who have expected poorer cancer-specific outcomes. The report by Belldegrun showed that RN was superior to PN for lesions larger than 7 cm (92% vs 66%, p < 0.01) [48]. However, the number of patients undergoing PN for tumors > 7 cm was only nine and also likely contained mostly patients with imperative indications. An additional study that was influential in establishing the 4 cm cut-off for PN was reported by Hafez et al., in which they demonstrated a worse DSS for patients with tumors > 4 cm undergoing PN [50]. However, this study did not have a RN comparison group. Tumor size is independently prognostic in RCC, and patients with larger tumors are likely to have poorer outcomes after RN as well, so this study did not directly show an advantage for PN over RN for tumors > 4 cm.

Renal functional outcomes

Studies showing that there is a difference in renal function between PN and RN There are no prospective studies addressing renal function after PN or RN. There are several retrospective reports that address renal function as a primary outcome, and they excluded patients without a normal contralateral kidney. In these reports, there has been a movement away from reporting renal function outcomes with serum creatinine values, instead using GFR which is a more meaningful reflection of renal function. Older series used changes in serum creatinine, which at least provided a relative measure between groups.

McKiernan et al. reported on 173 subjects undergoing RN and 117 undergoing PN, all with creatinine < 1.5 preoperatively and tumors < 4 cm [51]. No patients in the PN group developed a creatinine > 2.0 versus 9% in the RN group who did so. In a study by Zorn et al. of 97 patients with similar inclusion criteria and outcome measures, no one developed a serum creatinine > 1.5 after PN while 36% and 13% in the RN group developed creatinine of > 1.5 and 2.0, respectively [52]. Huang et al. reported on 662 patients with normal renal function and tumors < 4 cm undergoing elective PN or RN [53]. Five-year probabilities for the development of chronic kidney disease (GFR < 60 mL/min) for PN and RN were 23% and 77%, respectively. The risk of developing a GFR < 45 mL/min was 7% at 5 years for the PN cohort versus 43% for RN. Another study using estimated GFR as an outcome found the mean postoperative GFR after laparoscopic PN to be 79 mL/min versus 55 in the laparoscopic RN group (p < 0.01) despite equivalent preoperative renal function [54]. In a study using postoperative 24-hour creatinine clearance in 63 patients, the mean decline in renal function after PN was 6% versus 32% after RN [55].

Studies that show there is no difference in renal function between PN and RN The same studies demonstrating improved preservation of renal function for PN also show that patients with normal renal function undergoing RN do not have elevated rates of renal failure if the outcome being measured is long-term dialysis. In the report by McKiernan et al. of 290 patients undergoing RN or PN, no one from either group required dialysis, though the median follow-up time was not reported [51]. Similarly, no patient in the Huang study required dialysis at a median follow-up of at least 18 months, nor did any patient in the Zorn study after 6 months [52,53]. In the Clark study 1/37 patients developed renal failure after RN versus 0/26 after PN [55]. However, patients with preoperative renal insufficiency were not excluded from that study and there is little argument that patients with renal insufficiency benefit from nephron-sparing techniques.

Complications of PN

There is one prospective, randomized study comparing RN and PN for which complication data have been published (the follow-up for the study is ongoing, and oncological results require additional events before the two arms can be compared) [56]. The EORTC study of 541 patients included subjects with a normal contralateral kidney and a tumor $\leq$ 5 cm. Blood loss was higher in the PN group, with more patients undergoing RN losing < 500 cc than did those undergoing PN (96% vs 87%, p < 0.01). Severe blood loss (> 1 L) was also more frequent in the PN group (3.1% vs 1.6%). Urinary leaks occurred in 4.4% of PN. A large Veterans Administration-based analysis of 1885 RN and PN did not find any significant difference in short-term morbidity (15% vs 16%), mortality (2% vs 1.6%) or length of stay (8.1 vs 8.6 days) between the techniques [57]. However, the definition of morbidities included complications that the techniques have in common (need for transfusion > 4 U, ileus, wound infection, renal failure, prolonged hospital stay), and did not include complications that are specific to PN (urinary leak/urinoma). A drawback of this study was that the analysis of complications in the RN group was not limited to smaller tumors that were amenable to PN. It is possible that if the RN group included only smaller tumors, the difference in complication rates would be larger.

Stephenson et al. compared complications between PN and RN in 1049 patients [58]. They found that the overall complication rate did not significantly differ between techniques (19% vs 16%, p = 0.3), but the PN group did suffer more complications of a higher severity (requiring intervention, 4% vs 1.6%, p = 0.04). This difference was explained primarily by urine leaks, which occurred in 6.6% of PN. The rate of retroperitoneal hemorrhage after PN was 0.8% compared to 0.1% after RN, but the overall

percentage of patients requiring transfusion did not differ between groups (18% vs 15%, p = 0.36). A drawback of this study, similar to the VA study, was that the tumors in the RN group were larger on average (5.8 cm vs 2.1 cm, p < 0.01), which likely increased the RN complication rate. A large, single-institution series of open and laparoscopic PN reported complication rates without a direct comparison to RN. The rate of urine leakage was 2.3% for OPN and 3.1% for LPN [59]. For postoperative hemorrhage, it was 1.6% for OPN and 4.2% for LPN.

Implications for practice

In spite of the paucity of prospective studies comparing PN to RN, the vast majority of retrospective data have demonstrated PN to be equivalent to RN for lesions < 4 cm in terms of cancer-specific survival, and is also likely equivalent for lesions 4–7 cm. In studies not showing equivalence of PN for 4–7 cm tumors, many if not most patients underwent PN for imperative reasons. These patients will often fare worse due to the presence of previous or synchronous contralateral RCC which was often larger than the lesion for which the patient underwent PN. It is not known whether PN is a reasonable option for patients with tumors > 7 cm, though the limited data (with probable selection bias) suggest that it is not preferable. With respect to complications, PN has an overall complication rate similar to RN, but it probably has a somewhat higher rate of complications for smaller tumors due to the potential severe blood loss and the development of urine leaks.

Partial nephrectomy has clearly shown an advantage for the preservation of GFR compared to RN, which is not surprising. However, nearly all patients with a normal contralateral kidney have avoided the need for dialysis after RN. The benefits of a higher GFR have been demonstrated mainly in population-based studies. It is, therefore, only an indirect conclusion that patients undergoing PN will have better health outcomes than patients after RN. It is unknown if patients with lower GFR after RN are similar to patients with lower GFR due to reasons other than renal surgery.

Recommendations

• For tumors $\leq$ 4 cm, PN is preferable to RN due to equivalent cancer-specific survival and to improved preservation of renal function (strong recommendation, moderate-quality evidence, Grade 1B).

• For tumors 4–7 cm, PN also likely offers similar cancer-specific survival, but there is some evidence that RN might be preferable in these cases (weak recommendation, low-quality evidence, Grade 2C).

• For tumors > 7 cm, RN should be performed (weak recommendation, very low-quality evidence, Grade 2C).

Implications for research

As the data mature fully, the prospective phase III study from the EORTC group will certainly answer many questions presented above [56]. An important question regarding the benefit of PN over RN will be to determine if it increases OS. It is expected that the oncological outcomes of RN will be challenged by the beneficial renal (and its associated cardiovascular) outcomes of PN on OS. For now, we have only indirect evidence that PN can lead to improved OS.

Acknowledgments

Frédéric Pouliot is a urological oncology fellow at UCLA supported in part by the McLaughlin and the Conseil des Médecins, Dentistes et Pharmaciens fellowship scholarships, both from Laval University, the Québec Urological Association and the Canadian Institutes of Health Research fellowship scholarships.

References

1. Pantuck AJ, Zisman A, Belldegrun AS. The changing natural history of renal cell carcinoma. J Urol 2001;166(5):1611-23.
2. Chow WH, Devesa SS, Warren JL, et al. Rising incidence of renal cell cancer in the United States. JAMA 1999;281(17);1628-31.
3. Hock LM, Lynch J, Balaji KC. Increasing incidence of all stages of kidney cancer in the last 2 decades in the United States: an analysis of surveillance, epidemiology and end results program data. J Urol 2002;167(1):57-60.
4. Skinner DG, Colvin RB, Vermillion CD, et al. Diagnosis and management of renal cell carcinoma. A clinical and pathologic study of 309 cases. Cancer 1971;28(5):1165-77.
5. Jayson M, Sanders H. Increased incidence of serendipitously discovered renal cell carcinoma. Urology 1998;51(2):203-5.
6. Lee CT, Katz J, Shi W, et al. Surgical management of renal tumors 4 cm. or less in a contemporary cohort. J Urol 2000;163(3):730-6.
7. Clayman RV, Kavoussi LR, Soper NJ, et al. Laparoscopic nephrectomy: initial case report. J Urol 1991;146(2):278-82.
8. Brook NR, Harper SJ, Bagul A, et al. Laparoscopic donor nephrectomy yields kidneys with structure and function equivalent to those retrieved by open surgery. Transplant Proc 2005;37(2):625-6.
9. Oyen O, Andersen M, Mathisen L, et al. Laparoscopic versus open living-donor nephrectomy: experiences from a prospective, randomized, single-center study focusing on donor safety. Transplantation 2005;79(9):1236-40.
10. Simforoosh N, Basiri A, Tabibi A, et al. Comparison of laparoscopic and open donor nephrectomy: a randomized controlled trial. BJU Int 2005;95(6):851-5.
11. Wolf JS Jr, Merion RM, Leichtman AB, et al. Randomized controlled trial of hand-assisted laparoscopic versus open surgical live donor nephrectomy. Transplantation 2001;72(2):284-90.
12. Nanidis TG, Antcliffe D, Kokkinos C, et al. Laparoscopic versus open live donor nephrectomy in renal transplantation: a meta-analysis. Ann Surg 2008;247(1):58-70.
13. Baldwin DD, Dunbar JA, Parekh DJ, et al. Single-center comparison of purely laparoscopic, hand-assisted laparoscopic, and open radical nephrectomy in patients at high anesthetic risk. J EndoUrol 2003;17(3):161-7.
14. Busby E, Das S, Rao Tunuguntla HS, et al. Hand-assisted laparoscopic vs the open (flank incision) approach to radical nephrectomy. BJU Int 2003;91(4):341-4.
15. Dunn MD, Portis AJ, Shalhav AL, et al. Laparoscopic versus open radical nephrectomy: a 9-year experience. J Urol 2000; 164(4):1153-9.
16. Hemal AK, Kumar A, Kumar R, et al. Laparoscopic versus open radical nephrectomy for large renal tumors: a long-term prospective comparison. J Urol 2007;177(3):862-6.
17. Kawauchi A, Fujito A, Ukimura O, et al. Hand-assisted retroperitoneoscopic radical nephrectomy: initial experience. Int J Urol 2002;9(9):480-4.
18. Lee SE, Ku JH, Kwak C, et al. Hand assisted laparoscopic radical nephrectomy: comparison with open radical nephrectomy. J Urol 2003;170(3):756-9.
19. Makhoul B, de la Taille A, Vordos D, et al. Laparoscopic radical nephrectomy for T1 renal cancer: the gold standard? A comparison of laparoscopic vs open nephrectomy. BJU Int 2004;93(1):67-70.
20. Malaeb BS, Sherwood JB, Taylor GD, et al. Hand-assisted laparoscopic nephrectomy for renal masses > 9.5 cm: series comparison with open radical nephrectomy. Urol Oncol 2005;23(5):323-7.
21. Nakada SY, Fadden P, Jarrard DF, et al. Hand-assisted laparoscopic radical nephrectomy: comparison to open radical nephrectomy. Urology 2001;58(4):517-20.
22. Ono Y, Kinukawa T, Hattori R, et al. Laparoscopic radical nephrectomy for renal cell carcinoma: a five-year experience. Urology 1999;53(2):280-6.
23. Shuford MD, McDougall EM, Chang SS, et al. Complications of contemporary radical nephrectomy: comparison of open vs. laparoscopic approach. Urol Oncol 2004;22(2):121-6.
24. Oyen O, Line PD, Pfeffer P, et al. Laparoscopic living donor nephrectomy: introduction of simple hand-assisted technique (without handport). Transplant Proc 2003;35(2):779-81.
25. Godoy G, O'Malley RL, Taneja SS. Lymph node dissection during the surgical treatment of renal cancer in the modern era. Int Braz J Urol 2008;34(2):132-42.
26. Blom JH, van Poppel H, Marechal JM, et al. Radical nephrectomy with and without lymph-node dissection: final results of European Organization for Research and Treatment of Cancer (EORTC) Randomized Phase 3 Trial 30881 Eur Urol 2009;55(1):28-34.
27. Minervini A, Lilas L, Morelli G, et al. Regional lymph node dissection in the treatment of renal cell carcinoma: is it useful in patients with no suspected adenopathy before or during surgery? BJU Int 2001;88(3):169-72.
28. Pantuck AJ, Zisman A, Dorey F, et al. Renal cell carcinoma with retroperitoneal lymph nodes: role of lymph node dissection. J Urol 2003;169(6):2076-83.
29. Schafhauser W, Ebert A, Brod J, et al. Lymph node involvement in renal cell carcinoma and survival chance by systematic lymphadenectomy. Anticancer Res 1999;19(2C):1573-8.
30. Siminovitch JP, Montie JE, Straffon RA. Lymphadenectomy in renal adenocarcinoma. J Urol 1982;127(6):1090-1.
31. Robson CJ, Churchill BM, Anderson W. The results of radical nephrectomy for renal cell carcinoma. J Urol 1969;101(3): 297-301.

32. Joslyn SA, Sirintrapun SJ, Konety BR. Impact of lymphadenectomy and nodal burden in renal cell carcinoma: retrospective analysis of the National Surveillance, Epidemiology, and End Results database. Urology 2005;65(4):675-80.

33. Herrlinger A, Schrott KM, Schott G, et al. What are the benefits of extended dissection of the regional renal lymph nodes in the therapy of renal cell carcinoma? J Urol 1991;146(5):1224-7.

34. Canfield SE, Kamat AM, Sanchez-Ortiz RF, et al. Renal cell carcinoma with nodal metastases in the absence of distant metastatic disease (clinical stage TxN1-2M0): the impact of aggressive surgical resection on patient outcome. J Urol 2006;175(3 pt 1): 864-9.

35. Studer UE, Scherz S, Scheidegger J, et al. Enlargement of regional lymph nodes in renal cell carcinoma is often not due to metastases. J Urol 1990;144(2 pt 1):243-5.

36. Pantuck AJ, Zisman A, Dorey F, et al. Renal cell carcinoma with retroperitoneal lymph nodes. Impact on survival and benefits of immunotherapy. Cancer 2003;97(12):2995-3002.

37. Miller DC, Schonlau M, Litwin MS, et al. Renal and cardiovascular morbidity after partial or radical nephrectomy. Cancer 2008;112(3):511-20.

38. Go AS, Chertow GM, Fan D, et al. Chronic kidney disease and the risks of death, cardiovascular events, and hospitalization. N Engl J Med 2004;351(13):1296-305.

39. Frank I, Blute ML, Cheville JC, et al. Solid renal tumors: an analysis of pathological features related to tumor size. J Urol 2003;170(6 pt 1):2217-20.

40. Duchene DA, Lotan Y, Cadeddu JA, et al. Histopathology of surgically managed renal tumors: analysis of a contemporary series. Urology 2003;62(5):827-30.

41. Rabbani F, Herr HW, Almahmeed T, et al. Temporal change in risk of metachronous contralateral renal cell carcinoma: influence of tumor characteristics and demographic factors. J Clin Oncol 2002;20(9):2370-5.

42. Patard JJ, Shvarts O, Lam JS, et al. Safety and efficacy of partial nephrectomy for all T1 tumors based on an international multi-center experience. J Urol 2004;171(6 pt 1):2181-5, quiz 435.

43. Mitchell RE, Gilbert SM, Murphy AM, et al. Partial nephrectomy and radical nephrectomy offer similar cancer outcomes in renal cortical tumors 4 cm or larger. Urology 2006;67(2): 260-4.

44. Lerner SE, Hawkins CA, Blute ML, et al. Disease outcome in patients with low stage renal cell carcinoma treated with nephron sparing or radical surgery. J Urol 1996;155(6):1868-73.

45. Leibovich BC, Blute ML, Cheville JC, et al. Nephron sparing surgery for appropriately selected renal cell carcinoma between 4 and 7 cm results in outcome similar to radical nephrectomy. J Urol 2004;171(3):1066-70.

46. D'Armiento M, Damiano R, Feleppa B, et al. Elective conservative surgery for renal carcinoma versus radical nephrectomy: a prospective study. BJU 1997;79(1):15-19.

47. Butler BP, Novick AC, Miller DP, et al. Management of small unilateral renal cell carcinomas: radical versus nephron-sparing surgery. Urology 1995;45(1):34-40.

48. Belldegrun A, Tsui KH, de Kernion JB, et al. Efficacy of nephron-sparing surgery for renal cell carcinoma: analysis based on the new 1997 tumor-node-metastasis staging system. J Clin Oncol 1999;17(9):2868-75.

49. Barbalias GA, Liatsikos EN, Tsintavis A, et al. Adenocarcinoma of the kidney: nephron-sparing surgical approach vs. radical nephrectomy. J Surg Oncol 1999;72(3):156-61.

50. Hafez KS, Fergany AF, Novick AC. Nephron sparing surgery for localized renal cell carcinoma: impact of tumor size on patient survival, tumor recurrence and TNM staging. J Urol 1999;162(6):1930-3.

51. McKiernan J, Simmons R, Katz J, et al. Natural history of chronic renal insufficiency after partial and radical nephrectomy. Urology 2002;59(6):816-20.

52. Zorn KC, Gong EM, Orvieto MA, et al. Comparison of laparoscopic radical and partial nephrectomy: effects on long-term serum creatinine. Urology 2007;69(6):1035-40.

53. Huang WC, Levey AS, Serio AM, et al. Chronic kidney disease after nephrectomy in patients with renal cortical tumours: a retrospective cohort study. Lancet Oncol 2006;7(9):735-40.

54. Snow DC, Bhayani SB. Rapid communication: chronic renal insufficiency after laparoscopic partial nephrectomy and radical nephrectomy for pathologic t1a lesions. J EndoUrol 2008;22(2): 337-41.

55. Clark AT, Breau RH, Morash C, et al. Preservation of renal function following partial or radical nephrectomy using 24-hour creatinine clearance. Eur Urol 2008;54(1):143-9.

56. Van Poppel H, da Pozzo L, Albrecht W, et al. A prospective randomized EORTC intergroup phase 3 study comparing the complications of elective nephron-sparing surgery and radical nephrectomy for low-stage renal cell carcinoma. Eur Urol 2007;51(6):1606-15.

57. Corman JM, Penson DF, Hur K, et al. Comparison of complications after radical and partial nephrectomy: results from the National Veterans Administration Surgical Quality Improvement Program. BJU Int 2000;86(7):782-9.

58. Stephenson AJ, Hakimi AA, Snyder ME, et al. Complications of radical and partial nephrectomy in a large contemporary cohort. J Urol 2004;171(1):130-4.

59. Gill IS, Kavoussi LR, Lane BR, et al. Comparison of 1,800 laparoscopic and open partial nephrectomies for single renal tumors. J Urol 2007;178(1):41-6.

35 Treatment of metastatic kidney cancer

Przemyslaw W. Twardowski and Robert A. Figlin

City of Hope National Medical Center, Department of Medical Oncology and Therapeutics Research, City of Hope Comprehensive Cancer Center, Duarte, CA, USA

Introduction

With 50,000 new cases and 13,000 deaths in the United States every year, kidney cancer represents a major oncological therapeutic challenge [1]. Approximately one-third of patients present with metastases at initial diagnosis and between 20% and 40% relapse after nephrectomy. Several clinical prognostic factors stratify patients with metastatic disease to low-, intermediate- and high-risk groups with median survival ranging from 22 months in the low-risk patients to 12 months in the intermediate- and 5 months in the high-risk groups respectively (Table 35.1). Only a small number of patients with metastatic kidney cancer can be cured by existing therapies. Renal cell carcinoma (RCC) is generally resistant to chemotherapy [2,3]. Due to a possible immunological influence in well-documented cases of spontaneous regression of RCC metastases, attention has focused historically on the possible means of modifying biological response in these patients. In the 1980s and 1990s the immunocytokines interleukin-2 (IL-2) and interferon-alpha (IFN-alpha) became the standard systemic therapy for metastatic renal cell carcinoma based on documented durable responses in some patients.

Recent discoveries and better understanding of signaling pathways and targets important in the development and progression of renal cell carcinoma have resulted in significant expansion of therapeutic options of patients affected with this disease. Sunitinib malate, sorafenib tosylate, bevacizumab ± interferon-alpha, temsirolimus and everolimus have improved clinical outcomes in randomized clinical trials by inhibiting the vascular endothelial growth factor (VEGF), m-TOR and related pathways. Many other targeted agents are in clinical development, representing the main focus of clinical research in RCC (Table 35.2). The rapidly changing therapeutic landscape of metastatic RCC raises several important questions related to the appropriate selection and sequence of available agents, the role (if any) of immunotherapy and the relevance of surgical debulking of these patients.

Clinical question 35.1

Is there evidence that debulking nephrectomy provides clinical benefit in asymptomatic patients with metastatic renal cell carcinoma?

Background

Historically, the hypothesis that cytoreductive nephrectomy may play a role in therapy of metastatic kidney cancer

Table 35.1 Memorial Sloan Kettering Cancer Center (MSKCC) risk factor stratification scale

Factor	Poor prognosis
Karnofsky Performance Score	< 80 (WHO > 1)
Time from diagnosis to treatment	< 12 months
Hemoglobin	Below normal range
Lactate dehydrogenase	> 1.5 upper limit of normal
Calcium	> 10 mg/dL
Good risk	0 prognostic factors
Intermediate risk	1–2 prognostic factors
Poor risk	> 2 factors

WHO, World Health Organization

Evidence-Based Urology. Edited by Philipp Dahm, Roger R. Dmochowski.
© 2010 Blackwell Publishing.

Table 35.2 Agents in development for treatment of renal cell carcinoma

Agent	Mechanism of action	Manufacturer	Status in RCC
Everolimus	m-TOR inhibitor	Novartis	Phase III completed
Pazopanib	VEGFR, PDGFR, c-kit tyrosine kinase inhibitor	GSK	Phase III
Axitinib	VEGFR and PDGFR tyrosine kinase inhibitor	Pfizer	Phase II
Vatalanib	VEGFR, PDGFR, c-kit tyrosine kinase inhibitor	Novartis	Phase II
VEGF Trap	VEGF ligand inhibitor	Regeneron	Phase II

m-TOR, mammalian target of rapamycin; PDGFR, platelet-derived growth factor receptor; VEGF, vascular endothelial growth factor; VEGFR, vascular endothelial growth factor receptor

was based on observation of occasional "spontaneous" regressions of metastatic tumors after nephrectomy. Other possible advantages to debulking nephrectomy include prevention of complications during subsequent treatment and improving patient performance status by elimination of the source of additional metastases, hemorrhage, and discomfort. However, nephrectomy performed as a single treatment modality for metastatic disease does not appear to have significant effect on survival [4]. The renewed interest in debulking nephrectomy came to light in the context of immunotherapy for metastatic RCC and the hypothesis that persistence of a large primary tumor may generate immunosuppressive cytokines and negate the therapeutic benefits of immunostimulatory agents. More recently, the introduction of agents with more potent systemic activity against RCC led, yet again, to the re-emergence of the question of contribution of debulking nephrectomy to patient outcomes in the new era of targeted therapies.

Literature search

Potentially relevant studies were identified by a computerized search, restricted to English-language literature, of the Medline electronic database (source PubMed, 1966 to March 2009) using relevant text and keywords in combination as follows: "metastatic renal cancer and nephrectomy," "cytoreductive nephrectomy," "debulking nephrectomy." The reference lists of retrieved eligible articles were reviewed to identify additional relevant articles.

The evidence

Two prospective randomized clinical trials in patients with ECOG performance status of 0–1, Southwest Oncology Group (SWOG) 8949 [5] and European Organization for Research and Treatment of Cancer (EORTC) 30947 [6], reported statistically significant survival advantage for the combination of nephrectomy and IFN-alpha. Pooled analysis of these two trials demonstrated a median survival of 13.6 months for the combined arm versus 7.8 months for IFN-alpha alone which represented a 31% reduction in the risk of death (p = 0.002) in patients treated with nephrectomy and IFN-alpha [7]. Cytoreductive nephrectomy improved overall survival independently of patient performance status (0 or 1) and the site of metastases.

Comment

These two trials established debulking nephrectomy as a standard of care for patients who were considered candidates for systemic immunotherapy. The advent of antiangiogenic and targeted agents, as a preferred systemic therapy for metastatic RCC, raises several questions regarding the validity of the paradigm of cytoreductive nephrectomy as the vital component of therapeutic strategy for metastatic kidney cancer. It is uncertain whether the biological factors responsible for enhanced effects of immunotherapeutic agents after debulking surgery remain relevant in conjunction with antiangiogenic treatments. There are no prospective randomized trials addressing this issue but it is important to stress that the vast majority (> 90%) of patients treated on pivotal trials that established beneficial effect of antiangiogenic therapies in metastatic kidney cancer underwent prior cytoreductive nephrectomy.

Recommendations

A randomized clinical trial comparing the effectiveness of new targeted agents with or without debulking nephrectomy would address this valid scientific question but at this point it is not certain if such a study will be conducted. Until evidence to the contrary is established, it is prudent to incorporate cytoreductive surgery for all patients who are appropriate surgical candidates for that procedure. This represents a conditional recommendation for cytoreductive nephrectomy based on low-quality evidence according to Grade.

Clinical question 35.2

With the advent of targeted therapies in renal cell carcinoma, what are the clinical circumstances in which immunotherapy with high-dose IL-2 may be considered as the initial therapeutic option?

Background

Interleukin-2 is a cytokine which activates T cells and natural killer cells, stimulating them to produce a variety of other cytokines, such as IFN-gamma, granulocyte-macrophage colony stimulating factor, and tumor necrosis factor alpha, which in turn stimulate the activity of other cells in the immune system, such as the monocyte-macrophage lineage. It was first administered to patients with advanced RCC in the early 1980s. The initial reports of the efficacy of high-dose IL-2 (HDIL-2) in RCC demonstrated that a small fraction of patients achieved durable complete responses. Based on these results, the Food and Drug Administration (FDA) approved HDIL-2 therapy for advanced RCC in 1992.

Literature search

Potentially relevant studies were identified by a computerized search, restricted to English-language literature, of the Medline electronic database (source PubMed, 1966 to March 2009) using relevant text and keywords in combination as follows: "metastatic renal cancer and interleukin-2," "metastatic renal cancer and high-dose interleukin 2," "immunotherapy and kidney cancer." The reference lists of retrieved eligible articles were reviewed to identify additional relevant articles

The evidence

Consecutive series of patients treated with HDIL-2 in the Surgery Branch of the National Cancer Institute from September 1985 through December 1992 were reported by Rosenberg et al. in 1994 [8]. Two hundred and eighty-three patients with metastatic melanoma or metastatic renal cell cancer who had failed standard treatment for their cancers received IL-2 at a dose of 720,000 IU/kg intravenously every 8 hours for a maximum of 15 doses per cycle. Ten patients (7%) with metastatic renal cell cancer experienced complete regression and 20 patients (13%) had partial regression; 78% of patients with complete regression have remained in complete remission from 7 to 91 months after treatment. The response rates of these initial studies have been subsequently updated, demonstrating that some patients with complete responses have not relapsed and may be effectively cured [9].

Comment

High-dose IL-2 remains the only potentially curative treatment in selected patients with metastatic RCC. Unfortunately, HDIL-2 treatment is associated with significant toxicity requiring ICU monitoring. Capillary leakage is almost universal and leads to hypotension, renal toxicity,

altered mental status, fluid shifts, pulmonary edema, myocardial infarction, thrombocytopenia, infection, and mortality of 1–2%. Attempts to decrease the toxicity of HDIL-2 have so far been unsuccessful. Lowering the dose appears to reduce the effectiveness of therapy. A randomized clinical trial comparing HDIL-2 and low-dose IL-2 (LDIL-2) demonstrated no significant differences in overall and progression-free survival for the whole study population, but only HDIL-2 therapy resulted in durable complete responses in a small fraction of patients [10].

Recommendations

High-dose IL-2 can be considered as a first-line therapy for patients with excellent performance status and no underlying cardiopulmonary co-morbidities. Treatment should be administered only at tertiary centers with appropriate expertise in management of complications of HDIL-2 and ideally in the context of clinical trials evaluating predictive factors that would allow for the identification of patients who benefit the most from HDIL-2, thus justifying the risk of significant morbidity. This represents a conditional recommendation for HDIL-2 treatment in this select group of patients based on moderate-quality evidence (Grade 2B).

Clinical question 35.3

What are the current treatment options for the majority of patients with low- and intermediate-risk metastatic renal cell carcinoma?

Background

The inactivation of the von Hippel–Lindau (VHL) tumor suppressor gene leading to overexpression of hypoxia-regulated genes, including vascular endothelial growth factor (VEGF) and platelet-derived growth factor (PDGF), is of particular importance in RCC and especially in the clear cell histological variant (cRCC) (Figure 35.1). More detailed understanding of the role of tumor angiogenesis and multiple signaling pathways responsible for progression of kidney cancer resulted in the clinical development and FDA approval in RCC of sorafenib (Nexavar®) and sunitinib (Sutent®), both targeted agents that work via inhibiting specific receptor tyrosine kinase activities. Another antiangiogenic agent, bevacizumab (Avastin®, Genentech, San Francisco, CA) received regulatory approval in Europe. Sunitinib malate (Sutent®, Pfizer Inc. New York, NY) is a highly potent, selective inhibitor of multiple receptor tyrosine kinases (RTKs) including VEGFR-1, VEGFR-2, VEGFR-3, PDGFR-alpha, PDGFR-beta, c-kit, and Flt-3. Sorafenib tosylate (Nexavar®;

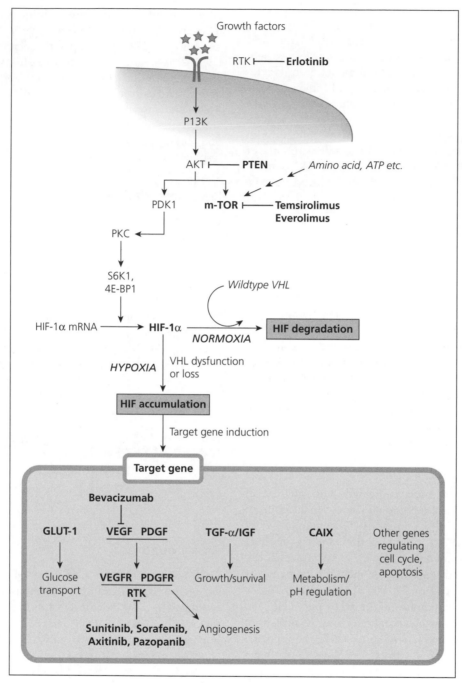

Figure 35.1 Signaling pathways in renal cell carcinoma and their inhibitors.

Bayer Pharmaceuticals, West Haven, CT, and Onyx Pharmaceuticals, Richmond, CA) is an oral, biaryl urea molecule that was designed as a c-Raf and b-Raf kinase inhibitor, but was also found to inhibit several RTKs including VEGFR-1, VEGFR-2, VEGFR-3, PDGFR-beta, Flt3, and c-KIT. Bevacizumab is a recombinant monoclonal antibody that binds and neutralizes circulating VEGF-A, and has demonstrated activity against metastatic RCC in several clinical trials.

Literature search

Potentially relevant studies were identified by a computerized search, restricted to English-language literature, of the Medline electronic database (source PubMed, 1966 to March 2009) using relevant text and keywords in combination as follows: "metastatic renal cancer and sunitinib," "metastatic renal cancer and sorafenib," "metastatic renal cancer and bevacizumab." The reference lists of retrieved eligible articles were reviewed to identify additional relevant articles.

The evidence

Sunitinib

Sunitinib received FDA regulatory approval in January 2006 based upon results from two phase II trials in patients with metastatic RCC progressing after prior therapy with IFN or IL-2 [11,12]. Subsequently, a large randomized multinational phase III trial was conducted to further evaluate the efficacy of sunitinib in previously untreated patients with metastatic RCC [13]. A total of 750 patients, predominantly with MSKCC good- and intermediate-risk clear cell RCC (see Table 35.1), were randomized to receive either sunitinib at 50 mg/daily, 4 weeks on, 2 weeks off, or subcutaneous IFN-alpha. The objective tumor response was 39% for patients receiving sunitinib versus 8% for patients receiving IFN ($p < 0.000001$) [14]. Median progression-free survival (PFS) was significantly greater for sunitinib-treated patients (11.0 months vs IFN 5.1 months; hazard ratio (HR) 0.538, $p < 0.000001$). Severe adverse events (grade 3–4 toxicities) were acceptable, with neutropenia (12%), thrombocytopenia (8%) and hypertension (8%) being noteworthy in the sunitinib arm, while fatigue was more common with IFN-alpha (12% vs 7%).

At the 2008 ASCO meeting, overall survival (OS) data were presented and despite cross-over interference, statistically significant survival advantage was noted among patients treated with sunitinib versus IFN-alpha (26.4 months versus 21.8 months, p value (Wilcoxon) = 0.0128) [15].

Sorafenib

Sorafenib received FDA regulatory approval in December 2005 as therapy for advanced RCC based upon the initial results of a phase III placebo-controlled randomized trial, known as TARGET (Treatment Approaches in RCC Global Evaluation Trial), conducted in 905 patients primarily with clear cell histology who had previously failed initial therapy with either IFN or IL-2 [16]. In a preliminary report, tumor control defined as stable disease (SD) or partial response (PR) with sorafenib given at 400 mg twice daily was achieved in 80% of patients, although only 2% attained a PR. Sorafenib significantly prolonged median PFS compared with placebo (24 versus 12 weeks, $p < 0.000001$) and median survival improvement was preliminarily reported (19.3 versus 15.9 months, HR 0.77, p = 0.015). Cross-over from the placebo to sorafenib arm

was allowed due to the magnitude of effect on PFS. With the placebo arm censored at the time of cross-over, there was a significant improvement in median survival for sorafenib (17.8 months) versus placebo (14.3 months; HR 0.78, p = 0.0287) [17]; however, due to the confounding effect of cross-over, median OS at the time of final analysis was not statistically significant (sorafenib 17.8 months, placebo 15.2 months; HR 0.88, p = 0.146) [18]. Adverse effects were manageable with grade 3–4 hand-foot syndrome, fatigue and hypertension observed in 5%, 2% and 1%, respectively.

In order to determine the efficacy of sorafenib in previously untreated patients with metastatic clear cell RCC, a randomized phase II trial of sorafenib versus IFN was conducted and the final results were reported [19]. In this trial, progressing patients on the IFN arm crossed over to sorafenib and patients on the sorafenib arm were dose escalated to 600 mg twice daily. Tumor regression was more common with sorafenib (68%) versus IFN (39%); however, no statistically significant difference in median PFS between treatment arms was demonstrated (sorafenib 5.7 months, IFN 5.6 months; HR 0.88, p = 0.504) [19]. On cross-over, more than half of patients responded to second-line sorafenib irrespective of response to previous IFN therapy, confirming the results seen in the phase III TARGET trial. Additionally, one-third of patients in this trial who responded to sorafenib (400 mg twice daily) experienced a further response on dose escalation following progression.

Bevacizumab

Two randomized phase III trials (CALGB-90206 and Roche B017705) of IFN-alpha with or without bevacizumab in previously untreated patients with metastatic RCC have been conducted, and the results from the phase III Roche B017705 (AVOREN) trial were reported [20]. In this randomized, controlled, double-blinded study, 649 patients with metastatic clear cell RCC were randomized 1:1 to receive either IFN (9 MIU three times weekly) and placebo or the combination of bevacizumab (10 mg/kg every 2 weeks) and IFN (9 MIU three times weekly. The treatment arms were well balanced for prognostic factors and all patients enrolled onto the study had previous nephrectomy. Side effects were similar between treatment arms, and bevacizumab-related side effects were generally mild and consistent with previous observations. The addition of bevacizumab to IFN significantly increased PFS (10.2 months versus 5.4 months; HR 0.63, $p < 0.0001$) and objective tumor response (CR and PR) (30.6% versus 12.4%; $p < 0.0001$). A trend toward improved OS was also observed (p = 0.0670). In this trial, only MSKCC prognostic scale (see Table 35.1) good- and intermediate-risk patients benefited, with poor-risk patients having no added improvement in PFS over IFN alone. These results support the antitumor activity of bevacizumab/IFN as a therapy for patients with metastatic clear cell RCC. Given the similar PFS reported in previous trials of bevacizumab [21,22], the added benefit of IFN is uncertain.

Comment

Sunitinib (Sutent®), Sorafenib (Nexavar®), and bevacicumab (Avastin®) have demonstrated clinically meaningful activity in patients with metastatic RCC. Their benefit is well documented in patients with clear cell histology and in the good- and intermediate-risk categories. Although antiangiogenic and targeted agents can induce long-term suppressive effects on kidney cancer growth, disease recurs after discontinuation of therapy and ultimately resistance develops in virtually all patients.

There have been no published clinical trials looking specifically at the effects of antiangiogenic compounds in nonclear cell histologies but the analysis of clinical trials that allowed treatment of various subtypes of RCC suggests that clinical benefit, although present, is inferior to the one observed in clear cell histology [23]. At this point sunitinib appears to be the most efficacious agent. The epidermal growth factor receptor (EGFR) inhibitor erlotinib demonstrated modest activity against papillary RCC (pRCC) [24].

Recommendations

Based on available evidence from phase III randomized clinical trials, sunitinib is the initial treatment of choice for the majority of patients with metastatic RCC of clear cell histology who fall into the good and intermediate prognostic groups. This represents a strong recommendation for sunitinib treatment based on moderate-quality evidence (Grade 1B). Combination of bevacizumab and interferon is also an acceptable first-line therapeutic option in these patients (Grade 1B). The beneficial role of sorafenib has been established in the setting of second-line therapy following prior exposure to immunotherapy (Grade 1B).

Clinical question 35.4

What are the applications for m-TOR inhibitors in patients with metastatic renal cell carcinoma?

Background

The m-TOR (mammalian target of rapamycin) pathway has a central role in the regulation of cancer cell growth (see Figure 35.1). m-TOR receives input from multiple signaling pathways, including growth factors, hormones, nutrients and other stimulants, or mitogens to stimulate protein synthesis by phosphorylating key translational regulators. The m-TOR enzyme also contributes to many other critical cellular functions, including protein degradation and angiogenesis, and appears to be of major importance in the molecular pathophysiology of RCC. Temsirolimus (Torisel®, Wyeth, Madison, NJ) is a specific inhibitor of m-TOR kinase, forming a complex that inhibits m-TOR, leading to decreased translation of several proteins regulating cell cycle and angiogenesis. Everolimus (Novartis, Basel, Switzerland) is an orally administered m-TOR inhibitor.

Literature search

Potentially relevant studies were identified by a computerized search, restricted to English-language literature, of the Medline electronic database (source PubMed, 1966 to March 2009) using relevant text and keywords in combination as follows: "metastatic renal cancer and m-TOR inhibitors," "metastatic renal cancer and temsirolimus," "metastatic renal cancer and everolimus." The reference lists of retrieved eligible articles were reviewed to identify additional relevant articles

The evidence

Temsirolimus

A phase II single-agent study of temsirolimus in patients with cytokine-refractory metastatic RCC was associated with encouraging PFS and overall survival [22]. A subsequent phase III trial of temsirolimus and interferon in patients with advanced RCC established the benefit of this compound in a subset of patients with high-risk metastatic RCC according to MSKCC prognostic criteria (see Table 35.1) [25]. Six hundred and twenty-six patients were randomized to receive IFN-alpha at escalating doses up to 18 MU subcutaneously three times a week or temsirolimus at 25 mg IV weekly or a combination of temsirolimus at 15 mg weekly with IFN-alpha at 6 MU three times a week. These patients did not have prior systemic therapy, almost all had prior nephrectomy and 80% had clear cell histology. At the time of second interim analysis performed in March 2006, patients treated with single-agent temsirolimus demonstrated statistically improved overall median survival compared to the IFN-treated group (10.9 versus 7.3 months, p = 0.0069), which represented a 49% increase. Patients treated with the combination of temsirolimus and interferon did not experience improved outcomes. Objective response of temsirolimus was 9% and clinical benefit (CR + PR + SD > 16 weeks) was 46% which was higher than the IFN group (7% and 29% respectively). Progression-free survival was improved from 1.9 to

3.7 months. Temsirolimus was better tolerated than IFN, with a 16% reduction in the proportion of patients with grade ≥ 3 adverse events.

Everolimus

The results of a phase III, randomized, double-blind, placebo-controlled trial of everolimus in patients with metastatic RCC whose disease had progressed on VEGF-targeted therapy were reported in 2008 [26]. Patients with metastatic disease which had progressed on sunitinib, sorafenib or both were randomly assigned in a 2:1 ratio to receive everolimus 10 mg once daily (N 272) or placebo (N 138), in conjunction with best supportive care. The results of the second interim analysis indicated a significant difference in efficacy between arms and the trial was thus halted early after 191 progression events had been observed. Median PFS was 4.0 months in the everolimus group (95% confidence interval (CI) 3.7–5.5) versus 1.9 (95% CI 1.8–1.9) months in the placebo group. Main side effects of everolimus included stomatitis (40%), rash (25%) and fatigue (20%) but they were mostly mild or moderate in severity. Pneumonitis (any grade) was detected in 22 (8%) patients in the everolimus group, of whom eight had pneumonitis of Grade 3 severity.

Comments

m-TOR inhibition is a valid strategy for the treatment of RCC. m-TOR inhibitors appear to be well tolerated even in patients with high-risk features and poor performance status. Based on the outcome of a randomized clinical trial, temsirolimus received FDA approval for the treatment of advanced RCC. Approval of everolimus is currently under review.

Recommendations

Temsirolimus at 25 mg IV weekly is an appropriate first-line therapy for patients with metastatic RCC and high-risk features.This represents a strong recommendaton for temsirolimus based on moderate-quality evidence (**Grade 1B**). Everolimus is the appropriate choice for patients who demonstrate disease progression on sunitinib and/or sorafenib (**Grade 1B**).

Conclusion

Kidney cancer represents one of the first common solid tumors for which rationally designed targeted agents (sunitinib, sorafenib, temsirolimus, bevacizumab) currently constitute the main therapeutic option. This is the direct result of very comprehensive understanding of molecular abnormalities responsible for the pathophysiology of this

Table 35.3 Proposed algorithm for RCC therapy based on phase III data

	Setting	Angiogenesis	Therapy
First-line therapy	Low + intermediate risk	Sunitinib Bevacizumab/ INF-alpha	HDIL-2 (highly selected patients)
	Poor risk	m-TOR inhibitor	
Second-line therapy	Prior cytokines Prior rTKI	Sorafenib m-TOR inhibitor	

Low, intermediate and poor risk as determined by MSKCC risk factor stratification (see Table 35.1). HDIL-2, high-dose interleukin-2; IFN, interferon; m-TOR, mammalian target of rapamycin; rTKI, receptor tyrosine kinase inhibitors

disease. As molecular pathways and targets important in the development and progression of RCC are being identified, the search for novel therapeutic compounds for this disease continues apace (see Table 35.2). Immunotherapy, which until recently represented the mainstay of therapy, is used less frequently, primarily in combination with antiangiogenic agents. High-dose IL-2 also continues to be used in patients with excellent performance status with an ongoing effort to appropriately select individuals who may benefit the most from this very toxic therapy.

Based upon the results of published phase III trials, a treatment algorithm which integrates these new targeted agents into the management of metastatic RCC begins to emerge (Table 35.3). Since progression eventually occurs with these targeted agents, mechanisms of resistance need to be elucidated and strategies to overcome this problem must be developed. Future research is needed to determine the most effective dosing schemes, the optimal sequencing and combination of these agents, as well as the development of biomarkers predictive of response that will enable the practicing oncologist to optimize and individualize therapy for patients with this disease.

References

1. Jemal A, Siegel R, Ward E, et al. Cancer statistics. CA Cancer J Clin 2007;57:43-66.
2. Yagoda A, Abi-Rached B, Petrylak D. Chemotherapy for advanced renal cell carcinoma: 1983–1993. Semin Oncol 1995;22:42-60.
3. Motzer RJ, Vogelzang NJ. Chemotherapy for renal cell carcinoma. In: Raghavan D, Scher HI, Leibel SA, et al. (eds) *Principles and Practice of Genitourinary Oncology.* Philadelphia, PA: Lippincott-Raven, 1997: 885-96.

4. Dekernion JB, Ramming KP, Smith RB. The natural history of metastatic renal cell carcinoma: a computer analysis. J Urol 1978;120:148-52.

5. Flanigan RC, Salmon SE, Blumenstein BA, et al. Nephrectomy followed by interferon α-2b compared with interferon α-2b alone for metastatic renal-cell cancer. N Engl J Med 2001;345:1655-9.

6. Mickisch GH, Garin A, van Poppel H, de Prijck L, Sylvester R. Radical nephrectomy plus IFN-α based immunotherapy compared with IFN-α alone in metastatic renal-cell carcinoma: a randomized trial. Lancet 2001;358:966-70.

7. Flanigan RC, Mickisch G, Sylvester R, Tangen C, van Poppel H. Crawford ED. Cytoreductive nephrectomy in patients with metastatic renal cancer: a combined analysis. JUrol 2004;171:1071-6.

8. Rosenberg SA, Yang JC, Topalian SL, et al. Treatment of 283 consecutive patients with metastatic melanoma or renal cell cancer using high-dose bolus interleukin 2. JAMA 1994;271:907-13.

9. Fisher RI, Rosenberg SA, Fyfe G. Long-term survival update for high-dose recombinant interleukin-2 in patients with renal cell carcinoma Cancer J Sci 2000;6(suppl 1):S55-S57.

10. Yang C, Sherry RM, Steinberg SM, et al. Randomized study of high-dose and low-dose interleukin-2 in patients with metastatic renal cancer. J Clin Oncol 2003;21:3127-32.

11. Motzer RJ, Rini BI, Bukowski RM, et al. Sunitinib in patients with metastatic renal cell carcinoma. JAMA 2006;295:2516-24.

12. Motzer RJ, Michaelson MD, Redman BG, et al. Activity of SU11248, a multitargeted inhibitor of vascular endothelial growth factor receptor and platelet-derived growth factor receptor, in patients with metastatic renal cell carcinoma. J Clin Oncol 2006;24:16-24.

13. Motzer RJ, Hutson TE, Tomczak P, et al. Phase III randomized trial of sunitinib malate (SU11248) versus interferon-alfa as first-line systemic therapy for patients with metastatic renal cell carcinoma. N Engl J Med 2007;356:115-24.

14. Motzer RJ, Figlin RA, Hutson TE, et al. Sunitinib versus interferon-alfa (INF-α) as first-line treatment of metastatic renal cell carcinoma (mRCC): updated results and analysis of prognostic factors. ASCO Annual Meeting Proceedings Part I. Vol 25, No. 18S (June 20 Supplement, 2007): 5024.

15. Figlin R. Overall survival with sunitinib versus interferon (IFN)-alfa as first-line treatment of metastatic renal cell carcinoma (mRCC). Paper presented at the 2008 ASCO Meeting, Genitourinary Cancer Session.

16. Escudier B, Eisen T, Stadler WM, et al. Treatment approaches in renal cancer global evaluation trial (TARGETs): a randomized, double-blind, placebo-controlled phase III Trial of sorafenib, an oral multi-kinase inhibitor in advanced renal cell carcinoma. N Engl J Med 2007;356(2):125-34.

17. Eisen T, Bukowski RM, Staehler M, et al. Randomized phase III trial of sorafenib in advanced renal cell carcinoma (RCC): impact of crossover on survival. ASCO Annual Meeting Proceedings Part I. Vol 24, No. 18S (June 20 Supplement, 2006): 4524.

18. Bukowski RM, Eisen T, Szczylik C, et al. Final results of the randomized phase III trial of sorafenib in advanced renal cell carcinoma: survival and biomarker analysis. ASCO Annual Meeting Proceedings Part I. Vol 25, No. 18S (June 20 Supplement, 2007): 5023.

19. Szczylik C, Demkow T, Staehler M, et al. Randomized phase II trial of first-line treatment with sorafenib versus interferon in patients with advanced renal cell carcinoma: final results. ASCO Annual Meeting Proceedings Part I. Vol 25, No. 18S (June 20 Supplement, 2007): 5025.

20. Escudier B, Koralewski P, Pluzanska A, et al. A randomized, controlled, double-blind phase III study (AVOREN) of bevacizumab/interferon-α2a vs placebo/interferon-α2a as first-line therapy in metastatic renal cell carcinoma. ASCO Annual Meeting Proceedings Part I. Vol 25, No. 18S (June 20 Supplement, 2007): 3.

21. Bukowski RM, Kabbinavar F, Figlin RA, et al. Bevacizumab with or without erlotinib. Proc Am Soc Clin Oncol 2006; 24, 18S: abstract 4523.

22. Yang JC, Haworth L, Sherry RM, et al. A randomized trial of bevacizumab, an antivascular endothelial growth factor antibody, for metastatic renal cancer. N Engl J Med 2003;349:427-34.

23. Choueiri T, Plantade E, Elson P, et al. Efficacy of sunitinib and sorafenib in metastatic papillary and chromophobe renal cell carcinoma. J Clin Oncol 2008;26(1):127-13.

24. Pan C, Hussey M, Lara P, et al. A phase II trial of the EGFR inhibitor erlotinib in patients with advanced papillary renal cell carcinoma – SWOG S0317. Proceedings of the ASCO Meeting, 2007, Abstract # 15516.

25. Hudes G, Carducci M, Tomczak P, et al. Temsirolimus, interferon alfa or both for advanced renal cell carcinoma. N Engl J Med 2007;356(22):2271-81.

26. Motzer RJ, Escudier B, Oudard S, et al., for the RECORD-1 Study Group. Efficacy of everolimus in advanced renal cell carcinoma: a double-blind, randomised, placebo-controlled phase III trial. Lancet 2008;372(9637):449-56.

36 Seminoma

Mark Shaw, Peter Chung and Padraig Warde

Department of Radiation Oncology, University of Toronto, and the Radiation Medicine Program, Princess Margaret Hospital, Toronto, Canada

Background

Testicular cancer is the most common solid malignancy in males between the ages of 20 and 35 and primary germ cell tumors (GCT) are by far the most common histological type. Approximately 60% of GCT are pure seminoma, 30% are nonseminomatous GCT (NGCT), and 10% are mixed tumors [1,2]. In the United States, 8000 new cases and 390 deaths from the disease have been projected for 2008 [3]. Following orchidectomy, most seminoma patients (70–80%) present with no radiological evidence of disease (stage I), 15–20% have infradiaphragmatic lymph node involvement (stage II) and 5% present with distant metastatic disease (stage III). Therefore, in the United States in 2008, there will be approximately 4800 cases of seminoma, approximately 4100 of which will have stage I disease.

Treatment options

Management options for stage I seminoma include radiotherapy, surveillance, and adjuvant chemotherapy. For the past 65 years, the standard management of patients with stage I seminoma has been adjuvant retroperitoneal radiotherapy. Although providing excellent long-term results with virtually 100% local control in the abdomen and pelvis, this approach has been associated with increased risk of late gonadal toxicity, development of second malignancies and an increased risk of cardiovascular disease [4-9]. Various approaches have been investigated in efforts to reduce radiation-induced long-term morbidity, including reducing the radiation dose and treatment volume, as well as alternative management

Evidence-Based Urology. Edited by Philipp Dahm, Roger R. Dmochowski.
© 2010 Blackwell Publishing.

strategies including surveillance (including risk-adapted surveillance) and adjuvant chemotherapy [10-13].

It has been suggested that more patients with stage I seminoma will die of their treatment than of their cancer, so the thrust of modern management is to maintain the current 100% cure rate while minimizing the burden of treatment [9]. This chapter will discuss management of stage I seminoma, and outline and grade the evidence for our recommendations [14].

Literature search

The Medline and EMBASE databases were searched for evidence using the following text, MeSH, and EMBASE subject headings: "testicular neoplasms," "testicular cancer," "neoplasms," "germ cell and embryonal," "seminoma," "germinoma," "dysgerminoma," and "germ cell tumor." These results were combined with the terms "radiotherapy," "surveillance," "watchful waiting," "chemotherapy," and "drug therapy" to provide a base pool of literature on the treatment of stage I seminoma, with the total results being limited to human studies published from 1981 through to September 2008.

Clinical question 36.1

Which patient, pathological and treatment factors are significant in selecting a management plan for a patient with stage I seminoma?

The evidence

A prognostic factor is a variable that can account for some of the heterogeneity associated with the expected course and outcome for a patient with a specific disease [15]. Thus, prognostic factors contribute to our best forecast of the behavior of cancer. This knowledge of outcome, or prognosis, forms an integral part of the decision-making process in medicine and formulating a management plan for any patient with stage I seminoma, or indeed any medical condition, requires a careful assessment of three principal groups of prognostic factors: host-related factors (factors inherent to the patient), tumor-related factors (the most common is pathological factors), and environment-related factors (principally treatment factors) [15].

In terms of selecting a management plan for a patient with stage I seminoma, two patient-related factors are of primary importance. First is the presence of co-existing illnesses that would largely preclude certain treatment options. Examples here would include inflammatory bowel disease or acquired immunodeficiency syndrome, which would rule out consideration of the use of adjuvant radiation therapy. In addition, the willingness or ability of the patient to be compliant to medical advice must be considered especially if surveillance with no adjuvant treatment is being considered as this approach entails multiple follow-up visits with repeated imaging over a 5–10-year time frame. Detection of disease recurrence at an early stage is important and while overall survival may not be affected because of the efficacy of salvage therapies, the type and therefore the morbidity of treatment are determined by the extent of disease at relapse.

Pathological prognostic factors for relapse have been studied in a number of surveillance series (Table 36.1). In the first series of surveillance patients, the Royal Marsden Hospital group reported on 103 patients and the only significant factor predicting relapse was the presence of lymphatic and/or vascular invasion (9% vs 17% relapse rate) [16]. On multivariate analysis in the Princess Margaret Hospital series of 201 patients, age and tumor size predicted for relapse, while small vessel invasion (SVI) approached statistical significance [17]. In a large Danish series of 261 patients, tumor size was the only significant predictive factor for disease recurrence [18]. A pooled analysis of four large surveillance series using individual patient data from four centers – Royal Marsden Hospital, Danish Testicular Cancer Study Group, Princess Margaret Hospital and the Royal London Hospital – has been performed [19]. Six hundred and thirty-eight patients were included in the study and on multivariate analysis, tumor size and rete testis invasion were identified as the only factors that predicted for relapse. An incremental rise in 5-year relapse rate was noted in the presence of zero, one or both of these risk factors (12.2%, 15.9% and 31.5% respectively; Figure 36.1). The hazard ratio (HR) for relapse with a tumor size > 4 cm was 2.0 (95% confidence interval (CI) 1.3–3.2) relative to baseline (tumor size < 4 cm and no rete testis invasion; see Table 36.1). The hazard ratio for rete testis involvement was 1.7 (95% CI 1.1–2.6) and with both adverse prognostic factors present, the hazard ratio for relapse was 3.4 (95% CI 2.0–6.1).

This prognostic model has not being validated in an independent dataset. However, a number of other reports give indirect support to the importance of tumor size and rete testis invasion as prognostic factors for relapse on surveillance. A recent retrospective review assessing factors predictive of metastasis at diagnosis indicated that tumor size > 6 cm and rete testis involvement predicted for the presence of more advanced disease at diagnosis [20]. In addition, a risk-adapted treatment study using tumor size > 4 cm and rete testis invasion as indicators for treatment was implemented in the second Spanish Germ Cell Co-operative Group (SGCCG) study [10]. Patients with no risk factors were managed with surveillance and 6% relapsed, similar to the expected percentage derived from the multi-institutional analysis prognostic model.

The most important treatment-related factor in selecting management for a patient with stage I seminoma is the late toxicity of adjuvant treatment, in particular radiation therapy. Other treatment-related factors include distance from the treatment center, which may influence the acceptability of surveillance as a management option.

Testicular germinal epithelium is extremely sensitive to ionizing radiation. Scatter dose to the contralateral testis may be significant and may cause severe depression of spermatogenesis and compromise future fertility. A radiation dose between 20 and 50 cGy may produce temporary aspermia, while higher doses may preclude recovery of spermatogenesis [21,22]. Although scrotal shielding should be used in every patient to reduce scattered radiation dose to the contralateral testis, it cannot ensure protection of spermatogenesis in all patients. A study of 451 consecutive testicular cancer patients in France demonstrated that the cumulative conception rates for patients who received radiotherapy were significantly lower compared with the rates for patients who received chemotherapy [23].

An increased risk of second nontesticular cancers after radiation therapy (RT) has been documented in a number of studies, and since this increased risk is expressed more than 10–15 years following RT, it is often not apparent in series with shorter follow-up [24]. Zagars et al. have reported an increased cancer-specific standardized mortality ratio (SMR) in 453 long-term survivors of radiation treatment for testicular seminoma [4]. A Dutch population-based study of 2707 testicular cancer survivors with a median follow-up of 17.6 years showed that the rate of second nontesticular cancers was 2.6-fold increased as compared to surgery alone [5]. A recent report combined 14 population-based registries including 10,534 patients with seminoma (all stages) treated with radiotherapy [7]. Compared with matched cohorts from corresponding registries, the overall relative risk of a second nontesticular malignancy was 2.0 (95% CI 1.8–2.2). For a 35-year-old patient with seminoma, the cumulative 40-year risk of a

Table 36.1 Prognostic factors for relapse in surveillance series

Study	Number	Follow-up (yrs)	Univariate prognostic factors for relapse			Multivariate prognostic factor for relapse
			Factor	Stratification	Relapse (%)	
DATECA [18]	261	4.0 (0.5–5.6)	Size	< 3.0 cm	6	Yes (tumor size > 6 cm)
				3.0–5.9 cm	18	
				> 6 cm	36	
			Histology	Spermatocytic	0	No
				Classic	16	
				Anaplastic	33	
			Necrosis	No	14	No
				Yes	23	
			Rete testis	No	14	No
				Yes	23	
PMH [17]	201	6.1 (1.3–12.3)	Size	< 6 cm	12	Yes (tumor size > 6 cm)
				> 6 cm	33	
			Age	> 34 years	9	Yes (age ≥ 34 years)
				≤ 34 years	21	
			Small vessel	No	14	No
				Yes	31	
RMH Horwich et al., 1992 [16]	103	5.2(1.2–11.8)	Small vessel	No	10	–
				Yes	20	
Pooled analysis [19]	638	7.0 (0.02–17.5)	Size	≤ 4 cm	13	Yes (tumor size > 4 cm)
				> 4 cm	24	
			Rete testis	No	14	Yes (rete testis invasion)
				Yes	24	
			Small vessel	No	14	No
				Yes	23	

second malignancy was 36%, compared with 23% in the normal population.

Data from the M.D. Anderson and Royal Marsden Hospitals suggest that long-term survivors of testicular seminoma treated postorchidectomy with radiotherapy are also at significant excess risk of death as a result of cardiac disease [4,9]. In the M.D. Anderson series of 453 patients treated between 1951 and 1999, the standardized cardiac mortality ratio for patients > 15 years after radiotherapy (infradiaphragmatic radiotherapy, no mediastinal radiotherapy) was 1.80 (95% CI 1.01–2.98) [4]. Huddart reported a similar increase in cardiac events in a cohort of 992 patients treated at the Royal Marsden Hospital with a risk ratio of 2.4 (95% CI 1.04–5.45) in those treated with infradiaphragmatic radiotherapy as compared to those managed by surveillance [9]. The etiology of this effect is currently unclear. While some have questioned the relevance of these data to the modern practice of radiotherapy, patients should be informed of this increased risk of cardiac death when deciding whether to undergo radiotherapy in the adjuvant setting [25].

The short follow-up and limited number of patients treated make it impossible to assess the frequency of significant long-term toxicity with adjuvant carboplatin in stage I seminoma. Like RT, chemotherapy (in particular high-dose carboplatin) has been associated with second malignancies and cardiovascular disease [5-7]. Whether one dose of carboplatin will lead to the same frequency of late toxicity as multiagent cisplatin-based therapy is unknown, but the lack of long-term data must not be interpreted as proof of safety. While it is encouraging that a recent report noted no increase in cardiovascular disease or secondary malignancies after one or two cycles of carboplatin for stage I seminoma compared with age-matched controls, the number of patients was small and the median follow-up was insufficient to allay fears regarding long-term problems [26].

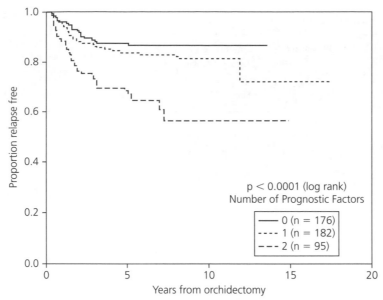

Figure 36.1 Relapse-free rate based on number of adverse prognostic factors. Reproduced from Warde et al. [19] with permission from the American Society of Clinical Oncology

Comment

Overall, the quality of evidence surrounding the patient, pathological and treatment factors that are important in selecting a management plan for a patient with a stage I seminoma is *low* and as such only a *weak* recommendation (as defined by the GRADE working group) can be made on which management strategy is best in this setting (Grade 1c) [14]. As agreed to at the most recent European Germ Cell Consensus Conference in 2007, surveillance should be the management option of choice in compliant patients but both adjuvant radiation therapy and adjuvant carboplatin should be discussed with each patient [27].

Clinical question 36.2

In patients with stage I seminoma, how does adjuvant radiotherapy of 30 Gy versus 20 Gy compare in terms of relapse rates?

The evidence

The minimum dose of radiation required to control occult seminomatous tumor has not been defined and one strategy that has been investigated to reduce the long-term toxicity of adjuvant radiation therapy in stage I seminoma is the reduction of radiation therapy dose. In most centers across the world, a dose of 25–35 Gy has traditionally been used in stage I seminoma.

The MRC conducted a RCT (TE18), using a noninferiority design, to assess the possibility of reducing radiotherapy

doses without compromising efficacy in stage I seminoma [12]. A total of 625 patients were randomized to a conventional dose of 30 Gy in 15 fractions over 3 weeks or a reduced dose of 20 Gy in 10 fractions over 2 weeks. The vast majority of patients in both groups received para-aortic strip irradiation only (88.1% in the 30 Gy group and 88.7% in the 20 Gy group). At publication, the median follow-up was 61 months and a total of 10 and 11 relapses, respectively, occurred in the 30 Gy and 20 Gy groups (HR 1.11, 90% CI 0.54–2.28). The 5-year relapse rates were 3% and 3.6% respectively for the 30 Gy and 20 Gy groups.

Following the closure of the TE18 study, a further 469 patients from another trial (TE19/30982) comparing adjuvant chemotherapy to adjuvant radiotherapy, who were randomized to receive radiotherapy, were further randomized with respect to dose (30 Gy versus 20 Gy) [28]. The median follow-up for this group was much shorter at 2.5 years but the combined TE18 and TE19 groups gave a sample size of 1094 patients. The observed 2-year relapse rates were similar at 3.2% and 2.5% respectively for the 30 Gy and 20 Gy groups.

Both TE18 and TE19 studies were updated and presented at the ASCO 2008 Annual Meeting [29]. With a median follow-up of 7 years, there were 27 relapses from 550 patients in the 30 Gy arm versus 16 relapses from 544 patients in the 20 Gy arm. The updated combined 5-year relapse rates were 4.9% versus 3%, for the 30 Gy and 20 Gy groups respectively. This difference was reflected in a HR of 0.59 (90% CI 0.35–0.99). This longer follow-up confirmed the original findings of noninferiority of 20 Gy compared to 30 Gy.

Acute toxicity in the MRC TE18 study was greater in the 30 Gy group, with moderate to severe lethargy (20%

versus 5%) and the proportion unable to work (46% versus 28%) both being significantly higher at 4 weeks (p < 0.001) yet returning to baseline by 12 weeks in both groups [12]. Nausea and vomiting were similar in both groups, as were reported episodes of dyspepsia.

Using the linear quadratic model to compare differing dose/fractionation schedules, commonly used regimens such as 25 Gy in 15–20 fractions over 3–4 weeks are similar to 20 Gy in 10 fractions over 2 weeks in terms of biologically effective doses for tumor control and late effects (assuming an alpha/beta ratio of 10 for tumor and an alpha/beta ratio of 2 for late responding tissue toxicity) (Table 36.2).

Comment

Using the GRADE Working Group recommendations, there is good evidence that 20 Gy is equivalent to 30 Gy in terms of relapse rates and the quality of evidence is high [14]. If adjuvant radiotherapy is used in stage I seminoma, 20 Gy/10 fractions over 2 weeks (or a biologically similar regimen) should be the treatment regimen of choice (**Grade 1A**).

Clinical question 36.3

In patients with stage I seminoma, how does retroperitoneal para-aortic irradiation versus para-aortic plus ipsilateral iliac and pelvic nodal irradiation "dogleg" compare in terms of relapse rates?

The evidence

The traditional management of stage I seminoma patients after orchidectomy has consisted of radiotherapy to the para-aortic and pelvic (retroperitoneal) lymph nodes using parallel-opposed anteroposterior fields and 18 MV linear accelerator photons. With left-sided tumours, the left renal hilum is included in the field by shaping the

left lateral border of the RT portal. This classic plan was called "hockey stick" in North America and "dogleg" in the United Kingdom and Europe. The radiation fields typically extended from the top of the T11 vertebral body (or T10) to the inguinal ligament.

The low incidence of pelvic lymph node involvement in stage I seminoma led to the investigation of adjuvant radiotherapy directed to the para-aortic lymph nodes alone. The advantages of such an approach include decreased scatter to the remaining testicle and a reduction in the integral radiation dose, presumably decreasing the risk of second malignancy. Reports from phase II trials and retrospective single-institution experiences have shown excellent results with few pelvic failures [30,31]. The MRC Testicular Study Group randomized 478 patients to traditional para-aortic and pelvic radiation or para-aortic irradiation alone [13]. Patients treated with para-aortic radiotherapy alone had a 4% relapse rate as compared to a 3.4% relapse rate in those treated to the para-aortic and pelvic lymph nodes. All patients who received para-aortic and pelvic radiotherapy relapsed in supradiaphragmatic sites, but four (1.6%) patients treated to the para-aortic lymph nodes alone failed with disease in the pelvis. This trial showed that treating the para-aortic nodes alone gives excellent results, but a small risk of pelvic failure remains.

Comment

Using the GRADE Working Group recommendations, there is good evidence that para-aortic RT is equivalent to para-aortic and ipsilateral pelvic RT in terms of relapse rates and the quality of evidence is high (**Grade 1A**) [14]. However, if this treatment approach is adopted, regular imaging with CT of the pelvic lymph nodes must be performed to ensure that if pelvic relapse occurs, it is detected at an early stage. Data from the Christie Hospital in Manchester, where no routine evaluation of the pelvis was carried out after para-aortic radiation alone, have shown that the median size of the pelvic lymph nodes at time of detection of relapse was 5 cm (range 2.5–9 cm) [30]. The advantage of para-aortic radiotherapy alone is therefore not clear, particularly in comparison to surveillance.

Clinical question 36.4

In patients with stage I seminoma, how does adjuvant chemotherapy versus adjuvant radiotherapy compare in terms of relapse rates?

The evidence

Another strategy that has been investigated to reduce the long-term toxicity of adjuvant radiation therapy in stage

Table 36.2 Biologically effective doses (BED) for tumor control and late normal tissue toxicity

Regimen	BED tumor control	BED late normal tissue effects
20 Gy in 10 fractions @2 Gy per fraction	24	40
25 Gy in 20 fractions @1.25 Gy per fraction	28.1	40.6
25 Gy in 15 fractions @1.67 Gy per fraction	29.2	45.8
20 Gy in 8 fractions @2.5 Gy per fraction	25	45

I seminoma is the use of adjuvant chemotherapy. The MRC UK has conducted a randomized phase III study of 1447 patients comparing adjuvant radiotherapy and a single course of carboplatin [28]. The initial publication from 2005, with a median follow-up of 4 years, reported 3-year relapse rates of 4.1% and 5.2% for radiotherapy and chemotherapy respectively (HR 1.28, 90% CI 0.85–1.93). An update of the study was presented at the ASCO 2008 Annual Meeting; with 6.5 years median follow-up, the 5-year relapse rates were 4% and 5.3% respectively for radiotherapy and chemotherapy (HR 1.25, 90% CI 0.83–1.89) [29]. Sixty-seven percent of those who relapsed in the carboplatin arm did so in the retroperitoneum alone. An unexpected finding in this study was a reduction in the observed number of second primary germ cell tumors in patients treated with adjuvant chemotherapy, with a 5-year event rate of 1.96% with radiotherapy versus 0.54% with chemotherapy.

Data from other single-institution series indicate that if adjuvant carboplatin is given in this setting, two courses of treatment may well be necessary. A prospective cohort study reported on eight relapses in 93 patients treated with a single cycle of carboplatin compared to no relapses in 32 patients treated with two cycles [32]. The dosing strategy for carboplatin used in this study was 400 mg/m^2. However, a more contemporary practice is carboplatin dosing based on an area under the curve (AUC) of 7 which is typically around 15% greater than using a m^2 dosing regimen [33]. This dosing schedule was used in the MRC TE19 and Spanish Germ Cell Cancer Co-operative Group trials [10,28]. Aparicio reported on the prospective treatment of patients with risk factors for recurrence (tumors > 4 cm and/or rete testis invasion) with two cycles of AUC7 carboplatin and the 5-year relapse rate was 3.8% [10]. As observed in the MRC TE19 study, most relapses were retroperitoneal, thus necessitating ongoing abdominopelvic CT imaging. No randomized study has compared one to two cycles of carboplatin.

Comment

Using the GRADE Working Group recommendations, there is good evidence that adjuvant radiotherapy and adjuvant chemotherapy are similar in terms of relapse rates and the quality of evidence is high (Grade 1A) [14]. The relapse pattern after adjuvant single-agent carboplatin mandates that continued cross-sectional imaging of the retroperitoneal lymph nodes is required (similar to surveillance), and the reduction in relapse rates is only from 15% with surveillance to 5% with adjuvant chemotherapy. Eighty-five percent of patients receive unnecessary treatment and the long-term toxicity of this strategy is unknown.

Conclusion

Testicular seminoma is initially managed with an inguinal orchidectomy which will cure 80–85% of men. Following surgery, subsequent treatment options include adjuvant radiotherapy, adjuvant chemotherapy and surveillance. Despite the differences in choice of subsequent management, when salvage options are taken into account, the overall cure rate of stage I seminoma approaches 100%. Retrospective studies have suggested that tumor size > 4 cm and rete testis invasion may be prognostic factors for relapse on surveillance but these factors are yet to be prospectively validated. When radiotherapy is the chosen adjuvant modality, a dose of 20 Gy in 10 fractions versus 30 Gy in 15 fractions yields equivalent freedom from relapse rates. Further dose/fraction modifications may improve the therapeutic ratio by decreasing acute and/or late toxicity whilst maintaining equivalent freedom from relapse rates. Para-aortic radiation only yields similar freedom from relapse rates compared to extended "dogleg" fields but is associated with greater relapses in the pelvis and ongoing abdominopelvic imaging is required. Adjuvant chemotherapy in the form of single-agent carboplatin yields similar relapse rates compared to adjuvant radiotherapy but the majority of relapses following chemotherapy occur in the retroperitoneal or pelvic lymph nodes and thus ongoing abdominopelvic imaging is required.

References

1. Shah MN, Devesa SS, Zhu K, McGlynn KA. Trends in testicular germ cell tumours by ethnic group in the United States. Int J Androl 2007;30(4):206-13; discussion 213-14.
2. Sokoloff MH, Joyce GF, Wise M. Testis cancer. J Urol 2007; 177(6):2030-41.
3. Jemal A, Siegel R, Ward E, Hao Y, Xu J, Murray T, Thun MJ. Cancer statistics, 2008. CA Cancer J Clin 2008;58(2):71-96.
4. Zagars GK, Ballo MT, Lee AK, Strom SS. Mortality after cure of testicular seminoma. J Clin Oncol 2004;22(4):640-7.
5. van den Belt-Dusebout AW, de Wit R, Gietema JA, et al. Treatment-specific risks of second malignancies and cardiovascular disease in 5-year survivors of testicular cancer. J Clin Oncol 2007;25(28):4370-8.
6. van den Belt-Dusebout AW, Nuver J, de Wit R, et al. Long-term risk of cardiovascular disease in 5-year survivors of testicular cancer. J Clin Oncol 2006;24(3):467-75.
7. Travis LB, Fossa SD, Schonfeld SJ, et al. Second cancers among 40,576 testicular cancer patients: focus on long-term survivors. J Natl Cancer Inst 2005;97(18):1354-65.
8. Robinson D, Moller H, Horwich A. Mortality and incidence of second cancers following treatment for testicular cancer. Br J Cancer 2007;96(3):529-33.
9. Huddart RA, Norman A, Shahidi M, Horwich A, Coward D, Nicholls J, Dearnaley DP. Cardiovascular disease as a long-term

complication of treatment for testicular cancer. J Clin Oncol 2003;21(8):1513-23.

10. Aparicio J, Germa JR, Garcia del Muro X, et al. Risk-adapted management for patients with clinical stage I seminoma: the Second Spanish Germ Cell Cancer Cooperative Group study. J Clin Oncol 2005;23(34):8717-23.

11. Daugaard G, Petersen PM, Rorth M. Surveillance in stage I testicular cancer. Apmis 2003;111(1):76-83; discussion 83-5.

12. Jones WG, Fossa SD, Mead GM, et al. Randomized trial of 30 versus 20 Gy in the adjuvant treatment of stage I testicular seminoma: a report on Medical Research Council Trial TE18, European Organisation for the Research and Treatment of Cancer Trial 30942 (ISRCTN18525328). J Clin Oncol 2005;23(6): 1200-8.

13. Fossa SD, Horwich A, Russell JM, et al. Optimal planning target volume for stage I testicular seminoma: a Medical Research Council randomized trial. Medical Research Council Testicular Tumor Working Group. J Clin Oncol 1999;17(4):1146.

14. Guyatt G, Vist G, Falck-Ytter Y, Kunz R, Magrini N, Schunemann H. An emerging consensus on grading recommendations? ACP J Club 2006;144(1):A8-9.

15. Gospodarowicz M, Mackillop W, O'Sullivan B, et al. Prognostic factors in clinical decision making: the future. Cancer 2001;91(8 suppl):1688-95.

16. Horwich A, Alsanjari N, A'Hern R, Nicholls J, Dearnaley DP, Fisher C. Surveillance following orchidectomy for stage I testicular seminoma. Br J Cancer 1992;65(5):775-8.

17. Warde P, Gospodarowicz MK, Banerjee D, et al. Prognostic factors for relapse in stage I testicular seminoma treated with surveillance. J Urol 1997;157(5):1705-9; discussion 1709-10.

18. Von der Maase H, Specht L, Jacobsen GK, et al. Surveillance following orchidectomy for stage I seminoma of the testis. Eur J Cancer 1993;29A(14):1931-4.

19. Warde P, Specht L, Horwich A, et al. Prognostic factors for relapse in stage I seminoma managed by surveillance: a pooled analysis. J Clin Oncol 2002;20(22):4448-52.

20. Valdevenito JP, Gallegos I, Fernandez C, Acevedo C, Palma R. Correlation between primary tumor pathologic features and presence of clinical metastasis at diagnosis of testicular seminoma. Urology 2007;70(4):777-80.

21. Fossa SD, Abyholm T, Normann N, Jetne V. Post-treatment fertility in patients with testicular cancer. III. Influence of radiotherapy in seminoma patients. BJU 1986;58(3):315-19.

22. Fossa SD, Abyholm T, Normann N, Jetne V. Post-treatment fertility in patients with testicular cancer. III. Influence of radiotherapy in seminoma patients. BJU 1986;58(3):315-19.

23. Huyghe E, Matsuda T, Daudin M, et al. Fertility after testicular cancer treatments: results of a large multicenter study. Cancer 2004;100(4):732-7.

24. Moller H, Friis S, Kjaer SK. Survival of Danish cancer patients 1943–1987. Male genital organs. APMIS 1993;33(suppl):122-36.

25. Horwich A. Radiotherapy in stage I seminoma of the testis. J Clin Oncol 2004;22(4):585-8.

26. Powles T, Robinson D, Shamash J, Moller H, Tranter N, Oliver T. The long-term risks of adjuvant carboplatin treatment for stage I seminoma of the testis. Ann Oncol 2008;19(3):443-7.

27. Krege S, Beyer J, Souchon R, et al. European consensus conference on diagnosis and treatment of germ cell cancer: a report of the second meeting of the European Germ Cell Cancer Consensus Group (EGCCCG): part I. Eur Urol 2008;53(3): 478-96.

28. Oliver RT, Mason MD, Mead GM, et al. Radiotherapy versus single-dose carboplatin in adjuvant treatment of stage I seminoma: a randomised trial. Lancet 2005;366(9482):293-300.

29. Mead GM, Fossa SD, Oliver RT, Fogarty PJ, Pollock SP. Relapse patterns in 2,466 stage 1 seminoma patients (pts) entered into Medical Research Council randomised trials. Available from: http://www.asco.org/ASCOv2/Meetings/Abstracts?&vmview=abst_detail_view&confID=55&abstract ID=30836.

30. Logue JP, Harris MA, Livsey JE, Swindell R, Mobarek N, Read G. Short course para-aortic radiation for stage I seminoma of the testis. Int J Radiat Oncol Biol Phys 2003;57(5):1304-9.

31. Classen J, Schmidberger H, Meisner C, et al. Para-aortic irradiation for stage I testicular seminoma: results of a prospective study in 675 patients. A trial of the German Testicular Cancer Study Group (GTCSG). Br J Cancer 2004;90(12):2305-11.

32. Dieckmann KP, Bruggeboes B, Pichlmeier U, Kuster J, Mullerleile U, Bartels H. Adjuvant treatment of clinical stage I seminoma: is a single course of carboplatin sufficient? Urology 2000;55(1):102-6.

33. Calvert AH, Egorin MJ. Carboplatin dosing formulae: gender bias and the use of creatinine-based methodologies. Eur J Cancer 2002;38(1):11-16.

37 Nonseminomatous germ cell tumor

Alana M. Murphy and James M. McKiernan
Department of Urology, Columbia University Medical Center, New York, NY, USA

Background

Testicular cancer is the most common malignancy in men age 15–35 years old. As a result of therapeutic advances over the past several decades and the integration of multimodal treatment, testicular cancer is now one of the most curable neoplasms. Nonseminomatous germ cell tumor (NSGCT) includes embryonal carcinoma, choriocarcinoma, teratoma and yolk sac tumor. Despite favorable long-term survival, the multimodal treatment of NSGCT is constantly evolving and incorporating new paradigms. This chapter aims to present evidence available for several controversies regarding the management of NSGCT.

Clinical question 37.1

How should the violated scrotum be managed?

Literature search

A search of Medline and PubMed databases was conducted to retrieve available publications pertaining to each clinical question. Each database search was limited to articles published between 1960 and 2008 and included only English-language reports. All clinical studies were eligible for inclusion and reports utilizing all levels of evidence were considered for inclusion. The reference list from all included publications was scrutinized to identify potentially relevant publications. Search terms included "testicular neoplasm," "germ cell tumor," "scrotal violation," "trans-scrotal

orchiectomy," "trans-scrotal biopsy" and "postorchiectomy complications."

The evidence

An inguinal orchiectomy with high ligation of the spermatic cord is the standard of care for managing a testicular mass that is suspicious for neoplasm. While this technique is undisputed, management of the violated scrotum is more controversial. Scrotal violation can occur during scrotal orchiectomy, percutaneous testicular biopsy, percutaneous fine-needle aspiration or inguinal-scrotal orchiectomy. Prior inguinal or scrotal surgery could also alter the normal lymphatic drainage of the testis [1]. Scrotal violation before or during orchiectomy leads to concern for higher rates of local and distant recurrence outside conventional retroperitoneal templates.

In the past two decades, three retrospective reviews and one meta-analysis have specifically examined the impact of scrotal violation on recurrence in patients with NSGCT (Table 37.1). The incidence of scrotal violation ranges from 5% to 17% [2-4].

A retrospective analysis by Leibovitch et al. noted that 11% of patients who underwent a hemiscrotectomy after scrotal violation were found to have residual tumor and 66% of these patients experienced local recurrence even after local resection [4]. The same study also noted that no patient treated with chemotherapy after scrotal violation experienced local recurrence. A retrospective study by Giguere et al. noted that 68% of patients with scrotal violation underwent hemiscrotectomy and were found to have no residual tumor [3]. Despite the absence of residual tumor, the authors reported a 17% recurrence rate in the group that underwent local excision versus 40% in patients with scrotal violation who did not undergo hemiscrotectomy. A more recent study by Aki et al. found no local recurrence after scrotal violation and no significant difference in recurrence rates between patients with scrotal violation and those who underwent a standard orchiectomy [5].

Evidence-Based Urology. Edited by Philipp Dahm, Roger R. Dmochowski.
© 2010 Blackwell Publishing.

Table 37.1 Management of the violated scrotum

Authors	Methods	Intervention	Participants	Outcomes	Results	Notes
Aki et al. [5]	retrospective review mean FU 45 months	orchiectomy	• 62 control patients with stage I NSGCT • 13 patients with stage I NSGCT + scrotal violation	• local + distant recurrence	• 3/35 (17%) scrotal violation • no local recurrence • no sig difference in relapse rate of scrotal violation patients (38%) vs control patients (27%)	• all patients had negative surgical margins • no mention of adjuvant therapy • scrotal violation before or during orchiectomy
Capelouto et al. [2]	meta-analysis 1958-1993 mean FU 22–116 months	orchiectomy	• 7 series, 1182 patients • 976 control patients with NSGCT • 206 patients with NSGCT, scrotal violation ± adjuvant therapy	• local + distant recurrence • overall survival	• 206/1,182 (17%) scrotal violation • no sig difference in distant recurrence or survival • sig difference in local recurrence rates of 0.4% for control vs 2.9% for scrotal violation patients • no sig difference in local recurrence when NSGCT patients isolated • no sig difference in local or distant recurrence or survival between scrotal violation patients who underwent surveillance vs adjuvant therapy	
Leibovitch et al.[4]	retrospective review median FU 33 months	orchiectomy + RPLND (2 delayed post-chemotherapy)	• 78 patients with NSGCT+ scrotal violation	• local + distant recurrence	• 78/1708 (4.5%) scrotal violation • 56 (72%) underwent hemiscrotectomy → tumor found in 6 (11%), gross tumor spillage noted in 5 • 5 (6.4%) had local recurrence → 4 after hemiscrotectomy • no patient treated with chemotherapy had local recurrence	• scrotal violation during orchiectomy
Giguere et al. [3]	retrospective review median FU 36 months	orchiectomy + RPLND pathological stage 1 → observation with salvage chemotherapy pathological stage II → 2 cycles chemotherapy or observation	• 35 patients with stage I or II NSGCT, scrotal violation and no adjuvant chemotherapy	• local + distant recurrence	• 47/462 (10%) scrotal violation • 15/22 (68%) patients with gross tumor contamination underwent hemiscrotectomy (no residual tumor) → 17% recurrence in post-hemiscrotectomy group vs 40% in patients without hemiscrotectomy • 8/35 (23%) recurrence in scrotal violation group vs. 21% in routine orchiectomy group • no scrotal recurrence	• scrotal violation during orchiectomy

Of note, all patients included in the study had negative surgical margins after orchiectomy. Despite these favorable results, the authors did not provide information regarding adjuvant treatment for patients with scrotal violation so few conclusions can be drawn from this study.

A meta-analysis by Capelouto et al. examined 206 cases of scrotal violation and found no difference in distant recurrence or survival between patients with scrotal violation and patients who underwent standard orchiectomy [2]. When NSGCT cases were isolated, there was also no significant difference in rates of local recurrence. The analysis also reported no significant difference in local or distant recurrence rates for patients with scrotal violation who received local adjuvant therapy and those who did not receive additional local treatment. The authors did not provide information regarding the presence or absence of residual tumor in hemiscrotectomy specimens.

Comment

The current literature indicates that patients with scrotal violation and clinical stage I NSGCT are not good candidates for surveillance. A conditional recommendation (**Grade 2C**) can be made to counsel these patients regarding adjuvant chemotherapy or retroperitoneal lymph node dissection (RPLND) with simultaneous hemiscrotectomy and excision of the spermatic cord remnant. Based on the current low-quality evidence, patients with scrotal violation are not necessarily at higher risk for local or distant recurrence if they receive adjuvant therapy.

Clinical question 37.2

What is the role of laparoscopy in primary RPLND?

Literature search

A Medline and PubMed search was conducted using the previously described methods. Search terms included "testicular neoplasm," "germ cell tumor," "laparoscopic RPLND" and "laparoscopic lymphadenectomy."

The evidence

Laparoscopic RPLND (L-RPLND) has been developed since the early 1990s in an effort to reduce perioperative morbidity while maintaining the diagnostic and therapeutic benefits of an open RPLND. The indications for L-RPLND mirror those for a primary open RPLND: stage I or IIA NSGCT, negative serum markers and absence of surgical contraindications. L-RPLND was initially accepted as a diagnostic tool and controversy still surrounds its ability to

match the therapeutic benefit of an open RPLND. Multiple reviews published in the last decade have addressed the role of L-RPLND (Table 37.2).

Several series have demonstrated that L-RPLND is associated with less perioperative morbidity. While operative times are typically longer with L-RPLND, studies by Poulakis et al. and Abdel-Aziz et al. reported that L-RPLND resulted in significantly less blood loss and shorter length of hospital stay [6,7]. Poulakis et al. also reported that patients who underwent L-RPLND had significantly less narcotic requirement, shorter time to oral intake and faster return to normal activity when compared to nonrandomized historical controls. In addition, open RPLND was associated with significantly higher rates of early and late postoperative complications. Open conversion was required in 2.7–6.9% of cases, primarily for intraoperative bleeding.

In order to provide comparable therapeutic benefit, L-RPLND should produce similar lymph node yields in comparison to the open technique. This comparison is difficult to assess, however, since many of the studies in the current literature did not perform L-RPLND as a completely therapeutic intervention. While one study noted that L-RPLND "is used for diagnostic purposes only," another reported that L-RPLND was not completed if grossly positive nodes were encountered during dissection [8,9]. The same study noted that lymph node yield was higher for patients with negative nodes (25 ± 3) compared to patients found to have positive nodes (14 ± 2). Another study that employed a similar template for both L-RPLND and open RPLND reported a significantly higher lymph node yield in the open group (33 ± 11) compared to the L-RPLND group (17 ± 10) [7]. Poulakis et al. reported no significant difference in the lymph node yield between open RPLND (11, range 6–15) and L-RPLND (10, range 7–16), but the lymph node yields reported in this study were considerably lower than other current series so no conclusion can be made based on these data [6].

In order to accurately compare the therapeutic efficacy of open and laparoscopic techniques, series would have to employ similar templates. Even when similar templates were employed, L-RPLND did not uniformly involve dissection of lymph nodes behind the great vessels [7]. The decision to forego dissection behind the great vessels during L-RPLND is based on a study by Holtl et al., which documented the lack of isolated retro-aortic or retro-caval lymph nodes [10]. While this study demonstrates that patients will likely be properly staged based on a laparoscopic dissection that does not include lymph nodes behind the great vessels, the authors make the supposition that all pathological stage II patients will receive adjuvant chemotherapy that will theoretically treat any residual retro-aortic or retrocaval GCT.

The therapeutic benefit of L-RPLND is also difficult to assess since the overwhelming majority of pathological

Table 37.2 Role of laparoscopic RPLND

Authors	Methods	Intervention	Participants	Outcomes	Results	Notes
Bhayani et al. [9]	retrospective review mean FU 72 months	L-RPLND	29 patients with clinical stage I NSGCT	operative + pathological parameters	• 2/29 (6.9%) required open conversion • mean OR time = 258 min (157-380) • mean EBL = 389 mL (75-3000) • mean node yield = 20 nodes (7-53) • mean node yield higher for negative nodes (25 ± 3) compared to positive nodes (14 ± 2) • 17/29 (59%) negative nodes → observation until failure (2 recurrences: chest at 3 months, serum markers at 5 months) • 12/29 (41%) positive nodes → chemotherapy (n = 10) or observation (n = 2) (1 observation patient salvaged with chemotherapy at 13 months for elevated serum markers) • complications: 2 hemorrhage, 1 retrograde ejaculation	• RPLND not completed if grossly positive nodes encountered • retro-aortic + retrocaval nodes not routinely removed • long-term FU • included pathological stage II patients who were initially observed after RPLND
LeBlanc et al. [11]	prospective study median FU 15 months	L-RPLND using extraperitoneal approach	20 patients with clinical stage I NSGCT+ 5 patients with clinical stage IIA NSGCT	operative + pathological parameters	• no patient required open conversion • mean OR time = 230 min (180-300) • EBL <50 mL for all cases • mean LOS = 1.2 days (1-3) • mean node yield = 9.8 (right) + 17.7 (left) • 10/25 (40%) positive nodes → chemotherapy • no recurrence	• 4/5 patients with clinical stage IIA had positive nodes • retro-aortic + retrocaval nodes not routinely removed

(Continued on p. 362)

Table 37.2 (Continued)

Authors	Methods	Intervention	Participants	Outcomes	Results	Notes
Janetschek et al. [8]	prospective study mean FU 43 months	lap RPLND	73 patients with clinical stage I NSGCT	operative + pathologic parameters	• 2/73 (2.7%) required open conversion • mean OR time = 297 min (150-630) • mean EBL = 156 mL (10-350) • mean LOS = 3.3 days (2-5) • 19/73 (26%) positive nodes → chemotherapy • 1 contralateral recurrence in pathological stage I group	• retro-aortic + retrocaval nodes dissected only in early cases • no mention of node yield
Poulakis et al. [6]	retrospective review mean lap FU 4 months mean open FU 26 months	L-RPLND (21) or open RPLND (29)	50 patients with clinical stage I NSGCT	operative + QOL parameters	• no lap case required open conversion • *mean OR time = 233 min (lap) vs. 203 min (open) • *mean EBL = 270 mL (lap) vs. 422 mL (open) • mean LOS = 2 days (lap) vs. 7 days (open) • sig more early + late complications in open group • lap group had sig less narcotic requirement, shorter time to oral intake + faster return to normal activity • no sig difference between mean node yield for lap (10, 7-16) vs. open (11, 6-15) • positive nodes in 4/21 (19%) lap + 7/29 (24%) open → chemotherapy (all NED at last FU)	• direct comparison with open RPLND
Nielsen et al. [13]	retrospective review mean FU 36 months	L-RPLND	120 patients with clinical stage I NSGCT	operative + pathological parameters	• 74/120 (62%) negative nodes → observation (7 recurrences → 1 elevated serum markers + 6 outside conventional RPLND template) • 46/120 (38%) positive nodes → 36 chemotherapy + 10 observation (2 recurrences in observation group → 1 elevated serum markers + 1 chest) • median node yield = 20	• included excision of retro-aortic + retrocaval nodes • included pathological stage II patients who were initially observed after RPLND

Reference	Study type / follow-up	Intervention	Patients	Parameters	Results	Comments
Abdel-Aziz et al. [7]	retrospective review; mean lap FU 12 months; mean open FU 15 months	L-RPLND (22) or open RPLND (6)	28 patients with clinical stage I NSGCT	operative + pathological parameters	• mean OR time = 313 min (lap) vs. 284 min (open) • *mean EBL = 159 mL (lap) vs. 254 mL (open) • *mean LOS = 1.2 days (lap) vs. 8.5 days (open) • node yield sig higher in open (33 ± 11) vs. lap (17 ± 10)	• similar modified template for lap + open • open group with sig more pT2 patients • included pathological stage II patients who were initially observed after RPLND
Holtl et al. [10]	retrospective review; mean FU 55 months	group 1 (29): clinical stage I, L-RPLND with retroaortic/retrocaval dissection; group 2 (64): clinical stage II, chemotherapy; group 3 (46): clinical stage I, L-RPLND without retroaortic/retrocaval dissection	75 patients with stage I NSGCT + 64 patients with stage II NSGCT	distribution of nodal metastases	• positive nodes in 7/22 (32%) lap + 0/6 open → 5 chemotherapy + 2 observation (all NED at last FU) • group 1: 10/29 (34%) positive nodes exclusively ventral to great vessels → chemotherapy • group 2: no patient with enlarged node(s) only dorsal to great vessels • group 3: 6/46 (13%) positive nodes → chemotherapy	• basis for excluding retro-aortic + retrocaval dissection • assumes that all patients upstaged from stage I to stage II will receive chemotherapy
Neyer et al. [12]	retrospective review; median FU 72 months	L-RPLND	136 patients with clinical stage I NSGCT	operative + pathologic parameters	• 7/136 (5%) required open conversion • mean OR time = 261 min (115-570) • median EBL = 50 mL (20-3000) • mean LOS = 4.1 days • 25/136 (18.4%) positive nodes → 2 cycles of adjuvant chemotherapy (NED at last FU) • 111/136 (81.6%) negative nodes → observation (8 relapsed → 6 chest + 1 elevated serum markers + 1 contralateral retroperitoneum)	

stage II patients in the L-RPLND studies receive adjuvant chemotherapy [6,8,10-12]. Despite this pervasive treatment algorithm, several studies have included patients with pathological stage II who have undergone surveillance. Studies by Bhayani et al., Nielson et al. and Abdel-Aziz et al. included a total of 14 patients with nodal involvement who were initially observed after L-RPLND [7,9,13]. With a mean follow-up ranging from 12 months to 72 months, two patients experienced relapse with serum tumor markers and one patient recurred in his chest. No retroperitoneal recurrences were noted.

Comment

The contemporary literature demonstrates that L-RPLND is a well-tolerated procedure with less perioperative morbidity than open RPLND when the procedure is performed by skilled laparoscopic surgeons. Despite this benefit, the literature has not demonstrated that the therapeutic efficacy of L-RPLND currently matches that of open RPLND. Ultimately, a randomized study of laparoscopic versus open RPLND utilizing similar templates is needed to definitively compare the two techniques. Until this study is complete, only a weak recommendation (Grade 2C) can be made to utilize an open technique for patients undergoing RPLND. In the meantime, more evidence regarding the efficacy of L-RPLND will come from patients with pathological stage II NSGCT who elect to undergo observation after RPLND.

Clinical question 37.3

What is the best management of the normal retroperitoneum following platinum-based chemotherapy?

Literature search

A Medline and PubMed search was conducted using the previously described methods. Search terms included "testicular neoplasm," "germ cell tumor," "postchemotherapy RPLND" and "induction chemotherapy."

The evidence

Patients with bulky retroperitoneal lymphadenopathy greater than 2 cm are customarily treated with induction chemotherapy as first-line therapy. Persistent elevation of serum markers is evidence of residual GCT and these patients are candidates for salvage chemotherapy. Patients who achieve serological remission after chemotherapy may or may not have residual retroperitoneal masses. Significant controversy surrounds the optimal management of patients with complete serological and radiographic remission after induction chemotherapy. Several retrospective studies have specifically examined patients with normal serum markers and imaging after chemotherapy or included these patients in their post-chemotherapy RPLND (PC-RPLND) analysis (Table 37.3).

A study of 101 patients by Fossa et al. reported that 51% had necrosis and fibrosis in PC-RPLND specimens, while 37% had mature teratoma and 12% had residual viable GCT [14]. Using univariate analysis, the authors found that lack of teratoma in the primary tumor, normal preoperative markers, complete response on imaging and smaller initial retroperitoneal masses were significant predictors of necrosis. If a patient had no teratoma in their primary tumor, normal preoperative markers and complete radiographic response to chemotherapy, then necrosis was correctly predicted in 79% of cases. A similar study by Oldenburg et al. reported that 7% of patients with residual retroperitoneal masses ≤ 20 mm had viable GCT and 26% had teratoma on PC-RPLND [15]. All patients with viable GCT had normal preoperative markers and 83% had residual masses ≤ 10 mm, which is considered within the normal range for a lymph node. Both studies demonstrate that viable GCT can be found on PC-RPLND despite favorable preoperative characteristics and a "normal" retroperitoneum on CT imaging.

A larger study by Debono et al. included 78 patients who were observed after they experienced complete serological and radiographic remission after induction chemotherapy [16]. These patients had a 6% recurrence rate with a median follow-up of 61 months. Despite salvage therapy, 80% of relapsed patients died of their disease.

Comment

The current literature does not support an absolute standard of care for patients with a normal retroperitoneum and complete serological remission after induction chemotherapy. In this regard, no definitive treatment recommendation can be made based on the available studies. While the majority of these patients will only have necrosis or fibrosis at the time of PC-RPLND, even patients with favorable preoperative characteristics can have residual viable GCT or teratoma in their retroperitoneum and will benefit from PC-RPLND. Such uncertainty stresses the need for lifelong follow-up for patients who elect observation.

Clinical question 37.4

What is the best management of the stage IS patient?

Table 37.3 Management of the normal retroperitoneum following platinum Based Chemotherapy

Authors	Methods	Intervention	Participants	Outcomes	Results	Notes
Fossa et al. [14]	retrospective review	induction chemotherapy followed by PC-RPLND	101 patients with stage ≥IIB NSGCT	histology of residual retroperitoneal mass	• histology: 51% necrosis/fibrosis + 37% mature teratoma + 12% viable GCT • univariate predictors of necrosis/fibrosis: no teratoma in primary tumor, normal preop markers, complete response on CT, smaller initial burden of RP disease • no teratoma + complete response + normal preop markers → necrosis/fibrosis correctly predicted in 79%	
Oldenburg et al. [15]	retrospective review	induction chemotherapy followed by PC-PRLND	87 patients with stage ≥II NSGCT and residual retroperitoneal masses 20 mm	histology of residual retroperitoneal mass	• histology: 67% necrosis/fibrosis + 26% teratoma + 7% viable GCT • no associated between RP histology and primary histology, initial size of RP mass and preop markers • 5/6 (83%) patients with viable GCT had masses ≤10 mm + 6/6 (100%) had normal preop markers	• single radiologist and pathologist
Debono et al. [16]	retrospective review median FU 61 months	induction chemotherapy → observation in cases of complete serologicak + radiographic remission	78 patients with stage ≥II NSGCT	recurrence	• 5/78 (6%) recurrence rate • recurrence: RP GCT (2), second testicular primary (1), bone/RP sarcoma (1), CNS • GCT (1) • 4/5 (80%) relapsed patients DOD	

Literature search

A Medline and PubMed search was conducted using the previously described methods. Search terms included "testicular neoplasm," "germ cell tumor," "stage IS," "tumor markers" and "elevated serum markers."

The evidence

Clinical stage IS NSGCT is defined by persistently elevated serum markers after orchiectomy with no radiographic evidence of metastatic disease or nodal involvement. Historically, these patients were treated with RPLND in the belief that the persistently elevated serum markers were indicative of occult disease in the retroperitoneum. Several small retrospective reviews provide evidence supporting the trend away from primary RPLND for clinical stage IS patients (Table 37.4).

A study by Saxman et al. included 30 patients with clinical stage IS NSGCT who were treated with primary RPLND [17]. With a median follow-up of 36 months, 24% of patients with no detected nodal involvement at the time of RPLND required chemotherapy for later disease progression. A significant limitation of the study is the omission of post-RPLND serum markers, which would allow detection of patients who experienced serological remission after surgery. In contrast to this surgical series, a study by Culine et al. included 20 patients with clinical stage IS NSGCT treated with induction chemotherapy [18]. All patients had normalization of serum markers after chemo-therapy. Although no direct comparison can be made to the Saxman et al. study, only 15% of patients treated with induction chemotherapy required later salvage therapy for radiographic recurrence.

Two nonrandomized studies compared patients with clinical stage IS NSGCT who were treated with either induction chemotherapy or primary RPLND. Davis et al. noted that 100% of patients treated with primary RPLND required chemotherapy for retroperitoneal recurrence or persistent elevation of serum markers, while only 25% of patients treated with induction chemotherapy required delayed RPLND for radiographic recurrence [19]. Similarly, Dash et al. reported that 100% of patients who did not receive adjuvant chemotherapy after RPLND required salvage chemotherapy for later recurrence [20]. In the group that received induction chemotherapy, all patients achieved serological remission. A total of seven patients (41%) underwent RPLND, three electively and four for radiographic recurrence. Of patients undergoing RPLND, five were found to have teratoma and one patient had viable GCT, further supporting the conclusion that absence of radiographic abnormality following chemotherapy does not guarantee an absence of retroperitoneal disease.

Comment

Although the literature lacks robust studies comparing RPLND and chemotherapy, the available evidence supports a conditional recommendation (**Grade 2C**) to avoid primary RPLND and to utilize induction chemotherapy for clinical stage IS patients. Persistently elevated serum markers after orchiectomy in a patient with a normal retroperitoneum are indicative of systemic disease and patients should be treated accordingly.

Clinical question 37.5

What is the best management of the high-risk stage I patient?

Literature search

A Medline and PubMed search was conducted using the previously described methods. Search terms included "testicular neoplasm," "germ cell tumor," "stage I," "embryonal carcinoma," "lymphovascular invasion" and "high risk."

The evidence

The goal of risk stratification of stage I NSGCT patients is to identify high-risk patients who will likely benefit from adjuvant therapy and low-risk patients who can avoid the associated toxicity of additional treatment. The presence of lymphovascular invasion (LVI) and a predominance of embryonal histology are the factors most commonly used to identify high-risk patients. Other high-risk factors include stage $\geq$ T2, the presence of malignant teratoma or undifferentiated histology in the primary tumor or the absence of yolk sac elements. While the literature provides guidelines to aid in identifying high-risk patients, the optimal treatment of these patients is still a question of significant debate (Table 37.5).

Several retrospective studies from North America have examined the role of RPLND in the treatment of high-risk clinical stage I patients [21-23]. Two studies included one treatment arm and demonstrated that predominance of embryonal histology and presence of LVI were associated with higher rates of upstaging to pathological stage II disease [22,23]. Although these studies also demonstrated good control of the retroperitoneum, no comparison was made to similar patients who underwent active surveillance or chemotherapy. A study by Al-Tourah et al. included high-risk patients who underwent either RPLND or surveillance and reported no significant difference in chemotherapy-free survival between the two groups [21]. Despite the inclusion of two treatment arms, no statistical comparison of high-risk features was included and the study was not randomized.

Table 37.4 Management of stage IS NSGCT

Authors	Methods	Intervention	Participants	Outcomes	Results	Notes
Davis et al. [19]	retrospective review mean FU 81 months	group 1 (11): primary RPLND group 2 (4): induction chemotherapy	• 15 patients with clinical stage IS NSGCT	recurrence	• group 1: 11/11 (100%) required chemotherapy for RP disease or persistent serum marker elevation • group 2: 1/4 (25%) required post-chemotherapy RPLND for recurrence	• excluded patients given adjuvant chemotherapy after RPLND • no clarification of which patients experienced serum marker normalization after RPLND
Saxman et al. [17]	retrospective review median FU 36 months	RPLND	• 30 patients with clinical stage IS NSGCT	recurrence	• 9/30 (30%) positive nodes • 5/21 (24%) patients with negative nodes required chemotherapy for later disease progression	
Culine et al. [18]	retrospective review FU range 14-112 months	induction chemotherapy	• 20 patients with clinical stage IS NSGCT	recurrence	• 100% patients achieved normal serum markers after chemotherapy • 3/20 (15%) recurrence (8-9 months post-chemotherapy)	• equal distribution of recurrences amongst chemotherapy regimens
Dash et al. [20]	retrospective review median FU 35 months	group 1 (7): primary RPLND group 2 (17): induction chemotherapy	• 24 patients with clinical stage IS NSGCT	recurrence	• group 1: 6/7 (86%) positive nodes, 3 patients received chemotherapy → NED at last FU, 4 patients observed → all required chemotherapy for recurrence • group 2: all patients had normal markers post-chemotherapy, 3 patients underwent elective PC-RPLND + 14 patients observed → 4 patients required later PC-RPLND for recurrence • PC-RPLND histology: 1 fibrosis, 5 teratoma, 1 viable GCT	

Table 37.5 Management of high-risk stage I NSGCT1

Authors	Methods	Intervention	Participants	Outcomes	Results	Notes
Albers et al. [29]	RCT	RPLND (191) or 1 cycle BEP (191)	382 patients with clinical stage I NSGCT	recurrence	• significant difference between relapse rate of 1% in BEP group vs 8% in RPLND group (p = 0.001)	• intention to treat analysis (17 lost from BEP + 18 lost from RPLND)
	median FU 56 months				• 2 year DFS 99.5% for BEP vs. 91.9% for RPLND	• powered to detect 7% reduction in recurrence with BEP vs RPLND
					• HR for recurrence with RPLND vs BEP = 7.937 (95% CI 1.8–34.4)	• largest RCT for adjuvant therapy in clinical stage I NSGCT
						• no comparison of embryonal component or LVI, not necessarily high-risk patients
						• all patients with nodal metastases treated with 2 cycles of adjuvant BEP
Stephenson et al [23]	retrospective review	RPLND	267 patients with clinical stage I-IIA NSGCT + embryonal predominance or LVI	pathological staging, recurrence	• 112/267 (42%) pathological stage II → 54% with low volume N1 disease, 50% received adjuvant chemotherapy	• no comparison to surveillance or chemotherapy
	median FU 53 months				• patients with both embryonal predominance + LVI had higher rate of pathological stage II disease compared to patients with either embryonal predominance or LVI (54% vs 37%, p = 0.009)	• no comparison to low-risk clinical stage I patients
					• estimated 52% of clinical stage I patients overtreated with RPLND (no recurrence in 5 years)	
Sweeney et al. [22]	retrospective review	RPLND	292 patients with clinical stage I NSGCT → 125/292 (43%) embryonal predominance	pathological staging, recurrence	• 66/292 (22%) pathological stage II → 32% embryonal predominant vs. 16% nonembryonal predominant (p = 0.002), 36% LVI vs 15% non-LVI (p<0.0001)	• "embryonal predominant" = >50% embryonal histology
	median FU 46 months				• recurrence rate significantly higher for embryonal predominant pathological stage I (21%) compared to nonembryonal predominant (3%, p<0.0001)	• "embryonal predominant" = most common histology
					• recurrence rate significantly higher for LVI pathological stage I (20%) compared to non-LVI (7%, p<0.001)	• good control of RP
					• 1/292 relapsed in retroperitoneum (embryonal predominant pathological stage I)	

Study	Study type / median FU	Intervention	Patient population	Outcome	Results	Comments
Al-Tourah et al. [21]	retrospective review; median FU 48 months	surveillance (72) or RPLND (32)	104 patients with embryonal predominant clinical stage I NSGCT → 46/104 (46%) LVI	pathological staging, recurrence	• surveillance: 24/72 (33%) recurrence → 10 biochemical recurrence + 10 RP mass + 4 chest metastasis (all salvaged with chemotherapy ± RPLND, 1 dead of stroke) • RPLND: 14/32 (44%) pathological stage II, no RP relapse for pathological stage I or II • no sig difference in 4 year chemotherapy-free survival between surveillance and RPLND groups	• "embryonal predominant" = ≥50% embryonal histology • initial therapy determined by patient • 13% recurrence rate during surveillance for nonembryonal predominant patients
Oliver et al. [26]	retrospective review; median FU 84 months	surveillance (234) or adjuvant chemotherapy with 1-2 cycles BEP (148) for high risk patients (i.e. LVI, malignant teratoma, absence of yolk sac elements, undifferentiated histology)	234 patients with clinical stage I NSGCT	recurrence	• surveillance group after 1986: 27% recurrence • adjuvant chemotherapy: 4% recurrence	• patients enrolled between 1978-2000, adjuvant chemotherapy not offered until 1986 • no indication of how patients relapsed
Bohlen et al. [24]	prospective study; median FU 93 months	adjuvant chemotherapy (2 cycles PVB before 6/87 → 2 cycles BEP after 6/87)	59 patients with clinical stage I NSGCT and ≥1 risk factors (embryonal histology, LVI, stage >T1)	recurrence, toxicity	• 2/59 (3%) completed only 1 cycle of chemotherapy due to toxicity (1 paralytic ileus, 1 suspected cardiotoxicity) • WHO grade 4 toxicity observed in 9/59 (15%) patients • most common toxicities included myelosuppression, nausea/vomiting and alopecia • 2/59 (3%) recurrence (1 ipsilateral pelvis, 1 metachronous second testicular primary)	• no quantification of embryonal component
Pont et al. [25]	prospective study; median FU 79 months	surveillance (42) or adjuvant chemotherapy with 2 cycles BEP (42) for patients with LVI	84 patients with clinical stage I NSGCT ± LVI	recurrence, toxicity	• adjuvant chemotherapy: 2/29 (7%) recurrence among patients with >2 years FU (1 retroperitoneum + 1 iliac fossa, no recurrence in patients with <2 years FU) • short-term toxicity of BEP: no WHO grade 4 toxicity, most common WHO grade 3 toxicity included transient neutropenia + alopecia • no patient developed ischemic heart disease, cerebrovascular disease or Raynaud's syndrome	• age-matched controls used from surveillance group to perform matched-pair analysis for toxicity • no long-term comparison of recurrence rates between adjuvant chemotherapy + surveillance groups

(Continued on p. 370)

Table 37.5 (Continued)

Authors	Methods	Intervention	Participants	Outcomes	Results	Notes
Cullen et al. [27]	prospective study	2 cycles BEP	114 patients with clinical stage I NSGCT and ≥3 high risk features (LVI, undifferentiated histology, absence of yolk sac elements)	recurrence, toxicity	• no long-term pulmonary sequelae, high-tone hearing loss or hematological malignancies in BEP group • 3/114 (3%) recurrence (1 RP/chest/liver, 1 metachronous second testicular primary, 1 groin)	• 1 patient with groin relapse not confirmed to have NSGCT upon final pathologic review
	median FU 48 months				• short-term toxicity of BEP: 4% WHO grade 3 leukopenia, 27% WHO grade 3 emesis, 11% peripheral neuropathy, 8% tinnitus • 1/114 died of cerebrovascular accident during second cycle	
Maroto et al. [28]	prospective study	surveillance (358) or adjuvant chemotherapy with 1-2 cycles BEP (231) for patients with ≥1 high risk features (embryonal histology, LVI, stage >T2)	589 patients with clinical stage I NSGCT	recurrence, toxicity	• recurrence rates: 17% non-LVI on surveillance, 55% +LVI on surveillance, 1.3% +LVI with adjuvant chemotherapy (majority of relapses limited to RP)	• 22 patients with LVI chose surveillance over chemotherapy → highest recurrence + lowest DFS
	median FU 40 months				• embryonal predominance and LVI were sig predictors of recurrence in multivariate model • most common toxicity included transient neutropenia and nausea/vomiting	
Westermann et al. [29]	prospective study	1 cycle BEP	40 patients with clinical stage I NSGCT with embryonal predominance and/or LVI	recurrence, toxicity	• 5/40 (13%) recurrence (1 chest recurrence, 2 metachronous second testicular primary, 2 unknown recurrence pattern)	• "embryonal predominant" = >50% embryonal histology
	median FU 96 months				• long-term toxicity minimal → 1 patient with NCI grade 2 peripheral neuropathy after salvage chemotherapy, 2 patients with intermittent tinnitus after 1 cycle of BEP (no cardiotoxicity)	• central pathology review

The role of adjuvant chemotherapy for high-risk patients is largely addressed by European studies. Studies using one or two cycles of platinum-based chemotherapy for high-risk patients reported favorable relapse rates of ≤ 7% [24-27]. The recurrence rates, which are comparable if not better than RPLND, are tempered by the potentially significant long-term toxicity documented in patients receiving platinum-based chemotherapy. In an effort to limit cumulative chemotherapy exposure, a recent study by Westermann et al. treated 40 high-risk patients with one cycle of BEP [29]. The recurrence rate of 13% was higher than recurrence rates when patients predominantly received two cycles of platinum-based chemotherapy, but long-term toxicity was minimal with a median follow-up of 96 months.

A recent randomized clinical trial by Albers et al. is a valuable addition to the literature [30]. Although the study was not limited to high-risk clinical stage I patients, the design allowed direct comparison of RPLND and one cycle of BEP. The authors reported a significant decrease in the recurrence rates after patients received one cycle of BEP compared to RPLND.

Comment

Surveillance is not appropriate for patients with clinical stage I NSGCT and high-risk features. However, evidence regarding the optimal treatment of these patients is not definitive despite the completion of a randomized clinical trial and no treatment recommendation can be made based on the available studies. The perioperative morbidity of RPLND is balanced by more accurate staging, control of the retroperitoneum and potential avoidance of chemotherapy and its associated toxicity. Adjuvant chemotherapy offers the advantage of providing systemic treatment with fewer cycles than salvage chemotherapy. The recent studies using one cycle of BEP reported favorable recurrence rates and the randomized trial by Albers et al. demonstrated clinical superiority of one cycle of BEP in direct comparison to RPLND. Adjuvant chemotherapy is certainly advisable in centers that lack the expertise to perform a diagnostic and potentially therapeutic RPLND.

References

1. Sayegh E, Brooks T, Sacher E, et al. Lymphangiography of the retroperitoneal lumph nodes through the inguinal route. J Urol 1966;95:102-7.
2. Capelouto CC, Clark PE, Ransil BJ, et al. A review of scrotal violation in testicular cancer: is adjuvant local therapy necessary? J Urol 1995;153:981-5.
3. Giguere JK, Stablein DM, Spaulding JT, et al. The clinical significance of unconventional orchiectomy approaches in testicular cancer: a report from the Testicular Cancer Intergroup Study. J Urol 1988;139:1225-8.
4. Leibovitch I, Baniel J, Foster RS, et al. The clinical implications of procedural deviations during orchiectomy for nonseminomatous testis cancer. J Urol 1995;154:935-9.
5. Aki FT, Bilen CY, Tekin MI, et al. Is scrotal violation per se a risk factor for local relapse and metastases in stage I nonseminomatous testicular cancer? Urology 2000;56:459-62.
6. Poulakis V, Skriapas K, de Vries R, et al. Quality of life after laparoscopic and open retroperitoneal lymph node dissection in clinical Stage I nonseminomatous germ cell tumor: a comparison study. Urology 2006;68:154-60.
7. Abdel-Aziz KF, Anderson JK, Svatek R, et al. Laparoscopic and open retroperitoneal lymph-node dissection for clinical stage I nonseminomatous germ-cell testis tumors. J Endourol 200620:627-31.
8. Janetschek G, Hobisch A, Peschel R, et al. Laparoscopic retroperitoneal lymph node dissection for clinical stage I nonseminomatous testicular carcinoma: long-term outcome. J Urol 2000;163:1793-6.
9. Bhayani SB, Allaf ME, Kavoussi LR. Laparoscopic RPLND for clinical stage I nonseminomatous germ cell testicular cancer: current status. Urol Oncol 2004;22:145-8.
10. Holtl L, Peschel R, Knapp R, et al. Primary lymphatic metastatic spread in testicular cancer occurs ventral to the lumbar vessels. Urology 2002;59:114-18.
11. LeBlanc E, Caty A, Dargent D, et al. Extraperitoneal laparoscopic para-aortic lymph node dissection for early stage nonseminomatous germ cell tumors of the testis with introduction of a nerve sparing technique: description and results. J Urol 2001;165:89-92.
12. Neyer M, Peschel R, Akkad T, et al. Long-term results of laparoscopic retroperitoneal lymph-node dissection for clinical stage I nonseminomatous germ-cell testicular cancer. J Endourol 2007;21:180-3.
13. Nielsen ME, Lima G, Schaeffer EM, et al. Oncologic efficacy of laparoscopic RPLND in treatment of clinical stage I nonseminomatous germ cell testicular cancer. Urology 2007;70:1168-72.
14. Fossa SD, Ous S, Lien HH, et al. Post-chemotherapy lymph node histology in radiologically normal patients with metastatic nonseminomatous testicular cancer. J Urol 1989;141:557-9.
15. Oldenburg J, Alfsen GC, Lien HH, et al. Postchemotherapy retroperitoneal surgery remains necessary in patients with nonseminomatous testicular cancer and minimal residual tumor masses. J Clin Oncol 2003;21:3310-17.
16. Debono DJ, Heilman DK, Einhorn LH, et al. Decision analysis for avoiding postchemotherapy surgery in patients with disseminated nonseminomatous germ cell tumors. J Clin Oncol 1997;15:1455-64.
17. Saxman SB, Nichols CR, Foster RS, et al. The management of patients with clinical stage I nonseminomatous testicular tumors and persistently elevated serologic markers. J Urol 1996;155:587-9.
18. Culine S, Theodore C, Terrier-Lacombe MJ, et al. Primary chemotherapy in patients with nonseminomatous germ cell tumors of the testis and biological disease only after orchiectomy. J Urol 1996;155:1296-18.
19. Davis BE, Herr HW, Fair WR, et al. The management of patients with nonseminomatous germ cell tumors of the testis with

serologic disease only after orchiectomy. J Urol 1994;152:111-13; discussion 114.

20. Dash A, Carver BS, Stasi J, et al. The indication for postchemotherapy lymph node dissection in clinical stage IS nonseminomatous germ cell tumor. Cancer 2008;112:800-5.

21. Al-Tourah AJ, Murray N, Coppin C, et al. Minimizing treatment without compromising cure with primary surveillance for clinical stage I embryonal predominant nonseminomatous testicular cancer: a population based analysis from British Columbia. J Urol 2005;174:2209-13, discussion 2213.

22. Sweeney CJ, Hermans BP, Heilman DK, et al. Results and outcome of retroperitoneal lymph node dissection for clinical stage I embryonal carcinoma-predominant testis cancer. J Clin Oncol 2000;18:358-62.

23. Stephenson AJ, Bosl GJ, Bajorin DF, et al. Retroperitoneal lymph node dissection in patients with low stage testicular cancer with embryonal carcinoma predominance and/or lymphovascular invasion. J Urol 2005;174:557-60; discussion 560.

24. Bohlen D, Borner M, Sonntag RW, et al. Long-term results following adjuvant chemotherapy in patients with clinical stage I testicular nonseminomatous malignant germ cell tumors with high risk factors. J Urol 1999;161:1148-52.

25. Pont J, Albrecht W, Postner G, et al. Adjuvant chemotherapy for high-risk clinical stage I nonseminomatous testicular germ cell cancer: long-term results of a prospective trial. J Clin Oncol 1996;14:441-8.

26. Oliver RT, Ong J, Shamash J, et al. Long-term follow-up of Anglian Germ Cell Cancer Group surveillance versus patients with Stage 1 nonseminoma treated with adjuvant chemotherapy. Urology 2004;63:556-61.

27. Cullen MH, Stenning SP, Parkinson MC, et al. Short-course adjuvant chemotherapy in high-risk stage I nonseminomatous germ cell tumors of the testis: a Medical Research Council report. J Clin Oncol 1996;14:1106-13.

28. Maroto P, Garcia del Muro X, Aparicio J, et al. Multicentre risk-adapted management for stage I nonseminomatous germ cell tumours. Ann Oncol 2005;16:1915-20.

29. Westermann DH, Schefer H, Thalmann GN, et al. Long-term followup results of 1 cycle of adjuvant bleomycin, etoposide and cisplatin chemotherapy for high risk clinical stage I nonseminomatous germ cell tumors of the testis. J Urol 2008;179:163-6.

30. Albers P, Siener R, Krege S, et al. Randomized phase III trial comparing retroperitoneal lymph node dissection with one course of bleomycin and etoposide plus cisplatin chemotherapy in the adjuvant treatment of clinical stage I Nonseminomatous testicular germ cell tumors: AUO trial AH 01/94 by the German Testicular Cancer Study Group. J Clin Oncol 2008;26:2966-72.

38 Pediatric urinary tract infections

Regina D. Norris[1] and John S. Wiener[2]
[1]University of Pittsburgh Medical Center, Children's Hosptial of Pittsburgh, Pittsburgh, PA, USA
[2]Departments of Surgery and Pediatrics, Duke Univesity Medical Center, Durham, NC, USA

Clinical question 38.1

How does one reliably diagnose a urinary tract infection in an infant or child?

Background

Urinary tract infection (UTI) is normally defined as the presence of microbial organisms in the urine. UTI afflicts approximately 4–6% of children who present to the emergency department for evaluation of fever. The signs and symptoms of UTI in the pediatric population are often nonspecific, particularly in the nonverbal and nontoilet trained; thus, the diagnosis is often difficult and requires a heightened level of suspicion on the part of the clinician. Diagnosis of a UTI first begins with a proper collection of urine specimen to minimize false-negative and false-positive findings on quantitative culture. The method of collection has a major impact on the result.

Literature search

A literature search was performed using the US National Library of Medicine and the National Institutes of Health PubMed database. The search terms with imposed limits were as follows: urinary tract infection AND diagnose NOT reflux NOT neurogenic NOT abscess NOT imaging NOT ultrasound Limits: Entrez Date from 1920/01/01 to 2008/07/31, Humans, English, All Child: 0–18 years. This search yielded a total of 42 articles which were reviewed to determine their relevance to our clinical question.

Evidence-Based Urology. Edited by Philipp Dahm, Roger R. Dmochowski.
© 2010 Blackwell Publishing.

The evidence

Several urine collection methods with varying diagnostic thresholds are available: an absorbent pad, sterile perineal bag, clean-catch mid-stream void, urethral catheterization, and suprapubic bladder aspiration. Both absorbent pad and perineal bag urine collection are used in the nontoilet trained and have a high parental acceptance rate, but these techniques are hampered by high susceptibility to contamination. In these instances, a negative culture excludes infection, but a positive culture is not necessarily diagnostic of UTI. Clean-catch mid-stream void collection is difficult in the infant or nontoilet-trained child as voiding habits are unpredictable, making for a time-consuming method. Even in toilet-trained children, the reliability of getting a true mid-stream specimen with proper wiping of the meatus and retraction of the labia/prepuce is uncertain. Urethral catheterization is considered to be a reliable method of collection but carries the risk of introducing urethral organisms into the sterile bladder and is often psychologically traumatic to child and parents. Suprapubic bladder aspiration is considered the gold standard as it bypasses routes of possible contamination common to the other modalities. However, the invasive nature of suprapubic bladder aspiration is often a source of angst for the parents, patient and, in some cases, the clinician. The success rate of obtaining a urine specimen via suprapubic bladder aspiration ranges from 23% to 90% [1-4]. The American Academy of Pediatrics currently recommends two options for the diagnosis of UTI in infants and young children (2 months to 2 years) with unexplained fever [5]. The first option is suprapubic bladder aspiration or urethral catheterization. The second option is to obtain a urine specimen by the most convenient means and perform a urinalysis; if the urinalysis suggests a UTI, then a culture specimen should be obtained via suprapubic bladder aspiration or urethral catheterization.

A number of papers have studied the method of urine collection in infants and children for the diagnosis of UTI; however, of these studies, only 13 were considered clinically relevant to the scope of this chapter (Table 38.1). These studies differ greatly in their design, with collection methods and the age of the cohort being the most variable. Upon examining the data from Pryles et al. [1], suprapubic aspiration approaches 100% specificity for excluding urinary tract infection. In this series, suprapubic aspiration was safe with complications of gross hematuria lasting less than 24 hours in 4/654 and bladder wall hematoma in 1/654, yielding a morbidity rate of 0.6%. Rare cases of bowel perforation and suprapubic abscess have been reported. The specificity of urethral catheterization for the exclusion of UTI approaches 100%. Potential complications include hematuria, catheter-induced UTI, and urethral trauma. Given the few reports documented in the literature, the rate of these complications is considered negligible. Ramage et al. [3] demonstrated that the specificity of clean-catch urine specimens can approach 95% for the diagnosis of UTI in infants. Higher contamination rates are seen in uncircumcised males versus girls. The specificity of bag urine specimen cultures range from 14% to 85% as demonstrated by Saccharow & Pryles [2], McGillivray et al. [6], and Falcão et al. [7]. Given that the sensitivity of a bag urine specimen is 100%, a negative specimen excludes the possibility of UTI.

The definition of true infection versus contamination based on bacterial culture colony count remains controversial. The mode of urine collection is the primary factor in defining a significant colony count. The current American Academy of Pediatrics criteria [5] for the diagnosis of UTI in febrile infants and children by urine culture are:

• suprapubic aspiration: the presence of any gram-negative bacilli or more than a few thousand of gram-positive cocci (99% probability of infection)
• urethral catheterization: $> 10^5$ colony count (95% probability of infection)
• clean catch:

male: $> 10^4$ colony-forming units – infection likely

female: 3 specimens $\geq 10^5$ colony count (95% probability)

2 specimens $\geq 10^5$ colony count (90% probability)

1 specimen $\geq 10^5$ colony count (80% probability)

$5 \times 10^4 - 10^5$ colony count – if suspicious, repeat

$10^4 - 5 \times 10^4$ – if symptomatic, repeat: if asymptomatic, infection unlikely

$< 10^4$ – infection unlikely

The clinician must consider other factors before diagnosing a UTI, such as clinical status of the patient, the number of different bacteria species isolated, findings on urinalysis, and the identification of the bacteria isolated.

Comment

We make a strong recommendation that suprapubic bladder aspiration or urethral catheterization be used as the modality of urine collection for the diagnosis of UTI

(Grade 1B). They should be considered in critically ill infants who require immediate antimicrobial therapy. These methods can be undertaken with little morbidity, but lack of clinician experience and parental angst may limit their use. In nontoxic-appearing, nontoilet-trained children, specimens obtained by bag collection or absorbent pad have a high contamination rate and should only be considered reliable when negative. If the urinalysis is positive, then urine should be obtained for culture by catheter or aspiration. Clean-catch specimens in toilet-trained children, particularly girls, are also prone to contamination and, likewise, must be interpreted with caution when positive.

Clinical question 38.2

Are there specific antibiotic duration treatment recommendations for acute urinary tract infections in children?

Background

Short-course antibiotic regimens ranging in duration from a single dose to 3 days are common practice in the treatment of uncomplicated UTI in adult women, but this practice has not been applied to the pediatric population. Concerns about renal scarring and pyelonephritis have prompted standard treatment recommendations from the American Academy of Pediatrics of 7–14 days of antibiotics for UTIs in children, although the optimal duration of treatment remains elusive [5].

Literature earch

A literature search was performed using the US National Library of Medicine and the National Institutes of Health PubMed database. The search terms with imposed limits were as follows: urinary tract infection AND antibiotic AND treatment AND duration NOT reflux NOT neurogenic NOT chronic NOT prophylaxis NOT recurrent NOT abscess NOT bacteruria Limits: Entrez Date from 1920/01/01 to 2008/07/31, Humans, English, All Child: 0–18 years This search yielded a total of 82 articles which were reviewed to determine their relevance to our clinical question. There were 23 articles relevant to our clinical question.

The evidence

A total of 23 studies have examined the duration of antibiotic therapy for the treatment of acute UTI in children, excluding those which studied children with recurrent UTI (Table 38.2). The overwhelming majority of studies

Table 38.1 Analysis of urine collection techniques to diagnose UTIS

Authors	Methods	Intervention	Participants	Outcomes	Results	Notes	Quality of evidence
Liaw [8]	Observational study of urine collection by absorbent pad, bags, and clean catch in nontoilet-trained children without suspected UTI	Urine collection by parents	44 parents of children aged 1–18 months	– Contamination rate – Parental opinion of 3 methods	– Insignificant (<10⁴/mL) or no growth: 70% pads, 66% bags, 75% clean catch – Contamination (>10⁴/mL of one or more organisms): 16% pads, 18% bags, 2% clean catch 8% grew 10⁵/mL, suggesting infection, but excluded by sterile f/u samples collected on the same day	– No child had a suspected UTI – Bags and pads were easy for parental use	Low
Schroeder [9]	Prospective study of predictors for choices for obtaining urine by urethral catheterization or bag	Urine collection in febrile infants	3066 eligible patients, 1384 infants enrolled aged 0–3 months with T >38°C	– Ability to successfully obtain urine by catheterization – Predictors of attempted catheterization	– 70% samples successfully obtained by catheterization – Practitioner age and female sex positive predictors of successful catheterization	Not randomized	Moderate
Farrell [10]	Observational study of urine collection by absorbent pad and bag urine specimens in nontoilet-trained children without confirmed UTI	Urine collection by bag and absorbent pad	20 nontoilet-trained children aged 2–27 months	– Urine WBC – Bacterial growth profile	– Poor agreement in presence or absence of WBC between pad and bag systems, κ statistic 0.2 – Moderate agreement in presence or absence of bacteriuria between pad and bag systems, κ statistic 0.5 – Poor agreement in proportion of bacterial growth between bag and absorbent pad, κ statistic 0.15	– Not randomized – Small sample size	Low
Hardy [11]	Observational study of urine collection in children with suspected UTI (clean catch vs bag vs suprapubic aspiration)	Urine collection by clean catch, bag, and suprapubic aspiration	30 children suspected of having UTI	Pure growth or contamination	– Bag specimens 4/30 pure growth, 22/30 contaminated – Clean catch 2/30 pure growth, 22/30 mixed growth – Suprapubic aspiration 4/30 pure growth, none contaminated	– Small sample size – Inpatients having routine screening	Low
Alam [12]	Observational study of urine collection in children without suspected UTI (clean catch vs bag vs absorbent pad)	Urine collection by clean catch, bag, and absorbent pad (most patients had all three)	191 children <3 years of age without suspected UTI	– Contamination – Inability to collect specimen	– Contamination found in: clean catch 14.7%; absorbent pad 29%; urine bag 26.6% – Specimen not collected by clean catch in 12%, by bag in 4%, and by pad in 4%	Excluded true UTIs	Low

(Continued on p. 376)

Table 38.1 (Continued)

Authors	Methods	Intervention	Outcomes	Participants	Results	Notes	Quality of evidence
McGillivray [6]	Prospective cross-sectional study (paired bag and catheter specimens)	Urine collection by both bag and catheterization in same visit	– Sensitivity and specificity of dipstick and microscopic evaluation – Positive urine culture >10^3 CFU/mL	303 nontoilet-trained children aged <3 years with suspected UTI in ED setting	UTI prevalence 27% – Dipstick sensitivity: 0.85 (bag) vs 0.71 (catheter) (p=0.003) – Dipstick specificity: 0.62 (bag) vs 0.97 (catheter) (p<0.001) – Combined dipstick and microscopic sensitivity: 0.95 (bag) vs 0.83 (catheter) (p=0.003) – Combined dipstick and microscopic specificity: 0.45 (bag) vs 0.95 (catheter) (p<0.001) – For each method, sensitivity rose and specificity fell with an increasing thershold for defining a positive culture	– Selective catheterization strategy would have led to catheterization of 138/255 in the 3–36 month age group – No bag specimens sent for culture – Studied different thresholds of CFU counts in cultures	Moderate
Lau [13]	Observational study of urine collection in children without suspected UTI	Urine collection by clean catch and catheterization	Positive urine culture (>10^3 CFU/mL)	98 infants (82 boys, 16 girls) aged <2 years without suspected UTI	– Boys (all uncircumcised): clean catch: mixed growth 56%, single contaminant 32%. Catheter: mixed growth 29%, single contaminant 37% – Girls: clean catch: no growth 31%. Catheter: no growth: 88%	– Small sample size – Blind catheter passage through the preputial space in males	Moderate
Falcão [7]	Retrospective study of efficacy of urine collection by bag specimen to detect neonatal UTI with suspected UTI	Urine collection by bag specimen. If positive, suprapubic bladder aspiration conducted to confirm the diagnosis	Positive urine culture – Bag specimens (>10^5 CFU/mL) – Suprapubic aspiration (any CFU/mL)	61 full-term newborns	Suprapubic aspiration confirmed diagnosis of UTI on bag specimen in 19/61 (31%) infants	Small sample size	Moderate
Rao [14]	RCT of single absorbent pad + alarm vs replacing absorbent pad every 30 minutes + alarm	Urine collection by absorbent pad	– UTI >10^5 CFU single organism/mL – Contamination rates (heavy mixed growth) between the collection methods	68 febrile children under 2 years of age	– UTI in 3/68 (4%) – Heavy mixed growth in 10/35 (29%) single pad vs 1/30 (3%) replacing pad	– Adequate randomization – Inadequate sample in 12 children – Small sample size	Moderate

	Study	Intervention	Population	Outcome	Results	Limitations	Quality
Pryles [1]	Prospective study of urine culture obtained via suprapubic aspiration and catheterization	Urine collection by suprapubic aspiration and catheterization	42 children aged 3 months to 10 years undergoing elective surgery	Development of UTI after urethral catheterization	– Suprapubic aspiration specificity for excluding UTI 100%, sensitivity could not be calculated – Catheterization specificity for excluding UTI 100%, sensitivity could not be calculated – Some difference noted in bacterial growth in first (92.5% correlation) vs second 5 mL (97.5% correlation) of collection	– No child had signs or symptoms of UTI – Small sample size	Moderate
Saccharow [2]	Prospective study of bag specimen vs suprapubic aspiration	Urine collection by suprapubic aspiration and bag	154 children aged 6 months to 12 years with recurrent UTI	– UTI prevalence – Contamination rates	– UTI prevalence of 8.3% – Sensitivity and specificity for bag specimens 77% and 68%, respectively – Morbidity of suprapubic aspiration C.6%	Subjects had history of recurrent UTI	Moderate to high
Ramage [3]	Prospective study of clean catch vs suprapubic aspiration	Urine collection by suprapubic aspiration and clean catch	49 infants aged <24 months with suspicion of UTI	– UTI prevalence – Sensitivity and specificity of clean catch	– UTI prevalence 32% – Sensitivity and specificity of clean catch of 88.9% and 95%, respectively	Small sample size	Low
Austin [4]	Prospective study of catheterization vs suprapubic aspiration	Urine collection by suprapubic aspiration vs clean catch	90 documented infection screens for sepsis in neonates in NICU	UTI as defined as pure growth of >10^8 colonies/L – Success of transurethral catheterization – Success of suprapubic aspiration	UTI prevalence of 6.3%. – Suprapubic aspiration was successful in 32 of 65 infants – Urethral catheterizations was successful in 33 of 43 infants – 18 catheterizations were attempted after unsuccessful suprapubic aspiration of which 12 were successful	– Small sample size – Method of collection left to the judgment of the clinician	Low

Table 38.2 Analysis of antibiotic regimens to treat pediatric UTIs

Authors	Methods	Intervention	Participants	Outcomes	Results	Notes	Quality of evidence
Bailey [19]	Randomized trial of single dose vs 7 d course of TMP-SMX	Antibiotic therapy with TMP-SMX	20 children aged 14 months to 11 years	Treatment failure	Single dose TMP-SMX as effective as 7 d course	– No placebo control – No double blinding – Small sample size – Compliance not studied	Low
Khan [20]	Randomized trial of 3 vs 10 d course of antibiotic therapy with ampicillin, sulfasoxizole, and cephalexin	Antibiotic therapy with ampicillin, sulfasoxizole, and cephalexin	32 children	Treatment failure	High rate of reinfection in 3 d course group	– No placebo control – No double blinding – Small sample size – Antibiotic therapy not standardized	Low
Avner [21]	Randomized trial of single dose vs 10 d of amoxicillin	Antibiotic therapy with amoxicillin	73 children aged 2.5–12 years, 24 excluded, yielding a study population of 49	Treatment failure	Cure rate: 63% (single dose) vs 92% (10 d)(p<0.01)	– No placebo control – Small sample size – 14 excluded b/c of negative or mixed urine culture results – Compliance not studied	Low
Copenhagen Study Group [22]	Randomized trial of 3 d SMX vs 10 d SMX vs 3 d pivmecillinamin	Antibiotic therapy with SMX or pivmecillinamin	333 girls enrolled; 264 evaluated	– Treatment failure at 1–10 d after treatment and at 1 month or more – Development of resistant organism	No difference in the actuarial percentage recurrence-free curves of the 3 treatment groups	– No 10 d comparison group for pivmecillinam – Up to 80 d f/u – Compliance not studied – No placebo control	Moderate
Gaudreault [23]	Randomized trial of single daily dose of TMP-sulfadiazine 4/17.5 mg/kg for 3 vs 10 d	Antibiotic therapy with TMP-sulfadiazine	40 children aged 2.5–18 years	– Treatment failure – Development of resistant organism	Both 3 & 10 d courses are effective in the treatment of uncomplicated UTI in children	– F/u = 38 d – Small sample size – Compliance not studied	Low
Helin [24]	Prospective study of TMP-sulfadiazine 4/16 mg/kg/d bid for 3 vs 10 d	Antibiotic therapy with TMP-sulfadiazine	43 children aged 3 months to 16 years	– Treatment failure at 3–7 d after completion of treatment – Reinfection during next 12 months	Recurrence in 22% treated for 3 d vs 35% for 10 d	– Mean f/u 11 months – Small sample size – Randomization unclear – Compliance not studied – No placebo control	Low

Helin [25]	Prospective study of cephalexin 25–50 mg/kg/d qid for 3 d vs nitrofurantoin 3–4 mg/kg/d qid for 10 d	Antibiotic therapy with cephalexin or nitrofurantoin	43 children (cephalexin N 19, nitroruantoin N 24)	Treatment failure	– Immediate cure rates were 90% (cephalexin) and 96% (nitrofurantoin) – Relapses: cephalexin (2), nitrofurantoin (1) – Reinfection in mean f/u of 7–8 months: cephalexin (2), nitrofurantoin (4) – Treatment with cephalexin for 3 d is a reasonable alternative	– Small sample size – Randomization unclear – Mean f/u 7–8 months – Compliance not studied – No placebo control	Low
Johnson [26]	RCT of 3 vs 10 d treatment for uncomplicated UTI and to determine the role of host factors, including vesicoureteral reflux, and of bacterial virulence factors, including adhesins, in treatment outcome	Antibiotic therapy with amoxicillin 20 mg/kg/d + clavulanic acid 5 mg/kg/d tid	37 children with uncomplicated UTI	– Treatment failure at 4 d – Treatment failure at 30–47 d – Development of resistant organisms	– Success rate: 55% (11/20) vs 82% (14/17) for 3 vs10 d treatment (p =0.09) – Among the 35 with E. coli, 100% of adhesin-negative isolates treated successfully vs 56% of adhesin-positive isolates (p=0.015)	– Small sample size – Mean f/u 33 ds – Urine collection method not standardized – Compliance not studied – No placebo	Low
Jojart [27]	RCT of 3 vs 14 d of nitrofurantoin compared to 3 vs 14 d of TMP-SMX	Antibiotic therapy with nitrofurantoin or TMP-SMX	– Nitrofurantoin 43 children – TMP-SMX 44 children – Age range: 1.5–9 years	Treatment failure at 1 month	Recurrence within 1 month in 9/43 patients in 3 d therapy and 8/44 in 14 d therapy	– Small sample size – Mean f/u 36 ds – Urine collection method not indicated – Multiple treatment groups without control	Low
Kornberg [28]	Randomized trial of 2 vs 10 d of cefuroxime	Antibiotic therapy with cefuroxime	50 children aged 2–11 years	Treatment failure at 3–5 d after treatment	Therapy successful in 8/12 (67%) in 2 d group vs 12/14 (86%) in 10 d group (not significantly significant)	– F/u 15 months – 50% withdrawal rate – Small sample size – No placebo control	Low
Lohr [15]	Double-blinded randomized trial of 3 vs 10 d of nitrofurantoin	Antibiotic therapy with nitrofurantoin	49 girls aged 2–18 years with a symptomatic UTI	– Treatment failure within 7 d of treatment – Reinfection during next 6 months	– Treatment failure: 2/23 (9%) in 10 d group vs 2/26 (8%) in 3 d group – Reinfection: 12 UTI in 7 patients (30%) in 10 d group vs 12 UTI in 6 patients (23%) in 3 d group – 3 d treatment is effective regimen for uncomplicated lower UTI	– F/u 6 months – Small sample size – Compliance not studied – No placebo control	Low

(Continued on p. 380)

Table 38.2 (Continued)

Authors	Methods	Intervention	Participants	Outcomes	Results	Notes	Quality of evidence
Madrigal [29]	Randomized trial of single dose, bid for 3 or bid for 7 d of TMP-SMX	Antibiotic therapy with TMP-SMX	132 children aged 3 months to 12 years	– Treatment within 12 d of treatment – Reinfection at 28–37 ds	– No significant difference in bacteriological cure rates for the single dose (93%) vs multidose regimens (96%) – Recurrence in the single dose (20.5%) vs 3 d (5.6%) and 7 d (8%) regimens was statistically significant (p=0.033) – Single dose of TMP-SMX is inadequate UTI treatment for infants and children	– F/u 44 ds – Compliance not studied – No placebo control	Low
Wientzen [30]	Randomized trial of 4 d vs 10 d of amoxicillin 30 mg/kg/d	Antibiotic therapy with amoxicillin	52 children aged 3 months to 16 years	– Treatment failure – Reinfection within 12 months	4 d and 10 d therapy equally effective	– F/u 12 months – Urine collection method not standardized – Multiple subgroup analyses – No placebo control	Low
Zaki [31]	Prospective study of nalidixic acid and TMP-SMX for 3 d vs 10 d	Antibiotic therapy with nalidixic acid or TMP-SMX	Nalidixic acid (16) TMP-SMX (19) Aged 6 months to 13 years	– Treatment failure at 2–3 d after treatment – Reinfection within 3 months	3 d and 10 d therapy equally effective for both nalidixic acid and TMP-SMX in uncomplicated UTI	– F/u 3 months – Small sample size – Urine collection method not specified	Low
McCracken [32]	Randomized trial of 1 vs 10 d of cefadroxil	Antibiotic therapy with cefadroxil	76 children aged 2 months to 16 years	– Treatment failure at 4–5 d – Reinfection at 20–29 d – Reinfection at 74–83 d	– Treatment failure at 4–5 d in 16/36 (1 d) vs 6/30 (10 d) – Reinfection at 20–29 d and at 74–83 d: 8.3% (1 d) vs 20% (10 d) – Total failure/reinfection rate: 50% (1 d) vs 35% (10 d) – Conventional 10 d therapy should be used in all infants and children with UTI	– F/u 3 months – Urine collection method not standardized – Small sample size – No placebo control	Low
Nolan [33]	Randomized trial of TMP (single dose) vs TMP-SMX for 7 d	Antibiotic therapy with TMP or TMP-SMX	106 children aged 2–16 years	Treatment failure at 2 d and 10 d after the start of treatment	Positive culture at 2 d: TMP (0/50) vs TMP-SMX for 7 d (2/56) – Positive culture at 10 d: TMP (10/44) vs TMP-SMX for 7 d (1/46)	– F/u 10 d – Different agents – No placebo control	Low
Grimwood [16]	Randomized trial of gentamicin (single dose) vs 7 d of culture-appropriate oral antibiotic therapy	Antibiotic therapy	45 children	Treatment failure/ reinfection within 6 weeks	Tendency for those not cured by single-dose treatment to relapse whereas those treated by conventional therapy tended to be reinfected	– Different agents utilized – Small sample size – No placebo control – Compliance not studied	Low

Study	Description	Treatment	Sample	Outcome measure	Results	Limitations	Quality
Stahl [34]	Randomized trial of single dose vs 10 d course of amoxicillin	Antibiotic therapy with amoxicillin	26 girls aged 2–17 years	– Treatment failure – Reinfection – Development of resistant organism	– Cure rate: 70 % (single-dose) vs 75% (10 d) – Relapse rates: 30% (single dose) vs 25% (10 d) – Reinfection rates 0% (single-dose) vs 12% (10 d) – Single dose of culture-proven antibiotic therapy of uncomplicated UTI was effective	– Small sample size – No placebo control – Compliance not studied	Low
Fine [35]	Randomized trial of amoxicillin single 3 g dose vs 250 mg tid for 10 d	Antibiotic therapy with amoxicillin	31 girls aged 12–18 years; 28 sexually active	Treatment failure at 2–5 d after completing therapy	– Negative f/u culture: 69% (single dose) vs 87% (10 d) -Resolution of symptoms in treatment failures in 80% (4/5) (single dose) vs 100% (2/2) (10 d)	– Small sample size – No placebo control – Compliance not studied	Low
Shapiro [36]	Double-blinded randomized trial of amoxicillin single dose (50 mg/kg) vs 10 d course (40 mg/kg/d given tid) in girls with suspected UTI	Antibiotic therapy with amoxicillin	35 girls aged 2–16 years	– Treatment failure – Reinfection within 12 months	– Cure rate: 78% (single dose) vs 88% (10 d) (p>0.26) – Reinfection rates similar – Single dose appeared equivalent to 10 d course	– Small sample size – Compliance not studied – No placebo control – Mean f/u 8.7 months	Low
Repetto [17]	Randomized trial of single dose of cefotaxime (50 mg/kg IM) vs 10 d treatment of antibiotic chosen by in vitro sensitivities	Antibiotic therapy with cefotaxime or multiple oral agents	37 children with uncomplicated UTI	Treatment failure at 2 d after therapy – Reinfection at 28 d after therapy	Sterile urine at 48 h: 100% cefotaxime vs 18/19 (10 d) (1 remained symptomatic with positive culture) – Recurrence at 28 d: 2/18 cefotaxime vs 0/18 (10 d) – Rates of cures and recurrence not statistically different (p>0.05)	– Small sample size – No placebo control – Compliance not studied – Different agents utilized	Low
Wallen [18]	Randomized trial of sulfasoxizole 150 mg/kg/d orally for 10 d vs amikacin 7.5 mg/kg single dose IM	Antibiotic therapy with sulfasoxizole or amikacin	54 girls aged 1–12 years	Treatment failure/ reinfection within 40 d of completing therapy	Positive culture at 40 d: amikacin 6/23 (26%) vs sulfasoxizole 4/21 (19%) (p>0.5) – A single dose of amikacin is as effective as a 10 d course of sulfasoxizole in the treatment of presumed first lower tract UTI in girls – 10 excluded from final analysis	– Different agents utilized – Small sample size – No placebo control – Compliance not studied	Low
Pitt [37]	Randomized trial of TMP-SMX single dose vs 7 d course	Antibiotic therapy with TMP-SMX	42 children aged 6 months to 12 years	Treatment failure at 2 d after starting therapy	One patient in the single-dose group had a recurrent infection on 7 – Single-dose and 7 d course TMP-SMX equally effective for symptomatic UTI	– Small sample size – No placebo control – Compliance not studied	Low

were confounded by poor design. Even considering the randomized controlled trials, the overall quality of the evidence is low. Allocation concealment was adequate in two of the trials while it was inadequate or unclear in the remaining studies. Lohr et al. [15] was the only double-blinded study in the cohort. In three of the studies [16-18], the design precluded blinding as the antimicrobials were administered via different routes. Finally, there is no mention of an intention-to-treat analysis in any of the studies.

Overall, the studies were very heterogeneous with regard to cohort age, gender, symptomatology (to differentiate cystitis from pyelonephritis), method of obtaining urine samples, and definition of treatment success. The choice of antibiotic choice and dosage was variable, and confirmation of patient compliance was often lacking. The follow-up periods were also highly variable. The definitions of treatment failure, relapse, and reinfection were not standardized, thus further hampering the ability to draw conclusions regarding adequate treatment.

Comment

In summary, there is no clear evidence available to recommend an optimal agent or duration of antimicrobial therapy for the treatment of pediatric UTI.

Clinical question 38.3

Do prophylactic antibiotics prevent recurrent urinary tract infections in children?

Background

Prophylactic antibiotics have long been a standard therapy for children with recurrent UTIs. However, the evidence supporting such practice is limited. The few reports examining prophylactic antibiotics are confounded by a paucity of controlled studies, variability in the agent used, inclusion of additional nonpharmacological interventions, and variability of host factors in subjects (anatomical anomalies, most specifically vesicoureteral reflux).

Literature search

The literature search was initiated with a review of the Cochrane database and utilization of the noted primary and secondary references. In addition, a PubMed search using the terms "prophylaxis," "prophylactic antibiotics," and "urinary tract infections" was conducted with no time frame restriction. Articles were then reviewed to determine which studies involved children (under age 18 years).

The evidence

Twenty-one studies have assessed the effect of long-term antibiotic usage to prevent UTIs in children (Table 38.3); however, the studies are very heterogeneous. Although the majority of studies used trimethoprim-sulfamethoxazole (TMP-SMX) and/or nitrofurantoin (NF) for prophylaxis, a total of 12 antimicrobial agents were utilized in these 21 studies, and the prophylactic dosages of the antimicrobials were not consistent between studies. Few took measures to assess patient compliance with therapy.

The majority of these studies were confounded by poor design. Five studies lacked controls [38-43] and another was an observational study of secondary data from 27 pediatric practices [44]. Four studies were randomized trials comparing one prophylactic regimen versus another, rather than a comparison against a control group of no prophylaxis [45-48]. The outcome of one study was the occurrence of UTIs after completion of a course of prophylactic antibiotics, not during the course [49]. Four studies were only interested in the occurrence of pyelonephritis (or febrile UTIs), not all UTIs [50-53]. Another study used an outcome of asymptomatic UTIs (positive urine culture without symptoms) which is now believed to be clinically irrelevant [54]. Three studies specifically studied only children with vesicoureteral reflux (VUR) [53,55,56] and in at least 11 other studies, a significant number of subjects had VUR or other anatomical abnormalities. Five studies were limited to girls [39,42,47,54,57] and only four studies included more than 25% of boys [50,52,53,55]. Nearly all studies were confounded by the inclusion of children of a wide age range from the neonatal period to post puberty. Many studies were further confounded by implementing behavioral therapy in addition to antibiotic prophylaxis to reduce UTI recurrences, and this could have been particularly misleading in those studies without controls.

On careful examination of the evidence, there are only two comparative trials (one cross-over and one unblinded randomized controlled trial) that studied the efficacy of prophylactic antibiotics in preventing symptomatic UTIs (not limited to pyelonephritis) in children; the number of subjects was exceedingly small in these two studies. Lohr et al. [57] noted statistically significantly fewer total and symptomatic UTIs in 18 girls on NF for 6 months in a cross-over study. Smellie et al. [58] found no recurrence of UTIs in 25 children randomized to TMP-SMX or NF for an average of 10 months compared to recurrences in 13/22 children in the control group. Two RCTs using pyelonephritis as an outcome measure enrolled greater than 200 children (most with VUR) and neither found statistically significantly fewer recurrences of pyelonephritis in children on prophylaxis [50,55]. Interestingly, there appeared to be statistically significantly fewer total UTIs in the treatment group in one study, and fewer episodes of cystitis in

Table 38.3 Analysis of antibiotic prophylaxis to prevent UTIs

Authors	Methods	Intervention	Participants	Outcomes	Results	Notes	Quality of evidence
Normand & Smellie [38]	Observational study of 6–12 months of antimicrobial prophylaxis in pts with no VUR and indefinitely in pts with VUR or other anatomical abnormality	– Sulfadimidine or sulfafurazole 0.25–1 g daily in 109 – Nitrofurantoin 2–4 mg/kg/d in 6 – Tetracycline in 1	116 children aged 3 weeks to 12 years; 25% boys	Positive urine culture (not defined)	– Of those with recurrent UTI (70), UTI rate dropped 2.4/yr to 0.26/yr with no recurrences in 41/70 – Of those with medical treatment only for VUR (24), UTI rate dropped 2.5/yr to 0.37/yr – Of those with medical treatment only for chronic pyelonephritis (12), UTI rate dropped 2.6/yr to 0.15/yr	– No control group – 57% had radiological abnormality (70% of these VUR) – At least 33 children had surgery as well	Low
Bergstrom [39]	Randomized study of treatment for 10 vs 60 d	Sulfasoxizole 200 mg/kg/d for 10 d then 100 mg/kg/d for 2 wks then 50 mg/kg/d for 2 months	279 girls aged 2 months to 16 years after 1st or 2nd uncomplicated UTI	Positive urine culture (>100 K colonies/mL of single organism)	– No sig difference in overall recurrence rate – Greater proportion of asymp (& fewer symp) UTI in long-term treatment group (p<0.05)	– UTI with resistant organisms higher in long-term group (95% vs 59%, p<0.01) – No difference among age groups	Moderate
Stansfeld [49]	Blinded RCT of TMP-SMX for 6 months vs no therapy following 2 weeks therapy for active UTI	TMP-SMX (dose not given)	50 children aged 6 months to 14 years; 3 boys in treatment group	UTI after cessation of therapy	No difference between groups (cure rates of 46% and 48%)	– Small sample size – only 45/50 completed study – Did not compare # UTIs during therapy – 36% had VUR	Very low
Savage et al. [54]	Blinded RCT of 10 week therapy of antimicrobial prophylaxis agents in girls with covert (asymptomatic) UTI followed for 4 years	TMP-SMX 100–200/20– 40 mg twice daily or nitrofurantoin 4 mg/kg/d	63 5-year-old girls	Positive urine culture	Stat sig fewer UTIs in treatment group in first 6 months ONLY	– Small sample size – Studied only asymptomatic UTIs – 25% of controls & 38% of study group had urological abnormalities	Low
Smellie et al. [40]	Observation study of antimicrobial prophylaxis for 6–24 months in children with history of UTI	TMP-SMX 10 mg/2 mg/kg/d	130 children aged 1–12 yrs, 13% boys	Positive urine culture	– No UTI in 73 pts without VUR (mean of 13.9 mo) – UTI noted in 6/57 girls with VUR (1 in 22 pt-yr) – 27/65 developed UTI after therapy (70% within 3 mo)	– No control group – 44% had VUR – All UTI resistant to TMP-SMX – Compliance noted in 50/54 tested – Side effects (3 sleepy,2 rash)	Very low
Lohr et al. [57]	Double-blind controlled cross-over trial of 6 months of antimicrobial prophylaxis	Nitrofurantoin (50 mg/d >20 kg; 25 mg/d <20 kg)	18 girls aged 3–13 yrs	Positive urine culture (>100 K colonies/mL of single organism)	– Total # UTI stat sig less in period on drug (35 vs 2, p<0.01) – Symptomatic UTI stat sig less in period on drug (14 vs 0, p<0.01)	– Very small sample size – 8/18 did not complete study – Compliance test excellent – 1 patient with VUR	Low

(Continued on p. 384)

Table 38.3 (Continued)

Authors	Methods	Intervention	Participants	Outcomes	Results	Notes	Quality of evidence
Smellie et al. [58]	Unblinded RCT of 6–12 months of antimicrobial prophylaxis	- TMP-SMX 10/2 mg/kd/d - Nitrofurantoin 1–2 mg/kg/d	47 children (42 girls, 5 boys) aged 2–12 yrs	Positive urine culture (not defined)	- No UTI in either treatment group during therapy vs 50% in control group - Two years after stopping therapy, 32% of treatment group and 64% of control group had further UTI (p=0.008)	- Small sample size - Behavioral therapy also initiated - No patients with VUR or abnormal IVP included	Very low
Carlsen et al. [45]	Randomized cross-over trial of antimicrobial prophylaxis comparing 6 mo of pivmecillinam vs nitrofurantoin	- One agent for 6 months then cross-over to other agent - Pivmecillinam 100 mg <6 yrs; 200 mg >6 yrs - Nitrofurantoin 1.5 mg/kg/d	24/35 children completed study (VUR in 15)	Positive urine culture	- No difference noted between agents (0.6 vs 0.4 UTI/pt yr)	- Small sample size - Side effects less on pivmecillinam (18% vs 56%) - No ages given - 63% had VUR	Very low
Smellie et al. [41]	Observational study of 6–12 months of antimicrobial prophylaxis in pts without VUR and indefinitely in pts with VUR comparing TMP alone vs TMP-SMX	- Trimethoprim 1–2 mg /kg/d - TMP-SM X 1–2/5–10 mg/kg/d	334 children aged 1–12 yrs, 20% boys	Positive urine culture (>100 K colonies/mL of single organism)	- TMP-SMX: 1 recurrence in 10 children (or 1 in 22 child-years on therapy) - TMP: 1 recurrence in 10 children (or 1 in 18 child-years on therapy)	- No control group - 50% had VUR - All recurrences in girls - All recurrences symptomatic	Low
Brendstrup et al. [46]	Double-blind RCT of nitrofurantoin vs trimethoprim for 6 months	- Trimethoprim 2–3 mg/kg/d - Nitrofurantoin 1–1.5 mg/kg/d	120 children aged 1–15 years; 3% male. 3 groups: abnormal imaging (30), normal imaging with VUR (30), normal with no VUR (60)	Positive urine culture (>100 K colonies/mL of single organism)	- Nitrofurantoin had higher recurrence-free rate (p=0.039) - Difference noted only in pts with abnormal imaging/VUR (p=0.02) vs normal/no VUR (p=0.88) - No difference noted between groups 3 months after treatment	- Side effects more common with nitrofurantoin (55% vs 27%, p<0.002) - Behavioral therapy also initiated (confounding)	Low
Smith & Elder [42]	Observational study of children with breakthrough UTIs on single-agent antimicrobial prophylaxis (nitrofurantoin or TMP-SMX) placed on combination therapy of both for 2–49 mo	Nitrofurantoin 2 mg/kg/d each morning + TMP-SMX 10 /2 mg/kd/ d each evening	31 girls aged 1–16 years	Positive urine culture (>100 K colonies/mL of single organism)	Reduction in incidence of breakthrough UTI from 17.4 to 3.7 UTIs per 100 pt-mo of therapy (p<0.001)	- Small sample size - 68% had VUR; 49% had voiding dysfunction; 26% had both (10% had neither)	Very low

(Continued on p. 386)

Study	Study description	Drug/dose	Population	Diagnostic criteria	Results	Comments	Quality
Lettgen & Tröster [47]	RCT of 6–12 months of cefixime vs nitrofurantoin	– Cefixime – Nitrofurantoin	60 girls aged 1–11 years	Documented UTI	No difference noted	Tolerance comparable between groups	Very low
Hellerstein & Nickell [43]	Retrospective review of children placed on prophylactic antibiotics	– TMP-SMX 5–10/1–2 mg/kd/d – Nitrofurantoin 1–2 mg/kg/d	58 girls and 8 boys aged birth to 6 years; 76% had VUR		– 72% of girls & 100% boys had no breakthrough UTI – Voiding dysfunction and abnormal upper tract associated with UTI, not VUR or constipation – 42% had UTI after cessation of prophylaxis	– Mixed cohorts – Small sample size – Length of prophylaxis period not defined	
Montini et al. [50]	RCT of 12 months of antimicrobial prophylaxis	– TMP-SMX 15 mg/kg/d – Amox/clavulanic acid 15 mg/kg/d	235 children aged 1–64 months with prior history of pyelonephritis; 35% boys	– Positive urine culture – Positive DMSA scan	– UTI recurrence stat sig less in treatment group (p=0.015) – Pyelonephritis recurrence or positive DMSA scan not stat sig diff	– Study limited to those with prior pyelonephritis – 75 in no treatment group – Randomization protocol not given – VUR % not given but evenly distributed among groups	Moderate
Belet et al. [48]	Nonblinded RCT of 6 mo of antimicrobial prophylaxis with TMP-SMX, cephadroxil, and cefprozil	– TMP-SMX 5–10 /1–2 mg/kd/d – Cephadroxil 5 mg/kg/d – Cefprozil 5 mg/kg/d	104 children aged 6 months to 15 years with no urological abnormalities; 16% boys	Positive urine culture (>100 K colonies/mL of single organism)	– No difference noted between agents in recurrence of symptomatic infections – Stat sig more asymptomatic UTIs on cefprozil	– Small sample size: only 80/104 completed study – # pts in each group were unbalanced – Age of pts between groups were stat sig diff	Very low
Garin et al. [51]	Multicenter RCT of 12 months of antimicrobial prophylaxis in pts with or without VUR after pyelonephritis	– TMP-SMX 5–10 /1–2 mg/kd/d – Trimethoprim 1.5 mg/kg/d	218 children aged 3 months to 17 years; 18% boys; only grades 1–3 VUR included	Positive urine culture	– In those with VUR, no stat sig diff in recurrence of pyelonephritis (7 in treatment vs 1 in control) or recurrence of total UTI (20.4% in treatment vs 24.4% in control) – In those not on prophylaxis, no stat sig diff between UTI in those with VUR (22.4%) vs those without VUR (23.3%) – In those on prophylaxis, no stat sig diff between UTI in those without VUR (8.8%) vs those without VUR (23.6%) (p=0.0633) – In those without VUR, cystitis in prophylaxis group was 2.2% vs 13.8% in control group, no stat analysis given	– Underpowered to look at differences between subgroups – Study designed to look mainly at those with VUR – No randomization of specific prophylactic antibiotics	Moderate

Table 38.3 (Continued)

Authors	Methods	Intervention	Participants	Outcomes	Results	Notes	Quality of evidence
Conway et al. [44]	Analysis of secondary data from 27 primary pediatric practices	19/83 received antimicrobial prophylaxis – TMP-SMX 61% – Amoxicillin 29% – Nitrofurantoin 7% – Other 3%	Of 611 children with first UTI, 83 children had recurrent UTI aged 6 yr or younger; 10% male	Positive urine culture	No difference noted in risk of recurrent UTI in those on antimicrobial prophylaxis (1.05 univariate, 1.01 multivariate)	– Very small sample size – No mechanism to check compliance – No recurrence in 9 pts on nitrofurantoin – Subject to errors in reporting	Low
Roussey-Kesler et al. [55]	Unblinded RCT of 18 mo of antimicrobial prophylaxis in children with VUR grades 1–3	TMP-SMX 10 mg/2 mg/kg/d	225 children aged 1 month to 3 years; 31% male	Positive urine culture (>100 K colonies/mL of single organism)	– No stat sig diff in total UTI between groups (treated 17% vs control 26%, p=0.13) – No stat sig diff in febrile UTI between groups (treated 13% vs control 16%, p=0.52) – Stat sig diff noted only for boys (p=0.013) vs girls (p=0.8), notably in grade 3 VUR	– May have been underpowered – Did not examine compliance	Moderate
Pennesi et al. [53]	Multicenter RCT of 24 months of antimicrobial prophylaxis in pts with VUR grades 2–4 after pyelonephritis	– TMP-SMX 5–10 /1–2 mg/kd/d – Nitrofurantoin 2 mg/kg/d	100 children aged 1–30 months, 48% male	– Positive urine culture – Positive DMSA scan	No difference noted in recurrence of pyelonephritis or development of renal scarring	– Only looked at pyelonephritis and not all UTI – All pts had VUR – No segregation of two drugs	Low
Montini et al. [52]	Multicenter RCT of 12 months of antimicrobial prophylaxis in pts following first febrile UTI	– TMP-SMX 15 mg/kg/d – Amox/clavulanic acid 15 mg/kg/d	338 children aged 1–101 months; 29% male; 38% with VUR grades 1–3	– Febrile UTI – New scars on DMSA	No difference in febrile UTIs or new renal scars	– No difference noted in those with VUR – One-half fewer positive urine cultures on routine follow-up in those on treatment – Inadequate recruitment to allow planned segregation of two drugs – Compliance verified in 71%	Moderate
Cheng et al. [56]	Multicenter retrospective study of breakthrough UTIs in children on prophylactic antibiotics for VUR	– TMP-SMX – Cephalexin – Cefaclor	324 children aged 0–11 years	Febrile and "a few afebrile" UTI with documented culture and sensitivity	– Breakthrough recurrence rate of 20–25% – Prevalence of E. coli in breakthrough UTI dropped from 82% to 44% – Antibiotic resistance much greater in those on cephalosporin prophylaxis compared to TMP-SMX	– All children had VUR – Retrospective study – Compliance not verified	Moderate

the prophylaxis arm of those without VUR in the second. The most recent large RCT used recurrence of febrile UTI and new scars on DMSA as primary and secondary endpoints and found no difference in those not on therapy and those on prophylaxis with either TMP-SMX or amoxicillin/clavulanic acid; however, those on prophylaxis had 50% fewer positive urinalysis/urine cultures collected on a monthly to bimonthly basis [52].

All antimicrobial agents were not equally effective in preventing UTIs. Brendstrup et al. [46] found that NF had a higher recurrence-free rate compared to trimethoprim alone, but this difference was noted only in children with abnormal imaging or VUR and only for the first 3 months of prophylaxis. Importantly, NF was associated with significantly greater side effects. Cheng et al. [56] noted development of greater resistance patterns with the use of cephalosporins in comparison to TMP-SMX.

Two recent RCT studies have questioned the utility of antimicrobial prophylaxis in the setting of VUR specifically [51,55], and in the United States, the nationwide NIH-funded Randomized Intervention in Vesicoureteral Reflex (RIVUR) trial is currently enrolling children in a RCT to attempt to answer the same question. The two published trials founded no overall statistically significant difference in the recurrence of UTIs in those on versus not on prophylaxis, but some subgroups did show benefit.

Comment

The evidence supporting the use of prophylactic antibiotics to prevent recurrent UTIs is limited and weak. The two studies with statistically significant higher recurrence-free rates in those on prophylactic antibiotics had very small sample sizes. All studies were confounded by the choice of antibiotic, the dosage utilized, confirmation of patient compliance, and the heterogeneity of subjects in terms of age and anatomical anomaly (specifically VUR). It is likely that certain antimicrobials may be superior for prophylaxis but may have greater side effects that could limit their utilization. Finally, no evidence is available to recommend an optimal agent or dosing regimen.

Clinical question 38.4

Are there nonantimicrobial measures to prevent recurrent urinary tract infection in children?

Background

Multiple nonantimicrobial measures have been employed in the prevention of UTI in children. These include behavioral interventions, as well as oral agents. Constipation has

been strongly linked to the occurrence of recurrent UTIs, so treatment of constipation has been employed to prevent recurrence of UTIs. Voiding dysfunction related to poor urinary sphincter relaxation is also a well-described risk factor for recurrent UTIs; therefore, behavioral intervention via pelvic floor biofeedback has been reported to reduce the recurrence of UTIs. The most widely touted nonantimicrobial oral agents for prevention of UTI are cranberry products.

Literature search

A literature search was performed using the US National Library of Medicine and the National Institutes of Health PubMed database. The search terms with imposed limits were as follows: urinary tract infection AND prevent NOT reflux NOT antibiotic NOT prophylaxis NOT imaging limits: Entrez Date from 1920/01/01 to 2008/07/31, Humans, English, All Child: 0–18 years This search yielded a total of 49 articles which were reviewed to determine their relevance to our clinical question. There were 11 articles relevant to our clinical question.

The evidence

Although constipation has been linked to recurrent UTIs in many descriptive manuscripts, there is a paucity of data looking at treatment of constipation as a measure to prevent recurrent UTIs. It is intuitive that constipation should be treated if noted in children with recurrent UTIs, but evidence of the efficacy of such treatment is limited to three studies with small sample size and/or poorly defined methods and outcomes [59-61].

Voiding dysfunction is frequently found in children with recurrent UTIs and can be manifested by urinary urgency/frequency, urinary incontinence, elevated postvoid residual urine volume, and abnormal urinary flow patterns/rates. Behavioral therapy to promote pelvic floor/voluntary sphincter relaxation and thus better bladder emptying at lower voiding pressures has been widely employed in children with both voiding dysfunction and a history of recurrent UTIs. The effect of biofeedback therapy upon the reduction in the recurrence of UTIs is difficult to glean from the literature. Most studies investigating this therapy have primary outcomes focused upon urodynamic data and voiding symptoms; the recurrence of UTIs was always a secondary outcome that was poorly meausured [62-67].

Few studies exist that evaluate the use of nonantimicrobials for UTI prevention in the pediatric population (Table 38.4). Foda et al. [68] performed a cross-over RCT of the administration cranberry cocktail and water over a 6-month period for the prevention of UTI in 40 children with neurogenic bladder managed by intermittent catheterization (IC). Daily cranberry juice had no effect on UTI

Table 38.4 Analysis of non-pharmacologic interventions to prevent UTIs

Authors	Methods	Intervention	Participants	Outcomes	Results	Notes	Quality of evidence
O'Regan [59]	Retrospective study	Aggressive treatment of constipation with enemas	47 girls with recurrent UTI and constipation, mean age 8.2 ± 2.5 years	– Recurrence of UTI – Resolution of constipation/ encopresis – Urodynamic parameters	– Absence of recurrent UTI in 44/47 – 2/3 with recurrent UTI did not comply with enema protocol – Urodynamics normalized in 12/12 studied	– No placebo group – Definition of UTIs not given – Mean f/u of 12 months	Low
Loening-Baucke [60]	Prospective study of recurrent UTIs following treatment of constipation	Disimpaction and maintainence therapy for constipation	Of 234 children, 3 boys and 11 girls had recurrent UTIs	– Recurrence of UTI – Ability to stop prophylactic antibiotics	– 8/14 were able to stop prophylactic antibiotics – No recurrence of UTI off antibiotics	– Small sample size – 7/14 had anatomical abnormalities – Mean f/u = 15 months – No control group	Low
Chrzan [61]	Retrospective study of patients with recurrent UTIs following treatment of constipation	Colonic washout enemas and oral laxatives (all on prophylactic antibiotics)	50 children aged 6–12 years	– Recurrence of UTI – Ability to stop prophylactic antibiotics	– 30/50 had no UTI and stopped antibiotics – 12/50 had no UTI but had voiding dysfunction – 8/50 had at least 1 UTI	– Retrospective – No control group – Poor definition of outcomes – Short f/u of 6 months	Low
DePaepe [62]	Prospective study of biofeedback for treatment of voiding dysfunction and recurrent UTIs	Physical therapy and biofeedback to teach pelvic floor relaxation	42 girls: 4 were less than 6 years; 38 were aged 6–14 years	– Recurrence of UTI – Attainment of urinary continence	– 35/42 had successful treatment of recurrent UTIs – 7/7 with recurrence of UTIs also had no resolution of incontinence – 4 had no recurrence of UTIs but remained incontinent	– Mixed cohort – No placebo group – Definition of UTIs not given – Confounded by additional behavioral interventions	Low
McKenna [63]	Study of interactive computer game biofeedback in patients with voiding dysfunction	Biofeedback of pelvic floor musculature using computerized video games	41 children aged 5–11 years; 20% boys	– Subjective symptoms – Recurrence of UTI	– Of 22 with recurrent UTI at initiation of study, only 3 (14%) had UTI after beginning study	– No placebo group – Definition of UTIs not given – Confounded by additional behavioral interventions – Mean f/u of 7 months – Unclear if prospective or retrospective	Low
Wiener [64]	Retrospective study of Kegel exercises without biofeedback	Family questionnaire following program of Kegel exercises and behavioral therapy	48 children aged 3–14 years	– Subjective symptoms – Frequency of UTI	– 56% reported improvement in frequency of UTIs	– No placebo group – UTI frequency based on parental recall – Confounded by additional behavioral interventions – Mean f/u of 4.7 years	Low

Study	Study description	Intervention	Population	Outcome measures	Results	Limitations	Quality
Chin-Peuckert [65]	Study of biofeedback in patients with voiding dysfunction	Biofeedback of pelvic floor musculature	77 children aged 3–17 years; 10% boys	– Subjective symptoms – Objective urodynamic findings – Ability to stop prophylactic antibiotics	– Prophylactic antibiotics stopped in 17/25 (68%)	– No placebo group – Definition of UTIs not given – Confounded by additional behavioral interventions – Cessation of antibiotics subjective – F/u not given – Not clear if prospective or retrospective	Low
Nelson [66]	Retrospective study of biofeedback in patients with voiding dysfunction	Biofeedback of pelvic floor musculature	81 children aged 4–17 years; 20% boys	– Subjective symptoms – Objective urodynamic findings – Recurrence of UTIs – Ability to stop prophylactic antibiotics	– 22/42 (52%) of patients able to stop prophylactic antibiotics – 17/22 (73%) of those off antibiotics had no UTI recurrence – 15/20 (75%) of those remaining on antibiotics had no UTI recurrence – Only urodynamic parameter difference between groups was in max. flow rate	– No placebo group – Definition of UTIs not given – Confounded by additional behavioral interventions – Cessation of antibiotics subjective – F/u of 9 months	Low
Kibar [67]	Prospective study of biofeedback for treatment of voiding dysfunction and recurrent UTIs	Biofeedback of pelvic floor musculature	78 children aged 5–14 years; 10% boys	– Subjective symptoms – Objective urodynamic findings – Recurrence of UTIs – Resolution of vesicoureteral reflux	33/41 (80%) had no documented UTI in f/u period	– No placebo group – Definition of UTIs not given – Confounded by additional behavioral interventions – Short f/u of 6 months	Low
Foda [68]	Cross-over RCT	Cranberry cocktail vs water for 6 months followed by the cross-over for 6 months	40 children aged 1–18 years with neurogenic bladder on IC	Positive urine culture	– Daily cranberry juice did not have a significant effect on the prevention of UTI	– Single-blind – 42.5% dropout rate – Small sample size – Inability to extrapolate to non-neurogenic population	Low
Schlager [69]	Cross-over RCT	Cranberry concentrate vs placebo for 3 months followed by crossover for 3 months	15 children aged 2–18 years with neurogenic bladder on IC	– Bacteriuria = >10^4 CFU/mL – UTI (bacteriuria + fever, abdominal pain, change in continence, or change in odor/color of urine)	– No change in prevalence of bacteriuria (75%) from consumption of placebo vs cranberry concentrate – 3 symptomatic infections occurred during the placebo and cranberry periods	– F/u 6 months – Inability to extrapolate to non-neurogenic population – Placebo controlled – Double-blinded – Small sample size	Low

recurrence. This study was hampered by a high dropout rate of greater than 40%, small sample size, and single-blind design. Schlager et al. [69] conducted a double-blind, placebo-controlled, cross-over RCT investigation of cranberry concentrate and placebo over a 3-month period in 15 children with neurogenic bladder managed by intermittent catheterization. There was no difference noted in frequency of bacteriuria (75%) or number of symptomatic UTIs between groups.

Comment

Recurrent UTIs often occur in the setting of constipation, voiding dysfunction, and neurogenic bladder. Measures to treat constipation and voiding dysfunction are intuitive in the management of children with recurrent UTIs if such symptoms are present; however, the efficacy of such therapy for the recurrence of UTIs has not been well evaluated. This does not mean that such therapy should not be utilized, but that it should be better studied.

The evidence for the use of nonantimicrobial oral agents in the prevention of recurrent UTI in the pediatric population is lacking; therefore, no recommendation can be made. The two studies detailed previously were hampered by small sample sizes precluding adequate statistical power, as well as by variability in the concentrations and pharmacokinetics of different cranberry formulations. Also, the data presented cannot be extrapolated to the non-neurogenic population.

References

1. Pryles CV Atkin MD Morse TS, et al. Comparative bacteriologic study of urine obtained from children by percutaneous suprapubic aspiration of the bladder and by catheter. Pediatrics 1959;24:983-91.
2. Saccharow L, Pryles CV. Further experience with the use of percutaneous suprapubic aspiration of the urinary bladder. Bacteriologic studies in 654 infants and children. Pediatrics 1969;43:1018-24.
3. Ramage IJ, Chapman JP, Hollman AS, et al. Accuracy of clean-catch urine collection in infancy. J Pediatr 1999;135:765-7.
4. Austin BJ, Bollard C, Gunn TR. Is urethral catheterization a successful alternative to suprapubic aspiration in neonates? J Paediatr Child Health 1999;35:34-6.
5. American Academy of Pediatrics. Practice parameter: the diagnosis, treatment, and evaluation of the initial urinary tract infection in febrile infants and young children. Pediatrics 1999;103:843-52.
6. McGillivray D, Mok E, Mulrooney E, et al. A head-to-head comparison: "clean-void" bag versus catheter urinalysis in the diagnosis of urinary tract infection in young children. J Pediatr 2005;147:451-6.
7. Falcão MC, Leone CR, d'Andrea RA, et al. Urinary tract infection in full-term newborn infants: value of urine culture by bag specimen collection. Rev Hosp Clin Fac Med Sao Paulo 1999;54(3):91-6.
8. Liaw LC, Nayar DM, Pedler SJ, et al. Home collection of urine for culture from infants by three methods: survey of parents' preferences and bacterial contamination rates. BMJ 2000;320:1312-13.
9. Schroeder AR, Newman TB, Wasserman RC, et al. Choice of urine collection methods for the diagnosis of urinary tract infection in young, febrile infants. Arch Pediatr Adolesc Med 2005;159:915-22.
10. Farrell M, Devine K, Lancaster G, et al. A method comparison study to assess the reliability of urine collection pads as a means of obtaining urine specimens from non-toilet-trained children for microbiological examination. J Adv Nurs 2002;37:387-93.
11. Hardy JD, Furnell PM, Brumfitt W. Comparison of sterile bag, clean catch and suprapubic aspiration in the diagnosis of urinary infection in early childhood. BJU 1976;48:279-83.
12. Alam MT, Coulter JB, Pacheco J, et al. Comparison of urine contamination rates using three different methods of collection: clean-catch, cotton wool pad and urine bag. Ann Trop Paediatr 2005;25:29-34.
13. Lau AY, Wong SN, Yip KT, et al. A comparative study on bacterial cultures of urine samples obtained by clean-void technique versus urethral catheterization. Acta Paediatr 2007;96:432-6.
14. Rao S, Houghton C, Macfarlane PI. A new urine collection method; pad and moisture sensitive alarm. Arch Dis Child 2003;88:836.
15. Lohr JA, Hayden GF, Kesler RW, et al. Three-day therapy of lower urinary tract infections with nitrofurantoin macrocrystals: a randomized clinical trial. J Pediatr 1981;99:980-3.
16. Grimwood K, Abbott GD, Fergusson DM. Single dose gentamicin treatment of urinary infections in children. N Z Med J 1988;24:539-41.
17. Repetto HA, MacLoughlin GJ. Single-dose cefotaxime in the treatment of urinary tract infections in children: a randomized clinical trial. J Antimicrob Chemother 1984;14(suppl B):307-10.
18. Wallen L, Zeller WP, Goessler M, Connor E, Yogev R. Single-dose amikacin treatment of first childhood E. coli lower urinary tract infections. J Pediatr 1983;103:316-19.
19. Bailey RR, Abbott GD. Treatment of urinary tract infection with a single dose of trimethoprim-sulfamethoxazole. Can Med Assoc J 1978;4:551-2.
20. Khan AJ, Kumar K, Evans HE. Three-day antimicrobial therapy of urinary tract infection. J Pediatr 1981;99:992-4.
21. Avner ED, Ingelfinger JR, Herrin JT, et al. Single-dose amoxicillin therapy of uncomplicated pediatric urinary tract infections. J Pediatr 1983;102:623-7.
22. Copenhagen Study Group of Urinary Tract Infections in Children. Short-term treatment of acute urinary tract infection in girls. Scand J Infect Dis 1991;23:213-20.
23. Gaudreault P, Beland M, Girodias JB, et al. Single daily doses of trimethoprim/sulphadiazine for three or 10 days in urinary tract infections. Acta Paediatr 1992;81:695-7.
24. Helin I. Short-term treatment of lower urinary tract infections in children with trimethoprim/sulphadiazine. Infection 1981;9:249-51.
25. Helin I. Three-day therapy with cephalexin for lower urinary tract infections in children. Scand J Infect Dis 1984;16:305-7.

26. Johnson CE, Maslow JN, Fattlar DC, et al. The role of bacterial adhesins in the outcome of childhood urinary tract infections. Am J Dis Child 1993;147:1090-3.

27. Jójárt G. Comparison of 3-day versus 14-day treatment of lower urinary tract infection in children. Int Urol Nephrol 1991;23:129-34.

28. Kornberg AE, Sherin K, Veiga P, et al. Two-day therapy with cefuroxime axetil is effective for urinary tract infections in children. Am J Nephrol 1994;14:169-72.

29. Madrigal G, Odio CM, Mohs E, et al. Single dose antibiotic therapy is not as effective as conventional regimens for management of acute urinary tract infections in children. Pediatr Infect Dis J 1998;7:316-19.

30. Wientzen RL, McCracken GH Jr, Petruska ML, et al. Localization and therapy of urinary tract infections of childhood. Pediatrics 1979;63:467-74.

31. Zaki M, Helin I. Nalidixic acid and trimethoprim/sulphamethoxazole as alternatives for short-term treatment of urinary infections. Ann Trop Paediatr 1986;6:205-7.

32. McCracken GH Jr, Ginsburg CM, Namasonthi V, et al. Evaluation of short-term antibiotic therapy in children with uncomplicated urinary tract infections. Pediatrics 1981;67:796-801.

33. Nolan T, Lubitz L, Oberklaid F. Single dose trimethoprim for urinary tract infection. Arch Dis Child 1989;64:581-6.

34. Stahl GE, Topf P, Fleisher GR, et al. Single-dose treatment of uncomplicated urinary tract infections in children. Ann Emerg Med 1984;13(pt 1):705-8.

35. Fine JS, Jacobson MS. Single-dose versus conventional therapy of urinary tract infections in female adolescents. Pediatrics 1985;75:916-20.

36. Shapiro ED, Wald ER. Single-dose amoxicillin treatment of urinary tract infections. J Pediatr 1981;99(6):989-92.

37. Pitt WR, Dyer SA, McNee JL, et al. Single dose trimethoprim-sulphamethoxazole treatment of symptomatic urinary infection. Arch Dis Child 1982;57:229-31.

38. Normand ICS, Smellie JM. Prolonged maintenance chemotherapy in the management of urinary infection in childhood. BMJ 1965;1:1023-6.

39. Bergström T, Lincoln K, Redin B, et al. Studies of urinary tract infections in infancy and childhood. Acta Paediatr Scand 1968;57:186-94.

40. Smellie JM, Grüneberg RN, Leakey A, et al. Long-term low-dose co-trimoxazole in prophylaxis of childhood urinary tract infection: clinical aspects. BMJ 1976;2:203-6.

41. Smellie JM, Grüneberg RN, Bantock HM, et al. Prophylactic co-trioxazole and trimethoprim in the management of urinary tract infection in children. Pediatr Nephrol 1988;2:12-17.

42. Smith EM, Elder JS. Double antimicrobial prophylaxis in girls with breakthrough urinary tract infections. Urology 1994;45:708-11.

43. Hellerstein S, Nickell E. Prophylactic antibiotics in children at risk for urinary tract infection. Pediatr Nephrol 2002;17:506-10.

44. Conway PH, Cnaan A, Zaoutis T, et al. Recurrent urinary tract infections in children: risk factors and association with prophylactic antimicrobials. JAMA 2007;298:179-86.

45. Carlsen NLT, Hesselbjerg U, Glenting P. Comparison of long-term, low-dose pivmecillinam and nitrofurantoin in the control of recurrent urinary tract infections in children: an open, randomized, cross-over study. J Antimicrob Chemother 1985;16:509-17.

46. Brendstrup L, Hjelt K, Petersen KE, et al. Nitrofurantoin versus trimethoprim prophylaxis in recurrent urinary tract infections in children: a randomized, double-blind study. Acta Paediatr Scand 1990;79:1225-34.

47. Lettgen B, Tröster K. Prophylaxis of recurrent urinary tract infections in children. Results of an open, controlled and randomized study about the efficacy and tolerance of cefixime compared to nitrofurantoin. Klin Padiatr 2002;214:353-8.

48. Belet N, Islek I, Belet U, et al. Comparison of trimethoprim-sulfamethoxazole, cephadroxil and cefprozil as prophylaxis for recurrent urinary tract infections in children. J Chemother 2004;16:77-81.

49. Stansfeld JM. Duration of treatment for urinary tract infections in children. BMJ 1975;2:65-6.

50. Montini G, Rigon L, Gobber D, et al. A randomized controlled trial of antibiotic prophylaxis in children with a previous documented pyelonephritis. Pediatr Nephrol 2004;19:70.

51. Garin EH, Olavarria F, Garcia Nieto V, et al. Clinical significance of primary vesicoureteral reflux and urinary antibiotic prophylaxis after acute pyelonephritis: a multicenter, randomized, controlled study. Pediatrics 2006;117:626-32.

52. Montini G, Rigon L, Zucchetta P, et al. Prophylaxis after first febrile urinary tract infection in children? A multicenter, randomized, controlled, noninferiority trial. Pediatrics 2008;122:1064-71.

53. Pennesi M, Travan L, Peratoner L, et al. Is antibiotic prophylaxis in children with vesicoureteral reflux effective in preventing pyelonephritis and renal scars? A randomized, controlled trial. Pediatrics 2008;121:e1489-194.

54. Savage DCL, Howie G, Adler K, et al. Controlled trial of therapy in covert bacteriuria of childhood. Lancet 1975;i:358-61.

55. Roussey-Kesler G, Gadjos V, Idres N, et al. Antibiotic prophylaxis for the prevention of recurrent urinary tract infections in children with low grade vesicoureteral reflux: results from a prospective randomized study. J Urol 2008;179:674-9.

56. Cheng CH, Tsai MH, Huang YC, et al. Antibiotic resistance patterns of community-acquired urinary tract infections in children with vesicoureteral reflux receiving prophylactic antibiotic therapy. Pediatrics 2008;122:1212-17.

57. Lohr JA, Nunley DH, Howards SS, et al. Prevention of recurrent urinary tract infections in girls. Pediatrics 1977;59:562-5.

58. Smellie JM, Katz G, Grüneberg RN. Controlled trial of prophylactic treatment in childhood urinary-tract infection. Lancet ii:175-178.

59. O'Regan S, Yazbeck S, Schick E. Constipation, bladder instability, urinary tract infection syndrome. Clin Nephrol 1985;23:152-4.

60. Loening-Baucke V. Urinary incontinence and urinary tract infection and their resolution with treatment of chronic constipation of childhood. Pediatrics 1997;100:288-32.

61. Chrzan R, Klijn AJ, Vijverberg AW, et al. Colonic washout enemas for persistent constipation in children with recurrent urinary tract infection based on dysfunction voiding. Urology 2008;71:607-10.

62. Depaepa H, Hoebeke P, Renson C, et al. Pelvic-floor therapy in girls with recurrent urinary tract infections and dysfunction voiding. BJU 1998;81(suppl 3):109-13.

63. McKenna PH, Herndon CDA, Connery S, et al. Pelvic floor muscle retraining for pediatric voiding dysfunction using interactive computer games. J Urol 1999;162:1056-63.

64. Wiener JS, Scales MT, Hampton J, et al. Long-term efficacy of simple behavioral therapy for daytime wetting in children. J Urol 2000;164:786-90.

65. Chin-Peuckert L, Pippi Salle JL. A modified biofeedback program for children with detrusor-sphincter dyssynergia: 5-year experience. J Urol 2001;166:1470-5.

66. Nelson JD, Cooper CS, Boyt MA, et al. Improved uroflow parameters and post-void residual following biofeedback therapy in pediatric patients with dysfunctional voiding does not correspond to outcome. J Urol 2004;172:1653-6.

67. Kibar Y, Ors O, Demir E, et al. Results of biofeedback treatment on reflux resolution rates in children with dysfunctional voiding and vesicoureteral reflux. Urology 2007;70:563-7.

68. Foda MM, Middlebrook PF, Gatfield CT, et al. Efficacy of cranberry in prevention of urinary tract infection in a susceptible pediatric population. Can J Urol 1995;2:98-102.

69. Schlager TA, Anderson S, Trudell J, et al. Effect of cranberry juice on bacteriuria in children with neurogenic bladder receiving intermittent catheterization. J Pediatr 1999;135:698-702.

39   Treatment of nocturnal enuresis

Alexander Gomelsky

Department of Urology, Louisiana State University Health Sciences Center, Shreveport, LA, USA

Background

Nocturnal enuresis (NE) is defined as the involuntary urine loss at night (typically by age 5) in the absence of organic disease [1]. The prevalence of NE at age 7 approaches 10% in some cross-sectional studies, and may be up to 0.5% in otherwise healthy adults aged 18–64 years [2,3]. NE is frequently classified into monosymptomatic (MNE; night-time symptoms only) and polysymptomatic (diurnal symptoms) subtypes [4,5]. While MNE is a heterogeneous condition and the pathophysiology is not well understood, several factors are thought to contribute to its development. Other than genetic factors and early life stressors, physiological disturbances often exist. The persistence of infantile spontaneous bladder contractions (leading to a decreased bladder capacity), an inability to produce or respond to physiological amounts of vasopressin (leading to nocturnal polyuria), and failure to arouse to the sensation of a full or contracting bladder have all been implicated in the development and persistence of NE [6]. Children with NE may be slow to attain full maturational control of one, or a combination, of these pathophysiological factors, thus displaying a variety of clinical patterns [7]. Hence, treatment has aimed to address each aforementioned mechanism by increasing bladder capacity, decreasing nocturnal urine production, and improving arousal and awakening.

The purpose of this chapter is to review the available evidence regarding the efficacy of treatment options for MNE. Due to length constraints, no assessment or comparison of treatment side effects has been performed. Grading of the quality of evidence and strengths of recommendations in this chapter is based on the guidelines proposed by the international Grading of Recommendations Assessment, Development, and Evaluation Working Group (Grade) [8].

Literature search

Potentially relevant studies were identified by a computerized search of the Medline electronic database (PubMed, 1966–2008). Relevant text and keywords were: enuresis OR nocturnal enuresis OR monosymptomatic nocturnal enuresis, AND randomized controlled trial OR controlled trial OR meta-analysis. The search was limited to the English-language literature. The Cochrane reviews represent a fertile starting point for an evidence-based evaluation of the treatment of NE. All seven Cochrane NE reviews were based on a previous systematic review performed by Lister-Sharpe et al. at the Centre for Reviews and Dissemination [9]. Relevant trials were identified from a specialized register of controlled trials identified from Medline, CINAHL, the Cochrane Central Register of Controlled Trials, and hand searching of journals and relevant conference proceedings. Details regarding review methods, including identification of primary studies, quality assessments, and data extraction, are described in detail in each Cochrane review.

There exist some challenges in interpretation of studies. While there is no shortage of randomized, controlled trials (RCTs) in the NE literature, few are methodologically sound. Thus, the conclusions of these trials must be tempered by shortcomings, such as high dropout rates and poor rates of adherence to therapeutic regimen. Additionally, many trials are small and, frequently, outcomes may be represented by findings of single trials. Furthermore, especially when medical therapy is involved, the initial response rates may not be representative of durable, long-term response rates. Outcome measures may be different, as well. Some of the outcomes considered in the Cochrane reviews were: change in the mean number of

Evidence-Based Urology. Edited by Philipp Dahm, Roger R. Dmochowski.
© 2010 Blackwell Publishing.

wet nights per week during treatment; number of children failing to attain 14 consecutive dry nights during treatment; mean number of wet nights per week when participants were followed up after treatment cessation; and number of children failing during treatment and/or relapsing after treatment cessation.

Clinical question 39.1

What is the evidence supporting behavioral and educational intervention for NE?

The evidence

While multiple modalities may be employed in the treatment of NE, simple and complex behavioral interventions are often a component of the initial therapeutic attempt. The various behavioral techniques are summarized in Box 39.1. Additionally, educational interventions, including different methods of providing information or teaching for children and their parents, may be used to supplement behavioral therapy. In a Cochrane review (updated February 19, 2004) encompassing 13 trials, 387 out of 702 children received a simple behavioral intervention [11]. A meta-analysis could not be performed as each outcome in each comparison was reported in a single trial. Five trials

BOX 39.1 Simple and complex behavioral interventions used in the treatment of NE [10–12]

Simple interventions

- Lifting — Taking the child to the toilet during the night (usually before bedwetting is expected, without necessarily waking the child)
- Waking reward systems — Star charts, for example, for each dry night achieved
- Retention control training — Increasing functional bladder capacity by delaying urination for extended periods of time during the day
- Stop-start training — Strengthening of the pelvic floor muscles

Complex interventions

- Dry bed training (DBT) — Waking routines, positive practice, cleanliness training, bladder training, and reward systems; may include enuresis alarms
- Full-spectrum home training (FSHT) — Combines a urine alarm triggered by wetting with cleanliness training, retention control training, and overlearning (stressing of the detrusor muscle by imbibing extra fluid at bedtime)

compared simple interventions (including retention control training, rewards, lifting or waking) with no active treatment (control group). Star charts (with or without lifting or waking) were associated with significantly fewer wet nights and lower failure rates during treatment [13-15]. Additionally, fewer children relapsed after achieving success with reward therapy than controls. There was insufficient evidence to support retention control training alone.

Eight trials compared a simple behavioral intervention with another behavioral intervention, such as cognitive therapy, dry bed training (DBT) and alarms with or without imipramine. Evidence from single small trials revealed that children undergoing cognitive therapy had lower failure or relapse rates than those children using star charts. Additionally, children using alarms achieved fewer wet nights after the end of treatment than those practicing retention control training, or those who were randomly awakened. Five small trials included a placebo, desmopressin, imipramine or amitriptyline in one arm. There was insufficient evidence to compare desmopressin with retention control training; however, amitriptyline was associated with better initial results than waking, lifting, star chart and placebo in one small trial [16]. There was no significant association after treatment cessation. In another trial, imipramine with or without fluid deprivation and avoidance of punishment was better than the simple intervention alone [17]. Additionally, children using imipramine, with or without the addition of an alarm, had fewer absolute numbers of wet nights per week than during random wakening, while children receiving placebo had more wet nights per week [18].

A recent Cochrane review (updated March 20, 2008) evaluated studies of complex behavioral and educational interventions for NE [12]. Of 1174 children from 18 included trials, 746 received a complex behavioral or educational intervention. In eight of these trials, children undergoing a complex intervention were compared with those undergoing no treatment. Children allocated to DBT or full-spectrum home training (FSHT) with an alarm had fewer wet nights and were more likely to become dry during treatment (relative risk (RR) for failure 0.17, 95% confidence interval (CI) 0.11–0.28) and after treatment cessation (RR for failure of relapse after stopping DBT was 0.25, 95% CI 0.16–0.39) than those in control groups. However, if treatment was performed without an alarm, the difference between complex intervention and no treatment groups was not significantly different in the dry rate during treatment (RR for failure 0.82, 95% CI 0.66–1.02) and the rate of relapse after treatment cessation. In five trials, children receiving complex interventions were compared with those receiving other behavioral interventions. DBT alone, a three-step program of retention control training, wakening, and parental reassurance, and FSHT were compared with alarm alone, DBT with alarm, three-step program supplemented with counseling and parental education, and FSHT with pelvic floor muscle training. An alarm (RR for failure or relapse 1.7, 95% CI 1.06–2.73), DBT with alarm (RR for failure or relapse 2.81, 95% CI 1.80–4.38) or a three-step program with counseling and educational reinforcement (RR for failure or relapse 2.07, 95% CI 1.16–3.72) were significantly better than a complex intervention alone in the number of wet nights during treatment, failure rates during treatment, and combined failure and relapse rates after treatment cessation.

In four trials comparing supplemented complex intervention and other behavioral interventions, failure rates during treatment were marginally better after concomitant DBT with alarm compared to treatment with an alarm only (RR 0.6, 95% CI 0.38–0.94). There was not enough evidence to suggest that any method of providing instruction to children or parents regarding the implementation of complex behavioral interventions was better than another, except that live delivery of FSHT was better than filmed delivery in two small trials (RR for failure during treatment 0.36, 95% CI 0.15–0.90). In one trial, a three-step program with supplemental counseling and educational reinforcement seemed to be better than imipramine alone (RR for failure and relapse 0.27, 95% CI 0.16–0.43) [19]. In a second trial, children receiving various behavioral interventions had more wet nights than those on desmopressin (weighted mean difference (WMD) 1.67, 95% CI 0.35–2.99); however, there were not enough children to statistically assess failure rates [20].

Clinical question 39.2

What is the evidence supporting alarm use for NE?

The evidence

The most common enuresis alarms consist of a sensor on a bed pad or pajamas which is triggered by wetness, thereby waking the child when they begin to urinate. Complementary techniques such as overlearning or giving extra fluids at bedtime to stress the detrusor are often added after a child successfully becomes dry using an alarm. Alarm interventions have been evaluated in a recent Cochrane review (updated February 22, 2005) that encompassed 56 trials [21]. A total of 3257 children were included, of whom 2412 used an alarm.

The majority of the trials used a pad-and-buzzer type of alarm to wake the children when wetting occurred, although a few used an electric shock to the child's skin. Seventeen trials compared an alarm with a no-treatment control group. In nine of these trials, standard alarm use was associated with over three fewer wet nights per week

when compared to controls (WMD –3.34, 95% CI –4.14 to –2.55). In 13 trials, RR of failure was less in the alarm group in every trial (107 of 316 (34%) did not achieve 14 dry nights vs 250 of 260 (96%) in controls; RR 0.38, 95% CI 0.33–0.45). While approximately half of the children failed or relapsed after stopping alarm treatment (45 of 81, 55%), nearly all the children in the control group relapsed (80 of 81, 99%) (RR 0.56, 95% CI 0.46–0.68). There were no data regarding the number of wet nights after treatment cessation. Adding overlearning (RR 1.92, 95% CI 1.27–2.92) or DBT (RR 2.0, 95% CI 1.25–3.20) to alarm treatment contributed to lower relapse rates.

Alarm use was compared with behavioral intervention in eight trials. In one trial, alarm use was associated with fewer wet nights than stop-start training, both during treatment (WMD –2.25, 95% CI –4.2 to –0.3) and after treatment cessation (WMD –2.6, 95% CI –4.53 to –0.67) [22]. Likewise, alarm use was associated with fewer wet nights than DBT during treatment (RR for failure to achieve 14 dry nights was 0.22, 95% CI 0.09–0.53) and after treatment cessation (RR 0.59, 95% CI 0.37–0.95). While alarm use was associated with fewer wet nights, when compared to lifting, waking or rewards, the difference was not significant.

Sixteen trials attempted to evaluate whether augmenting alarms with behavioral intervention was better than an alarm alone. In five of these trials, failure rates during treatment with alarms alone were better than alarms and retention control training (RR 0.37, 95% CI 0.18–0.76); however, failure or relapse rates after treatment cessation were not significantly different (RR 1.12, 95% CI 0.77–1.64). The addition of overlearning did not improve results over alarms alone; however, the addition of overlearning may be associated with lower relapse rates after treatment cessation (33 of 67 (49%) failed or relapsed after alarms alone vs 19 of 77 (25%) with overlearning; RR 1.92, 95% CI 1.27–2.92). The addition of DBT to alarm therapy in five trials did not result in a statistically significant improvement in failure or relapse rate over alarm alone. However, after the exclusion of a trial using different alarm models [23], the failure or relapse rate was reduced in the alarm plus DBT group (20 of 32 (63%) relapsing with alarm alone vs 20 of 72 (27%) with alarm plus DBT; RR 2.0, 95% CI 1.25–3.20). The addition of rewards for dry beds to alarm treatment was associated with lower failure rates during treatment, but using penalties for wet beds was less effective or counterproductive after treatment cessation.

Twenty trials included a comparison of alarms with medications. Alarms were better than placebo drug treatment in terms of fewer wet nights during and after treatment, and a lower failure rate during treatment (RR 0.68, 95% CI 0.48–0.97). Unfortunately, there were no follow-up data after treatment cessation. In a comparison of desmopressin and alarms, children had fewer wet nights during the first week of treatment with desmopressin

(WMD 2.1, 95% CI 0.99–3.21). By the end of the treatment period in three trials, however, children using alarms had fewer wet nights. This was not statistically significant. Although there was a lower failure rate during alarm treatment in four trials (RR 0.85, 95% CI 0.53–1.37), this also was not statistically significant. In two small trials, fewer children failed or relapsed after alarm treatment stopped (29 of 57 (51%) vs 46 of 62 (74%) after desmopressin; RR 0.53, 95% CI 0.14–2.06); however, this difference was also not statistically significant.

Although there were fewer wet nights during alarm treatment compared with imipramine, amitriptyline or clomipramine in four trial arms out of five, no relationship reached statistical significance. Fewer children failed during alarm treatment in three trials involving imipramine (61of 105 (58%) vs 82 of 103 (80%); RR for failure 0.59, 95% CI 0.3–1.09), but these differences were not statistically significant. After treatment cessation, fewer children failed or relapsed after alarms in one small trial (RR 0.58; 95% CI 0.36–0.94) and fewer had wet nights at follow-up in another. There was no clear evidence that adding a tricyclic to an alarm was better than the alarm alone.

Five trials compared alarms with cognitive therapy or psychotherapy, ritual shaming, and restricted diet. Although the number of wet nights during treatment was similar, more children achieved 14 dry nights during alarm treatment compared with cognitive or psychotherapy (RR for failure 0.68, 95% CI 0.52–0.90) and restricted diet. If a single trial with disproportionate patient allocation was removed from statistical evaluation, the significant difference in the chance of failure disappeared (RR 0.93, 95% CI 0.67–1.30) [24]. Children had fewer wet nights after alarm treatment than after ritual shaming. In addition to the Cochrane review, several other meta-analyses and systematic reviews have shown that alarm implementation is a highly efficacious treatment strategy for NE [25-29].

Clinical question 39.3

What is the evidence supporting desmopressin use for NE?

The evidence

A significant number of children with MNE are lacking the normal circadian variation in urine production typically seen with a concurrent nocturnal elevation in vasopressin. Subsequently, these children produce disproportionately large quantities of dilute urine at night. The high overnight urine production exceeds the child's bladder capacity, which may result in NE if the child does not wake up appropriately [30]. This imbalance is believed to be an important pathophysiological factor in NE. Arginine

vasopressin (AVP) is released by the pituitary gland in response to hyperosmolality or low effective circulating blood volume. In addition to being a potent vasoconstrictor, AVP enhances water reabsorption in the renal collecting ducts and distal tubules. An analog of AVP, desmopressin has greater antidiuretic properties than AVP but is a much less potent vasopressor. It is available in oral and intranasal preparations, with a half-life of 1.5–3.5 hours.

A Cochrane review (updated May 21, 2002) evaluated the outcomes of desmopressin in children with NE [31]. Forty-seven randomized trials involving 3448 children met the inclusion criteria, of whom 2210 received desmopressin. In 29 trials comparing 20 μg desmopressin with placebo, desmopressin use was associated with 1.34 fewer wet nights during treatment (95% CI 1.11–1.57). Other dosages of desmopressin were also associated with fewer wet nights during treatment. Additionally, 10 trials addressed the cure rate (defined as achieving 14 consecutive dry nights) in children taking either desmopressin or placebo. The trials consistently reported an increased chance of cure with desmopressin regardless of desmopressin dose (RR for failure with 20 μg in five trials was 0.84, 95% CI 0.79–0.91; RR for 40 μg in six trials was 0.81, 95% CI 0.74–0.88; RR for 60 μg in two trials was 0.94, 95% CI 0.89–0.99). However, data from four small trials suggest that wet nights per week after treatment cessation were no different in children taking desmopressin or placebo. Data from trials comparing dose–response effects and oral versus nasal administration were also inconclusive.

Data from four small trials reported no significant differences between desmopressin and alarms during treatment. However, the chance of failure or relapse after treatment cessation was lower after alarm use (40 of 62 (65%) vs 26 of 57 (46%); RR 1.42, 95% CI 1.05–1.91). Children had fewer wet nights during treatment when they used desmopressin combined with alarm, compared with alarms alone (WMD –0.83, 95% CI –1.11 to –0.55). However, there were no significant differences either in failure rates during treatment (RR for the number of children failing to achieve 14 dry nights 0.88, 95% CI 0.73–1.05) or in relapse rate after treatment cessation (105 of 213 (49%) vs 118 of 214 (55%); RR 0.91, 95% CI 0.76–1.08).

Seven trials compared desmopressin with other medications; however, the four trials comparing desmopressin with amitriptyline or imipramine were too small to provide definitive results. In two trials, more children achieved dry nights with desmopressin than imipramine during treatment (RR 0.44, 95% CI 0.27–0.73) but there was insufficient evidence about subsequent relapse. In two small trials, desmopressin performed better than indometacin (WMD for wet nights per week –1.45, 95% CI –2.37 to –0.53) and diclofenac (RR for failure to achieve 14 dry nights was 0.52, 95% CI 0.30–0.89) during treatment, but there was no information about relapse rates after treatment cessation.

There was insufficient information to evaluate the relative effects of behavioral or complementary treatments versus desmopressin.

Clinical question 39.4

What is the evidence supporting the use of tricyclics for NE?

The evidence

Several mechanisms have been proposed to explain the success of tricyclics in treating NE. Anticholinergic effects may reduce detrusor activity and increase bladder capacity. Additionally, tricyclics may relax smooth muscle due to sympathomimetic effects from blockade of norepinephrine reuptake. Furthermore, these drugs have been suggested to enhance arousal and suppress REM sleep [32], as well as stimulating vasopressin release to decrease urine production [33]. Tricyclics and similar drugs for NE have been evaluated in a Cochrane review (updated May 28, 2003) [34]. Fifty-eight randomized trials involving 3721 children met the inclusion criteria; however, most comparisons and outcomes were addressed in single trials.

Seventeen of 36 trials comparing a tricyclic with placebo provided useable numerical data. In 16 of 17 trials, there were fewer wet nights in children taking tricyclics. A meta-analysis constructed from three of these trials revealed a reduction of one wet night per week during tricyclic therapy (WMD −0.92, 95% CI −1.38 to −0.46). In 11 trials, more children became dry during tricyclic therapy (314 of 400 (79%) failed to achieve 14 dry nights on imipramine vs 391 of 413 (95%) on placebo; RR for failure 0.77, 95% CI 0.72–0.83). However, data from five trials suggest that this effect was not sustained after treatment cessation (190 of 199 (96%) relapsed after imipramine treatment vs 210 of 217 (97%) after placebo; RR 0.98, 95% CI 0.95–1.03). In small trials, desipramine and amitriptyline were also better than placebo, but the difference for mianserin, based on outcomes of a single small trial, did not reach statistical significance. Adding chlordiazepoxide to imipramine was counterproductive, but a combination of imipramine and oxybutynin was better than placebo (RR 0.43; 95% CI 0.23–0.78). Data from three small trials suggested that viloxazine was associated with fewer wet nights after treatment cessation, but the difference was not statistically significant after imipramine.

Seventeen trials compared a tricyclic with another tricyclic, or a drug of another class. As most comparisons or outcomes were addressed in single small trials, there was not enough information to assess the relative performance of imipramine against three other tricyclics. In one small trial, imipramine was associated with fewer wet nights and greater success in achieving 14 dry nights than mianserin (RR 0.63, 95% CI 0.44–0.92). In three trials, the number of wet nights during treatment was similar during treatment between imipramine and desmopressin; however, more children became dry with desmopressin than imipramine in one small trial (RR 2.22, 95% CI 1.30–3.79). After treatment cessation, almost all the children relapsed after both treatments and the numbers of wet nights were similar.

A tricyclic was compared with a behavioral intervention in 12, mainly small, trials. Approximately half of the children relapsed after alarm treatment ended, as compared to all the children after cessation of tricyclic treatment. In a single large trial, imipramine appeared to be better than placebo with a star chart (WMD for mean number of wet nights during treatment −0.80, 95% CI −1.33 to −0.27), but follow-up data were not available. The data were insufficient to judge how tricyclics compared with random wakening or shaming. In another large trial, imipramine was worse than a program of retention control training, wakening, and parental involvement, especially if supplemented with motivational therapy and a computer-based education program. During treatment, 22 of 36 (61%) children failed on imipramine vs 15 of 96 (16%) during the intervention (RR 3.91, 95% CI 2.30–6.66). At follow-up, 24 of 36 (67%) failed or relapsed after imipramine vs 18 of 96 (19%) after the interventional program (RR 3.56, 95% CI 2.21–5.72).

Clinical question 39.5

What is the evidence supporting other medications for NE?

The evidence

In 33 eligible RCTs, 1268 of 1700 children received one of 31 active drugs, excluding desmopressin or a tricyclic antidepressant [35]. Twenty-two of 26 trials comparing an active drug with placebo provided data for analysis. There were fewer wet nights during treatment in the groups of children receiving indometacin (WMD −3.06, 95% CI −3.89 to −2.23), diclofenac (WMD −4.21, 95% CI −5.76 to −2.66), and diazepam (WMD −4.87, 95% CI −6.25 to −3.49). Additionally, fewer children failed to achieve 14 dry nights during active treatment while taking indometacin (RR 0.36; 95% CI 0.16–0.79), diclofenac (RR 0.52; 95% CI 0.38–0.70), diazepam (RR 0.22; 95% CI 0.11–0.46), and atomoxetine (RR 0.81, 95% CI 0.70–0.94). No data regarding relapse rates after treatment cessation were provided.

In one small trial of 62 children, fewer children failed to achieve 14 dry nights during treatment after desmopressin than after diclofenac (RR 1.94, 95% CI 1.13–3.33). In another trial, children taking desmopressin had fewer wet nights during treatment than those on indometacin (WMD 1.45, 95% CI 0.53–2.37). No data regarding relapse rates after treatment cessation were provided. Limited data suggested that an alarm was better than various drugs during treatment. Four trials included a behavioral or other non-drug intervention for bed wetting. In one of four trials comparing a drug with a nondrug intervention, fewer children failed to achieve 14 dry nights during treatment using an alarm than those taking an amphetamine (RR 2.2, 95% CI 1.12–4.29). No data regarding relapse rates after treatment cessation were provided. The number of children in the remaining three trials was too small to draw definitive conclusions.

Clinical question 39.6

What is the evidence supporting complementary and miscellaneous interventions for NE?

The evidence

A Cochrane database totaling 15 RCTs reported the outcomes of complementary intervention in children with NE [36]. Out of 1389 children, 703 underwent a complementary intervention, including hypnosis, acupuncture, chiropractic, diet, faradization, and homeopathy. In one trial comparing imipramine and hypnosis, the number of children cured or improved was similar at the end of treatment; however, the failure or relapse rate after stopping imipramine (19 of 25, 76%) was lower than after stopping hypnosis (8 of 25, 32%; RR 0.42, 95% CI 0.23–0.78). Children undergoing psychological and supportive interventions appeared to have fewer wet nights during treatment than children taking desmopressin or untreated controls (RR 0.69, 95% CI 0.55–0.85). Additionally, fewer children undergoing psychological interventions failed during treatment than those undergoing reward therapy or those taking piracetam. In one small trial, fewer children failed or relapsed following psychotherapy than after alarm use (RR 0.28, 95% CI 0.09–0.85) and reward therapy (RR 0.29, 95% 0.09–0.90).

Fewer children undergoing acupuncture failed or relapsed after treatment cessation than those who had sham control acupuncture (RR 0.67, 95% CI 0.48–0.94). Additionally, fewer children undergoing active chiropractic adjustment failed or relapsed after treatment cessation than those undergoing sham adjustments (RR 0.74, 95% CI 0.60–0.91). However, each of these findings came from small single trials. Trials regarding the effects of diet and faradization on NE were limited by small numbers of enrolled children and high dropout rate.

In a recent, three-arm randomized, double-blind, double-dummy controlled trial, 151 children with MNE were treated with homotoxicological remedies, desmopressin or placebo [37]. At 3 months, the decrease in wet nights per week was significantly higher after homotoxicological remedies than placebo (30% vs 2.4%, p < 0.001); however, the decrease in wet nights after desmopressin was significantly higher than both (62.9%, p < 0.001).

Conclusion

The conclusions regarding the efficacy of simple behavioral interventions must be tempered by the small size of the trials. When compared with controls receiving no treatment, the implementation of reward systems, lifting, and waking was associated with significantly fewer wet nights and higher cure rates during treatment. Relapse rates were also lower. There was little evidence to evaluate the effects of retention control training on NE. The outcomes after a complex intervention such as DBT or FSHT with an alarm were better than those in no-treatment control groups. While an alarm alone was better than DBT alone, the combination of an alarm with DBT may be better than an alarm alone, thus suggesting that DBT may augment alarm effects. While there were few data to evaluate the effectiveness of providing educational information about enuresis, direct contact between families and therapists may enhance the effect of a complex intervention.

Alarms are quite effective for NE in children, with two-thirds of the children becoming dry during treatment as compared with no-treatment controls. Nearly half of the children who continued to use an alarm remained dry after treatment cessation, while almost all the controls became wet again. Avoiding penalties and the addition of overlearning and DBT to alarms may further reduce the relapse rate. There was not enough evidence to determine if alarms were significantly superior to behavioral interventions alone. In general, children who used an alarm along with other behavioral strategies were as likely to attain 14 consecutive dry nights and had similar relapse rates as children using alarms alone. However, the confidence intervals were all fairly wide.

Children using desmopressin appeared to have a more rapid effect in reduction of wet nights (one to two per week) than those children using alarms; however, alarms appeared to be as effective by the end of a treatment course. As only two small trials compared alarms and desmopressin directly, their relative effectiveness after treatment cessation was unclear and the benefits seen during treatment may not be sustained. While alarms were not significantly better than tricyclics during treatment, their use was associated with a lower relapse rate after treatment cessation. In all, it appears that one half of the children using alarms relapse after cessation of active treatment, as compared to most of the children who took tricyclics and desmopressin.

The data were limited and insufficient to derive conclusions on whether drugs other than desmopressin and tricyclics reduced bed wetting. There was limited evidence to suggest that desmopressin, imipramine, and alarms were better than various other drugs to which they were compared. Two additional trials suggested that imipramine and amitriptyline were better than behavioral measures. The evidence supporting the use of hypnosis, psychotherapy, acupuncture and chiropractic was provided in each case by single small trials and no meaningful conclusions regarding these therapeutic options can be drawn.

Implications for practice and recommendations

Simple behavioral interventions, such as rewards (e.g. star charts), waking, and lifting, are a reasonable and safe first-line intervention for children with NE, although there was not enough evidence to show that these techniques were better than other treatment modalities for NE (Grade 1C: strong recommendation FOR despite low-quality evidence, but favorable benefit/risk ratio). Complex interventions such as DBT or FSHT may result in better outcomes if an alarm is added to this therapeutic regimen. The use of complex intervention and alarms may result in better outcomes than alarms alone (Grade 2B: conditional recommendation FOR based on moderate-quality evidence).

Alarms are the mainstay of treatment for NE and should be used whenever possible. Results during and after alarm use are significantly better than no treatment. Alarm therapy produces more sustained benefits than medications (Grade 1B: strong recommendation FOR based on moderate-quality evidence).

Desmopressin clearly produces fewer wet nights per week during treatment, but is associated with a high rate of relapse after treatment cessation. Although not addressed in this review, desmopressin may be associated with fluid overload and should be used with caution in children [4] (Grade 2A: suggestion FOR the use of desmopressin when compared against placebo, but adverse event risk is present; Grade 2C: there is low-quality evidence to suggest desmopressin when compared with other medications).

Tricyclics may be more effective than placebo, but almost all children relapse after treatment cessation. Their use may be limited to those children for whom behavioral interventions, alarms, and desmopressin fail (Grade 2C: there is low-quality evidence to suggest use of tricyclics, especially in light of adverse event risk).

There is currently not enough evidence to support the use of other medications for NE (no recommendation can be made).

There is currently not enough evidence to support the use of hypnosis, psychotherapy or other complementary intervention for NE (no recommendation can be made).

Implications for research

While there is no shortage of RCTs addressing a variety of treatment regimens for NE in children, most of these trials may be limited in several ways. Widely different estimates of the treatment effects, or heterogeneity, across many of these studies suggest potentially real differences in underlying effects [8]. Additionally, the relatively small size of many trials may contribute to imprecision in the form of wide confidence intervals, thus lowering the quality of evidence. Consequently, all future studies may benefit from power calculations to determine necessary sample size. Furthermore, future trials should focus on children with MNE, without physical causes of bed wetting, and should include adequate assessment of baseline levels of wetting [11]. Finally, the difficulty in comparing interventions may be exacerbated by the lack of uniformity in outcome measures. The authors of the Cochrane reviews suggest that reportable outcomes include: the number of wet nights during treatment and after the end of treatment; the number of children failing to achieve 14 consecutive dry nights; adverse events; acceptability of treatment; compliance; and relapse rates after treatment cessation [11]. Further research is also needed to determine which interventions are appropriate for which groups.

References

1. American Psychiatric Association. *Diagnostic and Statistical Manual of Mental Disorder (DSM IV)*, 4th edn. Washington, DC: American Psychiatric Press, 1990.
2. Hellström AL, Hanson E, Hansson S, et al. Micturition habits and incontinence in 7-year-old Swedish school entrants. Eur J Pediatr 1990;149:434-7.
3. Hirasing RA, van Leerdam FJ, Bolk-Bennink L, et al. Enuresis nocturna in adults. Scand J Urol Nephrol 1997;31:533-6.
4. Pennesi M, Pitter M, Bordugo A, et al. Behavioral therapy for primary nocturnal enuresis. J Urol 2004;171:408-10.
5. Yeung CK, Chiu HN, Sit FK. Bladder dysfunction in children with refractory monosymptomatic primary nocturnal enuresis. J Urol 1999;162:1049-54.
6. Wolfish NM. Sleep arousal function in enuretic males. Scand J Urol Nephrol 1999;33(suppl):24-6.
7. Wolfish NM, Pivik RT, Busby KA. Elevated sleep arousal thresholds in enuretic boys: clinical implications. Acta Paediatr 1997;86:381-4.

8. Guyatt GH, Oxman AD, Vist GE, et al. GRADE: what is "quality of evidence" and why is it important to clinicians? BMJ 2008;336:995-8.

9. Lister-Sharpe D, O'Meara S, Bradley M, Sheldon TA. *A Systematic Review of the Effectiveness of Interventions for Managing Childhood Nocturnal Enuresis.* CRD Report 11. York: NHS Centre for Reviews and Dissemination, University of York, 1997.

10. Glazener CMA, Peto RE, Evans JHC. Effects of interventions for the treatment of nocturnal enuresis in children. Qual Saf Health Care 2003;12:390-4.

11. Glazener CMA, Evans JHC. Simple behavioural and physical interventions for nocturnal enuresis in children. Cochrane Database Syst Rev 2004;2:CD003637.

12. Glazener CMA, Evans JHC, Peto RE. Complex behavioural and educational interventions for nocturnal enuresis in children. Cochrane Database Syst Rev 2004;1:CD004668.

13. Baker BL. Symptom treatment and symptom substitution in enuresis. J Abnorm Psychol 1969;74:42-9.

14. Fava GA, Cracco L, Facco L. Positive reinforcement and enuresis. Ital J Psychol 1981;8:149-52.

15. Ronen T, Wozner Y, Rahav G. Cognitive intervention in enuresis. Child Family Behav Ther 1992;14:1-14.

16. Mehrotra SN, Liu L, Srivastava JR, et al. Evaluation of various methods in treatment of enuresis. Indian Pediatr 1980;17:519-22.

17. Bhatia MS, Dhar NK, Rai S, et al. Enuresis: an analysis of 82 cases. Ind J Med Sci 1990;44:337-42.

18. Fournier JP, Garfinkel BD, Bond A, et al. Pharmacological and behavioral management of enuresis. J Am Acad Child Adolesc Psychiatry 1987;26:849-53.

19. Iester A, Marchesi A, Cohen A, et al. Functional enuresis: pharmacological versus behavioral treatment. Childs Nerv Syst 1991; 7:106-8.

20. Fera P, Glashan R, Lelis MA, et al. Immediate outcome of DDAVP versus behavioral modification for treatment of monosymptomatic nocturnal enuresis: a prospective randomized study of 30 patients. Neurourol Urodyn 2004;23:555-6.

21. Glazener CMA, Evans JHC, Peto RE. Alarm interventions for nocturnal enuresis in children. Cochrane Database Syst Rev 2005;2:CD002911.

22. Bennett GA, Walkden VJ, Curtis RH, et al. Pad-and-buzzer training, dry-bed training, and stop-start training in the treatment of primary nocturnal enuresis. Behav Psychother 1985; 13:309-19.

23. Butler RJ, Forsythe WI, Robertson J. The body-worn alarm in the treatment of childhood enuresis. Br J Clin Pract 1990;44:237-41.

24. Sacks S, de Leon G, Blackman S. Psychological changes associated with conditioning functional enuresis. J Clin Psychol 1974; 30:271-6.

25. Hjalmas K, Arnold T, Bower W, et al. Nocturnal enuresis: an international evidence based management strategy. J Urol 2004; 171:2545-61.

26. Nijman RJ, Butler RJ, van Gool JD, et al. Conservative management of urinary incontinence in childhood. In: Abrams P, Cardozo L, Khoury S, Wein A (eds) *Incontinence*. Plymouth: Health Publication Ltd, 2002: 540-2.

27. Houts AC, Berman JS, Abramson H. Effectiveness of psychological and pharmacological treatments for nocturnal enuresis. J Consult Clin Psychol 1994;62:737-45.

28. Mellon MW, McGrath ML. Empirically supported treatments in pediatric psychology: nocturnal enuresis. J Pediatr Psychol 2000;25:193-214.

29. Moffatt MEK. Nocturnal enuresis: a review of the efficacy of treatments and practical advice for clinicians. J Dev Behav Pediatr 1997;18:49-56.

30. Neveus T, Lackgren G, Tuvemo T, et al. Enuresis-background and treatment. Scand J Urol Nephrol 2000;34(suppl):1-44.

31. Glazener CMA, Evans JHC. Desmopressin for nocturnal enuresis in children. Cochrane Database Syst Rev 2002;3:CD002112.

32. Kales A, Kales JD, Jacobson A, et al. Effects of imipramine on enuretic frequency and sleep stages. Pediatrics 1977;60:431-6.

33. Tomasi PA, Siracusano S, Monni AM, et al. Decreased nocturnal urinary antidiuretic hormone excretion in enuresis is increased by imipramine. BJU Int 2001;88:932-7 .

34. Glazener CMA, Evans JHC, Peto RE. Tricyclic and related drugs for nocturnal enuresis in children. Cochrane Database Syst Rev 2003;3:CD002117.

35. Glazener CM, Evans JH, Peto RE. Drugs for nocturnal enuresis in children (other than desmopressin and tricyclics). Cochrane Database Syst Rev 2003;4:CD002238.

36. Glazener CMA, Evans JHC, Cheuk DK. Complementary and miscellaneous interventions for nocturnal enuresis in children. Cochrane Database Syst Rev 2005;2:CD005230.

37. Ferrara P, Marrone G, Emmanuele V, et al. Homotoxicological remedies versus desmopressin versus placebo in the treatment of enuresis: a randomised, double-blind, controlled trial. Pediatr Nephrol 2008;23:269-74.

40 Treatment of Wilms' tumor

Puneeta Ramachandra[1] and Fernando Ferrer[2]
[1]Division of Urology, University of Connecticut Health Center, Farmington, CT, USA
[2]Department of Urology, Connecticut Children's Medical Center, Hartford, CT, USA

Introduction

Wilms' tumor or nephroblastoma, is the most common renal tumor in children, accounting for approximately 7.6 cases per million children under age 15 [1]. Overall, about 6% of all childhood cancers arise from the kidney, and about 95% of these cancers are nephroblastomas. These are embryonal tumors that develop from immature kidney remnants. Wilms' tumor (WT) was once thought to occur as a result of the classic single-gene, two-hit model described in retinoblastoma [2]; now at least 10 different genes have been shown to be involved [3].

The highest incidence is in the first four years of life, although children of any age and adults also may be affected. The median age at presentation is between 3 and 4 years of age [1]. While solitary, unilateral lesions are most common, bilateral tumors occur in 7% of patients (Figure 40.1). Approximately 12% of patients have multiple lesions within one kidney [5]. The incidence is nearly equal between boys and girls worldwide, but in the United States, frequency is slightly higher in girls [4]. Based on the data from the Surveillance, Epidemiology, and End Results (SEER) program, prognosis is excellent, with an overall 5-year survival of over 88% for cases diagnosed between 1996 and 2004 [1]. Significant progress has been made in the treatment of WT mainly as a result of large collaborative groups, such as the Children's Oncology Group (COG) and the International Society of Pediatric Oncology (SIOP), which have helped develop a multidisciplinary approach to therapy. Newer research emphasizes reducing morbidity of treatment for low-risk patients and improving efficacy of treatment for the subset of high-risk patients with poor survival.

Children with WT may present in many ways. Most commonly, an asymptomatic abdominal mass is found; however, other signs and symptoms at presentation include abdominal pain, gross hematuria, fever or acute abdomen due to tumor rupture. In less than 10% of patients, symptoms related to compression of adjacent structures may occur. These include varicocele, hepatomegaly, ascites, and congestive heart failure, resulting from extension into the inferior vena cava (IVC) or renal vein.

Wilms' tumor generally has a great deal of histological diversity. The classic triphasic pattern, which mimics the cell types in the developing kidney, is composed of varying amounts of three cell types: blastemal, epithelial, and stromal. Each of these components responds differently to therapy and may influence outcomes [6]. Tumors with unfavorable histologic features, or anaplasia, are associated with increased relapse and death rates [7].

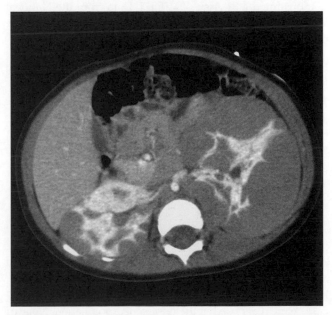

Figure 40.1 Multiple bilateral Wilms' tumors in a 2-year-old female

Evidence-Based Urology. Edited by Philipp Dahm, Roger R. Dmochowski.
© 2010 Blackwell Publishing.

Background

Wilms' tumor has been associated with many identifiable syndromes, divisible into those characterized by overgrowth and those not associated with overgrowth. Hemihypertrophy or overgrowth of a body segment can occur as part of the Beckwith–Wiedemann syndrome (BWS) or an isolated problem, termed isolated hemihypertrophy. The BWS is a rare disorder of developmental anomalies characterized by excessive growth at the organ or cellular levels, with features such as macroglossia, nephromegaly, and hepatomegaly, as well as hemihypertrophy. It is caused by dysregulation of genes at chromosome 11p15, which control prenatal and childhood growth. The WT 2 gene (*WT2*) has also been identified on this site. Other rare overgrowth syndromes such as Simpson–Golabi–Behmel syndrome and Perlman syndrome have also been reported to be associated with WT.

The incidence of tumors in this population is 10–20%, including WT, adrenocortical tumors, and hepatoblastoma. The risk of tumor declines with age and by age 10 approaches that of the general population. Patients with hemihypertrophy and BWS have a risk of developing WT of the order of 4–10%, with about 21% of those patients presenting with bilateral disease.[7] New evidence suggests that the risk of tumor development in BWS depends on the specific molecular mutation that causes BWS [8]. A prospective study of 168 patients with isolated hemihypertrophy demonstrated a 3% risk of WT [7]. Data from the National Wilms' Tumor Study Group indicate that the 90% of WT are diagnosed by age 7, and 99% are diagnosed by age 10 [9].

Literature search

An extensive search was performed on PubMed for relevant articles using the following terms: "hemihypertrophy," "Beckwith–Wiedemann syndrome," "Wilms' tumor," "nephroblastoma," "screening," and "surveillance." The references listed in identified publications were also reviewed. Three relevant studies were identified.

The evidence

A retrospective case series by Choyke and colleagues screened children with BWS or isolated hemihypertrophy and compared them to an unscreened group of patients [12]; 12 cases of WT were identified by screening and 59 cases were diagnosed in the unscreened population. None of the screened cases were late-stage WT, compared to 42% (25 cases) in the unscreened group. Three children in this series had a false-positive ultrasound and underwent invasive surgery for benign disease [10].

Another study from the UK by Craft et al. is a retrospective review of 41 patients with WT and BWS, isolated hemihypertrophy or aniridia [11]. This study did not show any difference in stage or outcome between patients who underwent tumor surveillance and those who did not.

Only one prospective, multicenter study, performed by Choyke and colleagues, has attempted to address the issue of tumor surveillance in isolated hemihypertrophy [12]. Of the 168 children in this study, 10 tumors developed, six of which were WT. Most study participants received an abdominal ultrasound every 6 months, but surveillance protocols varied amongst the study centers. One child developed a WT 5 months after the previous screening ultrasound, leading the authors to conclude that a screening interval of 6 months may be too long in these patients.

Comment

Based on the limited number of available studies, screening protocols appear to detect WT at earlier stages in children with BWS or isolated hemihypertrophy, potentially allowing these patients to undergo treatment with less morbidity. However, surveillance may lead to false-positive results, leading to unnecessary treatment, expense, and anxiety. Unfortunately, given the rarity of these overgrowth disorders and the low incidence of WT, a large, randomized controlled trial of surveillance is unlikely to occur.

Recommendations

Children with isolated hemihypertrophy should be screened with abdominal ultrasounds every 3–4 months until age 7. There is insufficient evidence to recommend screening beyond this age, given that 90% of WT are diagnosed by this age. Parents and families should be carefully counseled regarding the risk of tumor development and importance of adhering to surveillance protocols. Emerging evidence on epigenotyping of 11p15 in BWS and isolated hemihypertrophy patients may help delineate low-risk from high-risk individuals, but further clinical trials are needed in this area before screening recommendations can be amended.

Background

The term loss of heterozygosity (LOH) refers to the inactivation of one allele of a gene in which the other allele has already lost its normal function. One of the most notable recent findings in WT is the significance of LOH at chromosomes 1p and 16q reported in the National Wilms' Tumor Study Group (NWTSG) trials. Of the 232 patients enrolled in NWTS-3 and NWTS-4, LOH of chromosomes 1p or 16q was found in 11% and 17.2%, respectively. LOH of chromosome 16q was associated with a statistically significantly poorer 2-year relapse-free and overall survival, even when adjusted for tumor stage or histology. LOH of chromosome 1p was also associated with a lower overall and recurrence-free survival but the results were not statistically significant [13]. More extensive research has shed some light on this subject, allowing the use of LOH as a prognostic indicator in favorable histology WT (FHWT).

Literature search

A PubMed search was performed using the following terms: "loss of heterozygosity," "1p," "16q" and "Wilms' tumor." In addition we accessed the current COG protocol and reviewed the references listed.

The evidence

The NWTS-5 trial was designed to test the hypothesis that LOH of either chromosome 16q and/or 1p was associated with a worse prognosis in FHWT patients who were all treated with stage-specific treatment regimens. Of the 2021 WT patients enrolled in the study, 224 had LOH at chromosome 1p, and 360 had LOH at chromosome 16q. Patients with stage I or stage II FH tumors were at an increased risk of relapse or death with LOH at either one of the chromosomes. However, stage III/IV patients with LOH 1p alone did not have significantly worse outcomes than stage I/II patients when treated with stage-specific chemotherapy, suggesting that more aggressive chemotherapy may overcome the adverse effects of LOH.

Patients with LOH 16q alone had an almost identical overall survival as patients with no LOH (98.1% vs 98.4%, p = 0.60 in stage I/II and 92% vs 91.9%, p = 0.76 in stage III/IV). Most importantly, all FH patients with combined LOH (at *both* 1p and 16q) were at a statistically significantly higher risk of relapse and death than patients with single-chromosome LOH or no LOH. This included stage I and II FH patients, despite having received appropriate stage-specific chemotherapy (vincristine and dactinomycin) [14].

Based on NWTS-5 data, the newest COG protocol is designed to test the hypothesis that including additional chemotherapy (doxorubicin) for stage I/II FHWT patients who demonstrate LOH at both 1p and 16q will improve outcomes. These patients will now be considered "standard risk" instead of "very low risk" and will be receiving the same chemotherapeutic regimen as stage III FHWT patients who do not have combined LOH. Also, stage III FHWT patients with combined LOH will be considered "high risk" and may be treated with a high-risk protocol. Stage I and II patients with combined LOH had an equal incidence of recurrence in the abdomen and in the lungs, so abdominal radiation will not be added to their regimens.

Comment

The previous studies effectively demonstrate that LOH at chromosomes 1p or 16q can be used as an independent prognostic factor for WT. Together with stage, this may allow even further stratification of treatment intensity, at least for FH patients. The significance of LOH 1p alone was not clear from these studies, because the results were inconsistent across stages. Therefore, LOH 1p alone cannot be used as an independent prognostic factor, nor does it justify subjecting this subset of patients to the added morbidity of doxorubicin.

Recommendations

Stage I and II FHWT patients with LOH 1p and 16q should be considered standard risk and be treated with a chemotherapeutic regimen consisting of vincristine, dactinomycin, and doxorubicin. Doxorubicin should not be added in low-stage patients with no LOH or LOH at only 1 of the chromosomes.

Clinical question 40.3

How does histology of Wilms' tumor affect staging, outcome, and therapy?

Background

Histopathology and stage are the two most important predictors of outcome in WT. The staging system used by the COG is based on surgical findings and histopathology (Table 40.1). The recognition of certain unfavorable histological features, associated with increased risk of relapse and death from WT, has allowed for risk stratification. In 1978, Beckwith and Palmer identified anaplastic cells as those with nuclear enlargement three or more times the size of adjacent cells, nuclear hyperchromasia, and irregular mitotic figures [15]. Anaplasia is a feature of WT that is associated with resistance to chemotherapy and is further

Table 40.1 Stages of Wilms' tumor

Stage	Description
I	Tumor confined to the kidney, no intraoperative spillage, negative surgical margins
II	Tumor extends beyond kidney, surgical margins negative, no intraoperative spillage
III	Tumor spread outside the kidney but confined to abdomen, positive surgical margins or intraoperative tumor spillage
IV	Hematogenous metastasis or distal lymph node spread
V	Bilateral disease

Table 40.2 Experimental treatment protocols

Stage	Risk	Treatment
Stage I FH – < 2 yr, < 550 g	Very low risk	Nephrectomy/observation
Stage I, II FH – w/out LOH at 1p & 16q	Standard risk	Regimen DD-4A w/out XRT
Stage III FH – w/out LOH at 1p & 16q		Regimen DD-4A w/XRT
Stage III FH – w/out LOH at 1p & 16q	High risk	Regimen M
Stage IV FH	Higher risk	Regimen DD-4A × 2 cycles Local XRT after nephrectomy XRT to nonlung mets, followed by 6 wk eval prior to further therapy
Stage I–III focal AH Stage I diffuse AH	High risk	Regimen DD-4A
Stage IV focal AH Stage II–III diffuse AH Stage IV diffuse AH	High risk	Regimen UH-1 with XRT, followed by further therapy based on response of pulmonary lesions

AH, anaplastic histology; FH, favorable histology; LOH, loss of heterozygosity; Regimen DD-4A, VCN, AMD, DOX × 25 wks; Regimen M, VCN, AMD, DOX w/etoposide/CYCLO; Regimen UH-1, CYCLO, CARBO, etoposide × 30 wks; VCN, DOX, CYCLO × 30 wks; XRT, radiation therapy

divided into focal versus diffuse anaplasia which also has prognostic implications. Focal anaplasia denotes a very limited area of anaplastic nuclear changes within the primary tumor, whereas diffuse anaplasia indicates that anaplasia is present in more than one part of the tumor, an extrarenal site or a metastatic location [16]. In early NWTSG trials, unfavorable features, such as anaplasia, occurred in about 10% of patients, but accounted for 44% of all tumor deaths [17]. Accurate staging is crucial in determining appropriate treatment, and treatment outcome is highly correlated with tumor stage. Patients with WT can be stratified based on histology, namely favorable histology (FH) versus anaplastic (AH) WT.

Literature search

A PubMed literature search was performed using the following terms: "anaplastic Wilms' tumor," "favorable-histology Wilms' tumor," "anaplastic-histology Wilms' tumor," "anaplasia and prognosis," "Wilms' tumor histology." In addition, the current COG protocols were reviewed.

The evidence

In NWTS-3 and NWTS-4 patients with anaplastic WT were randomized to receive a three-drug chemotherapeutic regimen (vincristine, actinomycin D, and doxorubicin) with or without cyclophosphamide. Patients who had focal anaplasia had no difference in outcome, and these children had a similar prognosis as those with comparable stage, FH tumors. In patients with stage II–IV diffuse anaplasia, the addition of cyclophosphamide to the standard chemotherapeutic regimen improved 4-year relapse-free survival (27.2% vs 54.8%, p = 0.02) [18].

One of the primary objectives of NWTS-5 (1995–2002) was to further improve outcomes for patients with stage II–IV diffuse AHWT. Stage I AH patients received the same chemotherapy as stage I FH patients, while stage II–IV AH received a much more intensive regimen. Four-year recurrence-free survival rates for stage II, III, and IV diffuse AH were 82.6%, 67.4%, and 33.3% respectively. Although these rates are significantly improved from historical controls in prior studies, a considerable number of patients with diffuse AHWT experienced disease recurrence. In this study, stage I AH, 4-year recurrence-free survival was significantly lower than stage I FHWT (69.5% vs 92.4%, p < 0.001) [19]. This finding was in contrast to findings from earlier NWTS studies which had previously demonstrated a similar recurrence-free survival and overall survival between these two groups. The current ongoing COG trials are focusing on identifying novel treatment regimens for high-risk patients such as those with diffuse anaplasia. The experimental treatment protocols are summarized in Table 40.2.

Comment

Patients with stage I–IV AHWT have significantly worse outcomes than those with FHWT.

Recommendations

Compared to patients with FHWT, patients with anaplasia should be classified as high risk and should therefore receive a more intensive chemotherapeutic regimen. Specifics of these drug regimens are beyond the scope of this chapter.

Clinical question 40.4

What is the current treatment protocol for patients with bilateral Wilms' tumor?

Background

While unilateral WT is far more common, bilateral WT (BWT) occurs in 5–7% of all patients with WT. Patients with BWT are at increased risk of renal failure, and survival rates in this group of patients are inferior to similar stage patients with unilateral WT. In reviewing data from prior NWTSG studies, 9.1% of patients with BWT eventually developed renal failure. In most of these cases, renal failure was a result of a second (contralateral) nephrectomy for recurrent or persistent disease after initial nephrectomy for treatment of WT [20]. Therefore, total nephrectomy should be avoided if possible. For many years, the NWTSG has recommended that children with BWT should receive preoperative chemotherapy in order to allow partial nephrectomy in these patients.

Poor outcomes in BWT may be the result of various factors, such as understaging and undertreatment, increased incidence in unfavorable histology or anaplasia or delay in local control of disease. In this section, we will outline the major studies from prior years and give the rationale for the current ongoing Children's Oncology Group protocol for BWT.

Literature search

A PubMed search was performed using the following terms: "bilateral Wilms' tumor," "synchronous Wilms' tumor," and "outcomes." In addition, we accessed and reviewed the current ongoing Children's Oncology Group study protocol, including cited references.

The evidence

In prior studies, patients with BWT have had significantly worse outcomes than similar patients with unilateral WT. In NWTS-3 and -4, 344 patients with BWT had an 10-year relapse-free survival of only 65% and a 10-year overall survival of 78%, compared to unilateral stage I–IV FHWT (relapse-free survival (RFS) 86% and overall survival (OS) 92%). There was not much improvement in NWTS-5, where 158 BWT patients had a 4-year event-free survival of 61% and a 4-year OS of only 80%. Of the 145 patients enrolled in NWTS-2 and -3, total excision of tumor was possible in less than 40%, of whom 34 patients received only dactinomycin and vincristine. These 34 patients had a 100% 3-year survival [21]. In NWTS-4, local recurrence of tumor in the remnant kidney or tumor bed occurred in just over 8% of kidneys, despite successful removal of all gross tumor in 118 of 134 kidneys [22].

Progression of disease or lack of responsiveness to initial chemotherapy should prompt efforts to biopsy lesions, instead of prolonging chemotherapy. During NWTS-4, 38 of the 188 patients with BWT enrolled had evidence of progressive or nonresponsive disease [23]. Of these 38 patients, 15 were found to have pathologies which would not benefit from prolonged courses of chemotherapy, delaying definite surgery. Also, 27 BWT patients had diffuse anaplasia, identified in 0/7 patients who underwent a needle biopsy and only 3/9 patients undergoing wedge biopsy. In these cases chemotherapy was continued for a mean of 20 weeks after a needle biopsy and 39 weeks after wedge biopsy [24].

The current COG protocol aims for earlier biopsy or surgical resection for those patients who do not appear to be responding to chemotherapy in order to avoid prolonged inadequate or ineffective therapy. Upfront chemotherapy has been intensified, a second-look surgery is required at 6 weeks, and definitive surgery is done at 12 weeks. Following definitive surgery, chemotherapy is tailored based on histological response at definitive surgery. Open surgical biopsy at initial presentation is not required, because the likelihood of misdiagnosing a case of BWT is very low. Most benign entities and non-Wilms' malignancies present with unilateral lesions. As noted above, needle biopsies were not successful in detecting anaplasia in NWTS-4.

Preoperative "induction" chemotherapy will be done with a three-drug regimen called VAD (vincristine, dactinomycin, and doxorubicin) based on regimens used in both SIOP and the United Kingdom Children's Cancer Study Group WT Group [25]. These regimens have demonstrated good results with minimal toxicities [26]. The aim of intensifying chemotherapy preoperatively is to speed up the reduction in tumor size, so as not to delay performance of definitive surgery and allow more rapid assignment of appropriate postsurgical therapy. In NWTS-4, at least 114 of 188 patients were treated with a three-drug chemotherapy regimen, with the third drug being doxorubicin. In most cases, chemotherapy was intensified because of overwhelmingly inadequate response or progression on a two-drug regimen [23].

Those patients who demonstrate evidence of resistance to chemotherapy or no response on imaging may benefit from earlier biopsies than have been previously done. AH can occur in over 10% of BWT [22,25,27] and this subtype is known for its resistance to chemotherapy. Complete excision of AH tumors may improve survival [24] so earlier biopsy or definitive surgery may improve outcomes in these patients by limiting length of ineffective chemotherapy. Postsurgical chemotherapy can then be tailored to therapy targeting anaplastic histology.

Comment

Historically, patients with BWT have had worse outcomes than similar patients with unilateral WT. This may have been due to understaging, undertreatment or delay in definitive surgery. These patients are also at higher risk for renal failure if both kidneys need to be removed. The aim of therapy should be partial nephrectomies when feasible, facilitated by more intensive preoperative chemotherapeutic regimens. Early biopsy and early definitive surgery may also improve outcomes in this difficult group of patients.

Recommendations

Based on the above data, we recommend that all children with BWT be on current, ongoing COG protocol. Open biopsy is not needed to confirm the diagnosis of BWT if bilateral lesions are present on imaging studies. Intensive upfront chemotherapy should be given and assigned based on stage and histology, if known. A second-look surgery should be performed at 6weeks, with performance of partial nephrectomies, if possible. At this juncture, if surgery is still not feasible, chemotherapy is given for an additional 6 weeks. Definitive partial nephrectomies should not be delayed beyond 12 weeks when it is feasible to perform them. Postoperative chemotherapy or radiation is then assigned based on final histology and stage.

References

1. National Cancer Institute. Surveillance epidemiology and end results, 1975–2005. National Institutes of Health. Available at: http://seer.cancer.gov/statistics.
2. Knudson AG Jr, Strong LC. Mutation and cancer: a model for Wilms' tumor of the kidney. J Natl Cancer Inst 1972;48:313-24.
3. Breslow N, Beckwith JB, Perlman EJ, Reeve AE. Age distributions, birth weights, nephrogenic rests, and heterogeneity in the pathogenesis of Wilms tumor. Pediatr Blood Cancer 2006;47:260-7.
4. Breslow N, Olshan A, Beckwith JP, et al. Ethnic variation in the incidence, diagnosis, prognosis, and follow-up of children with Wilms' tumor. J Natl Cancer Inst 1994;86:49-51.
5. Breslow N, Beckwith JB, Ciol M, Sharples K. Age distribution of Wilms' tumor: report from the National Wilms' Tumor Study. Cancer Res 1988;48:1653-7.
6. Wierich A, Leuschner I, Harms D, et al. Clinical impact of histologic subtypes in localized non-anaplastic nephroblastoma treated according to the trial and study SIOP-9/GPOH. Ann Oncol 2001;12:311-19.
7. Scott RH, Stiller CA, Walker L, Rahman N. Syndromes and constitutional chromosomal abnormalities associated with Wilms tumour. J Med Genet 2006;43:705-15.
8. Rump P, Zeegers MP, van Essen AJ. Tumor risk in Beckwith–Wiedemann syndrome: a review and meta-analysis. Am J Med Genet A 2005;136:95-104.
9. Beckwith JB. Children at increased risk for Wilms tumor: monitoring issues. J Pediatr 1998;132:377-9.
10. Choyke PL, Siegel MJ, Craft AW, Green DM, DeBaun MR. Screening for Wilms tumor in children with Beckwith–Wiedemann syndrome or idiopathic hemihypertrophy. Med Pediatr Oncol 1999;32:196-200.
11. Craft AW, Parker L, Stiller C, Cole M. Screening for Wilms' tumour in patients with aniridia, Beckwith syndrome or hemihypertrophy. Med Pediatr Oncol 1995;24:231-4.
12. Hoyme HE, Seaver LH, Jones KL, et al. Isolated hemihyperplasia (hemihypertrophy): report of prospective multicenter study of the incidence of neoplasia and review. Am J Med Genet 1998;79:274-8.
13. Grundy PE, Telzerow PE, Breslow N, et al. Loss of heterozygosity for chromosomes 16q and 1p in Wilms' tumors predicts an adverse outcome. Cancer Res 1994;54:2331-3.
14. Grundy PE, Breslow N, Li S, et al. Loss of heterozygosity for chromosomes 1p and 16q is an adverse prognostic factor in favorable-histology Wilms tumor: a report from the National Wilms Tumor Study Group. J Clin Oncol 2005;23:7312-21.
15. Beckwith JB, Palmer NF. Histopathology and prognosis of Wilms tumor. Cancer 1978;41:1937-48.
16. Faria P, Beckwith JP, Mishra K, et al. Focal versus diffuse anaplasia in Wilms' tumor – new definitions with prognostic significance: a report from the National Wilms' Tumor Study Group. Am J Surg Pathol 1996;20:909-20.
17. Breslow NE, Churchill G, Beckwith JP, et al. Prognosis for Wilms' tumor patients with nonmetastatic disease at diagnosis – results of the Second National Wilms' Tumor Study. J Clin Oncol 1985;3:521-31.
18. Green DM, Beckwith JB, Breslow NE, et al. Treatment of children with stages II to IV anaplastic Wilms' tumor: a report from the National Wilms' Tumor Study Group. J Clin Oncol 1994;12:2126-31.
19. Dome JS, Cotton CA, Perlman EJ, et al. Treatment of anaplastic histology Wilms' tumor: results from the Fifth National Wilms' Tumor Study. J Clin Oncol 2006;24:2352-8.
20. Ritchey ML, Green DM, Thomas P, et al. Renal failure in Wilms tumor. Med Pediatr Oncol 1996;26:75-80.
21. Blute ML, Kelalis PP, Offord KP, et al. Bilateral Wilms' tumor. J Urol 1987;138:968-73.
22. Horwitz J, Ritchey ML, Moksness J, et al. Renal salvage procedures in patients with synchronous bilateral Wilms tumors: a report of the NWTSG. J Pediatr Surg 1999;31:1020-5.
23. Shamberger RC, Ritchey ML, Hamilton TE, et al. Bilateral Wilms tumors with progressive or nonresponsive disease. J Pediatr Surg 2006;41:652-7.

24. Hamilton TE, Green DM, Perlman EJ, et al. Bilateral Wilms tumor with anaplasia: lessons from the National Wilms Tumor Study Group. J Pediatr Surg 2006;41(10):1641-4.

25. Grundy RG, Hutton C, Middleton H, et al. Outcome of patients with Stage III or inoperable WT treated on the Second United Kingdom WT Protocol (UKWT2): a United Kingdom Children's Cancer Study Group (UKCCSG) study. Pediatr Blood Cancer 2004;42:311-19.

26. Kumar R, Fitzgerald R, Breatnach F. Conservative surgical management of bilateral Wilms tumor: results of the United Kingdom Children's Cancer Study Group. J Urol 1998;160: 1450-3.

27. Breslow NE, Churchill G, Beckwith JP, et al. Prognosis for Wilms' tumor patients with nonmetastatic disease at diagnosis – results of the Second National Wilms' Tumor Study. J Clin Oncol 1985;3:521-31.

Index

Note: page numbers in *italics* refer to figures, those in **bold** refer to tables

7